FROM THE EXPERTS IN ENDOCRINOLOGY

ENDO 2025
MEET THE PROFESSOR

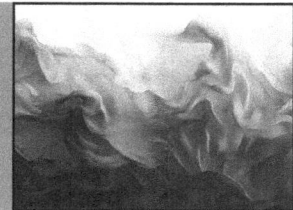

REFERENCE EDITION

ENDOCRINE
CASE MANAGEMENT

ENDO 2025

ENDOCRINE SOCIETY

ENDOCRINE
SOCIETY

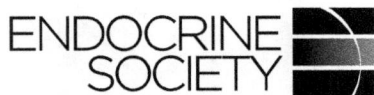

2055 L Street, NW, Suite 600
Washington, DC 20036
www.endocrine.org

Other Publications:
endocrine.org/publications

The Endocrine Society is the world's largest, oldest, and most active organization working to advance the clinical practice of endocrinology and hormone research. Founded in 1916, the Society now has more than 18,000 global members across a range of disciplines.

The Society has earned an international reputation for excellence in the quality of its peer-reviewed journals, educational resources, meetings, and programs that improve public health through the practice and science of endocrinology.

Clinical Practice Chair, ENDO 2025
Barbara Gisella Carranza Leon, MD

ENDO 2025
CONTENTS

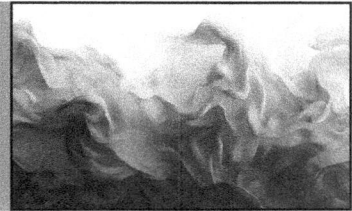

CARDIOVASCULAR ENDOCRINOLOGY

DIABETES AND VASCULAR DISEASE

GENERAL ENDOCRINOLOGY

NEUROENDOCRINOLOGY AND PITUITARY

PEDIATRIC AND ADOLESCENT ENDOCRINOLOGY

REPRODUCTIVE ENDOCRINOLOGY

THYROID BIOLOGY AND CANCER

TUMOR BIOLOGY

APPENDIX

ENDO 2025
FACULTY

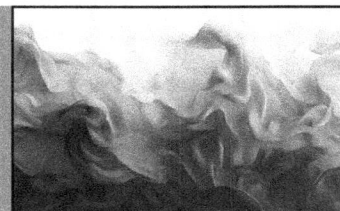

2025 Endocrine Case Management: Meet the Professor Faculty

José O. Alemán, MD, PhD
New York University Langone Health

Natasha M. Appelman-Dijkstra, MD, PhD
Leiden University Medical Center

Danit Ariel, MD, MS
Stanford University
School of Medicine

Wiebke Arlt, MD, DSc
Medical Research Council
Laboratory of Medical Sciences

Tânia Bachega, MD, PhD
São Paulo University
School of Medicine

Shichun Bao, MD, PhD
Vanderbilt University Medical Center

Andrew J. Bauer, MD
Children's Hospital of Philadelphia
and University of Pennsylvania
Perelman School of Medicine

Jérôme Bertherat, MD, PhD
Paris Cité University and
Cochin Hospital

Eveline Bruinstroop, MD, PhD
Amsterdam UMC

Mirjam Christ-Crain, MD, PhD
University Hospital Basel,
University of Basel

Stefano Cianfarani, MD
University of Rome, 'Bambino
Gesù' Children's Hospital,
and Karolinska Institute

Daniel A. Dumesic, MD
University of California Los Angeles
David Geffen School of Medicine

Grigoris Effraimidis, MD, PhD
University of Thessaly and University
General Hospital of Larissa

Ghada El-Hajj Fuleihan, MD, MPH
American University of Beirut

Rossella Elisei, MD
University Hospital of Pisa
and University of Pisa

Dana Erickson, MD
Mayo College of Medicine

Pouneh K. Fazeli, MD, MPH
University of Pittsburgh Medical
Center Presbyterian Hospital

Ian Ganly, MD, MS, PhD
Memorial Sloan Kettering
Cancer Center

Andrea Glezer, MD, PhD
University of São Paulo
Medical School Hospital

Aidar R. Gosmanov, MD, DMSc
Albany Medical College and Stratton
Veterans Affairs Medical Center

Claus H. Gravholt, MD, PhD
Aarhus University Hospital

A. G. (Onno) Holleboom, MD, PhD
Amsterdam UMC

Camilo Jimenez, MD
University of Texas MD
Anderson Cancer Center

Emmanuel Jouanneau, MD, PhD
Hospices Civils de Lyon, Claude
Bernard University, and Cancer
Research Center of Lyon

Randol Kennedy, MD
Duke University School of Medicine

Andrew T. Kraftson, MD
University of Michigan

Rayhan Lal, MD
Stanford University

Angela M. Leung, MD, MSc
University of California Los Angeles
David Geffen School of Medicine
and Veterans Affairs Greater Los
Angeles Healthcare System

Eva S. Liu, MD
Brigham and Women's Hospital
and Harvard Medical School

Marco Medici, MD, PhD, MSc
Erasmus Medical Center

Alyson K. Myers, MD
Montefiore Einstein

Michael W. O'Reilly, MD, PhD
Royal College of Surgeons in Ireland

Maria Papaleontiou, MD
University of Michigan

Melissa Putman, MD
Harvard Medical School and
Massachusetts General Hospital

Gerald Raverot, MD, PhD
Claude Bernard University,
Cancer Research Center of Lyon,
and Hospices Civils de Lyon

Tirissa J. Reid, MD, DABOM
Columbia University Vagelos College
of Physicians and Surgeons

Alan D. Rogol, MD, PhD
University of Virginia

Micol S. Rothman, MD
University of Colorado
School of Medicine

David Saxon, MD, MSc
University of Colorado School
of Medicine and Rocky
Mountain Regional Veterans
Affairs Medical Center

Ellen W. Seely, MD
Brigham and Women's Hospital
and Mass General Brigham

Afreen Shariff, MD
Duke University School of Medicine
and Duke Cancer Institute

Ashley Shoemaker, MD, MSCI
Vanderbilt University Medical Center

Marius N. Stan, MD
Mayo Clinic-Rochester

Michael Stowasser, MBBS, PhD
University of Queensland
Frazer Institute and Princess
Alexandra Hospital

Lisa R. Tannock, MD
Queen's University

Sonali Thosani, MD
MD Anderson Cancer Center

Selma Feldman Witchel, MD
University of Pittsburgh
Medical Center Children's
Hospital of Pittsburgh

Whitney W. Woodmansee, MD, MA
University of Florida

Annual Meeting Steering Committee (AMSC)

**Niki Karavitaki, MSc,
PhD – AMSC Chair**
University of Birmingham

**Barbara Gisella Carranza Leon,
MD – Clinical Practice Chair**
Vanderbilt University Medical Center

**Robin Peeters, MD, PhD –
Clinical Science Chair**
Erasmus Universiteit

**Monica Laronda, PhD –
Basic Science Chair**
Ann & Robert H. Lurie Children's
Hospital of Chicago

Annual Meeting Steering Committee Clinical Peer Reviewers

Ana Paula Abreu Metzger, MD, PhD

Olga Astapova, MD, PhD

Irina Bancos, MD

Laura Boucai, MD

Davide Calebiro, MD

Diane Donegan, MBBCh BAO, MRCPI

David A. Ehrmann, MD

Christa E. Flueck, MD

Oksana Hamidi, DO

Ole-Petter Hamnvik, MBBCh
BAO, MMSc, MRCPI

Edward Chiaming Hsiao, MD, PhD

Hebatullah M. Ismail, MD

Suzanne Jan De Beur, MD

Srividya Kidambi, MD

Katja Kiseljak-Vassiliades, DO

Raghavendra Mirmira, PhD, MD

Connie Baum Newman, MD

Gabrielle Page-Wilson, MD

Elizabeth N. Pearce, MD, MSc

Luca Persani, MD, PhD

Julie Refardt, MD, PhD

Yumie Rhee, MD, PhD

Laura Torchen, MD

Elena Tsourdi, MD

W. Edward Visser, MD, PhD

Jun Yang, MBBS, PhD

Elaine Wei-Yin Yu, MD

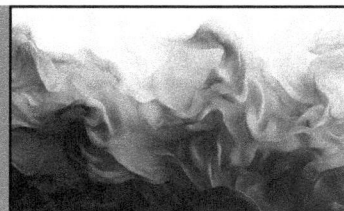

OVERVIEW

The *Endocrine Case Management: Meet the Professor* reference book is intended primarily for consultation relating to endocrinology. As a reference book, educational credits are not available. For information on educational products that include educational credit, please visit endocrine.org/store.

LEARNING OBJECTIVES

Endocrine Case Management: Meet the Professor will allow learners to assess their knowledge of all aspects of endocrinology, diabetes, and metabolism.

Completion of this educational activity enables learners to accomplish key objectives:

- Recognize clinical manifestations of endocrine and metabolic disorders and select among current options for diagnosis, management, and therapy.

- Identify risk factors for endocrine and metabolic disorders and develop strategies for prevention.

- Evaluate endocrine and metabolic manifestations of systemic disorders.

- Use existing resources pertaining to clinical guidelines and treatment recommendations for endocrine and related metabolic disorders to guide diagnosis and treatment.

TARGET AUDIENCE

Endocrine Case Management: Meet the Professor provides case-based education to clinicians interested in improving patient care.

STATEMENT OF INDEPENDENCE

The Endocrine Society has a policy of ensuring that the content and quality of this educational activity are balanced, independent, objective, and scientifically rigorous. The scientific content of this activity was developed under the supervision of the Endocrine Society's Annual Meeting Steering Committee.

DISCLOSURE POLICY

The faculty, committee members, and staff who are in position to control the content of this activity are required to disclose to the Endocrine Society and to learners any relevant financial relationship(s) of the individual or spouse/partner that have occurred within the last 12 months with any commercial interest(s) whose products or services are related to the content. Financial relationships are defined by remuneration in any amount from the commercial interest(s) in the form of grants; research support; consulting fees; salary; ownership interest (e.g., stocks, stock options, or ownership interest excluding diversified mutual funds); honoraria or other payments for participation in speakers' bureaus, advisory boards, or boards of directors; or other financial benefits. The intent of this disclosure is not to prevent planners with relevant financial relationships from planning or delivery of content, but rather to provide learners with information that allows them to make their own judgments of whether these financial relationships may have influenced the educational activity with regard to exposition or conclusion. The Endocrine Society has reviewed all disclosures and resolved or managed all identified conflicts of interest, as applicable.

The Endocrine Society has reviewed these relationships to determine which are relevant to the content of this activity and resolved any identified conflicts of interest for these individuals.

The following faculty reported relevant financial relationship(s) during the content development process for this activity:

José O. Alemán, MD, PhD Novo Nordisk (*consultant*)

Wiebke Arlt, MD, DSc Diurnal; Roche Diagnostics, Bayer Inc, Organon Laboratories, Crinetics, Spruce Bioscience, European Society of Endocrinology

Andrew J. Bauer, MD IBSA Pharm, Egetis Pharm (*consultant*)

Jérôme Bertherat, MD, PhD HRA Pharma, Recordati RD, Novo Nordisk

Eveline Bruinstroop, MD, PhD Aligos, Madrigal

Stefano Cianfarani, MD Novo Nordisk, Sandoz

Daniel A. Dumesic, MD Ferring Pharmaceuticals, Organon Laboratories, Spruce Biosciences Inc, Precede Biosciences Inc, Ferring Research Institute

Dana Erickson, MD Camurus, Crinetics (*advisory board*)

Pouneh K. Fazeli, MD, MPH Regeneron Pharmaceuticals, Crinetics (*research support and consultant*); Quest Diagnostics, Corcept, Chiesi (*consultant*)

Aidar R. Gosmanov, MD, DMSc Eli Lilly & Company (*research support paid to institution*), *BMJ Open Diabetes Research & Care* (*associate editor*)

A. G. (Onno) Holleboom, MD, PhD Merck, Novo Nordisk, Boehringer Ingelheim, Inventiva, Echosens

Camilo Jimenez, MD Merck, Exelixis, Inc (*research support*)

Randol Kennedy, MD Abbott Diabetes Care, Adaptyx Biosciences, Biolinq, Capillary Biomedical, Deep Valley Labs, Gluroo, Portal Diabetes, Tidepool, ProventionBio, Lilly, Sanofi

Eva S. Liu, MD Inozyme

Marco Medici, MD, PhD, MSc ACE Pharmaceuticals

Alyson K. Myers, MD Eli Lilly & Company, Travel Support for the ExCEL program

Melissa Putman, MD Anagram Therapeutics, Vertex Pharmaceuticals

Tirissa J. Reid, MD, DABOM UpToDate

Alan D. Rogol, MD, PhD Ascendis Pharma, Tolmar, Lumos Pharma, ALK Pharma, Comprehensive Drug Testing, United States Anti-Doping Agency, World Anti-Doping Agency

Afreen Shariff, MD Merck, Novartis Pharmaceuticals, Citrus Oncology, UpToDate

Ashley Shoemaker, MD, MSCI Soleno Therapeutics, Rhythm Pharmaceuticals

Marius N. Stan, MD Argenx, Genentech Inc, Ethyreal Bio, Lessen Inc, Merida, MingHui, Avilar, Viridian (*consultant*)

Selma Feldman Witchel, MD Neurocrine Biosciences Inc

The following faculty reported no relevant financial relationships:

Natasha M. Appelman-Dijkstra, MD, PhD; Danit Ariel, MD, MS; Tânia Bachega, MD, PhD; Shichun Bao, MD, PhD; Mirjam Christ-Crain, MD, PhD; Grigoris Effraimidis, MD, PhD; Ghada El-Hajj Fuleihan, MD, MPH; Rossella Elisei, MD; Ian Ganly, MD, MS, PhD; Andrea Glezer, MD, PhD; Claus H. Gravholt, MD, PhD; Emmanuel Jouanneau, MD, PhD; Andrew T. Kraftson, MD; Rayhan Lal, MD; Angela M. Leung, MD, MSc; Michael W. O'Reilly, MD, PhD; Maria Papaleontiou, MD; Gerald Raverot, MD, PhD; Micol S. Rothman, MD; David Saxon, MD, MSc; Ellen W. Seely, MD; Michael Stowasser, MBBS, PhD; Lisa R. Tannock, MD; Sonali Thosani, MD; and Whitney W. Woodmansee, MD, MA

The following AMSC peer reviewers reported relevant financial relationships:

Irina Bancos, MD Adrenas, HRA Pharma, Corcept, Recordati (*advisory board*); HRA Pharma, Corcept, Sparrow Pharmaceutics, Recordati (*consultant*); Elsevier (*writer*); Recordati, NIH (*funding for investigator-initiated award*); DynaMed (*reviewer*)

Barbara Gisella Carranza Leon, MD Novartis, IONIS Pharmaceutical Inc, NIH, FH Foundation, Regenxbio, Inc (*coinvestigator*); Maintenance of Certification Committee: American Board of Obesity Medicine (*member*)

Diane Donegan, MB BCh BAO, MRCPI Corcept, Recordati (*investigator*); Camarus (*advisory board*)

David A. Ehrmann, MD UpToDate (*editor*); NIH (*grant recipient*)

Christa E. Flueck, MD European Society Paediatric Endocrinology (*advisory board*); Novo Nordisk, Merck, Pfizer, Sandoz, Swiss National Science Foundation, European Society Paediatric Endocrinology (*grant recipient*); Novo Nordisk, Pfizer, EffRx (*consultant*); Sandoz (*speaker*); Hormone Research Paediatrics (*editor*)

Oksana Hamidi, DO Corcept Therapeutics, Crinetics Pharmaceuticals, Neurocrine Biosciences, Recordati Rare Diseases, Camurus (*advisory board*); Xeris Pharma (*speaker*)

Ole-Petter Hamnvik, MB BCh BAO, MMSc, MRCPI *New England Journal of Medicine* (*education editor*)

Edward Chiaming Hsiao, MD, PhD International FOP Association, FD/MAS Alliance, International Clinical Council on FOP (*advisory board*); *Endocrine Journal, Journal of Bone and Mineral Research* (*editor*); Clementia Pharmaceuticals/Ipsen Pharmaceuticals, Ultragenyx (*research investigator*)

Suzanne Jan De Beur, MD American Society of Bone and Mineral Research (*past president*); XLH Network, Current Osteoporosis Reports, Ultragenyx, Kyowa Kirin, Ascendis (*advisory board*); Bone Reports (*editorial board*); Mereo, Kyowa Kirin, Calcilytics (*researcher*); NIH, FDA (*grant reviewer*); PCORI (*investigator*)

Niki Karavitaki, MSc, PhD European Neuroendocrine Association (*advisory board*); HRA Pharma (*editor*); Recordati Rare Diseases, HRA Pharma, Pfizer, Ipsen, Conselient Health (*speaker*)

Srividya Kidambi, MD TOPS Inc (*medical editor and director*)

Katja Kiseljak-Vassiliades, DO HRA Pharma (*advisory board*)

Raghavendra Mirmira, PhD, MD *Journal of Clinical Endocrinology and Metabolism* (*editor*); Veralox Therapeutics (*advisory board*); Veralox Therapeutics, HiberCell, Inc (*investigator-initiated award*)

Connie Baum Newman, MD Food and Drug Association (FDA) for Endocrinologic and Metabolic Diseases (*advisory committee and consultant*); Federation of Medical Women of Canada (*honorarium*)

Gabrielle Page-Wilson, MD Strongbridge Biopharma, Recordati Rare Diseases, Inc, Xeris BioPharma (*advisory board*); Xeris BioPharma (*consultant*)

Elizabeth N. Pearce, MD, MSc Iodine Global Network (*management council*); *Journal of Clinical Endocrinology and Metabolism*, DynaMed-thyroid (*editor*); National Dairy Council, Merck China Symposium (*speaker*); American Thyroid Association (*Guidelines Task Force*); World Health Organization (*advisory panel*)

Luca Persani, MD, PhD Merck, Egetis, Sandoz (*advisory board*); Merck (*speaker*); *Journal of Clinical Endocrinology and Metabolism*, European Thyroid Association, European Thyroid Journal, Pituitary Society, Pituitary (*editor*)

Yumie Rhee, MD, PhD American Society of Bone and Mineral Research (*ambassador*); Korean Endocrine Society, Korean Society of Bone and Mineral Research (*committee*); JCEM Case Reports (*editor*)

Laura Torchen, MD Levo therapeutics, IBSA Pharma (*investigator*)

Elena Tsourdi, MD Amgen, Kyowa Kirin, UCB, Alexion, Ascendis (*clinical studies*); Amgen, UCB, Ascendis (*advisory boards and lectures*); UCB, Takeda, Ascendis (*educational grants*)

W. Edward Visser, MD, PhD Egetis Therapeutics (*royalties [institution]*)

Elaine Wei-Yin Yu, MD Amgen (*grant recipient*)

The following AMSC members reported no relevant financial relationships:

Ana Paula Abreu Metzger, MD, PhD; Olga Astapova, MD, PhD; Laura Boucai, MD; Davide Calebiro, MD; Hebatullah M. Ismail, MD; Julie Refardt, MD, PhD; and **Jun Yang, MBBS, PhD**

DISCLAIMERS
The information presented in this activity represents the opinion of the faculty and is not necessarily the official position of the Endocrine Society.

USE OF PROFESSIONAL JUDGMENT:
The educational content in this activity relates to basic principles of diagnosis and therapy and does not substitute for individual patient assessment based on the health care provider's examination of the patient and consideration of laboratory data and other factors unique to the patient. Standards in medicine change as new data become available.

DRUGS AND DOSAGES:
When prescribing medications, the physician is advised to check the product information sheet accompanying each drug to verify conditions of use and to identify any changes in drug dosage schedule or contraindications.

POLICY ON UNLABELED/OFF-LABEL USE
The Endocrine Society has determined that disclosure of unlabeled/off-label or investigational use of commercial product(s) is informative for audiences and therefore requires this information to be disclosed to the learners at the beginning of the presentation. Uses of specific therapeutic agents, devices, and other products discussed in this educational activity may not be the same as those indicated in product labeling approved by the Food and Drug Administration (FDA). The Endocrine Society requires that any discussions of such "off-label" use be based on scientific research that conforms to generally accepted standards of experimental design, data collection, and data analysis. Before recommending or prescribing any therapeutic agent or device, learners should review the complete prescribing information, including indications, contraindications, warnings, precautions, and adverse events.

ACKNOWLEDGMENT OF COMMERCIAL SUPPORT

The activity is not supported by educational grant(s) or other funds from any commercial supporters.

PUBLICATION DATE: June 2025

COMMON ABBREVIATIONS IN MEET THE PROFESSOR

ACTH = corticotropin

ACE inhibitor = angiotensin-converting enzyme inhibitor

ALT = alanine aminotransferase

AST = aspartate aminotransferase

BMI = body mass index

CNS = central nervous system

CT = computed tomography

DHEA = dehydroepiandrosterone

DHEA-S = dehydroepiandrosterone sulfate

DNA = deoxyribonucleic acid

DPP-4 inhibitor = dipeptidyl-peptidase 4 inhibitor

DXA = dual-energy x-ray absorptiometry

FDA = Food and Drug Administration

FGF-23 = fibroblast growth factor 23

FNA = fine-needle aspiration

FSH = follicle-stimulating hormone

GH = growth hormone

GHRH = growth hormone–releasing hormone

GLP-1 receptor agonist = glucagonlike peptide 1 receptor agonist

GnRH = gonadotropin-releasing hormone

hCG = human chorionic gonadotropin

HDL = high-density lipoprotein

HIV = human immunodeficiency virus

HMG-CoA reductase inhibitor = 3-hydroxy-3-methylglutaryl coenzyme A reductase inhibitor

IGF-1 = insulinlike growth factor 1

LDL = low-density lipoprotein

LH = luteinizing hormone

MCV = mean corpuscular volume

MIBG = *meta*-iodobenzylguanidine

MRI = magnetic resonance imaging

NPH insulin = neutral protamine Hagedorn insulin

PCSK9 inhibitor = proprotein convertase subtilisin/kexin 9 inhibitor

PET = positron emission tomography

PSA = prostate-specific antigen

PTH = parathyroid hormone

PTHrP = parathyroid hormone–related protein

SGLT-2 inhibitor = sodium-glucose cotransporter 2 inhibitor

SHBG = sex hormone–binding globulin

T$_3$ = triiodothyronine

T$_4$ = thyroxine

TPO antibodies = thyroperoxidase antibodies

TRH = thyrotropin-releasing hormone

TRAb = TSH-receptor antibodies

TSH = thyrotropin

VLDL = very low-density lipoprotein

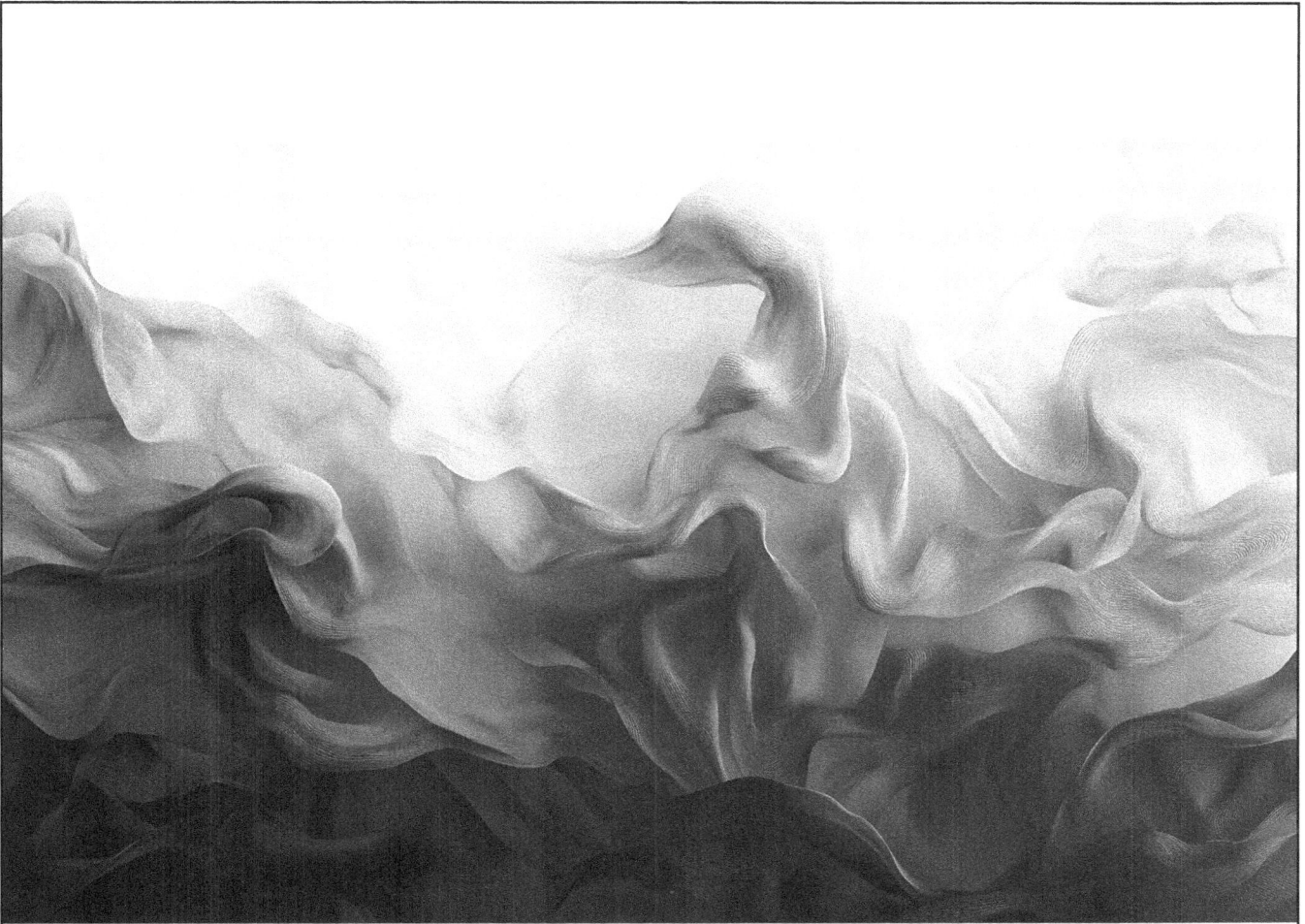

ADIPOSE TISSUE, APPETITE, OBESITY, AND LIPIDS

Weight-Loss Pharmacotherapy in the Spectrum of Obesity Care

José O. Alemán, MD, PhD. Laboratory of Translational Obesity Research, NYU Langone Health, New York, NY; Department of Medicine, Margaret Corbin Campus of the VA New York Harbor Health Care System, New York, NY; Holman Division of Endocrinology, Diabetes and Metabolism, New York University Langone Health, New York, NY; Email: jose.aleman@va.gov

Educational Objectives

After reviewing this chapter, learners should be able to:

- Recognize obesity as a chronic disease with relevant comorbidities.

- Describe FDA-approved and in-development obesity pharmacotherapy as an adjunct to lifestyle intervention for weight loss.

- Discuss the spectrum of obesity care, including dietary, pharmacologic, and surgical therapies.

Significance of the Clinical Problem

The prevalence of obesity in adults in the United States increased to more than 40% in recent years.[1] Obesity contributes to metabolic complications, such as type 2 diabetes, dyslipidemia, hypertension; increased risk of mechanical complications, such as osteoarthritis and obstructive sleep apnea; and comorbid diseases, including several major cancers.[2] Weight loss of 5% to 10% reduces obesity-related complications and improves quality of life.[3] Lifestyle interventions are currently the first-line therapy for weight loss; however, weight loss is difficult to maintain with lifestyle intervention alone.[4] The emergence of various pharmacotherapies for weight loss has significantly changed the landscape of obesity management over the past decade. Most approved first-generation antiobesity medications result in 5% to 10% total body weight loss (TBWL).[5] However, newer second-generation drugs, such as the GLP-1 agonist semaglutide, induce up to 17.4% weight loss from baseline in individuals without diabetes.

Similar to lifestyle interventions, of those who achieve at least 10% TBWL, many struggle to maintain this weight loss achieved with antiobesity medications.[6] Bariatric surgery induces more durable weight loss than pharmacotherapy or lifestyle interventions alone. More recently, endoscopic bariatric surgery, such as intragastric balloons and endoscopic sleeve gastroplasty, has offered a less-invasive option for weight loss.[7] Similar to other interventions for weight loss, there remains a common issue of weight regain or weight-loss plateau after surgical interventions. Studies have examined the benefit of combination therapy with antiobesity pharmacotherapy and endoscopic interventions, which results in more effective weight loss.[6] There are currently 6 FDA-approved medications for the long-term treatment of obesity, including orlistat, phentermine/topiramate, naltrexone/bupropion, liraglutide, semaglutide, and tirzepatide. Their effectiveness in treating postbariatric weight regain remains an active area of investigation. Herein, we present the pivotal trial evidence for each approved obesity pharmacotherapy agent, as well as the emerging data of its combination with available bariatric procedures.

Practice Gaps

- Six medications are FDA-approved for the long-term treatment of obesity, including orlistat, phentermine/topiramate, naltrexone/bupropion, liraglutide, semaglutide, and tirzepatide, yet their effectiveness in combination or sequence is not established.

- New drugs, such as retatrutide and orforglipron, are currently being evaluated for their efficacy in weight-loss management causing weight loss of similar magnitude to that of procedures.

- Surgical options, such as bariatric surgery, induce more durable weight loss than pharmacotherapy or lifestyle interventions alone. Recently, endoscopic bariatric surgery has offered a less-invasive option for weight loss. These procedures remain underused despite known longer-term effectiveness in weight loss and maintenance.

- The addition of pharmacotherapy has been shown to be a promising tool to address the common issue of weight regain or weight-loss plateau after surgical bariatric interventions. The choice of optimal pharmacotherapy to support weight-loss procedures remains unknown.

- The optimal timing of obesity pharmacotherapy with surgical and endoscopic interventions requires further investigation.

Discussion

Orlistat

Orlistat was FDA-approved for the treatment of obesity in 1999.[8] It is widely available, both as an over-the-counter medication at a dosage of up to 60 mg 3 times daily and at prescription dosages up to 120 mg 3 times daily. Orlistat can address weight-loss plateaus after weight-loss surgeries, such as adjustable gastric banding. The drug was associated with weight loss in a nonrandomized intervention study of 38 patients experiencing a weight-loss plateau after adjustable gastric banding, with a mean weight loss of 9 ± 3 kg in study participants compared with 3 ± 2 kg in the placebo group after 8 months of treatment with orlistat, 120 mg 3 times daily.[9] It was thought that perhaps orlistat was effective particularly for the high-calorie liquid diet required after bariatric procedures, which is often high in fat. Due to orlistat's mechanism, it also interferes with the absorption, and therefore effectiveness, of drugs, such as warfarin, amiodarone, cyclosporine, levothyroxine, and fat-soluble vitamins, which modifies their effectiveness. The only contraindications include pregnancy, breastfeeding, and cholestasis. However, despite these adverse effects, drug interactions, and some contraindications, orlistat remains a widely used, easily accessible therapy for weight loss.

Phentermine and Phentermine/Topiramate

Phentermine and phentermine/topiramate are currently approved for weight-loss management in the United States and came to the market as combination therapy in 2012.[10] Phentermine and phentermine/topiramate have been studied as adjunct therapy for weight loss for bariatric surgery and have been shown to be viable options for weight loss in patients with weight regain or weight-loss plateau after bariatric surgery. In a retrospective study of patients who had undergone Roux-en-Y gastric bypass or laparoscopic adjustable gastric banding, patients on phentermine lost 6.45 kg (12.8% excess weight loss), and those on phentermine/topiramate lost 3.81 kg (12.9% excess weight loss) at 90 days post surgery, but this study was limited by a short-term follow-up period.[11] An open-label trial of patients with a BMI of 50 kg/m² or higher who planned to undergo laparoscopic sleeve gastrectomy were prescribed phentermine/topiramate 7.5/46-15/92 mg or no therapy for at least 3 months preoperatively and 2 years postoperatively. Investigators found that the combination therapy group (phentermine/topiramate + laparoscopic sleeve gastrectomy) lost more than twice as much weight compared with control participants in the preoperative period (28.1 kg vs 12.3 kg) and lost 11.2% more initial weight than control participants 2 years after surgery.[12] Also, after 2 years of treatment, a higher proportion of patients in the phentermine/topiramate plus laparoscopic sleeve gastrectomy group achieved a BMI of less than 40 kg/m² than participants who had laparoscopic sleeve gastrectomy alone, thus favoring adjunct therapy for longer-term weight loss after laparoscopic sleeve gastrectomy.

Naltrexone/Bupropion

Naltrexone and bupropion are both FDA approved as monotherapies for indications other than weight loss but were approved by the US FDA in 2014 as combination therapy for long-term weight management in patients with obesity.[13] While the efficacy of combination therapy has been studied as pharmacotherapy, to date, there are no studies of the individual efficacies of naltrexone, bupropion, or combination therapy in the postbariatric surgery population. Randomized controlled trials of obesity pharmacotherapy often exclude patients with a history of bariatric surgery as a control. Given the proposed mechanism of naltrexone/bupropion for weight loss as a mediator of appetite in the hypothalamus, perhaps it would be useful adjunct therapy for patients experiencing weight regain, inadequate weight loss, or weight-loss plateau due to dietary indiscretion after bariatric or endoscopic bariatric surgery.

Liraglutide

The development of GLP-1 receptor agonists dramatically changed the landscape of weight loss pharmacotherapy. Liraglutide, a GLP-1 receptor agonist with 97% homology for human GLP-1, given as a once-daily subcutaneous injection, was approved by the US FDA for the treatment of type 2 diabetes in 2013 and for weight loss at a higher dosage in 2014.[14] While liraglutide alone has shown efficacy for weight loss, it has also been demonstrated as a useful adjunct to bariatric surgeries and more recently for endoscopic

bariatric procedures. The first placebo-controlled trial of adjunctive GLP-1 agonist therapy in patients with diabetes after bariatric surgery found a significant mean weight change from baseline to week 26 for patients receiving liraglutide, 1.8 mg daily, compared with placebo.[15] There was also a significant reduction in hemoglobin A_{1c} between the groups, favoring liraglutide. A retrospective study of patients with previous bariatric surgery who experienced weight recidivism (>10% weight regain from lowest postsurgical weight), inadequate weight loss (<20% weight loss from initial assessment or presurgical weight), and weight-loss plateau (patient desired further weight loss) found that those who had been on high-dosage liraglutide had median weight loss of 7.1% at 16 weeks and 9.7% at 28 weeks of therapy.[16]

GLP-1 receptor agonists have variably been shown to be effective adjunctive therapy for weight loss among patients who have undergone endoscopic bariatric interventions. Endoscopic bariatric procedures, such as endoscopic sleeve gastroplasty and intragastric balloons, face the same challenges of weight regain and inadequate weight loss as surgical bariatric procedures. A retrospective study of 26 matched patients who underwent endoscopic sleeve gastroplasty were offered liraglutide 5 months after endoscopic sleeve gastroplasty and found a significant total body weight loss after 7 months of treatment (1 year after endoscopic sleeve gastroplasty) compared with weight loss in patients who declined treatment (24.72% vs 20.51%, $P <$ .001).[17] While liraglutide plus endoscopic sleeve gastroplasty showed promising results, a study of liraglutide after intragastric balloon found that combination therapy did not decrease the risk of weight regain 6 months after balloon removal.[14] This study of 108 patients who received intragastric balloons alone vs intragastric balloons plus liraglutide 1 month after intragastric balloons insertion found higher mean weight loss after combination therapy. However, after adjusting for covariates, the intragastric balloon alone group had higher mean body weight loss at time of intragastric balloon removal and higher odds of treatment success 6 months after intragastric balloon removal. Of note, significantly more patients in the intragastric balloon alone group tolerated the therapy for 6 months (54 vs 46%; P = .038), but there were otherwise no significant differences between the groups regarding gastrointestinal symptoms, pain, early intragastric balloon removal or migration, or small-bowel obstruction. Liraglutide was discontinued 1 month after intragastric balloon removal. Although this study did not find decreased weight regain with combination therapy, perhaps the timing of the initiation and termination of liraglutide could have yielded different results.

Semaglutide

Semaglutide, a newer GLP-1 receptor agonist classified as second generation due to increased magnitude of weight loss, is given as a weekly subcutaneous injection for both diabetes and weight management. It was FDA approved for type 2 diabetes in 2017 and for chronic weight management in adults with obesity or overweight with at least 1 weight-related condition in June 2021. Semaglutide has been extensively studied as an adjunct therapy for patients who have undergone bariatric surgery and have weight regain or weight-loss plateau after surgery. A Swiss study reviewed patients who experienced weight regain after surgery who received 6 months of GLP-1 receptor agonist therapy with either semaglutide or liraglutide. Of patients who had a mean weight regain of 15.1% and received semaglutide (1.0 mg subcutaneously weekly or 14 mg orally daily) for at least 6 months, nearly one-quarter had total body weight loss of 15% or more. Combined with results from a liraglutide group, the authors concluded that two-thirds of weight regain after bariatric surgery can be safely lost with GLP-1 receptor agonist therapy.[18] Another study of patients with weight regain or insufficient weight loss found significant weight loss during semaglutide treatment with a mean of –10.3 kg at 6 months.[18] The mean time from surgery to initiation of semaglutide was 64.7

months with no difference between Roux-en-Y gastric bypass or sleeve gastrectomy. The timing of the initiation of adjunct pharmacotherapy is an important factor in determining how to optimize the use of obesity drugs, such as semaglutide, for weight-loss recidivism after bariatric surgery. Of note, the patients in those studies received a maximum dosage of semaglutide, 1.0 mg subcutaneously weekly, as it had not yet been approved for obesity at that time. Perhaps the higher dosage of semaglutide that is now approved for weight loss (2.4 mg weekly) would yield even greater weight-loss results in this patient population.

Tirzepatide

Tirzepatide is the first dual gastric inhibitory peptide (GIP) and GLP-1 co-agonist approved in the United States for the treatment of type 2 diabetes and obesity in the absence of diabetes.[19] GIP is also an incretin hormone that, like GLP-1, provides glucose-dependent insulin secretion from pancreatic β cells. Both GIP and GLP-1 are thought to play a role in appetite and satiety. The safety profile is comparable to that of other GLP-1 receptor agonists, with the most common adverse effects being a dose-dependent increase in mild to moderate and transient gastrointestinal events, such as nausea, diarrhea, and vomiting and rare fatal adverse effects, severe hypoglycemia, acute pancreatitis, and cholelithiasis or cholecystitis.[20] The SURMOUNT-1 trial of tirzepatide among patients with obesity who did not have diabetes demonstrated an average weight loss of 15%, 19.5%, and 20.9% over 72 weeks of treatment with tirzepatide, 5 mg, 10 mg, and 15 mg, respectively (vs 3.1% in the placebo group). In this trial, more than 35% of participants in the highest-dosage tirzepatide group had more than 25% weight reduction.[21] For comparison, bariatric surgery has been shown to result in estimated weight reduction up to 30% at 1 year after surgery. The integration of lifestyle, GLP-1 receptor agonists (liraglutide, semaglutide, tirzepatide), and endoscopic interventions and surgery after 12 months will be a key point of clinical comparison. Tirzepatide was approved for weight loss in 2022 as a new class of antiobesity medications, and it is a valuable addition to available weight-loss pharmacotherapies and may be an effective adjunct therapy for surgical and endoscopic weight-loss interventions.

Summary

Our multidisciplinary group at the Margaret Corbin (Manhattan) Campus of the VA New York Harbor Healthcare System initiated care for veterans with obesity and excess weight complications in 2017, and since this time has integrated obesity pharmacotherapy with endoscopic bariatric therapies into combined therapy. In our initial 1-year follow-up cohort study, we observed that weight-loss outcomes were significantly greater in the combined cohort compared with outcomes in the bariatric endoscopy-only cohort. In comparison, all weight-loss parameters were significantly greater in the combined therapy cohort at 12 months compared with parameters in the obesity pharmacotherapy cohort. This difference, specifically percentage change in BMI and percentage excess weight loss, was sustained at 24 months. In a cohort of 58 patients who underwent outpatient intragastric balloons or endoscopic sleeve gastroplasty and had at least 12 months of follow-up data, 43% of patients were also trialed on obesity pharmacotherapy with phentermine/topiramate, bupropion/naltrexone, liraglutide, or semaglutide. At 1-year follow-up after endoscopic bariatric therapies, there was no difference in TBWL, change in BMI, or excess weight loss between intragastric balloons and endoscopic sleeve gastroplasty cohorts. By year 3, excess weight loss was significantly greater in patients who had undergone endoscopic sleeve gastroplasty (40.4% ± 31.6%) compared with patients who had received intragastric balloons (17.4% ± 19.8%) (P = .025). These promising longitudinal results suggest combination of obesity pharmacotherapy and bariatric endoscopy results in greater sustained

weight loss than each modality alone, and that it address the chronic nature of obesity and weight management requiring multimodal therapies.

Optimal timing for pharmacotherapy initiation with bariatric intervention (both surgical and endoscopic) remains unclear. In a prospective study of 1000 consecutive patients undergoing endoscopic sleeve gastroplasty, the greatest rate of weight loss was observed within the first 6 months following the procedure. Average percentage TBWL at 1-, 3-, 6-, 9-, 12-, and 18-month follow-up was 8.9% ± 2.9%, 10.5% ± 4.5%, 13.7% ± 6.8%, 15.2% ± 8.3%, 15.0% ± 7.7%, 14.8% ± 8.5%, respectively, with a plateau in weight loss observed at 9 months after the procedure.[22] Obesity medications could be considered during this deceleration in weight loss following endoscopic sleeve gastroplasty before any weight regain. This finding is corroborated by a study by Badurdeen et al, in which patients who had undergone endoscopic sleeve gastroplasty and opted to take liraglutide 5 months after the procedure had superior weight loss compared with those who underwent endoscopic sleeve gastroplasty alone.[17] GLP-1 receptor agonist initiation at the onset of endoscopic bariatric intervention may increase adverse effects, such as nausea and abdominal pain. However, in a recent study of 58 patients randomly assigned to either semaglutide or placebo just 1 month after endoscopic sleeve gastroplasty, those in the semaglutide cohort had approximately 7% higher TBWL compared with TBWL in the placebo group, and there were no serious adverse effects.[17]

A qualitative study of 16 patients examining weight-loss patterns after gastric bypass described patterns that may help inform the optimal timing of pharmacotherapy. In the "honeymoon" period immediately after surgery and continuing for 6 to 12 months, weight loss was significant and rapid. This was followed by a weight "stabilization" period, followed by a "work begins" period when patients needed to implement cognitive and behavioral effort to maintain weight loss. Participants who regained weight reported a return to previous dietary habits, including lack of portion control, snacking, and emotional eating.[23] Pharmacotherapies that specifically decrease appetite, such as GLP-1 receptor agonists, phentermine/topiramate, and naltrexone/bupropion, may play a role in ameliorating these habits to prevent weight regain in the months to years following bariatric surgery. Further studies are needed to determine the optimal timing of combining pharmacotherapy with bariatric interventions to maximize weight loss and tolerability.

Clinical Case Vignettes

Case 1

A 61-year-old man with class 3 obesity (BMI = 42 kg/m^2) complicated by type 2 diabetes, hypertension, hyperlipidemia, and severe osteoarthritis presents for an initial weight management evaluation. His medical history is relevant for laparoscopic sleeve gastrectomy 6 years before his initial visit, causing weight loss from a peak weight of 392 lb (177.8 kg) to a nadir weight of 224 lb (101.6 kg). Over the ensuing 6 years, he slowly regained weight to his current 320 lb (145.2 kg). Social history is relevant for master's degree education and no toxic habits. His father has obesity and type 2 diabetes. His current medications include insulin glargine, 40 units daily; insulin lispro, 18 units before each meal; metformin, 1000 mg orally twice daily; atorvastatin; tamsulosin; omeprazole; lisinopril; amlodipine; atenolol; hydrochlorothiazide; aspirin; and naproxen as needed.

On physical examination, his pulse rate is 76 beats/min and blood pressure is 140/83 mm Hg. His height is 68 in (172.7 cm), and weight is 318 lb (144.2 kg) (BMI = 41.6 kg/m^2). Waist circumference is 51 in (129.5 cm). He has android fat distribution without acanthosis or dark striae.

Laboratory test results:

Hemoglobin A$_{1c}$ = 7.1% (54 mmol/mol)
TSH = 3.07 mIU/L
LDL cholesterol = 61 mg/dL (SI: 1.58 mmol/L)
Triglycerides = 73 mg/dL (SI: 0.82 mmol/L)
Creatinine = 0.6 mg/dL (SI: 53.0 μmol/L)

Results of dexamethasone-suppression testing are negative for hypercortisolism.

On the basis of published randomized controlled trials, which of the following FDA-approved medications for type 2 diabetes would provide the greatest improvement from baseline in glycemic control (by hemoglobin A$_{1c}$) and adjunct weight loss after 1 year of treatment?

A. Metformin, 1 g twice daily
B. Tirzepatide, 15 mg weekly
C. Semaglutide, 1 mg weekly
D. Liraglutide, 1.8 mg daily

Answer: B) Tirzepatide, 15 mg weekly

Several FDA-approved medications for type 2 diabetes provide weight-loss benefit, as demonstrated by their pivotal diabetes trials, and have a separate indication approval for patients with obesity but no diabetes. Of the medications listed, tirzepatide (Answer B) is associated with the greatest glycemic improvement and weight loss. In the 1995 SURPASS-4 trial comparing once-weekly subcutaneous tirzepatide with daily subcutaneous insulin glargine, people with type 2 diabetes (mean hemoglobin A$_{1c}$, 8.52%), BMI ≥25 kg/m^2, and high cardiovascular risk, the mean reduction in hemoglobin A$_{1c}$ with tirzepatide, 10 and 15 mg, over 25 weeks was greater than with insulin glargine (−2.43 and −2.58 percentage points, respectively, vs −1.44 percentage points with insulin glargine). Subsequently, in the SURPASS-2 study comparing tirzepatide with semaglutide weekly in 1878 patients with type 2 diabetes who were not reaching glycemic goals with metformin monotherapy, the reduction in hemoglobin A$_{1c}$ was superior with tirzepatide (−2 to −2.3 percentage points vs −1.86 percentage points with semaglutide). Overall, small differences in glycemic efficacy favor tirzepatide over subcutaneous semaglutide (1 mg) or liraglutide. Weight-loss outcomes in the pivotal diabetes trials showed tirzepatide resulted in greater weight loss than subcutaneous semaglutide (1 mg). In turn, weight loss was generally greater with subcutaneous semaglutide (–6 kg) than 1.8 mg liraglutide (–3.5 kg).

Interestingly, the use of liraglutide for postbariatric weight regain has been studied rigorously in patients following Roux-en-Y gastric bypass. Lofton et al conducted a 56-week, double-blind, placebo-controlled study in 132 participants who achieved 25% TBWL status post Roux-en-Y gastric bypass and regained 10% TBWL after reaching nadir weight. Eighteen to 120 months after Roux-en-Y gastric bypass, participants were randomized assigned to receive liraglutide, 3.0 mg daily, or placebo with lifestyle counseling regularly for 56 weeks. Trial recruitment was limited; 53.4% of the placebo group and 65% of the liraglutide group completed the trial due to the COVID-19 pandemic. The percentage change in TBWL from baseline to 56 weeks was 28.8% (8.5, 229.2 to 9.7) and 1.1% (3.5, 27.9 to 5.99) in the liraglutide and placebo groups, respectively. In the liraglutide and placebo groups, 76% and 17% of participants achieved 5% TBWL at 56 weeks, while 51% and 26.0% of the liraglutide group achieved 10% and 15% TBWL, respectively. None of the placebo group lost 10% TBWL. Twenty-one percent of participants receiving liraglutide surpassed postoperative nadir weight. No participants on placebo met this goal. Studies for semaglutide and tirzepatide as treatment for postbariatric weight regain are ongoing.

Case 1, Continued

This patient was treated with weight-centric management of type 2 diabetes at a time when liraglutide, 1.8 mg weekly, was the most effective medication providing weight and glycemic benefit in type 2 diabetes. Implementation of strict caloric restriction to 1500 calories daily, a low-carbohydrate diet, and liraglutide, 1.8 mg daily, resulted in clinically significant weight loss of 20% from baseline weight to a recent nadir weight of 255 lb (115.7 kg) and freedom from insulin. Weight-loss maintenance required the addition of phentermine-topiramate, 7.5/46 mg

daily, as well as resistance exercise to build muscle mass. He returns now, after 1 year of combined therapy, with concerns of increased appetite and weight regain.

Which of the following treatment options is most likely to result in weight-loss maintenance over the next 6 months?
A. Orlistat, 120 mg 3 times daily
B. Endoscopic sleeve gastroplasty
C. Semaglutide, 1 mg weekly
D. Naltrexone/bupropion, 32/360 mg daily

Answer: B) Endoscopic sleeve gastroplasty

Bariatric endoscopy is emerging as an alternative reversible procedure simulating bariatric surgery that overlaps in efficacy with second-generation antiobesity medications, such semaglutide and tirzepatide. Since 2015, several endoscopic bariatric and metabolic therapies have been approved by the US FDA for use in patients with BMI greater than 30 kg/m², which could potentially address the treatment gap for patients with lower weights. These therapies fall into 2 categories: space-occupying devices (gastric balloons and transpyloric shuttle) and gastric remodeling (endoscopic gastroplasty [US FDA approved for tissue apposition]), used for remodeling of the stomach anatomy to achieve weight loss. The reported weight loss with the available endoscopic bariatric and metabolic therapies ranges from about 10% (gastric balloons)[7] to 16% (endoscopic gastroplasty)[24] with a low rate of serious adverse events.

Peak reported weight loss for endoscopic bariatric and metabolic therapies occurs after 6 months of device placement or tissue apposition. A detailed meta-analysis of endoscopic sleeve gastroplasty collated available primary evidence in assessing effectiveness of endoscopic sleeve gastroplasty of 16% weight loss from baseline at 6 months.[24] In contrast, peak weight loss for antiobesity medications occurs at 52 weeks or later, as reported in the STEP trials of semaglutide.[25] In this study, weight loss with semaglutide at 28 weeks approximated 12% from baseline, and weight loss of 14.9% was reported from baseline at the formal 68-week study end point. The effectiveness of other antiobesity medications is commonly reported 1 year after intervention, with orlistat inducing 2.9% to 3.4% weight loss and naltrexone/bupropion inducing 4.8% weight loss below those of endoscopic sleeve gastroplasty. A final consideration with endoscopic bariatric and metabolic therapies, such as sleeve gastroplasty, is the possibility of weight regain, which often requires antiobesity medication support beyond 6 months after the procedure.

Key Learning Points

- The number of safe and effective options for the pharmacotherapy treatment of obesity is increasing rapidly. New and improved weight loss drugs continue to emerge, and several new multiagonist and multihormonal therapies will hopefully be approved for obesity in the near future and push the treatment envelope towards higher adiposity with complications (*Figure*).

- Understanding the individual mechanisms, tolerability, and efficacy of each of these weight-loss drugs is essential to inform how they may best be used not only as monotherapy, but also how they may be powerful adjuncts to endoscopic and surgical bariatric procedures.

- Some studies have already demonstrated the utility of the combination of bariatric surgery and pharmacotherapy for optimizing weight loss. With the increased use of less-invasive bariatric procedures, such as endoscopic surgeries, more studies are needed to evaluate the role of weight-loss drugs as adjunct therapy with such procedures.

- The optimal timing of adjunct obesity pharmacotherapy also requires further investigation to help provide patients with the most effective, tolerable, and long-lasting weight loss achievable.

Figure. Spectrum of Care for Obesity According to BMI

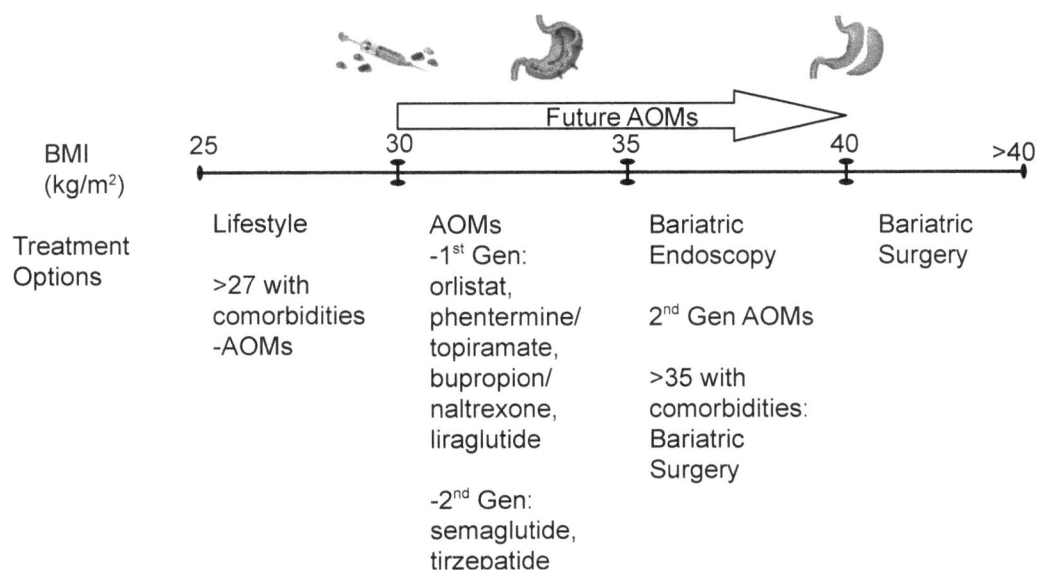

The spectrum of care for obesity by BMI reflects increasing overlap between AOMs and procedures, including bariatric endoscopy and bariatric surgery.

[Color—Print (Color Gallery page CG3) or web & ePub editions]

References

1. Centers of Disease Control and Prevention. *Adult Obesity Prevalence Maps*. US Department of Health and Human Services; 2023.

2. Aleman JO, Eusebi LH, Ricciardiello L, Patidar K, Sanyal AJ, Holt PR. Mechanisms of obesity-induced gastrointestinal neoplasia. *Gastroenterology*. 2014;146(2):357-373. PMID: 24315827

3. Mertens IL, Van Gaal LF. Overweight, obesity, and blood pressure: the effects of modest weight reduction. *Obes Res*. 2000;8(3):270-278. PMID: 10832771

4. Dombrowski SU, Knittle K, Avenell A, Araujo-Soares V, Sniehotta FF. Long term maintenance of weight loss with non-surgical interventions in obese adults: systematic review and meta-analyses of randomised controlled trials. *BMJ*. 2014;348:g2646. PMID: 25134100

5. Apovian CM, Aronne LJ, Bessesen DH, et al. Pharmacological management of obesity: an endocrine Society clinical practice guideline. *J Clin Endocrinol Metab*. 2015;100(2):342-362. PMID: 25590212

6. Dave N, Dawod E, Simmons OL. Endobariatrics: a still underutilized weight loss tool. *Curr Treat Options Gastroenterol*. 2023;21(2):172-184. PMID: 37284352

7. Popov VB, Ou A, Schulman AR, Thompson CC. The impact of intragastric balloons on obesity-related co-morbidities: a systematic review and meta-analysis. *Am J Gastroenterol*. 2017;112(3):429-439. PMID: 28117361

8. Lucas E, Simmons O, Tchang B, Aronne L. Pharmacologic management of weight regain following bariatric surgery. *Front Endocrinol (Lausanne)*. 2022;13:1043595. PMID: 36699042

9. Zoss I, Piec G, Horber FF. Impact of orlistat therapy on weight reduction in morbidly obese patients after implantation of the Swedish adjustable gastric band. *Obes Surg*. 2002;12(1):113-117. PMID: 11868286

10. Bray GA, Fruhbeck G, Ryan DH, Wilding JP. Management of obesity. *Lancet*. 2016;387(10031):1947-1956. PMID: 26868660

11. Schwartz J, Chaudhry UI, Suzo A, et al. Pharmacotherapy in conjunction with a diet and exercise program for the treatment of weight recidivism or weight loss plateau post-bariatric surgery: a retrospective review. *Obes Surg*. 2016;26(2):452-458. PMID: 26615406

12. Ard JD, Beavers DP, Hale E, Miller G, McNatt S, Fernandez A. Use of phentermine-topiramate extended release in combination with sleeve gastrectomy in patients with BMI 50 kg/m(2) or more. *Surg Obes Relat Dis*. 2019;15(7):1039-1043. PMID: 31147285

13. Yanovski SZ, Yanovski JA. Naltrexone extended-release plus bupropion extended-release for treatment of obesity. *JAMA*. 2015;313(12):1213-1214. PMID: 25803343

14. Mosli MM, Elyas M. Does combining liraglutide with intragastric balloon insertion improve sustained weight reduction? *Saudi J Gastroenterol*. 2017;23(2):117-122. PMID: 28361843

15. Miras AD, Perez-Pevida B, Aldhwayan M, et al. Adjunctive liraglutide treatment in patients with persistent or recurrent type 2 diabetes after metabolic surgery (GRAVITAS): a randomised, double-blind, placebo-controlled trial. *Lancet Diabetes Endocrinol*. 2019;7(7):549-559. PMID: 31174993

16. Rye P, Modi R, Cawsey S, Sharma AM. Efficacy of high-dose liraglutide as an adjunct for weight loss in patients with prior bariatric surgery. *Obes Surg*. 2018;28(11):3553-3558. PMID: 30022424

17. Badurdeen D, Hoff AC, Hedjoudje A, et al. Endoscopic sleeve gastroplasty plus liraglutide versus endoscopic sleeve gastroplasty alone for weight loss. *Gastrointest Endosc*. 2021;93(6):1316-1324.e1. PMID: 33075366

18. Lautenbach A, Wernecke M, Huber TB, et al. The potential of semaglutide once-weekly in patients without type 2 diabetes with weight regain or insufficient weight loss after bariatric surgery-a retrospective analysis. *Obes Surg*. 2022;32(10):3280-3288. PMID: 35879524

19. Nauck MA, D'Alessio DA. Tirzepatide, a dual GIP/GLP-1 receptor co-agonist for the treatment of type 2 diabetes with unmatched effectiveness regrading glycaemic control and body weight reduction. *Cardiovasc Diabetol*. 2022;21(1):169. PMID: 36050763

20. Seino Y, Fukushima M, Yabe D. GIP and GLP-1, the two incretin hormones: Similarities and differences. *J Diabetes Investig*. 2010;1(1-2):8-23. PMID: 24843404

21. Jastreboff AM, Aronne LJ, Ahmad NN, et al; SURMOUNT-1 Investigators. Tirzepatide once weekly for the treatment of obesity. *N Engl J Med*. 2022;387(3):205-216. PMID: 35658024

22. Alqahtani A, Al-Darwish A, Mahmoud AE, Alqahtani YA, Elahmedi M. Short-term outcomes of endoscopic sleeve gastroplasty in 1000 consecutive patients. *Gastrointest Endosc*. 2019;89(6):1132-1138. PMID: 30578757

23. Lynch A. "When the honeymoon is over, the real work begins:" Gastric bypass patients' weight loss trajectories and dietary change experiences. *Soc Sci Med*. 2016;151:241-249. PMID: 26820572

24. Hedjoudje A, Abu Dayyeh BK, Cheskin LJ, et al. Efficacy and safety of endoscopic sleeve gastroplasty: a systematic review and meta-analysis. *Clin Gastroenterol Hepatol*. 2020;18(5):1043-1053. e4. PMID: 31442601

25. Wilding JPH, Batterham RL, Calanna S, et al. Once-weekly semaglutide in adults with overweight or obesity. *N Engl J Med*. 2021;384(11):989-1002. PMID: 33567185

Metabolic Dysfunction-Associated Steatotic Liver Disease: Tips for Endocrinologists

Eveline Bruinstroop, MD, PhD. Department of Endocrinology and Metabolism, Amsterdam Gastroenterology Endocrinology and Metabolism Institute, Amsterdam UMC, Amsterdam, The Netherlands; Email: e.bruinstroop@amsterdamumc.nl

A. G. (Onno) Holleboom, MD, PhD. Department of Vascular Medicine, Amsterdam Gastroenterology Endocrinology and Metabolism Institute, Amsterdam UMC, Amsterdam, The Netherlands; Email: a.g.holleboom@amsterdamumc.nl

Educational Objectives

After reviewing this chapter, learners should be able to:

- Describe the importance and methods of screening for metabolic dysfunction-associated steatotic liver disease (MASLD) in patients with diabetes and obesity.

- Take MASLD into account while managing diabetes.

- Identify the horizon for medical treatment of fibrotic metabolic dysfunction-associated steatohepatitis (MASH).

Significance of the Clinical Problem

MASLD has become the most common liver disease, driven by the worsening epidemic of obesity and diabetes. The overall global prevalence of MASLD is 30% in the general population, with 3% of all children affected.[1] MASLD starts with the increased accumulation of fat within the liver (steatosis), which can lead to necroinflammation of hepatocytes and activation of nonparenchymal cells, a condition known as MASH. In patients with type 2 diabetes, the prevalence of MASLD worldwide is 65%. A greater proportion (15%) of patients with diabetes progress from MASH to the advanced fibrotic stages of the disease compared with patients who do not have diabetes, and this can ultimately culminate in liver-related complications. Half of patients with advanced fibrosis eventually develop cirrhosis.[1,2] Complications include decompensated cirrhosis and hepatocellular carcinoma, both of which are rising in prevalence. Currently, MASH is the reason for liver transplantation in 27% of the patients without hepatocellular carcinoma. In patients with hepatocellular carcinoma, however, MASH is the most common indication for liver transplantation.[3]

Most patients with diabetes and obesity never progress to end-stage liver disease. Yet, it has been shown that managing MASLD is important, even in patients with milder and less progressive forms of MASLD. Indeed, each incremental step along MASLD progression is associated with a concomitant increase in the risk of atherosclerotic cardiovascular events and mortality, independent of common drivers of MASLD and atherosclerotic cardiovascular disease.[3,4] In addition, MASLD and type 2 diabetes have a reciprocal relationship in that type 2 diabetes and hyperinsulinemia drive lipid accumulation and lipogenesis in the liver, while hepatic insulin resistance driven by lipotoxicity can in turn trigger gluconeogenesis and thus hyperglycemia, giving rise to or compounding type 2 diabetes.[5,6]

Therefore, in addition to screening for dyslipidemia, oculopathy, nephropathy, and neuropathy, MASLD should be screened for and treated as appropriate in patients with type 2 diabetes and obesity. This is also highlighted in the recommendations for screening in the American Diabetes Association 2023 guideline (Chapter 4: Comprehensive Medical Evaluation and Assessment of Comorbidities: Standards of Care in Diabetes): "Adults with type 2 diabetes or prediabetes, particularly those with obesity or cardiometabolic risk factors/established cardiovascular disease, should be screened/risk stratified for MASLD with clinically significant fibrosis using a calculated fibrosis-4 index even if they have normal liver enzymes."[7]

Practice Gaps

- Uncertainty about which screening tests should be used for MASLD.

- Difficulty discerning which diabetes treatments may also have benefit for MASLD.

- Lack of familiarity with the 3 pillars of treatment for MASLD.

Discussion
Which Screening Tests Should I Use?

It is important to estimate organ damage due to MASLD (ie, the presence of significant fibrosis). Therefore, tests have been developed aimed at ruling out advanced liver fibrosis corresponding to

Figure. Screening Strategy for MASLD

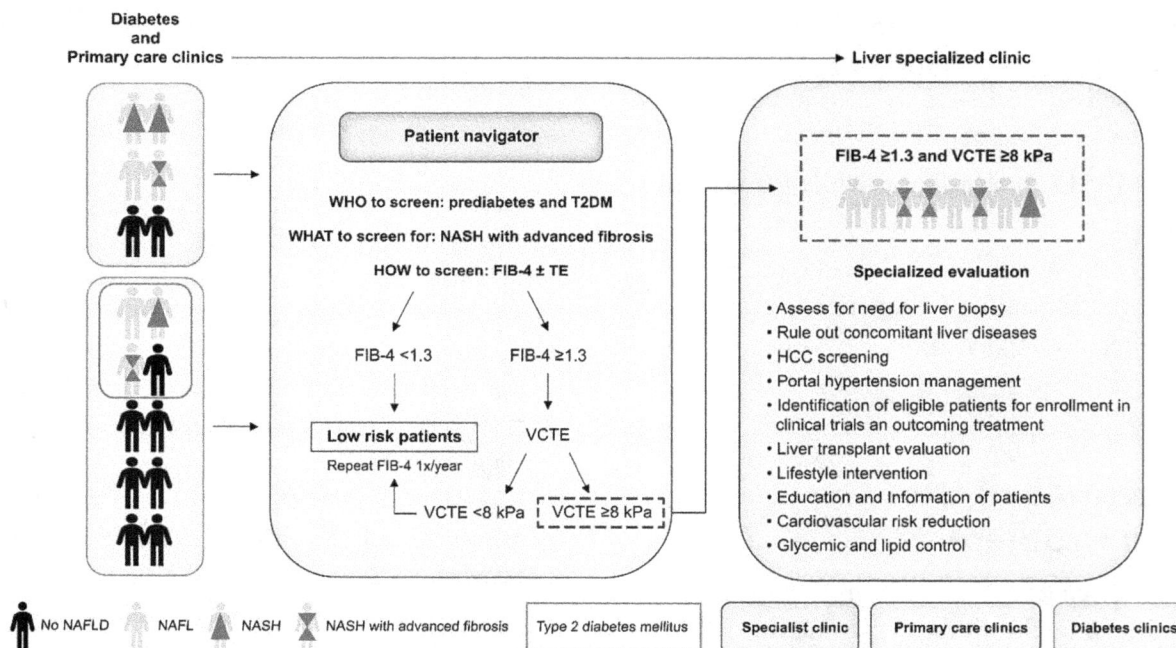

Screening strategy for MASLD, formerly known as nonalcoholic fatty liver disease (NAFLD) and nonalcoholic steatohepatitis (NASH). The strategy is based on a 2-tier testing approach starting with FIB-4 and, when necessary, vibration-controlled transient elastography (VCTE). Patients with high suspicion of advanced fibrosis should be referred to a specialized liver clinic for further evaluation.[10]

Reprinted with permission from Vieira Barbosa J &, Lai M. Hepatol Commun, 2020; 5(2): 158-167. © The Authors. Published by Wiley Periodicals LLC on behalf of American Association for the Study of Liver Diseases.

[Color—Print (Color Gallery page CG3) or web & ePub editions]

a histological stage of severe liver fibrosis (ie, F3 stage and higher). F3 stage designates the presence of bridging fibrosis between portal tracts.

Several noninvasive approaches have been developed for ruling out advanced MASLD fibrosis, without the need for liver biopsy. The most commonly used is the Fibrosis-4 score (FIB-4), where broadly available parameters, including age, AST and ALT levels, and platelet count, are used to calculate a score (age * AST / [0.001 * platelets * sqr(ALT)]).[8,9] Several calculators are available online and some laboratories and medical centers directly report this score to enhance ease of use. Dependent on the FIB-4 score (lower cutoff = 1.3), additional screening may be required (*Figure, preceding page*).

Which Diabetes Treatments May Benefit Patients With Different Stages of MASLD?

Several clinical trials have investigated the efficacy of known antidiabetes drugs on MASLD (*Table*).

What Are the 3 Pillars of MASLD Treatment?

The cornerstone of MASLD treatment remains lifestyle intervention with the aim of an 8% to 10% weight reduction. There is some histological evidence that combined lifestyle intervention (hypocaloric diet and aerobic exercise) inducing weight loss can improve MASLD, including steatohepatitis and fibrosis,[19,20] but most of the evidence for these interventions is based on liver imaging (ultrasonography or MRI) gauging steatosis only.

The thyroid hormone receptor β-agonist resmetirom was the first drug to receive FDA approval in 2024 for the treatment of MASLD with advanced fibrosis in the United States. Several additional pharmaceutical agents that are in late-stage development for fibrotic MASLD and cirrhotic MASH include the GLP-1 receptor agonist semaglutide and dual hormone agonists, such as tirzepatide, survodutide, and

Table. Clinical Trials Investigating Efficacy of Antidiabetes Drugs on MASLD

Medication	Effects on MASLD
Pioglitazone, 30 mg	Reduction in steatosis and inflammation, no improvement fibrosis stage[11]
GLP-1 receptor agonist (semaglutide, 2.4 mg)	Reduction in steatosis, MASH, and fibrosis (interim analyses)[12,13]
GLP-1 receptor agonist (liraglutide, 1.8 mg)	Reduction in steatosis, MASH[14]
GLP-1/GIP (tirzepatide)	Reduction in steatosis, MASH[15]
SGLT-2 inhibitors	No histopathological studies, possible reduction in steatosis[16-18]

efinopegdutide. Also promising are the FGF-21 analogues efruxifermin and pegozafermin (which, among many other effects, deflect ingested carbohydrates away from liver), the fatty acid synthase inhibitor denifanstat, and the pan-peroxisome proliferator–activated receptor agonist lanifibranor.[22]

In addition, the BRAVES trial found significant histological reductions in fibrotic MASLD at bariatric surgery, including both Roux-en-Y gastric bypass and sleeve gastrectomy.[21] This prospective evidence is supported by a large meta-analysis of bariatric procedures for clinical obesity and MASLD.[23]

Clinical Case Vignettes
Case 1

A 67-year-old woman with type 2 diabetes and obesity (BMI = 33 kg/m²) is referred after not achieving glycemic goals (hemoglobin A_{1c} = 9% [75 mmol/mol]) with a combination of metformin and sulfonylureas. Laboratory assessment showed no signs of chronic kidney disease, and there are no clinical signs of retinopathy or polyneuropathy.

Following the American Diabetes Association guidelines, the patient is also screened for MASLD.

By using the FIB-4 score based on age, AST, ALT, and blood platelet counts, the aim is to rule out which of the following?

A. Significant steatosis (>5% intrahepatic fat content)

B. Liver fibrosis of any stage (F1-F4)

C. Advanced liver fibrosis (stage F3 and higher)

D. Decompensated liver cirrhosis

Answer: C) Advanced liver fibrosis (stage F3 and higher)

A FIB-4 score less than 1.3 has a high negative predictive value for advanced fibrosis (≥F3), whereas a positive result should prompt further investigation. Although FIB-4 may be inferior to other serum-based fibrosis markers (ELF, FIBROSpect II) and imaging-based elastography methods, it is recommended as a first-line assessment for general practitioners and endocrinologists based on its simplicity and minimal cost. Disadvantages of the FIB-4 score include low accuracy in patients 35 years or younger and the possible requirement of different cutoffs for subgroups of patients with various conditions, including diabetes.[8,9] FIB-4 is not a test to identify steatosis, which can be measured qualitatively with ultrasonography and quantified by controlled attenuation parameter or magnetic resonance spectroscopy. The test is validated specifically for advanced fibrosis and does not rule out earlier signs of fibrosis (F1 and F2), which can be present on liver histology. Also, it does not rule out the presence of decompensated liver cirrhosis, which depends mainly on clinical factors, such as ascites.

Case 1, Continued

The patient has the following laboratory results documented:

> AST = 25 U/L (SI: 0.42 μkat/L)
> ALT = 32 U/L (SI: 0.53 μkat/L)
> Platelet count = 170 × 10³/μL (SI: 170 × 10⁹/L)

With these values combined with age, the FIB-4 score can be calculated.

Based on the patient's FIB-4 score, which of the following is the best next step?

A. There is a low risk of advanced liver fibrosis with currently no need for further investigation; reassess FIB-4 score in 2 to 3 years

B. There is an indeterminate risk of advanced liver fibrosis; recommend performing a liver stiffness measurement by vibration-controlled transient elastography

C. There is a high risk of advanced liver fibrosis; recommend liver biopsy

Answer: A) There is a low risk of advanced liver fibrosis with currently no need for further investigation; reassess FIB-4 score in 2 to 3 years

The FIB-4 score is 1.05, which represents a low risk of advanced liver fibrosis (<1.3).[7,8] No further action is currently needed, and the FIB-4 score can be reassessed in 2 to 3 years. A FIB-4 score of 2.67 or higher is considered to indicate a high risk of advanced liver fibrosis. Scores between 1.3 and 2.67 signal indeterminate risk. The American Diabetes Association guideline recommends patients with either an indeterminate risk or high risk score receive a liver stiffness measurement by vibration-controlled transient elastography, which is a well-validated ultrasound-based test for fibrosis. A liver stiffness measurement less than 8.0 kPa excludes advanced fibrosis with a good negative predictive value.[7]

Case 2

A 67-year-old woman with type 2 diabetes and obesity (BMI = 33 kg/m²) is referred after not achieving glycemic goals (hemoglobin A_{1c} = 9% [75 mmol/mol]) with a combination of metformin and sulfonylureas. Screening for MASLD showed an indeterminate FIB-4 score.

Laboratory test results:

> AST = 40 U/L (SI: 0.67 μkat/L)
> ALT = 32 U/L (SI: 0.53 μkat/L)
> Platelet count = 170 × 10³/μL (SI: 170 × 10⁹/L)

Liver stiffness is determined to be 7.0 kPa with a controlled attenuation parameter of 310 dB/min.

The measurements from this test indicate which of the following?

A. No signs of MASLD

B. Presence of steatosis

C. Presence of steatosis and fibrosis

Answer: B) Presence of steatosis

A liver stiffness value less than 8.0 kPa indicates no presence of advanced fibrosis. Controlled attenuation parameter is a feature that is implemented in the FibroScan device, which can also quantify liver steatosis by attenuation of the ultrasound beam as it passes through the liver. Different cut offs have been applied with values of 288 dB/min or higher generally considered indicative of steatosis.[8] Overall, the results are consistent with the presence of MASLD with steatosis but lack of fibrosis.

Case 2, Continued

Which of the following is the best next step to improve this patient's glycemic control, obesity, and MASLD?

A. Combined pharmacological treatments targeting not only glycemic control but also obesity, MASLD, and cardiovascular risk

B. Lifestyle interventions aimed at 8% to 10% weight loss

C. Bariatric surgery

D. All of the above

Answer: D) All of the above

To improve glycemic control, obesity, and MASLD progression, lifestyle measures, pharmacological interventions, and surgical options should be explored (Answer D). The cornerstone of MASLD treatment remains lifestyle intervention with the aim of 8% to 10% weight reduction. Several trials have been performed investigating the effects of known diabetes medications on MASLD (*Table*), including pioglitazone, GLP-1 receptor agonists, GLP-1/GIP dual agonists, and SGLT-2 inhibitors. The interim analyses from the phase 3 ESSENCE trial with 2.4-mg semaglutide once weekly showed significant improvements in histological activity and fibrosis markers after 72 weeks of treatment.[13] Significant histological reductions of fibrotic MASLD after bariatric surgery have also been shown.[19]

Case 3

A 67-year-old woman with type 2 diabetes and obesity (BMI = 33 kg/m^2) is referred after not achieving glycemic goals (hemoglobin A_{1c} = 9% [75 mmol/mol]) with a combination of metformin and a sulfonylurea. Laboratory assessment shows no signs of chronic kidney disease, and she has no clinical signs of retinopathy or polyneuropathy. Screening for MASLD shows a high FIB-4 score.

Laboratory test results:

> AST = 50 U/L (SI: 0.84 μkat/L)
> ALT = 44 U/L (SI: 0.73 μkat/L)
> Platelet count = 100 × 10^3/μL (SI: 100 × 10^9/L)

Liver stiffness measurement is 18.0 kPa, which indicates advanced fibrosis.

Should the patient be referred to a hepatologist?

A. Yes

B. No

Answer: A) Yes

Patients with advanced liver fibrosis should be referred to an hepatologist to (1) exclude other causes of fibrosis; (2) consider performing liver biopsy; (3) perform follow-up for potential progression to (decompensated) cirrhosis and consider hepatocellular carcinoma screening; and (4) consider treatment of liver fibrosis.

Case 3, Continued

Which of the following registered treatments for advanced liver fibrosis is currently available?

A. Semaglutide

B. Tirzepatide

C. Resmetirom

D. Lanifibranor

Answer: C) Resmetirom

The thyroid hormone receptor β-agonist resmetirom (Answer C) is currently the only conditionally FDA-registered treatment for MASLD. However, other drugs are currently in development in clinical trials, including semaglutide (Answer A), tirzepatide (Answer B), and lanifibranor (Answer D).

Key Learning Points

- Patients with diabetes should be screened for MASLD with the FIB-4 score based on age, AST, ALT, and platelet count.

- When choosing pharmacological treatment(s) for diabetes, the presence of MASLD and obesity should be taken into account.

- Patients with advanced liver fibrosis should be referred to a hepatologist for further diagnosis, follow-up, and treatment.

- Optimal diabetes management remains important in patients with MASLD and should focus on lifestyle, pharmacological treatment, and possible surgical treatment.

References

1. Younossi ZM, Golabi P, Paik JM, Henry A, Van Dongen C, Henry Linda. The global epidemiology of nonalcoholic fatty liver disease (NAFLD) and nonalcoholic steatohepatitis (NASH): a systematic review. *Hepatology.* 2023;77(4):1335-1347. PMID: 36626630

2. McPherson S, Hardy T, Henderson E, Burt AD, Day CP, Anstee QM. Evidence of NAFLD progression from steatosis to fibrosing-steatohepatitis using paired biopsies: implications for prognosis and clinical management. *J Hepatol.* 2015;62(5):1148-1155. PMID: 25477264

3. Younossi ZM, Stepanova M, Al Shabeeb R, et al. The changing epidemiology of adult liver transplantation in the United States in 2013-2022: The dominance of metabolic dysfunction-associated steatotic liver disease and alcohol-associated liver disease. *Hepatol Commun.* 2023;8(1):e0352. PMID: 38126928

4. Younossi ZM, Golabi P, Price JK, et al. The global epidemiology of nonalcoholic fatty liver disease and nonalcoholic steatohepatitis among patients with type 2 diabetes. *Clin Gastroenterol Hepatol.* 2024;22(10):1999-2010.e8. PMID: 38521116

5. Simon TG, Roelstraete B, Hagström H, Sundström J, Ludvigsson JF. Non-alcoholic fatty liver disease and incident major adverse cardiovascular events: results from a nationwide histology cohort. *Gut.* 2022;71(9):1867-1875. PMID: 34489307

6. Donnelly KL, Smith CI, Schwarzenberg SJ, Jessurun J, Boldt MD, Parks EJ. Sources of fatty acids stored in liver and secreted via lipoproteins in patients with nonalcoholic fatty liver disease. *J Clin Invest.* 2005;115(5):1343-1351. PMID: 15864352

7. Ter Horst KW, Gilijamse PW, Versteeg RI, et al. Hepatic diacylglycerol-associated protein kinase Cε translocation links hepatic steatosis to hepatic insulin resistance in humans. *Cell Rep.* 2017;19(10):1997-2004. PMID: 28591572

8. ElSayed NA, Aleppo G, Aroda VR, et al; on behalf of the American Diabetes Association. 4. Comprehensive medical evaluation and assessment of comorbidities: standards of care in diabetes-2023. *Diabetes Care.* 2023;46(Suppl 1):S49-S67. PMID: 36507651

9. Rinella ME, Neuschwander-Tetri BA, Siddiqui MS, et al. AASLD practice guidance on the clinical assessment and management of nonalcoholic fatty liver disease. *Hepatology.* 2023;77(5):1797-1835. PMID: 36727674

10. Vali Y, van Dijk AM, Lee J, et al; LITMUS investigators. Precision in liver diagnosis: varied accuracy across subgroups and the need for variable thresholds in diagnosis of MASLD. *Liver Int.* 2025;45(2):e16240. PMID: 39865358

11. Vieira Barbosa J, Lai M. Nonalcoholic fatty liver disease screening in type 2 diabetes mellitus patients in the primary care setting. *Hepatol Commun.* 2020;5(2):158-167.

12. Sanyal AJ, Chalasani N, Kowdley KV, et al; NASH CRN. Pioglitazone, vitamin E, or placebo for nonalcoholic steatohepatitis. *N Engl J Med.* 2010;362(18):1675-1685. PMID: 20427778

13. Newsome PN, Buchholtz K, Cusi K, et al; NN9931-4296 Investigators. A placebo-controlled trial of subcutaneous semaglutide in nonalcoholic steatohepatitis. *N Engl J Med.* 2021;384(12):1113-1124. PMID: 33185364

14. Newsome PN, Sanyal A, Kliers I, et al. Phase 3 ESSENCE trial: semaglutide in metabolic dysfunction-associated steatohepatitis (MASH) [AASLD abstract 5018]. Presented at: The Liver Meeting; November 15-19, 2024; San Diego, CA.

15. Armstrong MJ, Gaunt P, Aithal GP, et al. Liraglutide safety and efficacy in patients with non-alcoholic steatohepatitis (LEAN): a multicentre, double-blind, randomised, placebo-controlled phase 2 study. *Lancet.* 2016;387(10019):679-690. PMID: 26608256

16. Loomba R, Hartman ML, Lawitz EJ, et al; SYNERGY-NASH Investigators. Tirzepatide for metabolic dysfunction-associated steatohepatitis with liver fibrosis. *N Engl J Med.* 2024;391(4):299-310. PMID: 38856224

17. Kuchay MS, Krishan S, Mishra SK, et al. Effect of empagliflozin on liver fat in patients with type 2 diabetes and nonalcoholic fatty liver disease: a randomized controlled trial (E-LIFT Trial). *Diabetes Care.* 2018;41(8):1801-1808. PMID: 29895557

18. Harrison SA, Manghi FP, Smith WB, et al. Licogliflozin for nonalcoholic steatohepatitis: a randomized, double-blind, placebo-controlled, phase 2a study. *Nat Med.* 2022;28(7):1432-1438. PMID:

19. Ong Lopez AMC, Pajimna JAT. Efficacy of sodium glucose cotransporter 2 inhibitors on hepatic fibrosis and steatosis in non-alcoholic fatty liver disease: an updated systematic review and meta-analysis. *Sci Rep.* 2024;14(1):2122. PMID: 38267513

20. Vilar-Gomez E, Martinez-Perez Y, Calzadilla-Bertot L, et al. Weight loss through lifestyle modification significantly reduces features of nonalcoholic steatohepatitis. *Gastroenterology.* 2015;149(2):367-378.e5. PMID: 25865049

21. Verrastro O, Panunzi S, Castagneto-Gissey L, et al. Bariatric-metabolic surgery versus lifestyle intervention plus best medical care in non-alcoholic steatohepatitis (BRAVES): a multicentre, open-label, randomised trial. *Lancet.* 2023;401(10390):1786-1797. PMID: 25865049

22. Ratziu V, Francque S, Sanyal A. Breakthroughs in therapies for NASH and remaining challenges. *J Hepatol.* 2022;76(6):1263-1278. PMID: 35589249

23. Lee Y, Doumouras AG, Yu J, et al. Complete resolution of nonalcoholic fatty liver disease after bariatric surgery: a systematic review and meta-analysis. *Clin Gastroenterol Hepatol.* 2019;17(6):1040-1060.e11. PMID: 30326299

Atypical and Secondary Etiologies of Obesity

Andrew T. Kraftson, MD. Department of Internal Medicine, University of Michigan, Ann Arbor, MI; Email: andrewkr@med.umich.edu

Educational Objectives

After reviewing this chapter, learners should be able to:

- Identify the patient population that should be screened for atypical or secondary etiologies of obesity.

- Describe the differential diagnosis for atypical and secondary etiologies of obesity.

- Identify and incorporate appropriate screening and confirmatory testing for atypical etiologies of obesity in clinical practice.

Significance of the Clinical Problem

Obesity is a common condition that can present in myriad ways. There are often some fundamental commonalities that characterize conventional obesity, but occasionally there are cases that provoke the question, "Could there be an atypical cause of the weight issue?" To understand when atypical causes should be considered, it is helpful to provide some background.

Obesity is characterized by excess adipose tissue caused by various genetic, epigenetic, biologic, psychosocial, environmental, and behavioral factors.[1] It is a complex, systemic, chronic illness marked by a fluctuating, remitting, and reactivating course. Additionally, obesity poses a higher risk of developing other medical issues that are referred to as obesity-related diseases. While our scientific understanding of obesity has advanced, many questions remain about the best way to define obesity and how to apply this definition to clinical care.[2] As obesity is the most common chronic condition in adults, classification and treatment guidelines have a large magnitude of impact on many stakeholders in myriad clinical, psychosocial, and economic ways. Scientific and technological advancements have paved the way for expanding obesity treatment options; however, these treatments come with their own health risks and economic costs. Consequently, it has become increasingly important to have effective obesity screening and classification tools to guide public health policies and individualized care.

Within this context, we risk homogenizing obesity and missing atypical and/or secondary causes of the condition when weight and BMI are exclusively used to define and classify obesity. Unlike the most prevalent, multifactorial form of obesity, excess weight can result from various hormonal, metabolic, psychological, iatrogenic, and/or genetic etiologies. Identifying these exceptional cases is clinically important because the effects on medical management can be significant. However, widespread biochemical, dynamic, genetic, or radiographic screening for these uncommon causes would be economically wasteful, be of low clinical yield, and could have detrimental consequences. As such, there is a pressing need to increase clinical awareness, improve history/physical examination skills, and develop practical guidelines to facilitate focused, appropriate, and accurate screening for atypical and/or secondary etiologies of obesity.

Practice Gaps

- Most health care providers have limited training in obesity medicine.

- It is essential for clinicians to consider atypical and secondary forms of obesity based on clinical history and physical examination findings.

- There is a need to conduct testing/screening for atypical and secondary forms of obesity in a focused, clinically appropriate, and economically sensitive manner.

- It is important to understand how testing results will influence further evaluation of obesity and management decisions.

Discussion

Rather than the broad, multifactorial way that conventional forms of obesity develop, atypical forms of obesity are distinguished by their discrete pathophysiologic disruptions in the weight regulatory system. This chapter's discussion focuses on clearly identifiable atypical and secondary forms as summarized in *Figure 1*.

In clinical practice, most patients are coping with the common form of multifactorial, polygenic obesity. However, clinicians are confronted by consultations that can lead to either over testing or undertesting for atypical/secondary causes of obesity, such as concerns for hormonal causes of obesity, discrepancies between caloric intake and weight, insurance requirements for medication,

Figure 1. Atypical and Secondary Etiologies of Obesity

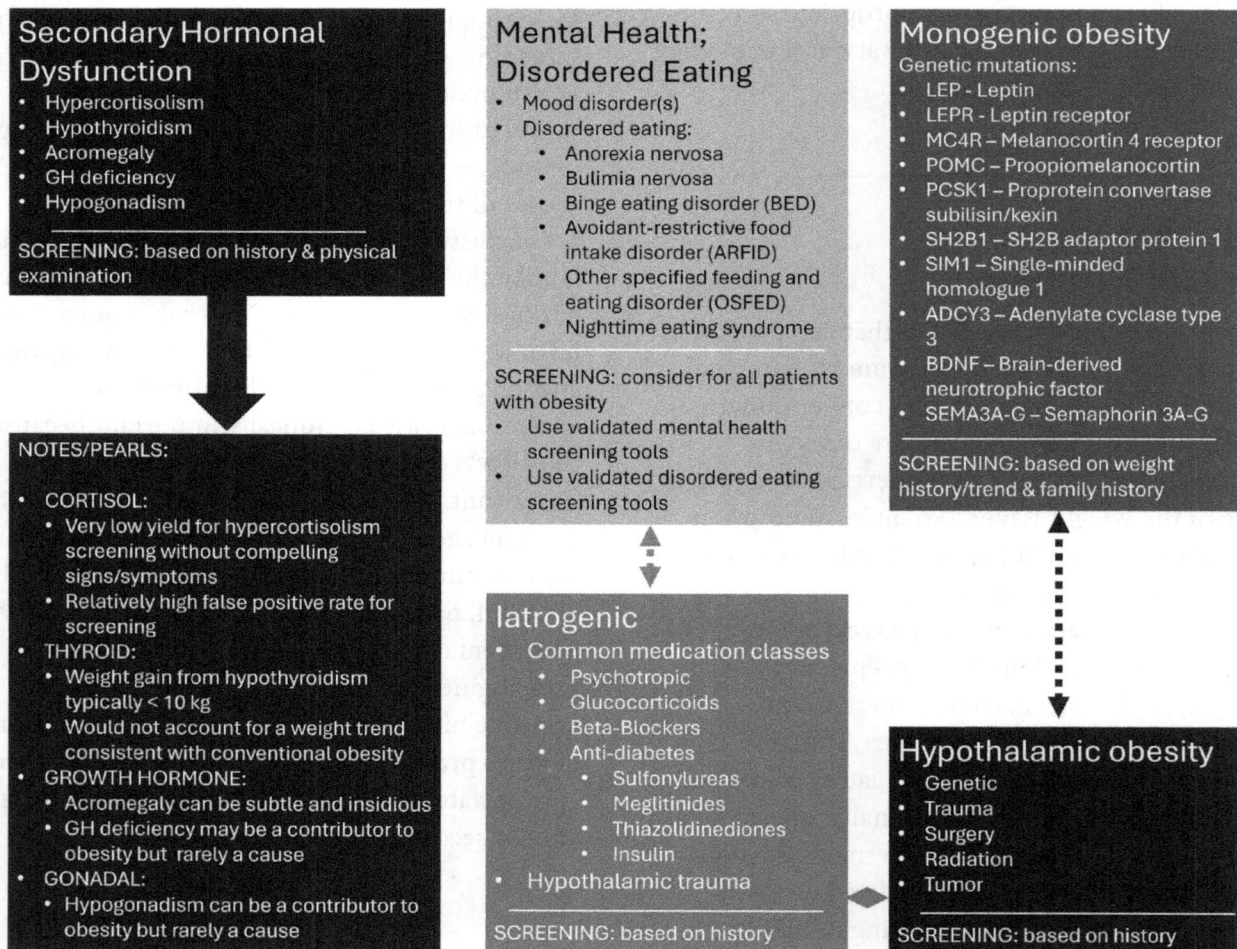

Secondary Hormonal Dysfunction
- Hypercortisolism
- Hypothyroidism
- Acromegaly
- GH deficiency
- Hypogonadism

SCREENING: based on history & physical examination

NOTES/PEARLS:
- CORTISOL:
  - Very low yield for hypercortisolism screening without compelling signs/symptoms
  - Relatively high false positive rate for screening
- THYROID:
  - Weight gain from hypothyroidism typically < 10 kg
  - Would not account for a weight trend consistent with conventional obesity
- GROWTH HORMONE:
  - Acromegaly can be subtle and insidious
  - GH deficiency may be a contributor to obesity but rarely a cause
- GONADAL:
  - Hypogonadism can be a contributor to obesity but rarely a cause

Mental Health; Disordered Eating
- Mood disorder(s)
- Disordered eating:
  - Anorexia nervosa
  - Bulimia nervosa
  - Binge eating disorder (BED)
  - Avoidant-restrictive food intake disorder (ARFID)
  - Other specified feeding and eating disorder (OSFED)
  - Nighttime eating syndrome

SCREENING: consider for all patients with obesity
- Use validated mental health screening tools
- Use validated disordered eating screening tools

Iatrogenic
- Common medication classes
  - Psychotropic
  - Glucocorticoids
  - Beta-Blockers
  - Anti-diabetes
    - Sulfonylureas
    - Meglitinides
    - Thiazolidinediones
    - Insulin
- Hypothalamic trauma

SCREENING: based on history

Monogenic obesity
Genetic mutations:
- LEP - Leptin
- LEPR - Leptin receptor
- MC4R – Melanocortin 4 receptor
- POMC – Proopiomelanocortin
- PCSK1 – Proprotein convertase subilisin/kexin
- SH2B1 – SH2B adaptor protein 1
- SIM1 – Single-minded homologue 1
- ADCY3 – Adenylate cyclase type 3
- BDNF – Brain-derived neurotrophic factor
- SEMA3A-G – Semaphorin 3A-G

SCREENING: based on weight history/trend & family history

Hypothalamic obesity
- Genetic
- Trauma
- Surgery
- Radiation
- Tumor

SCREENING: based on history

[Color—Print (Color Gallery page CG4) or web & ePub editions]

or pressure from medical personnel or patients to initiate obesity treatments.

While many are familiar with common, established obesity clinical practice guidelines,[3,4] there may be some practical elements of history taking that need to be bolstered.

Weight History

As illustrated *Figure 2*, the weight history can illuminate various trends that could increase or decrease pretest probability of atypical or secondary forms of obesity.

Genetics

The weight history can be the early clue of possible genetic forms of atypical obesity.[5] Conventional forms of obesity are polygenic in nature. However, atypical forms of obesity can be the result of monogenic defects. Regardless of any other factors, childhood onset of severe obesity (ie, BMI ≥97th percentile) should prompt consideration of monogenic forms of obesity.

Medical History

In addition to the standard elements of a comprehensive obesity-related history, questioning can be refined to improve identification of possible atypical cases of obesity.

Signs, Symptoms, and Physical Examination Findings

Sudden weight changes can be indicative of atypical causes of obesity. Questions should be asked to identify signs/symptoms of hormonal dysfunction, change in mental status, and/or initiation of weight-positive medications.

Similarly, patients should receive a physical examination to screen for atypical obesity causes, taking care to distinguish between physical findings that are specific vs nonspecific.

In the absence of compelling history or physical findings, secondary hormonal dysfunction becomes much less likely, which makes most hormonal screening (beyond thyroid testing) low yield and not cost-effective.

Figure 2. Various Weight Trends

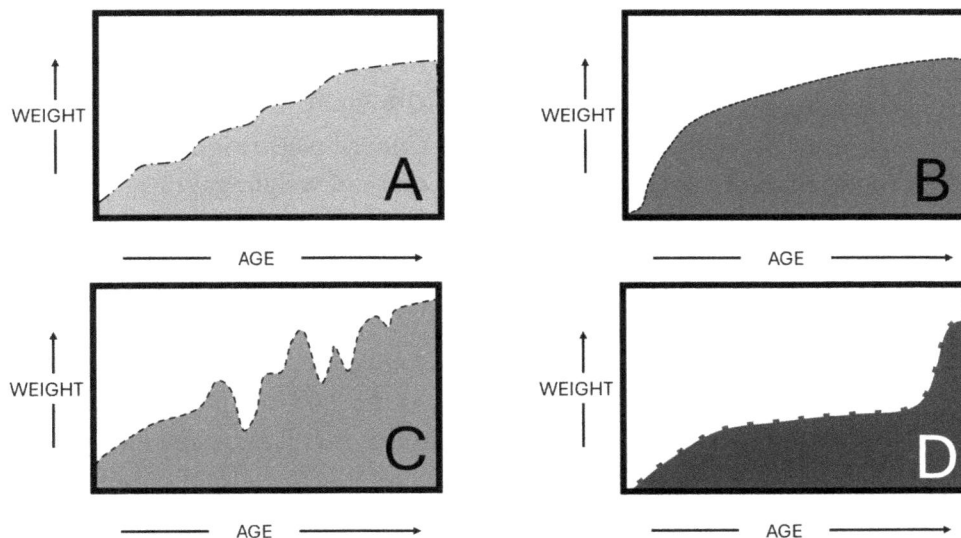

A: gradual weight gain associated with typical, polygenic obesity
B: early-onset, significant obesity associated with monogenic obesity
C: gradual weight gain with repeated weight loss attempts associated with typical obesity
D: sudden onset weight escalation associated with a medical change

[Color—Print (Color Gallery page CG4) or web & ePub editions]

Mental Health

The connection between obesity and mental health is complex and incompletely understood.[6] However, it is critical to assess mental health status and pharmacotherapy. Testing for hypercortisolism should be avoided in the absence of other compelling indications.[7]

Medications

Although iatrogenesis is well-understood to contribute to excess weight, the important (but time-consuming) step of medication review should not be forgotten (*Figure 1*).[8]

Eating Patterns, Hunger, and Cravings

Learning about eating patterns and individual experiences with hunger and cravings can have diagnostic and therapeutic value.[9,10] Monogenic forms of obesity are more likely to cause hyperphagia, which is defined as pathological, insatiable hunger,[11] whereas binge-eating disorder is marked by pronounced eating, even in the absence of hunger, and is associated with a diminished sense of control over eating.[12]

Response to Obesity-Modifying Treatments

It is useful to compare the patient's clinical outcomes with expected treatment response.[13–16] If responses are markedly discrepant from projections, this may prompt screening for atypical and secondary forms of obesity. However, discrepancies between reported caloric intake and weight trajectory do not automatically necessitate a workup for atypical obesity.[17]

Clinical Case Vignettes

Case 1

A 59-year-old woman with a history for obesity, gastroesophageal reflux disease, and dyslipidemia presents to the weight management program for consideration of total meal replacement for 12 weeks, partial meal replacement for another 4 to 12 weeks, and then individualized dietary and behavioral recommendations thereafter. Weight history reveals normal childhood weight. At age 18 years, she weighed 140 lb (63.5 kg) (BMI = 24.8 kg/m²). In her 20s, weight was stable in the range of 140 to 150 lb (63.5-68.0 kg). Pregnancy-related weight gain was easily lost. However, she had gradual weight gain since age 40 years and current weight is 197 lb (89.4 kg) (BMI = 34.9 kg/m²). After 12 weeks in the program, her weight is 166 lb (75.3 kg). She feels good and is ready to transition to the partial meal replacement plan (3 meal replacement products + 1 conventional meal). At the 18-week dietitian-only appointment, her weight is 163 lb (73.9 kg). but the patient notes some fatigue and hair loss. At the 24-week physician visit, her weight is 176 lb (79.8 kg), despite reported adherence to the partial meal replacement diet.

Without any other information provided, which of these statements is most likely true?

A. Total meal replacement therapy is not a good fit for her given inadequate weight loss at 3 months

B. Partial meal replacement therapy is not a good fit for her given weight regain seen at 6 months

C. Symptoms are likely consequences of rapid weight loss, including muscle weakness from sarcopenia and hair loss from telogen effluvium

D. Clinical picture is concerning for an atypical cause of weight gain

E. Clinical picture is consistent with a common response to the transition from total meal replacement to partial meal replacement

Now, for more information:

At the 24-week physician visit, the patient mentions that fatigue and hair loss have worsened. The hair loss includes the scalp but also arms, legs, and axillae. She notes whole-body swelling, facial puffiness, and ruddy complexion. She finds it difficult to rise from sitting or to climb stairs. On examination, her blood pressure is 186/92 mm Hg (compared with 121/58 mm Hg at the visit 12 weeks ago). She has facial plethora and round facies, hair thinning/loss, and notable proximal muscle weakness of her upper legs.

With this additional information, <u>now</u> which of the previous answer options is most likely true?
Answer: D) Clinical picture is concerning for an atypical cause of weight gain

This patient had a good response to treatment with meal replacement therapy. While some degree of weight regain is expected during the dietary transition process, the rapidity and magnitude of weight gain despite reported dietary adherence is concerning (Answer D). However, the signs, symptoms, and physical exam findings are the keys to the case. Given the clinical picture, screening for hypercortisolism was conducted, and the patient was found to have a pituitary macroadenoma. Surgical pathology results were consistent with an ACTH-producing tumor.

　　With or without the supplemental information, Answer A would be incorrect since 15% weight loss represents a good response to meal replacement therapy. Answer B would also be incorrect since some degree of weight regain commonly occurs in the transition from total to partial meal replacement. Therefore, without the supplemental history, Answer E could have been correct. While mild muscle weakness and hair loss can occur with meal replacement–associated weight loss, it would not fit with the clinical picture presented with the supplemental information. Of note, this particular patient had DXA at baseline and at 12 weeks (as part of research), and only a modest loss of lean body mass was seen (from 36,300 g down to 35,400 g). Telogen effluvium is common with rapid weight loss but would not be associated with loss of arm, leg, or axillary hair.

Case 2

A 27-year-old woman presents to the postbariatric endocrinology clinic for a second opinion and transfer of care due to weight regain. Two years ago, the patient underwent sleeve gastrectomy for treatment of obesity complicated by multiple conditions, including type 2 diabetes. Presurgical weight was 366 lb (166.0 kg) (height = 69 in [175.3 cm]; BMI = 54 kg/m^2). Based on a prediction model, expected 12-month nadir weight was projected to be 273 lb (123.8 kg). Postsurgical weights were as follows:

> 6 months: 292 lb (132.4 kg)
> 12 months: 294 lb (133.4 kg)
> 24 months: 324 lb (147.0 kg)

On self-assessment, she considers dietary adherence to be high and estimates that she consumes 1200 to 1500 calories per day. She describes issues with both satiation and satiety despite surgery. However, she feels uncomfortable if she eats more than 1.5 cups at a sitting. No evidence of an eating disorder was found on screening. Clinically, she feels fine, and her mental health is stable aside from frustration about her weight. Physical examination findings are notable for generalized obesity and negative for features of hypercortisolism or unusual fat distribution. She is tearful when discussing weight struggles.

Which of the following is most likely to be true?

A. Imaging should be ordered to evaluate stomach size given her high degree of hunger

B. Hypothyroidism is the most likely reason that the nadir weight projection was not achieved and that weight regain occurred

C. Obtaining a complete weight history could help guide next steps in evaluation and management

D. Screening for hypercortisolism should be conducted next

E. No additional evaluation is needed, and caloric intake should be reduced to 800 to 1000 calories per day

Answer: C) Obtaining a complete weight history could help guide next steps in evaluation and management

Taking a complete weight history (Answer C) can provide valuable information. In this case, the patient revealed that weight issues started before age 5 years. Additionally, she had an extensive family history of obesity. She was referred for genetic testing and found to have an *MC4R* pathogenic variant and was able to participate in a clinical trial of setmelanotide.

Gastric enlargement is not a common cause of increased hunger after bariatric surgery (thus, Answer A is incorrect). Additionally, she describes good portion control consistent with expectations after sleeve gastrectomy.

Hypothyroidism (Answer B) is not a common cause of primary nonresponse to bariatric surgery, nor is it a common cause of weight regain. Furthermore, hypothyroidism would not explain her lifelong weight issues.

There are no signs/symptoms of hypercortisolism, and screening for this condition (Answer D) would be of low yield and obtaining a weight history should be done before testing.

Further restricting calories (Answer E) despite likely high hunger levels would be both ineffective and punitive.

Case 3

A 53-year-old man is followed up in postbariatric endocrinology clinic. Twelve months after surgery, he exceeded projections by 10 lb (4.5 kg) when he reached a nadir weight of 206 lb (93.4 kg) (down from 285 lb [129.3 kg]). By 36 months after surgery, his weight was 228 lb (103.4 kg). Despite the gain, he felt satisfied with his weight and the "easy" routine and declined the offer of obesity-modifying medication. Thyroid function was checked and was normal. Forty-eight months after surgery, he was surprised to learn that his weight was 192 lb (87.1 kg) despite no obvious dietary changes. On extensive questioning, his only pertinent symptom was fatigue and examination findings were unremarkable. Workup was initiated for unintentional causes of weight loss, and he was found to have Graves disease. Methimazole was started, and he became euthyroid. Over the next 2 years, he had gradual weight gain to 260 lb (117.9 kg).

He is now wondering whether methimazole can be stopped. His current regimen is 10 mg daily, and he has missed a few doses in the past month. His current TSH concentration is 0.22 mIU/L (reference range, 0.3-5.5 mIU/L). He is encouraged to continue methimazole at the dosage of 10 mg daily (and to take it more consistently), and his TSH concentration is 2.2 mIU/L 8 weeks later. His weight has been fluctuating between 260 and 265 lb (117.9-120.2 kg).

Which of the following is true?

A. Methimazole is the iatrogenic cause of his weight issue and the dosage should be lowered to see if weight control can be improved

B. His weight gain is likely multifactorial in nature and is less likely to be due to an atypical form of obesity

C. Methimazole should be discontinued, and definitive thyroid treatment should be pursued since either radioactive iodine ablation or thyroidectomy would have superior weight outcomes

D. Testing for a monogenic form of obesity would be the best next step in evaluation

E. Testing for hypercortisolism is contraindicated in this situation

Answer: B) His weight gain is likely multifactorial in nature and is less likely to be due to an atypical form of obesity

Before the onset of Graves disease, the patient was experiencing weight regain in the setting of some laxity in his dietary routine and a trajectory that is commonly seen 3 years after surgery. He had significant weight loss associated with hyperthyroidism that was subsequently addressed. With resolution of hyperthyroidism, it is expected that weight can be modestly higher than the pre-Graves baseline.[18] Afterwards, gaining 13% weight beyond the pre-Graves baseline in a period of 2 years would not necessarily be considered pathological.

Given the clinical picture and laboratory test results, it is unlikely that either thyroid disease or methimazole (Answers A and C) is a major determinant of the patient's weight. Additionally, neither radioactive iodine ablation nor thyroidectomy is weight-negative when compared with methimazole.

Considering the patient's history of normal weight in childhood and early adulthood, it is unlikely that he has a monogenic form of obesity (Answer D).

While it is unlikely that he has hypercortisolism (Answer E) in the absence of suggestive signs/symptoms, there are no contraindications for screening, and it would be reasonable to consider.

Figure 3. Screening for Atypical and Secondary Forms of Obesity.[5,7,12,18-24]

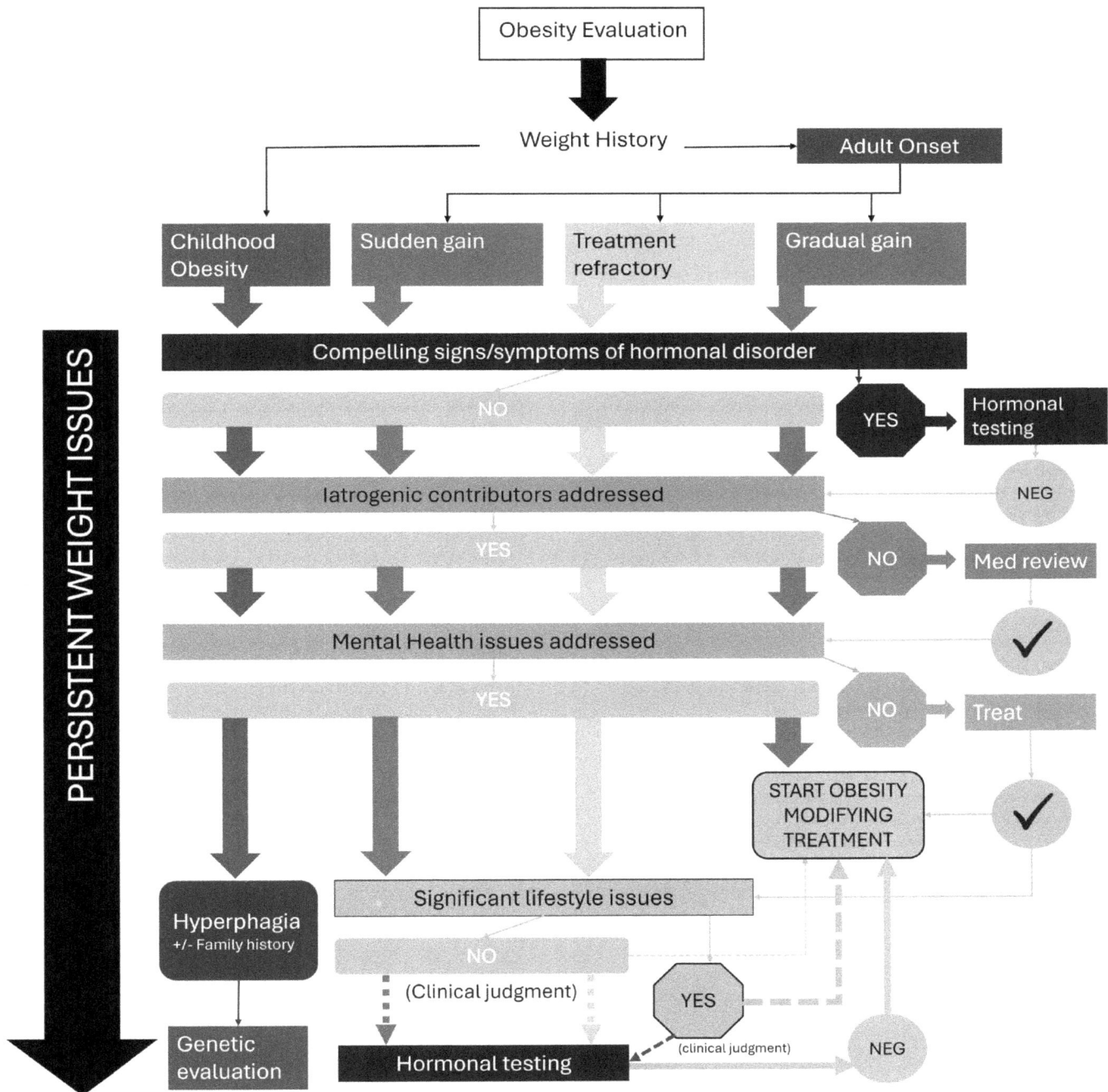

[Color—Print (Color Gallery page CG5) or web & ePub editions]

Key Learning Points

- Obesity is the most common chronic illness in adults and is caused by multifactorial, polygenic factors in most cases.

- Atypical and secondary forms of obesity are clinically important and are managed differently than conventional forms of obesity.

- Because atypical and secondary forms of obesity are both important and uncommon, there is a risk of over screening and underscreening.

- A comprehensive medical and weight history can result in screening that is both medically appropriate and cost-effective.

- A summary of the approach to atypical and secondary obesity screening is shown in *Figure 3, preceding page*.

References

1. Apovian CM. Obesity: definition, comorbidities, causes, and burden. *Am J Manag Care.* 2016;22(Suppl 7):s176s-185. PMID: 27356115

2. Rubino F, Cummings DE, Eckel RH, et al. Definition and diagnostic criteria of clinical obesity. *Lancet Diabetes Endocrinol.* 2025;13(3):221-262. PMID: 39824205

3. Elmaleh-Sachs A, Schwartz JL, Bramante CT, Nicklas JM, Gudzune KA, Jay M. Obesity management in adults: a review. *JAMA.* 2023;330(20):2000-2015. PMID: 38015216

4. Garvey WT, Mechanick JI, Brett EM, et al; Reviewers of the AACE/ACE Obesity Clinical Practice Guidelines. American Association of Clinical Endocrinologists and American College of Endocrinology comprehensive clinical practice guidelines for medical care of patients with obesity. *Endocr Pract.* 2016;22(Suppl 3):1-203. PMID: 27219496

5. Mahmoud R, Kimonis V, Butler MG. Genetics of obesity in humans: a clinical review. *Int J Mol Sci.* 2022;23(19):11005. PMID: 36232301

6. Taylor VH, McIntyre RS, Remington G, Levitan RD, Stonehocker B, Sharma AM. Beyond pharmacotherapy: understanding the links between obesity and chronic mental illness. *Can J Psychiatry.* 2012;57(1):5-12. PMID: 22296962

7. Baid SK, Rubino D, Sinaii N, Ramsey S, Frank A, Nieman LK. Specificity of screening tests for Cushing's syndrome in an overweight and obese population. *J Clin Endocrinol Metab.* 2009;94(10):3857-3864. PMID: 19602562

8. Kumar RB, Aronne LJ. Iatrogenic obesity. *Endocrinol Metab Clin North Am.* 2020;49(2):265-273. PMID: 32418589

9. Morton GJ, Cummings DE, Baskin DG, Barsh GS, Schwartz MW. Central nervous system control of food intake and body weight. *Nature.* 2006;443(7109):289-295. PMID: 16988703

10. Berridge KC, Robinson TE. Liking, wanting, and the incentive-sensitization theory of addiction. *Am Psychol.* 2016;71(8):670-679. PMID: 27977239

11. Heymsfield SB, Avena NM, Baier L, et al. Hyperphagia: current concepts and future directions proceedings of the 2nd International Conference on Hyperphagia. *Obesity (Silver Spring).* 2014;22(0 1):S1-S17. PMID: 24574081

12. Herman BK, Deal LS, DiBenedetti DB, Nelson L, Fehnel SE, Brown TM. Development of the 7-Item Binge-Eating Disorder Screener (BEDS-7). *Prim Care Companion CNS Disord.* 2016;18(2):10.4088/PCC. PMID: 27486542

13. Rothberg AE, McEwen LN, Kraftson AT, Fowler CE, Herman WH. Very-low-energy diet for type 2 diabetes: an underutilized therapy? *J Diabetes Complications.* 2014;28(4):506-510. PMID: 24849710

14. Lean ME, Leslie WS, Barnes AC, et al. 5-year follow-up of the randomised Diabetes Remission Clinical Trial (DiRECT) of continued support for weight loss maintenance in the UK: an extension study. *Lancet Diabetes Endocrinol.* 2024;12(4):233-246. PMID: 38423026

15. Salminen P, Grönroos S, Helmiö M, et al. Effect of laparoscopic sleeve gastrectomy vs Roux-en-Y gastric bypass on weight loss, comorbidities, and reflux at 10 years in adult patients with obesity: the SLEEVEPASS randomized clinical trial. *JAMA Surg.* 2022;157(8):656-666. PMID: 35731535

16. Kraftson A, Cain-Nielsen AH, Lockwood A, et al. Predicting early weight loss failure using a bariatric surgery outcomes calculator and weight loss curves. *Obes Surg.* 2022;32(12):3932-3941. PMID: 36253661

17. Lichtman SW, Pisarska K, Berman ER, et al. Discrepancy between self-reported and actual caloric intake and exercise in obese subjects. *N Engl J Med.* 1992;327(27):1893-1898. PMID: 1454084

18. Kyriacou A, Kyriacou A, Makris KC, Syed AA, Perros P. Weight gain following treatment of hyperthyroidism-a forgotten tale. *Clin Obes.* 2019;9(5):e12328. PMID: 31267667

19. Luppino FS, de Wit LM, Bouvy PF, et al. Overweight, obesity, and depression: a systematic review and meta-analysis of longitudinal studies. *Arch Gen Psychiatry.* 2010;67(3):220-229. PMID: 20194822

20. Clutter WE. Screening for Cushing's syndrome in an era of epidemic obesity. *Mo Med.* 2011;108(2):104-106. PMID: 21568231

21. Laurberg P, Knudsen N, Andersen S, Carlé A, Pedersen IB, Karmisholt J. Thyroid function and obesity. *Eur Thyroid J.* 2012;1(3):159-167. PMID: 24783015

22. Thomas V, Rallapalli S, Kapoor N, Kalra S. Weight gain and thyroid in women: the coexisting confounders. *J Pak Med Assoc.* 2022;72(9):1871-1873. PMID: 36280997

23. Kelly DM, Jones TH. Testosterone and obesity. *Obes Rev.* 2015;16(7):581-606. PMID: 25982085

24. Feltner C, Peat C, Reddy S, et al. Screening for eating disorders in adolescents and adults: evidence report and systematic review for the US Preventive Services Task Force. *JAMA.* 2022;327(11):1068-1082. PMID: 35289875

Treatment of Obesity in Patients With Complex Comorbidities

Tirissa J. Reid, MD, DABOM. Department of Medicine, Division of Endocrinology, Diabetes, and Metabolism, Columbia University Vagelos College of Physicians & Surgeons, New York, NY; Email: tjr2122@cumc.columbia.edu

Educational Objectives

After reviewing this chapter, learners should be able to:

- Explain how complex medical conditions can exacerbate weight gain and make weight loss more difficult.

- Identify which antiobesity medications (AOMs) may be contraindicated in patients with specific psychiatric diagnoses and symptoms.

- Recognize that in patients with eating disorders and obesity, the therapeutic goals must be modified to primarily focus on achieving remission of the eating disorder and minimizing the focus on weight loss.

Significance of the Clinical Problem

Patients with complex medical histories, complex medication regimens, and clinically tenuous status are often excluded from clinical trials for AOMs, which limits knowledge regarding the appropriateness and efficacy of AOMs in these populations. Patients who are pre– or post–organ transplant and those with severe psychopathology are included in this group. In these patients, weight management often takes a back seat to treating more acute symptoms. Additionally, patients with a history of an eating disorder are typically excluded from clinical trials for AOMs. Given that there are currently no large-scale clinical trials evaluating the efficacy of AOMs in any of these populations, clinicians lack informed guidance regarding the management of obesity in these settings.

Practice Gaps

- The efficacy of AOMs in patients pre– and post–organ transplantation is unknown. Given their tenuous clinical status, these patients have not been included in trials for AOMs, and clinical guidelines do not provide guidance for clinical management of this population.

- There are no studies guiding the use of AOMs in patients with significant psychopathology, as they are typically excluded from these medication trials. In addition, guidance for the clinical management of this population is lacking in clinical guidelines.

- Patients with eating disorders and obesity are excluded from AOM clinical trials, so efficacy and guidance regarding their use is lacking.

Discussion

Patients with complex medical histories, eating disorders, or severe psychopathology are often excluded from clinical trials for AOMs. At the same time, we know that many patients in these groups are at greater risk for obesity, whether due to their underlying disorders or medication adverse effects.

Patients Requiring Organ Transplantation

Patients requiring organ transplantation have an increased risk for obesity due to a variety of factors. Before transplantation, patients may often experience fatigue and debility to some degree, which significantly limits physical activity and may lead to weight gain. Patients with severe pulmonary disease often require frequent treatment with high-dose steroids, which are known promote weight gain by increasing appetite and worsening insulin resistance.

In patients who have already received an organ transplant, there are factors that increase the risk for obesity. These factors include long-term use of steroids or other immunosuppressive medications that may have weight gain as an adverse effect, as well as significant continued physical limitations.

In addition, we know that elevated BMI is a relative contraindication to transplantation for a variety of organs, as there is some evidence of increased rates of graft dysfunction and mortality in these patients. While there are data regarding the efficacy of metabolic and bariatric surgery in some transplant recipients, there remain patients who are too clinically frail to withstand additional surgery or who are unwilling to undergo bariatric surgery. Data regarding appropriate and effective AOM options in this group of patients are lacking.[1]

Patients With Psychiatric Conditions

While patients with psychiatric conditions, such as anxiety or depression, are not automatically excluded from clinical trials for AOMs, those with symptoms that are not fully controlled or those who are on multiple medications are not included. This makes sense in that it allows for precise determination of new symptoms related to the medication being tested. Complex medication regimens also increase the possibility of interactions with medications being tested in clinical trials. While these reasons are understandable, it leaves a paucity of data regarding how to most effectively treat obesity in these patients, even though they may be at increased risk for weight gain.

Patients with anxiety or depression may avoid outdoor activities, which then limits physical activity. Increased weight may also result from increased stress, anxiety affecting sleep, or, in cases of depression, psychomotor slowing leading to dramatically reduced physical activity.[2] Many common psychiatric medications have weight gain as an adverse effect. Even newer generations of antidepressants have clinically significant weight gain as an adverse effect (in up to 40% of patients).[3] One small study of 244 patients with obesity and mental health diagnoses were treated with AOMs for 52 weeks.[4] While the results showed these medications were effective, resulting in a 12% mean total body weight loss, there was also some worsening psychopathology noted with certain medications (depression increased for some on topiramate). Further studies are needed to expound upon the risk/benefits of antiobesity pharmacotherapy in these patients, particularly given that this study concluded in 2018, before the FDA approval of weekly incretin agonists for the treatment of obesity.

Patients With Eating Disorders

Studies have found 40% to 50% of patients with eating disorders also have obesity depending on the patient population examined.[5] Some patients with eating disorders present seeking weight management. There are some data on the efficacy of lifestyle interventions[6] and bariatric surgery in patients with treated eating disorders.[7] In patients with untreated eating disorders, interventions targeting weight loss, such as lifestyle intervention or AOMs, are not recommended as first-line therapies. Providers should be familiar with the recommended treatment paradigm to apply when treating patients with an eating disorder, such as bulimia nervosa, and obesity.[8] While weight loss is not recommended as the primary therapeutic objective in patients with untreated eating disorders, there are situations where a patient may need to lose weight to improve a weight-related comorbidity or qualify for a necessary surgery, such as orthopedic operation. In these cases, little is known regarding the appropriate choice of AOM, as these patients are typically excluded from clinical trials of AOMs.[9]

Further research is needed to assess the safety and efficacy of AOMs in patients with obesity and complex medical conditions to help guide clinician management.

Clinical Case Vignettes

Case 1

A 50-year-old woman with Hermansky-Pudlak syndrome, interstitial lung disease, type 2 diabetes, and class 2 obesity (status post sleeve gastrectomy 3 years ago) presents for assistance with weight loss to qualify for lung transplantation. Before her first pregnancy at age 20 years, her weight was 115 lb (52.2 kg) and height was 61 in (154.9 cm), (BMI = 21.7 kg/m^2). Over 30 years, her weight increased to 275 lb (124.7 kg) (BMI = 52.0 = kg/m^2) and was accelerated during 2 pregnancies (60 lb [27.2 kg] and 30 lb [13.6 kg]) and steroid tapers for pulmonary disease.

From a peak weight of 275 lb (124.7 kg), she lost 45 lb (20.4 kg) with lifestyle changes and 23 lb (10.4 kg) with metformin and liraglutide. However, she discontinued both medications due to adverse effects of diarrhea and vomiting. She lost 33 lb (15.0 kg) with sleeve gastrectomy, but regained weight after surgery to 188 lb (85.3 kg) (BMI = 35.5 kg/m^2). Intensified lifestyle changes have not resulted in weight loss. A goal weight of 160 lb (72.6 kg) is necessary to meet criteria for lung transplantation listing. Her current medications are levofloxacin and a multivitamin.

On physical examination, she has albinism and central obesity.

Laboratory test results:

Hemoglobin A$_{1c}$ = 6.8% (51 mmol/mol)
TSH, normal
Creatinine, normal

Her insurer does not cover AOMs, and she reports limited disposable income. She is not willing to try another incretin agonist because of the severe adverse effects she experienced with liraglutide.

Of the following medications approved by the US FDA to treat diabetes, which would be the best addition to her medication regimen to help the patient reach her weight-loss goal?

A. Pioglitazone
B. Glyburide
C. Sitagliptin
D. Acarbose
E. Dapagliflozin

Answer: E) Dapagliflozin

Common chronic medications used to treat diabetes have distinct effects on weight.[10] In addition to understanding their potential to improve glycemic control, providers should become familiar with their effects on weight. In patients with obesity, providers should aim to minimize the use of medications that promote weight gain and preferentially use medications that are weight neutral or promote weight loss.[11]

Dapagliflozin (Answer E) and other SGLT-2 inhibitors have been shown to cause weight loss.[12]

Pioglitazone (Answer A) has the potential to increase weight, given its adverse effect of edema. Glyburide and all sulfonylureas cause weight gain by increasing insulin secretion.

Sitagliptin (Answer C) and other DPP-4 inhibitors are weight-neutral and are not the best options for this patient who is hoping to lose weight.

Acarbose (Answer D) has been shown to be weight-neutral or cause only mild weight loss.

Case 2

A 26-year-old woman with class 3 obesity and weight-related comorbidities of obstructive sleep apnea and prediabetes presents for assistance with weight loss. Medical history also includes depression, severe anxiety, attention deficit–hyperactivity disorder, and Tourette syndrome. She has been overweight since age 15 years when she started aripiprazole, followed by rapid weight gain for 1 year and gradual weight gain thereafter. Previous weight-loss attempts include in-person intensive lifestyle interventions, visits with a dietitian, and lifestyle intervention via phone app, which is ongoing. Total weight loss has not exceeded 5% with any intervention. Her psychiatrist has adjusted her medications to prevent further weight gain, and aripiprazole was recently discontinued. Current medications are atomoxetine (selective norepinephrine reuptake inhibitor for attention deficit–hyperactivity disorder), escitalopram, buspirone, clonazepam, clonidine, and ethinyl estradiol/norgestimate. Family history includes obesity in several first-degree relatives. Review of systems is notable for loud snoring, heat intolerance, and excess facial hair. Menses are regular.

On physical examination, her height is 62 in (157.5 cm) and weight is 282 is lb (127.9 kg) (BMI = 51.6 kg/m^2). She does not appear acromegalic or cushingoid. Her Ferriman-Gallwey score is 8. She has no acne or reddish-purplish striae. She has acanthosis nigricans in the axillae and multiple skin tags. Her mood and affect are normal.

Laboratory test results:

> Hemoglobin A$_{1c}$ = 6.1% (43 mmol/mol)
> TSH, normal
> Liver enzymes, normal
> Creatinine, normal
> IGF-1 normal

Which of the following AOMs would be most appropriate to start in this patient?

A. Phentermine

B. Liraglutide

C. Naltrexone/bupropion

D. Tirzepatide

E. Phentermine/topiramate

Answer: D) Tirzepatide

Phentermine (Answer A), phentermine/topiramate (Answer E), and naltrexone/bupropion (Answer C) all have the possible adverse effect of anxiety and should not be used in a patient with severe

anxiety.[13] They also increase the risk of serotonin syndrome when used together with a selective serotonin reuptake inhibitor.

Liraglutide (Answer B) and tirzepatide (Answer D) may be used concomitantly with selective serotonin reuptake inhibitors or serotonin norepinephrine reuptake inhibitors without increasing the risk for serotonin syndrome, and they are not associated with anxiety as an adverse effect. Given its greater mean weight loss and less frequent dosing, tirzepatide is preferred over liraglutide,[14] and tirzepatide is also FDA-approved to treat moderate-to-severe obstructive sleep apnea in patients with obesity.

Case 3

A 38-year-old woman with a history of bulimia (in partial remission), depression, anxiety, class 3 obesity, and weight-related comorbidities (polycystic ovary syndrome, hypertension, gastroesophageal reflux disease, and osteoarthritis) presents for assistance with weight loss to improve her knee pain and eliminate antihypertensive medication. She recalls being overweight since age 10 years, with further weight gain exacerbated by depression and antidepressant medications.

Previous weight-loss attempts have included multiple structured commercial lifestyle interventions, increased physical activity, and visits with a dietitian. Current medications are hydrochlorothiazide, clonazepam, lamotrigine, vortioxetine (selective serotonin reuptake inhibitor), and venlafaxine (selective norepinephrine reuptake inhibitor—tapering off).

On physical examination, her height is 69 in (175.3 cm) and weight is 280 lb (127.0 kg) (BMI = 41.3 kg/m^2). Acanthosis nigricans is present in the axillae and on the neck. She has central obesity.

Laboratory test results:

> Hemoglobin A$_{1c}$ = 5.9% (41 mmol/mol)
> Fasting insulin = 34 µIU/mL (SI: 236.1 pmol/L)

She would like to initiate medication therapy but is not amenable to using an injection.

In addition to a referral to a behavioral therapist well-versed in treating patients with eating disorders, which of the following medications is most appropriate for this patient to assist her in reaching her health goals?

A. Phentermine

B. Phentermine/topiramate

C. Off-label metformin

D. Naltrexone/bupropion

E. Tirzepatide

Answer: C) Off-label metformin

In patients with eating disorders, the main goal of therapy is to achieve complete remission of the eating disorder; weight loss is not the primary goal. There are instances where weight loss may also be important, such as reducing pain due osteoarthritis. Cognitive behavioral therapy has been shown to be the most effective treatment for bulimia. There is insufficient evidence to determine which AOMs are best in patients with eating disorders, as this patient population is typically excluded from clinical trials. If weight loss is desired, it is important to focus any therapies, including medications, on the goal of improving health. In this patient with bulimia in partial remission, phentermine (Answer A), phentermine/topiramate (Answer B), and naltrexone/bupropion (Answer D) are all contraindicated, due to the potential to heighten the already elevated seizure risk with bulimia. These same medications also have the risk of worsening anxiety. This patient has stated that she will not use an injection, so incretin agonists, such as tirzepatide (Answer E), are not an option. While metformin is not FDA-approved to treat polycystic ovary syndrome, prediabetes, or weight loss, it is sometimes used off-label (Answer C) for each of these conditions. This patient has a known history of polycystic ovary syndrome and prediabetes and physical examination signs and laboratory evidence consistent with insulin resistance. The Diabetes Prevention Program trial demonstrated that metformin is able to assist with modest weight loss in patients who have an elevated BMI and prediabetes.[15] Another study found that metformin was able to effect a 6.4% placebo-subtracted weight loss in comparison with placebo in patients with obesity, with greater weight loss in patients who had severe insulin resistance, making this a good option for this patient.[16]

Key Learning Points

- Medication-induced weight gain is common in pre– and post–organ transplant recipients. Other mechanisms of weight gain in these patients include deconditioning pretransplantation, as their clinical status deteriorates prior to transplant.

- Common long-term medications used to treat comorbid disorders can be used to assist with weight loss.

- Patients with severe psychiatric comorbidities and obesity often have contraindications to multiple AOMs due to medication interactions or possible AOM adverse effects, such as anxiety. Incretin therapies are often used in these patients without exacerbating psychiatric conditions and without increasing the risk for serotonin syndrome in patients on selective serotonin reuptake inhibitors.

- Goals of therapy in patients with current, or history of, eating disorders and obesity should not focus on weight loss, but instead on improvements in health and other comorbidities, using proven interventions. Interdisciplinary care is key. Several AOMs are contraindicated in patients with bulimia nervosa, including phentermine and naltrexone/bupropion (due to the bupropion component).

References

1. Ghanem OM, Pita A, Nazzal M, et al; SAGES & ASTS. Obesity, organ failure, and transplantation: a review of the role of metabolic and bariatric surgery in transplant candidates and recipients. *Surg Endosc.* 2024;38(8):4138-4151. PMID: 38951240

2. Christensen SM, Varney C, Gupta V, Wenz L, Bays HE. Stress, psychiatric disease, and obesity: an Obesity Medicine Association (OMA) clinical practice statement (CPS) 2022. *Obes Pillars.* 2022;4:100041. PMID: 37990662

3. Uguz F, Sahingoz M, Gungor B, Aksoy F, Askin R. Weight gain and associated factors in patients using newer antidepressant drugs. *Gen Hosp Psychiatry.* 2015;37(1):46-48. PMID: 25467076

4. Tham M, Chong TWH, Jenkins ZM, Castle DJ. The use of anti-obesity medications in people with mental illness as an adjunct to lifestyle interventions - Effectiveness, tolerability and impact on eating behaviours: a 52-week observational study. *Obes Res Clin Pract.* 2021;15(1):49-57. PMID: 33257207

5. da Luz FQ, Hay P, Touyz S, Sainsbury A. Obesity with comorbid eating disorders: associated health risks and treatment approaches nutrients. 2018;10(7):829. PMID: 29954056

6. McDonald JB, Rancourt D. Treating bulimia nervosa and achieving medically required weight loss: a case study. *Cognitive Behavioral Pract.* 2023;30(1):146-159.

7. Hilbert A, Staerk C, Strömer A, et al. Nonnormative eating behaviors and eating disorders and their associations with weight loss and quality of life during 6 years following obesity surgery. *JAMA Netw Open.* 2022;5(8):e2226244. PMID: 35951326

8. Ralph AF, Brennan L, Byrne S, et al. Management of eating disorders for people with higher weight: clinical practice guideline. *J Eat Disord.* 2022;10(1):121. PMID: 35978344

9. Camacho-Barcia L, Giel KE, Jiménez-Murcia S, et al. Eating disorders and obesity: bridging clinical, neurobiological, and therapeutic perspectives. *Trends Mol Med.* 2024;30(4):361-379. PMID: 38485648

10. Domecq JP, Prutsky G, Leppin A, et al. Clinical review: drugs commonly associated with weight change: a systematic review and meta-analysis. *J Clin Endocrinol Metab.* 2015;100(2):363-370. PMID: 25590213

11. Barenbaum SR, Kumar RB, Aronne LJ. Management of medication-induced weight gain. *Gastroenterol Clin North Am.* 2023;52(4):751-760. PMID: 37919025

12. Akhanli P, Hepşen S, Arslan İE, et al. Impact of 24-week dapagliflozin treatment on body weight, body composition, and cardiac risk indicators of patients with type-2 diabetes mellitus. *Turk J Med Sci.* 2023;53(5):1178-1184. PMID: 38813008

13. Yanovski SZ, Yanovski JA. Long-term drug treatment for obesity: a systematic and clinical review. *JAMA.* 2014;311(1):74-86. PMID: 24231879

14. Henderson K, Lewis, Sloan CE, Bessesen DH, Arterburn D. Effectiveness and safety of drugs for obesity. *BMJ.* 2024;384:e072686. PMID: 38527759

15. Knowler WC, Barrett-Connor E, Fowler SE, et al; Diabetes Prevention Program Research Group. Reduction in the incidence of type 2 diabetes with lifestyle intervention or metformin. *N Engl J Med.* 2002;346(6):393-403. PMID: 11832527

16. Seifarth C, Schehler B, Schneider HJ. Effectiveness of metformin on weight loss in non-diabetic individuals with obesity. *Exp Clin Endocrinol Diabetes.* 2013;121(1):27-31. PMID: 23147210

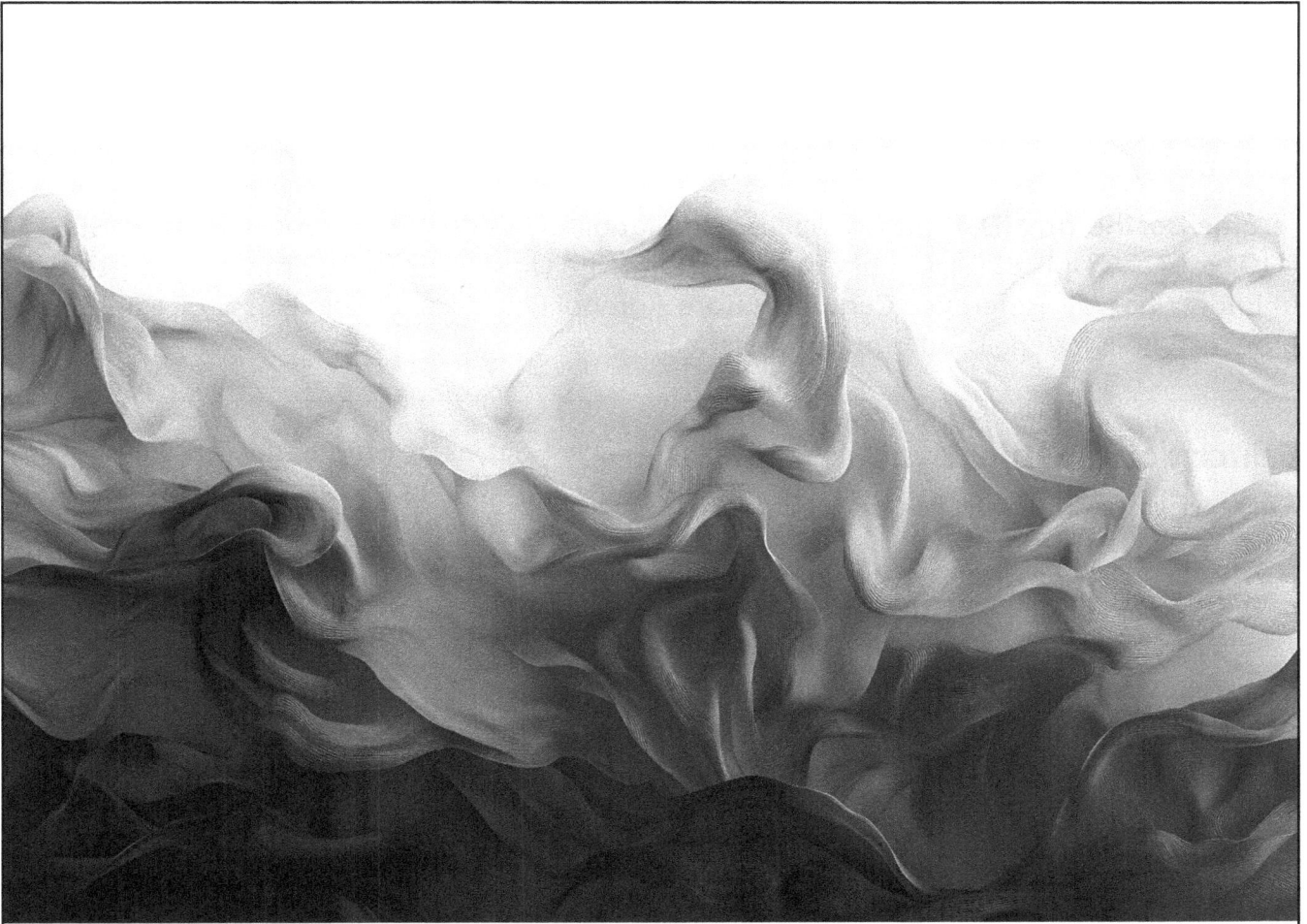

ADRENAL

How to Manage Bilateral Adrenal Masses

Jérôme Bertherat, MD, PhD. Genomics and Signaling of Endocrine Tumors Team, INSERM U1016, CNRS UMR8104, Cochin Institute, Paris Cité University, Paris, France; Department of Endocrinology, Reference Center for Rare Adrenal Diseases, Cochin Hospital, Paris, France; Email: Jerome.bertherat@aphp.fr

Educational Objectives

After reviewing this chapter, learners should be able to:

- Describe the various causes of bilateral adrenal masses.

- Perform the diagnostic workup of bilateral adrenal masses.

- Guide the management of bilateral adrenal masses.

Significance of the Clinical Problem

Bilateral adrenal masses are most often discovered incidentally, during evaluation of adrenal incidentalomas. Adrenal incidentalomas are common in the general population (1% to 5%, or even higher in individuals approaching age 70 years), and 10% to 15% of incidentalomas are bilateral.[1] More rarely, these bilateral masses are revealed by symptoms of steroid or catecholamine hypersecretion. Occasionally, bilateral lesions are discovered during the investigation of adrenal insufficiency. The diagnostic approach seeks to establish the nature of the adrenal lesions, primarily on the basis of imaging characteristics. Most often, the lesions are of the same type on both sides, but sometimes there may be a lesion of a different type on each side. Rigorous imaging analysis is therefore essential for initial characterization. At the same time, hormonal investigations are designed to assess the possibility of hypersecretion, primarily of cortisol, or more rarely of aldosterone or catecholamines.[2] Hormonal testing also helps identify adrenal insufficiency, especially when the adrenal glands are the site of metastases or infectious or inflammatory infiltration.

Practice Gaps

- Adrenal incidentalomas are bilateral in 10% to 15% of cases. However, the bilateral nature in asymmetric forms can be underdiagnosed, and systematic analysis of the contralateral adrenal gland is important for adrenal incidentaloma management.

- Multidisciplinary expertise is important for proper diagnosis and management of bilateral adrenal masses.

- Although it is important to not miss malignancy (especially metastasis) in patients with bilateral adrenal incidentalomas, they are most frequently benign adrenocortical lesions.

- Distinguishing mild forms of bilateral macronodular adrenal hyperplasia (PBMAH) from bilateral adrenocortical adenomas on imaging is often difficult; however, clinical management based on assessment of cortisol autonomous secretion and comorbidities is similar.

- The management of patients with mild autonomous cortisol secretion and benign bilateral adrenocortical lesions on the basis of comorbidities should be discussed on an individual basis and cannot yet be fully supported by evidence-based medicine.[3]

- There is lack of awareness that bilateral pheochromocytomas occur most often in patients with genetic etiologies and require a systematic genetic consultation.[4] In PBMAH, a genetic cause (most often an *ARMC5* variant) is identified in about 20% of affected patients.[5,6]

Discussion

The various etiologies of bilateral adrenal masses are listed in *Table 1*. The most frequent lesions are benign bilateral adrenocortical lesions. These may be bilateral adenomas or PBMAH. Bilateral pheochromocytoma is very often genetic in origin. PBMAH is genetic in 20% to 25% of cases. In a syndromic setting, bilateral lesions may also be observed, for example, in persons with multiple endocrine neoplasia type 1 (adrenocortical tumors), von Hippel–Lindau syndrome, or multiple endocrine neoplasia type 2 (pheochromocytomas).

The diagnostic approach to bilateral adrenal incidentalomas is similar to that of unilateral incidentalomas. CT is the most commonly used initial imaging to characterize the lesions. Benign adrenal cortical lesions most often have a spontaneous density of less than 10 Hounsfield units on CT. However, a higher spontaneous density does not rule out a benign lesion. In this context, MRI can provide additional information. If a malignant lesion is suspected, [18]FDG PET may be useful, and in the case of bilateral metastases, the primary tumor may also be visualized.

Endocrine investigations begin with a search for clinical evidence of hypercortisolism, hyperaldosteronism, or pheochromocytoma. The search for signs of adrenal insufficiency, particularly if imaging or clinical findings suggest metastatic malignancy (solid tumor or hemopathy), is important because it can represent a therapeutic emergency.

Biological investigations include an electrolyte panel and blood glucose measurement to check for hypokalemia and diabetes. Autonomous cortisol secretion is evaluated with a 1-mg dexamethasone-suppression test, with a normal serum cortisol cutoff value of 1.8 µg/dL or less (≤50 nmol/L).

Table 1. Etiology of Bilateral Adrenal Masses

Similar lesions on both sides
Bilateral adrenocortical adenoma
• Nonfunctioning
• Mild autonomous cortisol secretion
• Overt Cushing syndrome
• Primary aldosteronism
• Adrenal sex steroid excess (extremely rare)
Macronodular bilateral adrenal hyperplasia
• Mild autonomous cortisol secretion
• Overt Cushing syndrome
• Primary aldosteronism
• Nonfunctioning
• Adrenal sex steroid excess (extremely rare)
Micronodular bilateral adrenal hyperplasia and primary pigmented nodular adrenocortical disease
Cushing disease
Ectopic ACTH syndrome
Congenital adrenal hyperplasia

Different or similar lesions on both sides
• Adrenocortical adenoma
• Myelolipoma
• Cyst
• Hemorrhage
• Ganglioneuroma
• Schwannoma
• Pheochromocytoma
• Adrenocortical carcinoma
• Adrenal metastases
• Adrenal lymphoma
• Adrenal sarcoma
• Adrenal neuroblastoma
• Hemangioma
• Infiltrative infectious disease (tuberculosis, histoplasmosis, cryptococcosis)
• Infiltrative inflammatory disease (sarcoidosis, amyloidosis, Erdheim-Chester disease, etc)

In patients with incidentalomas and no specific signs of Cushing syndrome, a serum cortisol value greater than 1.8 µg/dL (>50 nmol/L), usually repeated after few months to reduce false-positive results, is classified as mild autonomous cortisol secretion (MACS). This warrants screening for comorbidities (diabetes, hypertension, osteoporosis, obesity, etc). If the adrenal masses are not typical of bilateral benign adrenocortical lesions, evaluation for pheochromocytoma should be done by measuring plasma or urinary metanephrines. If arterial hypertension or hypokalemia is present, aldosterone and renin should be measured. In the absence of autonomous cortisol secretion, adrenal insufficiency should be ruled out with a cosyntropin-stimulation test. If adrenal insufficiency or autonomous cortisol secretion is detected, ACTH measurement is useful to confirm the adrenal primary nature of adrenal insufficiency (high ACTH) or cortisol autonomous secretion (low ACTH). In the case of mild or overt Cushing syndrome, the differential diagnosis between an ACTH-independent cause and an ACTH-dependent cause is important because management differs (*Table 2*).

Clinical Case Vignettes

Case 1

Bilateral adrenal masses are found on CT (*Figure 1, following page*) performed for lumbar pain in a 73-year-old man. On the right adrenal gland, a 16-mm nodule is identified with an unenhanced density of 12 Hounsfield units. On the left adrenal gland, a 25-mm nodule is identified with an unenhanced density of 24 Hounsfield units. His medical history is relevant for hypertension treated for 5 years, type 2 diabetes, sleep apnea, and transient stroke. Current medications

Table 2. Differential Diagnosis of Bilateral Benign Similar Adrenocortical Masses

Characteristics	Bilateral macronodular adrenal hyperplasia	Bilateral adrenal adenomas	ACTH-dependent nodular hyperplasia	Partial glucocorticoid resistance syndrome
Clinical presentation	• Mild or overt clinical signs or comorbidities of Cushing syndrome • Bilateral incidentalomas	• Bilateral incidentalomas • Mild or overt clinical signs or comorbidities of Cushing syndrome	Overt clinical symptoms and comorbidities of Cushing syndrome are typical in chronic Cushing disease or ectopic ACTH syndrome leading to nodular adrenal hyperplasia	• Possible arterial hypertension • Possible hirsutism • Possible fatigue • No signs of overt Cushing syndrome
Imaging	Bilateral enlargement of both adrenal glands and macronodules with internodular hyperplasia	Bilateral nodules without internodular hyperplasia	Bilateral enlargement of both adrenal glands	• Bilateral nodular hyperplastic adrenals • Rarely very large
Hormonal characteristics	• Normal or high urinary free cortisol • Low/suppressed ACTH • Normal or elevated 17-hydroxyprogesterone • Normal or low DHEA-S • Partial or lack of cortisol suppression after dexamethasone-suppression test • Possible elevated aldosterone-to-renin ratio	• Normal or high urinary free cortisol • Low/suppressed ACTH • Normal 17-hydroxy-progesterone • Partial or lack of cortisol suppression after dexamethasone-suppression test	• High urinary free cortisol • Normal/high ACTH • Higher DHEA-S • Partial suppression after dexamethasone-suppression test • Response to desmopressin/CRH in Cushing's disease, less frequent in benign neuroendocrine tumors with ectopic ACTH	• High urinary free cortisol • Normal/high ACTH • Possible elevated adrenal androgens • Possible altered aldosterone-to-renin ratio • Reduced cortisol suppression after dexamethasone-suppression test

Adapted from Bertherat J et al. Endocrine Review, 2023; 44(4): 567–628. © The Authors. Published by Oxford University Press on behalf of the Endocrine Society.

include metformin, insulin, amlodipine, hydrochlorothiazide, valsartan, bisoprolol, and acetylsalicylate.

On physical examination, his weight is 187.4 lb (85 kg) (BMI = 29 kg/m^2). His blood pressure is 124/75 mm Hg.

Laboratory test results:

Sodium = 139 mEq/L (SI: 139 mmol/L)
Potassium = 4.6 mEq/L (SI: 4.6 mmol/L)
Creatinine = 1.10 mg/dL (SI: 97 μmol/L)
Hemoglobin A$_{1c}$ = 6.4% (46 mmol/mol)
Serum cortisol after 1 mg dexamethasone = 1.3 μg/dL (SI: 35 nmol/L)
Aldosterone = 8.3 ng/dL (8.3-23.6 ng/dL) (SI: 229 pmol/L [33-655 pmol/L])
Renin = 11 μIU/mL (3-40 μIU/mL)
Urinary metanephrine = 770 μg/24 h (49-217 μg/24 h) (SI: 3851 nmol/d [250-1100 nmol/d])
Urinary normetanephrine = 842 μg/24 h (92-440 μg/24 h) (SI: 4595 nmol/d [500-2400 nmol/d])

Which of the following is the best recommendation?

A. ^{18}FDG PET

B. ^{18}F FDOPA PET

C. Replacing hydrochlorothiazide with spironolactone

D. Biopsy

E. Simple follow-up with a CT in 6 months

Answer: B) ^{18}F FDOPA PET

The imaging findings and the urinary metanephrine and normetanephrine measurements, which show a moderate but likely significant increase, are suggestive of pheochromocytoma. In this patient with an apparently sporadic presentation, performing ^{18}F FDOPA PET (Answer B) would be the best next step to evaluate for pheochromocytoma.

Case 1, Continued

An ^{18}F FDOPA PET is performed (*Figure 2, following page*).

Figure 1.

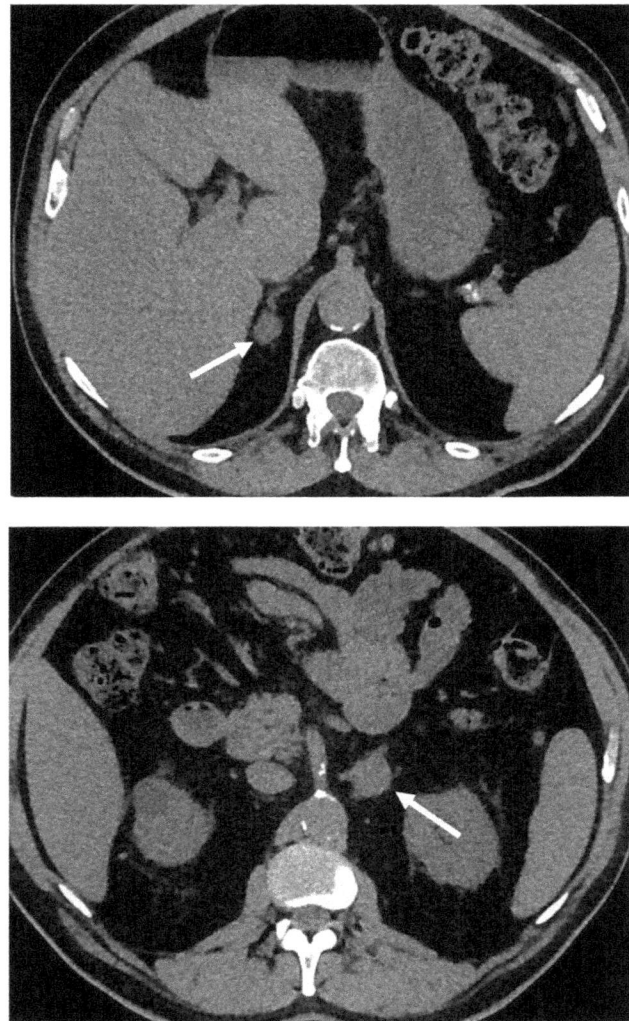

[Color—Print (Color Gallery page CG6) or web & ePub editions]

Which of the following is the most likely diagnosis?

A. Left pheochromocytoma

B. Right adrenal cancer

C. Primary bilateral macronodular adrenal hyperplasia

D. Bilateral adrenal adenomas

E. Bilateral myelolipoma

Answer: A) Left pheochromocytoma

The ^{18}F FDOPA PET shows unilateral uptake in the left adrenal gland (SUV 3.6) and no

Figure 2.

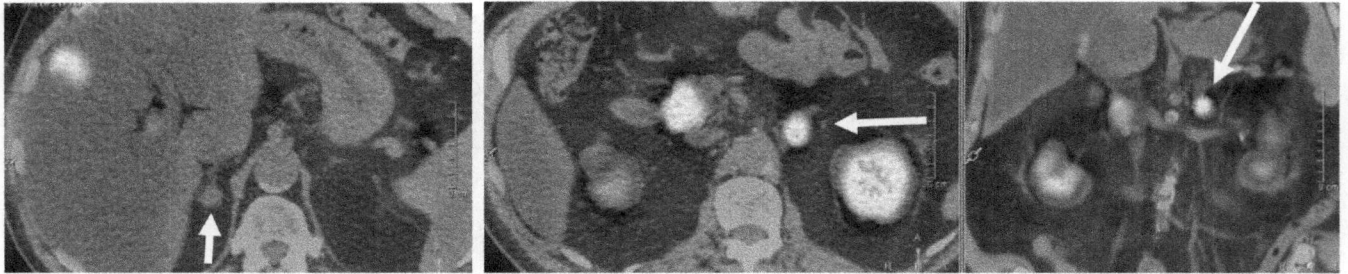

[Color—Print (Color Gallery page CG6) or web & ePub editions]

Figure 3.

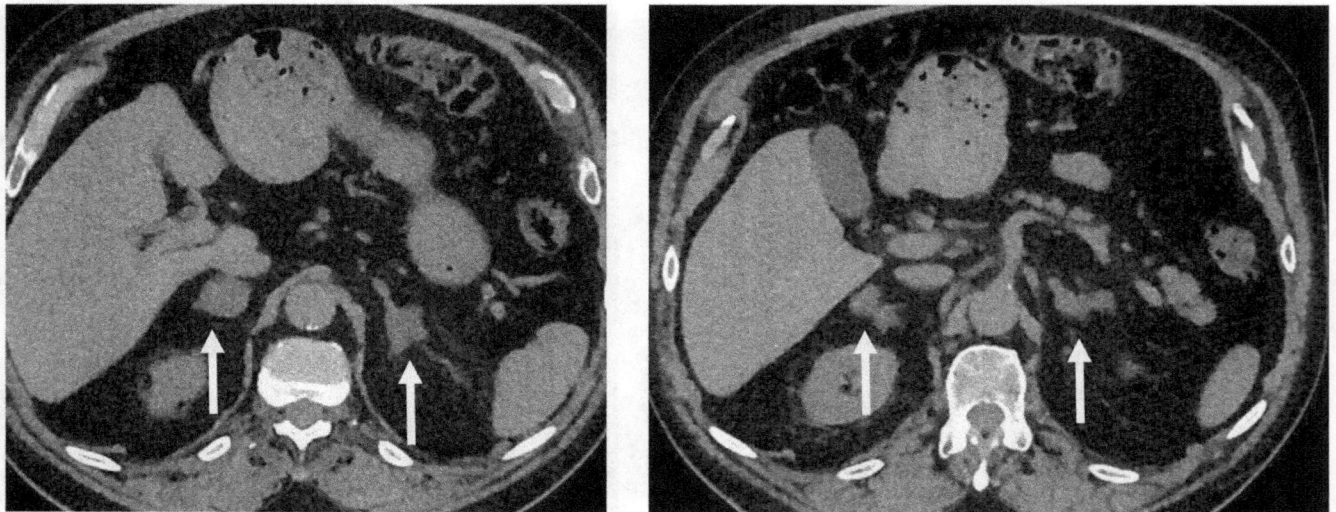

[Color—Print (Color Gallery page CG6) or web & ePub editions]

contralateral or extra-adrenal tracer uptake. This is highly suggestive of a pheochromocytoma (Answer A). After left laparoscopic adrenalectomy, pathologic examination confirmed a pheochromocytoma and chromogranin A immunostaining was positive (preoperative chromogranin A circulating level was 2 times normal). Based on CT imaging characteristics and results of the dexamethasone-suppression test, the right adrenal nodule was classified as a benign, nonsecreting adenoma.

Case 2

Bilateral multiple adrenal nodules are found on CT performed for abdominal pain in a 68-year-old man (*Figure 3*).

The 2 main nodules in the right adrenal gland have unenhanced density less than 10 Hounsfield units, while the additional smaller nodules have a density between 10 and 15 Hounsfield units. The nodules in the left adrenal gland have an unenhanced density less than 10 Hounsfield units. Medical history is relevant for hypertension treated for 15 years and cardiac arrythmia. Current medications are amlodipine, perindopril, indapamide, atenolol, fluindione, and potassium supplementation.

On physical examination, his weight is 240 lb (109 kg) (BMI = 32 kg/m²). Blood pressure is 157/92 mm Hg. There is truncal obesity and facial erythrosis. There are no catabolic signs.

Laboratory test results:

Sodium = 144 mEq/L (SI: 144 mmol/L)
Potassium = 3.5 mEq/L (SI: 3.5 mmol/L)
Creatinine = 1.2 mg/dL (SI: 107 μmol/L)
Glucose = 106.3 mg/dL (SI: 5.9 mmol/L)
Hemoglobin A_{1c} = 6% (42 mmol/mol)
Cortisol after 1 mg dexamethasone = 3.8 μg/dL
    (>1.8 μg/dL) (SI: 106 nmol/L [>50 nmol/L])
Urinary free cortisol = 34.8 μg/24 h (54.4 μg/24 h)
    (SI: 96 nmol/d [<142 nmol/d])
Morning cortisol = 17.9 μg/dL (4.5-24.0 μg/dL)
    (SI: 495 nmol/L [124-662 nmol/L])
ACTH = 9.1 pg/mL (<59.1 pg/mL) (SI: <2 pmol/L
    [<13 pmol/L])
Late-night salivary cortisol = 0.40 μg/dL
    (<0.14 μg/dL) (SI: 11.0 nmol/L [<3.9 nmol/L])
Aldosterone = 14.2 ng/dL (1.2-23.6 ng/dL)
    (SI: 393 pmol/L [33-655 pmol/L])
Renin = 46 μIU/mL (3-40 μIU/mL)

Which of the following is the most likely diagnosis?

A. Adrenal bilateral metastasis of a lung cancer

B. Nonclassic congenital adrenal hyperplasia

C. Bilateral adrenal cancer

D. Primary bilateral macronodular adrenal hyperplasia

E. Carney complex

Answer: D) Primary bilateral macronodular adrenal hyperplasia

The nodules are benign adrenocortical lesions, not cancer. Hormonal investigations demonstrate mild autonomous cortisol secretion, which is present in most cases of incidentally discovered primary bilateral macronodular adrenal hyperplasia (Answer D). Nonclassic congenital adrenal hyperplasia would not be associated with low ACTH and mild autonomous cortisol secretion. Carney complex can cause overt Cushing syndrome due to bilateral micronodular adrenal hyperplasia in children and young adults.

Case 2, Continued

Genetic analysis reveals an *ARMC5* pathogenic variant.

Which of the following is the best advice?

A. Bilateral adrenalectomy

B. Pasireotide

C. Brain MRI

D. Adrenal imaging in all first-degree relatives

E. 1-mg dexamethasone-suppression test in all first-degree relatives

Answer: C) Brain MRI

An *ARMC5* pathogenic variant is found in about 20% of index patients with primary bilateral macronodular adrenal hyperplasia. About half of *ARMC5* index patients diagnosed today have been initially evaluated for bilateral adrenal incidentalomas. An *ARMC5* pathogenic variant can be associated with meningioma, thus justifying brain imaging (Answer C). The finding of an *ARMC5* pathogenic variant in an index patient offers the possibility of genetic familial screening. Adrenal evaluation (imaging and hormonal assays) would only be recommended in relatives carrying the *ARMC5* pathogenic variant. Treatment of mild autonomous cortisol secretion in primary bilateral macronodular adrenal hyperplasia is based on the evaluation of comorbidities (diabetes, hypertension, obesity, osteoporosis). Among the therapies that can be discussed on an individual basis are unilateral adrenalectomy (but not bilateral adrenalectomy, at least not as first-line treatment) or steroidogenesis inhibitors.

Case 3

A 69-year-old man presents with moderate weight loss (11.0 lb [5 kg]) in a 4-month period and unusual asthenia with dizziness. He has a 12-year history of hypertension treated with amlodipine and enalapril/hydrochlorothiazide and a 4-year history of type 2 diabetes treated with metformin.

On physical examination, his temperature is 97.9°F (36.6°C), pulse rate is 88 beats/min, and blood pressure is 107/66 mm Hg. His weight is 165.3 lb (75 kg) (BMI = 22.7 kg/m²).

Laboratory test results:

Sodium = 131 mEq/L (SI: 131 mmol/L)
Potassium = 4.7 mEq/L (SI: 4.7 mmol/L)
Creatinine = 0.75 mg/dL (SI: 66 μmol/L)
Hemoglobin = 12.9 g/dL (SI: 129 g/L)

Leukocyte count = 5600/μL (SI: 5.6 × 10⁹/L)
C-reactive protein = 11 mg/L (SI: 104.8 nmol/L)
Hemoglobin A_{1c} = 6.5% (48 mmol/mol)
Liver enzymes, normal
TSH = 2.4 mIU/L

Figure 4.

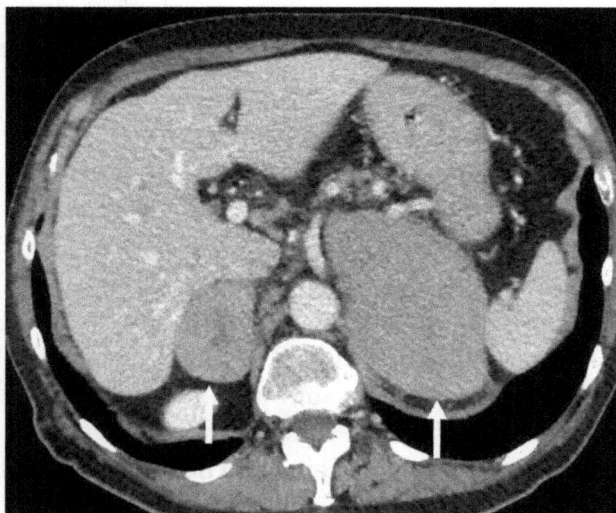

A

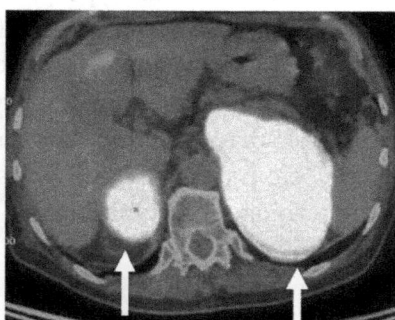

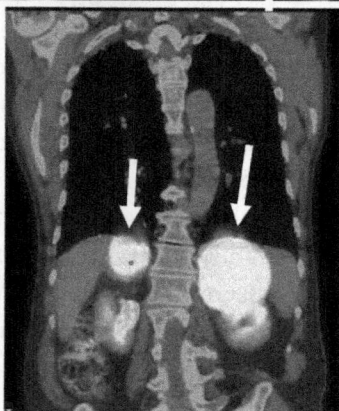

B

[Color—Print (Color Gallery page CG7) or web & ePub editions]

Whole-body CT reveals bilateral adrenal masses (right, 56 × 43 mm; left, 128 × 85 mm) (*Figure 4A*). An ¹⁸FDG PET shows high uptake (SUV = 11-18) in both adrenal masses and no other abnormal lesions (*Figure 4B*).

Which of the following should be recommended now?

A. Morning circulating ACTH and serum cortisol measurement

B. Chromogranin A measurement

C. Corticotropin-releasing hormone test

D. Immediate adrenal biopsy

E. Adrenal vein sampling

Answer: A) Morning circulating ACTH and serum cortisol measurement

This patient has signs suggestive of adrenal insufficiency, and basal ACTH and cortisol measurements (Answer A) are important to confirm this diagnosis. If the results demonstrate elevated ACTH and low cortisol, this would be enough evidence to start rapidly substitutive therapy with hydrocortisone. If this is not the case, cosyntropin-stimulation testing would be advised.

Chromogranin A (Answer B) is a marker of neuroendocrine tumor including pheochromocytoma, but its specificity and sensitivity precludes its use as a first-line investigation.

Corticotropin-releasing hormone testing (Answer C) would only be indicated in the setting of ACTH-dependent Cushing syndrome.

Adrenal vein sampling (Answer E) would only be relevant if unilateral adrenalectomy for steroid excess (mostly primary aldosteronism) were being discussed.

Adrenal biopsy (Answer D) cannot be performed before the results of metanephrine/normetanephrine assays to rule out pheochromocytoma.

Case 3, Continued

The following laboratory test results are documented:

ACTH = 59.1 pg/mL (<2.9 pg/mL) (SI: 42 pmol/L [<13.0 pmol/L])

Cortisol = 8.8 µg/dL (SI: 243 nmol)

Cortisol post cosyntropin-stimulation test = 10.3 µg/dL (>18.5 µg/dL) (SI: 283 nmol/L [>510 nmol/L])

Renin = 179 µIU/mL (2.8-39.9 µIU/mL)

Aldosterone = 1.2 ng/dL (1.2-2.4 ng/dL) (SI: 32 pmol/L [32.5-65.5 pmol/L])

Urinary normetanephrine = 460.4 µg/24 h (125.4-483.9 µg/24 h) (SI: 2514 nmol/d [677-2642 nmol/d])

Urinary metanephrine = 70.0 µg/24 h (43.0-260.0 µg/24 h) (SI: 355 nmol/d [218-1318 nmol/d])

Which of the following should be recommended?

A. Adrenalectomy

B. Replace amlodipine with spironolactone

C. Plan an outpatient consultation in 1 week to prescribe glucocorticoid substitutive therapy

D. Adrenal biopsy

E. 1-mg dexamethasone-suppression test

Answer: D) Adrenal biopsy

This patient has a clinically significant primary adrenal insufficiency, and glucocorticoid and mineralocorticoid therapy should be started immediately. The diuretic (hydrochlorothiazide) should be stopped, and the indication for the antihypertensive drug should be reevaluated. Diuretics are not recommended for patients with primary adrenal insufficiency. Adrenal biopsy (Answer D) is indicated since pheochromocytoma has been excluded and this patient is likely to have adrenal destruction by an infiltrative malignant tumor. The biopsy confirmed the diagnosis of high-grade B-cell lymphoma, and the patient was immediately started on cytotoxic chemotherapy.

Key Learning Points

- Bilateral adrenal masses are most frequently found incidentally.

- Rigorous imaging analysis is the initial key step to ascertain the nature of the masses and should determine whether the nature of the lesion is similar on both sides.

- The most frequent cause is benign bilateral adrenocortical lesions (adenomas or primary bilateral macronodular adrenal hyperplasia) causing mild autonomous cortisol secretion.

- Management of benign bilateral adrenocortical lesions causing mild autonomous cortisol secretion is based on comorbidities, which are common and sometimes uncontrolled in these patients.

- Patients with bilateral infiltrative lesions (infectious, inflammatory, or malignant) should be screened for adrenal insufficiency.

References

1. Fassnacht M, Tsagarakis S, Terzolo M, et al. European Society of Endocrinology clinical practice guidelines on the management of adrenal incidentalomas, in collaboration with the European Network for the Study of Adrenal Tumors. *Eur J Endocrinol.* 2023;189(1):G1-G42. PMID: 37318239

2. Sweeney AT, Hamidi O, Dogra P, et al. Clinical review: the approach to the evaluation and management of bilateral adrenal masses. *Endocr Pract.* 2024;30(10):987-1002. PMID: 39103149

3. Pelsma ICM, Fassnacht M, Tsagarakis S, et al. Comorbidities in mild autonomous cortisol secretion and the effect of treatment: systematic review and meta-analysis. *Eur J Endocrinol.* 2023;189(4):S88-S101. PMID: 37801655.

4. Taïeb D, Nölting S, Perrier ND, et al. Management of phaeochromocytoma and paraganglioma in patients with germline SDHB pathogenic variants: an international expert Consensus statement. *Nat Rev Endocrinol.* 2024;20(3):168-184. PMID: 38097671

5. Bertherat J, Bourdeau I, Bouys L, Chasseloup F, Kamenický P, Lacroix A. Clinical, pathophysiologic, genetic, and therapeutic progress in primary bilateral macronodular adrenal hyperplasia. *Endocr Rev.* 2023;44(4):567-628. PMID: 36548967

6. Bouys L, Vaczlavik A, Cavalcante IP, et al; COMETE and ENSAT Networks. The mutational landscape of ARMC5 in primary bilateral macronodular adrenal hyperplasia: an update. *Orphanet J Rare Dis.* 2025;20(1):51. PMID: 39910635

Management of Metastatic Pheochromocytomas and Paragangliomas

Camilo Jimenez, MD. Department of Endocrine Neoplasia and Hormonal Disorders, University of Texas MD Anderson Cancer Center, Houston, Texas; Email: cjimenez@mdanderson.org

Educational Objectives

After reviewing this chapter, learners should be able to:

- Identify clinical predictors of metastases.

- Describe the current evidence-based pharmacotherapeutic agents used to treat individuals living with metastatic pheochromocytomas and paragangliomas (MPPGLs).

- Identify emerging therapies for patients with MPPGLs.

Significance of the Clinical Problem

Pheochromocytomas and paragangliomas (PPGLs) are rare neuroendocrine tumors. Approximately 1000 new cases of PPGLs are diagnosed annually in the United States. Of these, 25% are metastatic. The World Health Organization acknowledges that all PPGLs have the potential to metastasize and recommends that these tumors be classified as nonmetastatic or metastatic, rather than using the traditional classifications of benign or malignant. The risk of metastases is increased in patients with sympathetic extraadrenal tumors, pheochromocytomas larger than 5 cm, pheochromocytomas with periadrenal fat infiltration, and PPGLs associated with germline pathogenic variants in the gene encoding succinate dehydrogenase subunit B (*SDHB*).[1,2] Metastases most frequently happen in regional and distant lymph nodes (80%), the skeleton (72%), and the liver and lungs (50%). Patients with MPPGLs are at risk of complications due to their frequently large tumor burden, tumor location, speed of progression of the disease, and excessive secretion of catecholamines–mainly norepinephrine. MPPGLs are an orphan disease. The diagnosis of MPPGLs is frequently delayed, therapeutic options are limited, and for most part systemic therapies are not curative. In addition, medications are very expensive and are often not covered by private or public insurance plans, as most of them are not approved by regulatory agencies. High-specific-activity iodine-131 (^{131}I) MIBG (HSA ^{131}I-MIBG) is to date the first and only FDA-approved medication to treat MPPGLs.[3] Unfortunately, HSA ^{131}I-MIBG was discontinued in clinical practice due to its high manufacturing cost, sophisticated administration, lack of familiarity of most providers with its prescription, and a substantial amount of misleading information published in scientific literature.[4,5]

Practice Gaps

- There is a lack of awareness among many health care providers regarding the diagnosis and treatment of MPPGLs.

- It is crucial for clinicians to tailor treatments for patients with MPPGLs in an individualized manner.
- There is a lack of awareness of the complexity of the treatment of MPPGLs.

Discussion

MPPGLs have a very heterogeneous nature, and their clinical behavior is difficult to predict. The results of different populational studies indicate that the overall survival rates of patients with MPPGLs vary from 30% to 60% at 5 years after initial diagnosis.[6,7] Progression-free survivorship rate at 1 year is 50%.[8] Although most MPPGLs progress over time, some exhibit very fast progression leading to elevated mortality rates in a matter of a few weeks or months after their initial discovery. Other MPPGLs exhibit slow progression over time. These tumors will require intervention or systemic therapy at some point during their course. Conversely, there are some MPPGLs that will exhibit minimal or no progression over time; these patients are frequently asymptomatic. If symptomatic, their symptoms are usually mild and easy to control with supportive measures, such as the use of α- and β-adrenergic blockers. Furthermore, these patients may achieve a normal lifespan and subsequently they may not need systemic therapies, as currently the available treatments are not curative and are frequently associated with adverse events that may alter the individual's quality of life.[7,8] Together the last 2 groups of patients contribute to the higher progression-free survival rates that are seen, in general, in patients with MPPGLs when compared with progression-free survival rates associated with other cancers. Symptom severity, the presence of complications such as skeletal-related events (eg, pathologic fractures), and close follow-up help to determine the aggressiveness of the disease.[9,10] Although some retrospective studies have suggested that the presence of germline pathogenic variants in the *SDHB* gene predict a very aggressive outcome, other studies have failed to demonstrate this

and have shown that patients with apparently sporadic MPPGLs frequently exhibit a worse prognosis when compared with prognosis of *SDHB* carriers.[11-13] Currently, the speed of progression, the severity of symptoms, the presence of comorbidities, and the patient's performance status determine how and when to treat MPPGLs.[14]

Systemic therapies for patients with progressive MPPGLs include chemotherapy, tyrosine kinase inhibitors, radiopharmaceuticals, and hypoxia-inducible factor 2α inhibitors. Medications are classified as effective, active, and emerging therapies depending on the evidence derived from prospective studies dedicated to patients with MPPGLs. Medications that are considered effective are those that have prospectively demonstrated improved clinical outcomes when compared with either placebo or standard of care (randomized prospective clinical trials) and have demonstrated acceptable toxicity. Medications that are considered active are those that have demonstrated improved clinical outcomes with acceptable toxicity. Treatment outcomes have not been compared with either placebo or standard of care (single-arm prospective clinical trials). Emerging therapies are currently being evaluated in prospective clinical trials from which the final results have not been published yet. These medications have not yet been demonstrated to be active and/or safe.

Systemic therapies include chemotherapy (cyclophosphamide, vincristine, and dacarbazine or temozolomide), tyrosine kinase inhibitors (cabozantinib, sunitinib), radiopharmaceuticals (HSA ^{131}I-MIBG, low-specific-activity (LSA) ^{131}I-MIBG, ^{177}Lu-DOTATATE), and hypoxia-inducible factor 2α inhibitors (belzutifan).

Cyclophosphamide, vincristine, and dacarbazine chemotherapy has been demonstrated to be active against MPPGLs. It works fast and is associated with tumor size reduction, disease stabilization, improvement of symptoms of catecholamine excess, and perhaps improvement of survivorship.[15,16] Toxicity is substantial and includes bone marrow suppression, neuropathy, and gastrointestinal disease.[16,17] Temozolomide is an emerging therapy evaluated in a clinical trial.

Tyrosine kinase inhibitors have been demonstrated to be effective (sunitinib) or active (cabozantinib) against MPPGLs.[18,19] These medications also work fast and are associated with tumor size reduction, disease stabilization, and improvement of symptoms of catecholamine excess. Toxicity includes hypertension, catecholamine crisis, and fatigue.[18-20]

Radiopharmaceuticals works slowly. They are mainly associated with disease stabilization and improvement of symptoms of catecholamine excess and slow improvement of biomarkers.[3,21] Tumor size reduction has been described with MIBG.[3,22] Adverse effects include bone marrow suppression and catecholamine crisis.[22] HSA ^{131}I-MIBG is an exception, as it does not cause hypertension or catecholamine crisis.[3] HSA ^{131}I-MIBG is an active medication against MPPGLs. LSA ^{131}I-MIBG and ^{177}Lu-DOTATATE are emerging therapies.

Belzutifan is a small molecule that potently inhibits hypoxia-inducible factor 2α.[23] Thanks to the actions of belzutifan, pathways involved in tumor angiogenesis, inflammation, cell proliferation, and tumor spread might be mitigated. Most patients experience anemia due to inhibition of the synthesis of erythropoietin in the kidneys; in many patients, the anemia is asymptomatic and does not require intervention.[24] Occasionally, patients require supportive treatment with red blood cell transfusion or recombinant erythropoietin. A few patients experience transient and frequently asymptomatic hypoxia, which is usually corrected with exercise. Belzutifan is currently being evaluated in a phase 2 clinical trial. A lot of excitement exists regarding belzutifan, as it targets the "heart" of most MPPGLs.

Clinical Case Vignettes
Case 1

A 43-year-old man has abdominal pain, and abdominal CT reveals a 12-cm paraganglioma. His blood pressure is normal. He has no symptoms of catecholamine excess. He undergoes surgical resection. Genetic testing reveals a pathogenic variant in the *SDHB* gene. One year after surgery, he is found to have multiple abdominal nodules, the largest of which measures 3 cm. He has mild abdominal discomfort. Plasma normetanephrines are normal. DOTATATE PET reveals multiple peritoneal and retroperitoneal implants. The patient is treated with ^{177}Lu-DOTATATE. Three months after finishing this therapy, the largest nodule has decreased 10% in size when compared with baseline imaging studies. The other nodules are stable, and there are no new lesions. The patient is asymptomatic. Seven months after finishing treatment with ^{177}Lu-DOTATATE, he reports abdominal distention and pain and difficulty breathing while on his back. CT reveals diffuse tumor enlargement, new peritoneal nodules, ascites, pronounced collateral circulation, and a 7-cm mass that encases the iliac vessels.

Which of the following is the best therapeutic approach for this patient?

A. Cyclophosphamide, vincristine, and dacarbazine chemotherapy

B. Cabozantinib

C. Sunitinib

D. Repeat therapy with ^{177}Lu-DOTATATE

E. Observation

Answer: A) Cyclophosphamide, vincristine, and dacarbazine chemotherapy

The patient has disease that has progressed rapidly over a short period. The disease exploded shortly after finishing therapy with ^{177}Lu-DOTATATE. The patient has a large tumor burden, and his symptoms are overwhelming. The best approach is to treat the patient with cyclophosphamide, vincristine, and dacarbazine chemotherapy (Answer A). Chemotherapy works rapidly, and tumor responses can be impressive. Although cabozantinib and sunitinib work fast as well, the vascular encasement and the collateral circulation represent a relative contraindication to antiangiogenic medications. Cabozantinib and sunitinib might predispose to fistula formation and bleeding.

Case 2

A 48-year-old man presented with palpitations, panic attacks, and hypertension 10 years ago. Plasma normetanephrines were elevated. Abdominal CT revealed a 7-cm right pheochromocytoma. The patient underwent surgical resection. His symptoms subsided and blood pressure normalized. No additional follow-up was provided. The patient presented 6 months ago with lower back pain. Blood pressure was 150/100 mm Hg. MRI demonstrated 3 osteolytic lesions in the lumbar spine with no evidence of cord compression. CT identified 5 metastatic lesions to the liver. The largest lesion measured 2.5 cm. Plasma normetanephrines were elevated. FDG-PET confirmed the findings observed on CT and MRI. MIBG scan demonstrated MIBG uptake in all lesions. The bone lesions were treated with stereotactic beam radiation therapy. He started α-adrenergic blockade, and blood pressure normalized. Imaging studies obtained 3 months after radiation therapy revealed stable disease. Six months later, some of the liver lesions had increased in size. The largest lesion measured 3 cm.

The patient has noticed occasional palpitations. He has excellent performance status. FDG-PET shows decreased glucose uptake in the bone lesions but no new lesions. Plasma normetanephrines are increased when compared with baseline studies 6 months ago.

Which of the following is the best therapeutic approach for this patient?

A. Cyclophosphamide, vincristine, and dacarbazine chemotherapy

B. Cabozantinib

C. Sunitinib

D. MIBG

E. Observation

Answer: D) MIBG

This patient has disease that has progressed slowly over a period of 6 months. He does not have a large tumor burden. The best approach is to treat this patient with a radiopharmaceutical medication, such as MIBG (Answer D). MIBG works slowly but progressively over time, and responses can be durable. The patient was treated with HSA ^{131}I-MIBG. The symptoms of catecholamine excess disappeared. He discontinued antihypertensive medications. The tumors decreased in size by 35% when compared with baseline. The patient has been asymptomatic and with stable disease for 5 years.

Case 3

A 36-year-old man presents with a 3-cm right neck paraganglioma. The patient is asymptomatic. Genetic testing reveals a pathogenic variant in the *SDHD* gene. DOTATATE PET reveals 6 small skeletal lesions. Plasma normetanephrines are normal. Bone biopsy confirms a metastatic paraganglioma. DOTATATE PET 3 months later shows stable disease. DOTATATE PET 12 months later shows no tumor changes. The patient is asymptomatic.

Which of the following is the best therapeutic approach for this patient?

A. Cyclophosphamide, vincristine, and dacarbazine chemotherapy

B. Cabozantinib

C. Sunitinib

D. MIBG

E. Observation

Answer: E) Observation

This patient would benefit from observation (Answer E). Although he has a metastatic paraganglioma, the disease is asymptomatic and is not progressive. Some patients with MPPGLs exhibit indolent outcomes. These patients may never exhibit disease progression. For patients with stable disease, it is better to just watch and wait, as current systemic therapies are not curative and are associated with adverse effects. It is not clear why in some patients with MPPGLs the disease stops growing; these are fortunate individuals. Nevertheless, long-term follow-up is recommended in these situations.

Key Learning Points

- The indication for systemic therapy is determined by the speed of disease progression and the severity of the clinical symptoms.

- In most patients, it is not possible to predict a response to therapy based on tumor genotype.

- Patients with MPPGLs that secrete adrenaline and/or noradrenaline must have a normal blood pressure in preparation for treatment with chemotherapy, tyrosine kinase and selective RET inhibitors, and radiopharmaceuticals (eg, LSA ^{131}I-MIBG and ^{177}Lu-DOTATATE).

References

1. Ayala-Ramirez M, Feng L, Johnson MM, et al. Clinical risk factors for malignancy and overall survival in patients with pheochromocytomas and sympathetic paragangliomas: primary tumor size and primary tumor location as prognostic indicators. *J Clin Endocrinol Metab.* 2011;96(3):717-725. PMID: 21190975

2. Jimenez C, Ma J, Roman Gonzalez A, et al. TNM staging and overall survival in patients with pheochromocytoma and sympathetic paraganglioma. *J Clin Endocrinol Metab.* 2023;108(5):1132-1142. PMID: 36433823

3. Pryma DA, Chin BB, Noto RB, et al. Efficacy and safety of high-specific-activity ^{131}I-MIBG therapy in patients with advanced pheochromocytoma or paraganglioma. *J Nucl Med.* 2019;60(5):623-630. PMID: 30291194

4. Jha A, Taieb D, Carrasquillo JA, et al. High-specific-activity-^{131}I-MIBG versus ^{177}Lu-DOTATATE targeted radionuclide therapy for metastatic pheochromocytoma and paraganglioma. *Clin Cancer Res.* 2021;27(11):2989-2995. PMID: 33685867

5. Nastos K, Cheung VTF, Toumpanakis C, et al. Peptide receptor radionuclide treatment and (131)I-MIBG in the management of patients with metastatic/progressive phaeochromocytomas and paragangliomas. *J Surg Oncol.* 2017;115(4):425-434. PMID: 28166370

6. Hamidi O, Young WF Jr, Iniguez-Ariza NM, et al. Malignant pheochromocytoma and paraganglioma: 272 patients over 55 years. *J Clin Endocrinol Metab.* 2017;102(9):3296-3205. PMID: 28605453

7. Jimenez C, Rohren E, Habra MA, et al. Current and future treatments for malignant pheochromocytoma and sympathetic paraganglioma. *Curr Oncol Rep.* 2013;15(4):356-371. PMID: 23674235

8. Hescot S, Leboulleux S, Amar L, V et al. One-year progression-free survival of therapy-naive patients with malignant pheochromocytoma and paraganglioma. *J Clin Endocrinol Metab.* 2013;98(10):4006-4012. PMID: 23884775

9. Jimenez C, Baudrand R, Uslar T, Bulzico D. Perspective review: lessons from successful clinical trials and real-world studies of systemic therapy for metastatic pheochromocytomas and paragangliomas. *Ther Adv Med Oncol.* 2024;16:17588359241301359. PMID: 39574494

10. Sukrithan V, Perez K, Pandit-Taskar N, Jimenez C. Management of metastatic pheochromocytomas and paragangliomas: when and what. *Curr Probl Cancer.* 2024;51:101116. PMID: 39024846

11. Amar L, Baudin E, Burnichon N, et al. Succinate dehydrogenase B gene mutations predict survival in patients with malignant pheochromocytomas or paragangliomas. *J Clin Endocrinol Metab.* 2007;92(10):3822-3828. PMID: 17652212

12. Roman-Gonzalez A, Zhou S, Ayala-Ramirez M, Shen C, Waguespack SG, Habra MA, et al. Impact of surgical resection of the primary tumor on overall survival in patients with metastatic pheochromocytoma or sympathetic paraganglioma. *Ann Surg.* 2018;268(1):172-178. PMID: 28257320

13. Hescot S, Curras-Freixes M, Deutschbein T, et al. Prognosis of malignant pheochromocytoma and paraganglioma (MAPP-Prono Study): a European Network for the Study of Adrenal Tumors retrospective study. *J Clin Endocrinol Metab.* 2019;104(6):2367-2374. PMID: 30715419

14. Fischer A, Del Rivero J, Wang K, Nolting S, Jimenez C. Systemic therapy for patients with metastatic pheochromocytoma and paraganglioma. *Best Pract Res Clin Endocrinol Metab.* 2025;39(1):101977. PMID: 39880697

15. Averbuch SD, Steakley CS, Young RC, et al. Malignant pheochromocytoma: effective treatment with a combination of cyclophosphamide, vincristine, and dacarbazine. *Ann Intern Med.* 1988;109(4):267-273. PMID: 3395037

16. Ayala-Ramirez M, Feng L, Habra MA, et al. Clinical benefits of systemic chemotherapy for patients with metastatic pheochromocytomas or sympathetic extra-adrenal paragangliomas: insights from the largest single-institutional experience. *Cancer.* 2012;118(11):2804-2812. PMID: 22006217

17. Niemeijer ND, Alblas G, van Hulsteijn LT, Dekkers OM, Corssmit EP. Chemotherapy with cyclophosphamide, vincristine and dacarbazine for malignant paraganglioma and pheochromocytoma: systematic review and meta-analysis. *Clin Endocrinol (Oxf).* 2014;81(5):642-651. PMID: 25041164

18. Baudin E, Goichot B, Berruti A, et al. Sunitinib for metastatic progressive phaeochromocytomas and paragangliomas: results from FIRSTMAPPP, an academic, multicentre, international, randomised, placebo-controlled, double-blind, phase 2 trial. *Lancet.* 2024;403(10431):1061-1070. PMID: 38402886

19. Jimenez C, Habra MA, Campbell MT, et al. Cabozantinib in patients with unresectable and progressive metastatic phaeochromocytoma or paraganglioma (the Natalie Trial): a single-arm, phase 2 trial. *Lancet Oncol.* 2024;25(5):658-667. PMID: 38608693

20. Jimenez C, Fazeli S, Roman-Gonzalez A. Antiangiogenic therapies for pheochromocytoma and paraganglioma. *Endocr Relat Cancer.* 2020;27(7):R239-R254. PMID: 32369773

21. Jimenez C, Chin BB, Noto RB, et al. Biomarker response to high-specific-activity I-131 meta-iodobenzylguanidine in pheochromocytoma/paraganglioma. *Endocr Relat Cancer.* 2023;30(2):e220236. PMID: 36472300

22. Gonias S, Goldsby R, Matthay KK, et al. Phase II study of high-dose [131I]metaiodobenzylguanidine therapy for patients with metastatic pheochromocytoma and paraganglioma. *J Clin Oncol.* 2009;27(25):4162-4168. PMID: 19636009

23. Toledo RA, Jimenez C, Armaiz-Pena G, Arenillas C, Capdevila J, Dahia PLM. Hypoxia-inducible factor 2 alpha (HIF2alpha) inhibitors: targeting genetically driven tumor hypoxia. *Endocr Rev.* 2023;44(2):312-322. PMID: 36301191

24. Jonasch E, Donskov F, Iliopoulos O, et al. Belzutifan for renal cell carcinoma in von Hippel-Lindau disease. *N Engl J Med.* 2021;385(22):2036-2046. PMID: 34818478

Evaluation and Management of Postmenopausal Androgen Excess

Michael W. O'Reilly, MD, PhD. Androgens in Health and Disease Research Group, Academic Division of Endocrinology, Department of Medicine, Royal College of Surgeons in Ireland (RCSI), Dublin, Ireland; Email: michaelworeilly@rcsi.com

Wiebke Arlt, MD, DSc. Medical Research Council Laboratory of Medical Sciences, London, United Kingdom; Email: w.arlt@lms.mrc.ac.uk

Educational Objectives

After reviewing this chapter, learners should be able to:

- Describe the presentation pattern, clinical signs, and symptoms of androgen excess in postmenopausal women, including red-flag symptoms for underlying neoplastic disease.

- Identify biochemical signatures that assist clinicians in distinguishing adrenal vs ovarian pathology in women with androgen excess.

- Guide the biochemical workup and imaging approach in patients presenting with postmenopausal androgen excess, including dynamic testing.

Significance of the Clinical Problem

Androgen excess is defined as clinical or biochemical evidence of increased production of androgenic steroids in women. It is observed in up to 10% of women of reproductive age and less commonly in postmenopausal women.[1] Androgen excess typically manifests clinically as hirsutism or acne, but more severe and prolonged exposure can lead to overt virilization, including clitoromegaly, deepening of the voice, female-pattern hair loss, or polycythemia. Most adolescents and women of reproductive age who present with androgen excess have underlying polycystic ovary syndrome (PCOS).[2] However, other primary underlying pathologies must be excluded in a subset of patients harboring red-flag clinical features, such as severe androgen excess, rapidly progressive symptoms or signs, or presentation in the postmenopausal phase of life. In particular, postmenopausal patients have a significantly increased likelihood of underlying neoplastic ovarian, adrenal, or pituitary disease compared with the likelihood in women of reproductive age, regardless of the severity of androgen excess.[3]

A detailed clinical history, targeted physical examination, and evaluation of the pattern and severity of biochemical disturbances are critical to rationalize the requirement and strategy for further biochemical, radiological, and, where appropriate, genetic investigations. Although androgen excess in women with PCOS is closely correlated with adverse metabolic health outcomes throughout their lifetime, severe biochemical disturbances or overt virilization are rarely observed in PCOS.

This chapter will review the presentation, evaluation, and management of androgen excess in postmenopausal women. We will examine biochemical signals that signpost towards ovarian, adrenal, or potentially neoplastic or malignant disease, as well as nuances to distinguish adrenal from ovarian pathology and lateralization of unilateral tumors.

Practice Gaps

- There is limited awareness among clinicians regarding careful biochemical phenotyping in postmenopausal patients presenting with androgen excess.

- Clinicians may be uncomfortable with biochemical thresholds for increased testosterone or other androgen levels above which adrenal, ovarian, or other imaging should be triggered.

- Dynamic investigations such as GnRH analogue/GnRH antagonist testing or dexamethasone-suppression testing are underused in clinical practice, as clinicians may be uncomfortable interpreting their findings. There is also underuse of diagnostic tests such as ovarian and adrenal vein sampling, which can be highly valuable in selected cases.

Discussion

A detailed list of the causes of androgen excess in both premenopausal and postmenopausal women are listed in the *Table, following page.* Clinical features of androgen excess in women include hirsutism, acne, and alopecia. A focused history should include assessment of the severity and duration of symptoms, as well as rapidity of onset.[4] Clinical examination should assess for acanthosis nigricans and skin tags, which are clinical features of severe insulin resistance, as well as cushingoid features such as violaceous striae, bruising, and proximal muscle weakness. Adipose tissue distribution should be examined to look for signs of lipodystrophy. Examination of external genitalia may not be indicated unless the patient reports specific clinical signs such as clitoromegaly or other features of overt virilization.

Patients with clinical and biochemical features of severe androgen excess and with a detected adrenal or ovarian tumor on cross-sectional imaging can generally proceed to surgical intervention without delay, particularly in the case of suspected adrenocortical carcinoma. However, incidental adnexal masses occur frequently in postmenopausal women, with a prevalence of 3.3% to 18.0% in asymptomatic women. Similarly, adrenal incidentalomas are detected in at least 5% of the general population, most of which are benign and nonfunctioning. While androgen-producing adrenal tumors are typically apparent on imaging, ovarian tumors may remain radiologically occult because of their small size.[6] Therefore, an incidental adrenal adenoma may not be the source of androgen excess.

As LH is the central regulator of ovarian androgen synthesis, a GnRH-suppression test can be used to confirm an ovarian source of androgen production in cases where this is clinically or biochemically suspected (eg, isolated or predominant increase in serum testosterone). GnRH analogues induce a prolonged stimulation of GnRH receptors in pituitary gonadotroph cells, leading to desensitization and subsequent downregulation of these receptors. The net effect is to suppress gonadotropins, with subsequent suppression of testosterone in cases of gonadotropin-dependent ovarian testosterone secretion. This response is typically observed in ovarian hyperthecosis, but it is also common in virilizing ovarian tumors.[7] This test is not of diagnostic utility if gonadotropin suppression is already evident at baseline, as this finding confirms gonadotropin-independent androgen excess, as observed in poorly controlled congenital adrenal hyperplasia, adrenocortical carcinoma, and a proportion of patients with virilizing ovarian tumors. GnRH analogue or antagonists can also be used as long-term therapy in patients with ovarian androgen excess who are not candidates for surgery or would like to avoid this intervention.

In exceptional cases, when uncertainty persists after dynamic testing and cross-sectional imaging, simultaneous ovarian and adrenal vein sampling may aid in localizing the source of androgen excess. In this interventional radiology procedure, the adrenal and ovarian veins are

Table. Causes of Androgen Excess in Women

Condition	Prevalence or incidence	Virilization	Rapidity of onset	Supportive biochemical features	Other features
Polycystic ovary syndrome	8%-13% of premenopausal women	Not observed	Insidious, often since puberty	Mild-to-moderate elevations of serum T, typically <145 ng/dL (SI: <5 nmol/L) Elevated A4 and DHEA-S observed in the mild-to-moderate range depending on assay	Oligomenorrhea/ amenorrhea Increased AMH Increased metabolic risk with variable degrees of insulin resistance clinically depending on BMI
Ovarian hyperthecosis	9.3% of postmenopausal women with androgen excess	Often present	Insidious	Increased serum T ranging from mild to severe elevations (sometimes >290 ng/dL (SI: >10 nmol/L) Adrenal androgens usually normal >50% suppression of serum T on GnRH analogue test	Bilateral enlarged ovaries/ increased ovarian volume on ultrasonography Histology shows ovarian stromal hyperplasia with cellular luteinization May be observed in patients with insulin resistance and T2D
Virilizing ovarian tumor	2.7% of postmenopausal women with androgen excess	Present in 50%	Variable	Increased serum T usually >145 ng/dL (SI: >5 nmol/L) T >290 ng/dL (SI: >10 nmol/L) more likely VOT than OHT A4 and/or E2 may also be increased Adrenal androgens (eg, DHEA-S) usually normal Inhibin B and AMH may be increased Variable suppression with GnRH analogue test with significant overlap with OHT; no suppression if fully autonomous or suppressed gonadotropins	Difficult to visualize on imaging; asymmetry may be suggestive. MRI has higher PPV (78%) and NPV (100%) than ultrasonography for detecting VOTs MRI has 83% sensitivity and 80% specificity for distinguishing VOT from OHT Role for FDG-PET in selected cases if other imaging equivocal or negative
Nonclassic congenital adrenal hyperplasia	1%-10% in women with androgen excess depending on population studied	Virilization at birth in classic cases only; overt virilization unusual in nonclassic	Insidious, often since puberty	Increased 17-OHP as diagnostic hallmark; typically >290 ng/dL (SI: >10 nmol/L) at baseline Variable elevation of serum A4 and T DHEA-S is usually low in treated patients	Basal morning follicular phase 17-OHP >145 ng/dL (SI: >5 nmol/L) progress to cosyntropin-stimulation test Stimulated 17-OHP on cosyntropin-stimulation test >990 ng/dL (SI: >30 nmol/L) is diagnostic
Adrenocortical carcinoma	1 to 2 cases per million population per year	Often present	Usually rapid (3-6 months)	Severe elevation in serum T (>145 ng/dL [SI: >5 nmol/L] may be observed; T rarely elevated in isolation Severe but variable elevations in DHEA-S and/or A4 Clinical and biochemical cortisol excess (ACTH-independent) with failed overnight dexamethasone-suppression test may be observed Increased adrenal steroid precursors on steroid metabolome analysis	Unilateral adrenal mass should be visible on cross-sectional imaging

Condition	Prevalence or incidence	Virilization	Rapidity of onset	Supportive biochemical features	Other features
Cushing disease	1.8- to .2 cases per million population per year 1% of premenopausal women with androgen excess, and 4% of postmenopausal women with androgen excess	Seldom present	Variable	Highly variable; serum T/DHEA-S/A4 may be normal or elevated Failed overnight dexamethasone-suppression test with detectable or elevated ACTH levels at baseline May coexist with gonadotropin deficiency	Discriminant features: violaceous abdominal striae, proximal muscle weakness, osteoporosis Nonspecific features: abdominal obesity, interscapular fat pad, bruising, hypertension
Severe insulin resistance[5]	Not clearly defined; may be congenital or acquired Most common in severe obesity but also seen in lean people or those with mild obesity and lipodystrophy or insulin-signaling defects	May be present in severe cases	Most commonly insidious from puberty; exacerbated by weight gain Rarely can be acute and fulminant in acquired autoimmune insulin resistance (type B IR)	Serum T ranges from normal to extremely elevated (>576 ng/dL [SI: >20 nmol/L]) Severely increased plasma insulin and HOMA-IR and suppressed plasma adiponectin Usually high triglycerides, low HDL cholesterol, evidence of fatty liver (if not, then consider INSR pathogenic variant or anti-INSR antibodies)	Ovulatory dysfunction, polycystic ovarian morphology Acanthosis nigricans Often family history of T2D Lipodystrophy or centripetal obesity Wide range of syndromic features
Acromegaly	Prevalence: 2.8-13.7 cases per 100,000 Incidence: 0.2-1.1 cases per 100,000 per year	Seldom present	Insidious onset	Elevated IGF-1; failure to suppress growth hormone below 0.4 ng/mL on oral glucose tolerance testing Often biochemical evidence of androgen excess in women	Coarsening of facial features; enlarged hands; interdental separation; thyroid goiter; evidence of cardiomyopathy in advanced cases

Abbreviations: A4, androstenedione; AMH, antimullerian hormone; E2, estradiol; INSR, insulin receptor; NPV, negative predictive value; OHT, ovarian hyperthecosis; PCOS, polycystic ovary syndrome; PPV, positive predictive value; T, testosterone; T2D, type 2 diabetes; VOT, virilizing ovarian tumor.

Reprinted from Elhassan YS et al. Clinical Endocrinology, 2025, 1-27. https://doi.org/10.1111/cen.15265 © The Authors. Clinical Endocrinology is published by John Wiley & Sons Ltd.

cannulated simultaneously; peripheral, adrenal and ovarian venous effluent sampling is undertaken to demonstrate differential gradients in androgen levels.[8] However, in postmenopausal women in whom fertility preservation is not a consideration, it is not essential to lateralize the source of ovarian androgen excess, and bilateral oophorectomy can be considered.

The primary objective of imaging in the workup of patients with severe androgen excess is to identify structural culprit adrenal or ovarian pathology and also to distinguish between incidental and clinically relevant lesions.

When ovarian disease is suspected, pelvic MRI and transvaginal ultrasonography should be performed. FDG-PET can be considered if these are negative. Cross-sectional adrenal imaging should be performed in those with biochemical evidence of adrenal androgen excess (increased androstenedione or DHEA-S) or in those with evidence of ACTH-dependent Cushing syndrome.

A targeted history and exam are required to identify those patients who harbor non-PCOS pathology, particularly among those presenting with atypical or red-flag features such as rapid symptoms onset or overt virilization. Systematic

Figure. Clinical Algorithm for Evaluation and Management of Androgen Excess

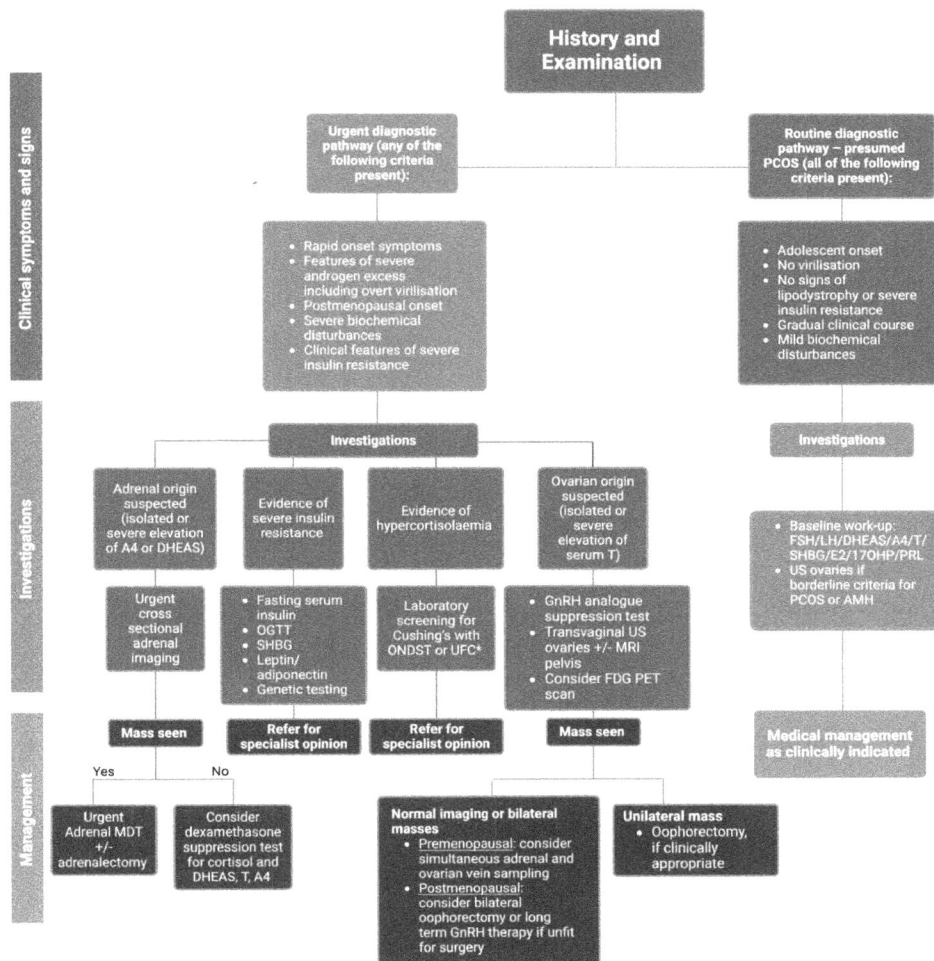

Reprinted from Elhassan YS et al. Clinical Endocrinology, 2025, 1-27. https://doi.org/10.1111/cen.15265 © The Authors. Clinical Endocrinology is published by John Wiley & Sons Ltd.

[Color—Print (Color Gallery page CG7) or web & ePub editions]

interrogation of circulating serum testosterone and adrenal androgen precursors, in tandem with other markers, such as 17-hydroxyprogesterone and gonadotropins, can identify signature patterns suspicious for underlying adrenal, pituitary, and ovarian disease and guide imaging strategies accordingly. Serum testosterone concentrations below 145 ng/dL (<5 nmol/L) measured using liquid chromatography–tandem mass spectrometry in premenopausal women typically do not warrant further evaluation in women with clinical features otherwise consistent with PCOS. However, in postmenopausal women, any degree of androgen excess should be investigated promptly due to the age-related decline in androgens in normal physiological circumstances.

Clinical Case Vignettes
Case 1

A 59-year-old woman presents with a 6-month history of hirsutism, weight gain, and abdominal striae. She has developed hypertension, and her hemoglobin A_{1c} is elevated at 6.5% (47 mmol/mol). She reports increasing breathlessness and ankle edema.

On physical examination, she has violaceous striae, bruising, and facial plethora. Her blood pressure is 158/97 mm Hg.

Laboratory test results:

Serum testosterone = 118.1 ng/dL (SI: 4.1 nmol/L)
DHEA-S = >1000 μg/dL (SI: >27.1 μmol/L)
Androstenedione = 1613 ng/dL (SI: 56.3 nmol/L)
17-Hydroxyprogesterone = 406.9 ng/dL
   (SI: 12.3 nmol/L)
FSH = <1.0 mIU/mL (SI: <1.0 IU/L)
LH = <1.0 mIU/mL (SI: <1.0 IU/L)
Estradiol = <25.1 pg/dL (SI: <92.1 pmol/L)
ACTH = <5 pg/mL (SI: <1.1 pmol/L)
Cortisol = 56.7 μg/dL (SI: 1565 nmol/L)

Which of the following is this patient's most likely diagnosis?

A. PCOS

B. Adrenocortical carcinoma

C. Virilizing ovarian tumor

D. Congenital adrenal hyperplasia

Answer: B) Adrenocortical carcinoma

This patient has preferential elevation of adrenal androgens. The increase in serum testosterone in this context is likely due to peripheral conversion of androstenedione and other precursors. She has clinical features of Cushing syndrome. Her biochemistry confirms adrenal androgen excess along with evidence of ACTH-independent hypercortisolism. The best next step in her evaluation is adrenal imaging, as well as CT of the chest/thorax/abdomen. An adrenal mass in the presence of adrenal androgen excess is diagnostic of adrenocortical carcinoma (Answer B) until proven otherwise.[9]

Elevation of 17-hydroxyprogesterone may also be observed in the setting of malignant adrenal neoplasms. This presentation is not consistent with late-onset congenital adrenal hyperplasia, either in terms of the rapidity of clinical onset or the clinical and biochemical evidence of adrenal hypercortisolism. Pharmacotherapy to control cortisol excess, hyperandrogenism, and hypertension are required urgently. Agents such as mitotane, spironolactone, metyrapone,

or ketoconazole are effective in this setting. Definitive treatment may consist of adrenalectomy or cytotoxic chemotherapy or a combination of both, depending on the extent of the primary disease.

Case 2

A 68-year-old woman presents with a 3- to 4-year history of facial hirsutism, requiring frequent topical cosmetic interventions. Symptoms include frontotemporal alopecia, altered body odor, deepening of the voice, and changes in the size and appearance of external genitalia. Medical history includes hypertension, chronic kidney disease, and osteoporosis. She had no fertility concerns during her reproductive years, with 5 uneventful pregnancies. She underwent vaginal hysterectomy for uterine prolapse 9 years ago (with ovarian preservation).

Initial laboratory test results:

Serum testosterone = 1190 ng/dL (SI: 41.3 nmol/L)
Androstenedione = 264.7 ng/dL (SI: 9.24 nmol/L)
DHEA-S = 107.4 μg/dL (SI: 2.9 μmol/L)
Gonadotropins, values in the postmenopausal range
Hematocrit = 50.4% (SI: 0.504)
Hemoglobin = 16.4 g/dL (SI: 164 g/L)

An overnight dexamethasone-suppression test is performed to exclude glucocorticoid excess, which reveals appropriate suppression of serum cortisol to less than 1.8 μg/dL (SI: <50 nmol/L).

Which of the following is this patient's most likely diagnosis?

A. PCOS

B. Adrenocortical carcinoma

C. Virilizing ovarian tumor

D. Severe insulin resistance

Answer: C) Virilizing ovarian tumor

This patient's most likely diagnosis is a virilizing ovarian tumor (Answer C). The pattern of androgen elevation is consistent with an ovarian source, with predominant elevation of testosterone and normal adrenal androgens. The severity of the testosterone elevation (up to

40-fold higher than expected postmenopausal levels) would be extremely unusual in the setting of ovarian hyperthecosis. In premenopausal women, serum testosterone levels with severe insulin resistance syndromes may be significantly elevated (sometimes >570 ng/dL [>20 nmol/L]). However, onset in the postmenopausal phase of life would be considered very unusual. Intriguingly, despite the severity of the testosterone elevation, gonadotropins are not suppressed, a finding not unusual even in virilizing ovarian tumors, although they tend to be lower than levels observed with ovarian hyperthecosis. Baseline suppression of gonadotropins is predictive of malignant potential with virilizing ovarian tumors in a number of case series.[10]

This patient's serum testosterone suppressed fully 28 days after GnRH analogue injection, consistent with a gonadotropin-dependent ovarian source. Typical GnRH preparations include triptorelin, 3 mg administered via intramuscular injection, with measurement of gonadotropins and serum testosterone at baseline and again after 28 days. Alternative options include using GnRH antagonists such as cetrorelix at a dose of 3 mg via subcutaneous injection, although some of these preparations may not be available or approved for use in all centers or countries. GnRH antagonists have the added advantage of avoiding the early surge in gonadotropins and testosterone in the first 7 days after administration that can be seen with GnRH analogues. Importantly, these prolonged tests are not likely to be appropriate for patients in whom malignancy is highly suspected and prompt treatment is required. Examples include patients with large adrenal or adnexal masses or with suppression of gonadotropins at baseline.

Imaging in this case revealed a right-sided, 3-cm ovarian mass. Theoretically, GnRH testing should distinguish between ovarian hyperthecosis and virilizing ovarian tumors due to autonomous androgen secretion in the context of virilizing ovarian tumors. However, real-world data highlight significant overlap in serum testosterone response to GnRH analogues in patients with ovarian hyperthecosis and virilizing ovarian tumors. In malignant lesions, testosterone secretion is less likely to remain under gonadotropin regulation, so, in theory, failure to suppress testosterone after GnRH raises the clinical suspicion of a malignancy.

As this patient was postmenopausal and had an incidental ovarian finding, bilateral oophorectomy was performed. Subsequent histology identified a 2-cm lipid-rich tumor with a low mitotic count, consistent with a benign ovarian steroid cell tumor. Her symptoms fully resolved after surgery. In women of reproductive age, selective ovarian vein sampling could be considered in the context of fertility preservation to lateralize the source of neoplastic testosterone secretion. Testosterone levels normalized within 4 weeks of bilateral oophorectomy.

Case 3

A 67-year-old multiparous woman is referred with a 15-year history of hirsutism. Symptom onset was during the sixth decade of life. She was previously evaluated at another institution, without definitive pathology identified. The patient removes hair on a daily basis. Additional symptoms of androgen excess include frontal hair thinning. There are no symptoms concerning for overt virilization or glucocorticoid excess. Her medical history is notable for primary hypothyroidism and hypertension. She has 4 biological children.

On physical examination, her BMI is 48.2 kg/m². There are no overt features of insulin resistance or Cushing syndrome. Initial testing confirms biochemical androgen excess.

Laboratory test results:

> Serum testosterone = 216 ng/dL (SI: 7.5 nmol/L)
> Serum androstenedione = 501.4 ng/dL
>   (SI: 17.5 nmol/L)
> DHEA-S = 107.4 μg/dL (SI: 2.9 μmol/L)

Which of the following is this patient's most likely diagnosis?

A. PCOS

B. Adrenocortical carcinoma

C. Virilizing ovarian tumor

D. Ovarian hyperthecosis

Answer: D) Ovarian hyperthecosis

Ovarian hyperthecosis (Answer D) results from hyperplasia of androgen-secreting theca cells in the ovary. It is thought that some of the steroidogenically inactive ovarian stromal cells differentiate into theca-like cells capable of producing androgens. Thus, they are spread through the ovarian stroma and are not purely associated with the ovarian follicles. These theca cells produce androgens under the influence of LH. This condition usually occurs after menopause, when LH concentrations are high and the ovaries have few, if any, remaining follicles able to aromatize androgens to estrogen. The cause of ovarian hyperthecosis is unknown, but genetic factors may be implicated. High insulin levels are also associated with this condition. Although androgens can increase insulin concentrations, hyperinsulinemia is likely to be the primary driver of hyperthecosis, albeit potentiated by positive feedback from increased androgens.

Ovarian hyperthecosis is often associated with significant elevations of serum testosterone, with relative preservation of adrenal androgens such as DHEA-S. Androstenedione may be elevated, as it can also arise from ovarian theca cells. It is commonly associated with insulin resistance, obesity, and metabolic disorders. Imaging, such as MRI, can be helpful to distinguish ovarian hyperthecosis from virilizing ovarian tumors. Testosterone levels suppress in response to GnRH analogues. Definitive treatment in postmenopausal women involves bilateral oophorectomy, although GnRH analogue therapy could be considered in patients who prefer not to undergo surgery or are not good surgical candidates.

Key Learning Points
Clinical Evaluation

- Postmenopausal women who present with clinical features or suspicion of androgen excess should be assessed for hirsutism, acne, female-pattern hair loss, and virilization.

- Older patient age and rapid onset and progression of symptoms should be considered predictive factors for underlying non-PCOS pathology.

- Assessment for syndrome-specific clinical features should be undertaken (eg, Cushing syndrome, severe insulin resistance).

- Women with a suspicion for neoplastic androgen excess should be urgently referred to a center with relevant expertise.

Biochemical Evaluation

- Testosterone, SHBG, androstenedione, DHEA-S, 17-hydroxyprogesterone, estradiol, LH, FSH, and free testosterone should be measured in all women presenting clinical features or suspicion of androgen excess.

- Samples for the investigation of androgen excess should be collected in the morning following an overnight fast.

- In postmenopausal women, any biochemical evidence of androgen excess should trigger urgent ovarian and/or adrenal imaging.

- Caution must be used in applying absolute cutoffs for serum androgens above which investigations such as adrenal and pelvic imaging should be triggered. This is due to the wide variability in assay methods in clinical laboratories across centers and countries.

- Androgen measurement with liquid chromatography–tandem mass spectrometry should be undertaken when possible because of the limitations with immunoassays, including cross-reactivity at low circulating androgen concentrations. In centers where immunoassays are used, a second sample should be run by liquid chromatography–tandem mass spectrometry if the immunoassay-based androgen measurement does not align with the clinical picture.

- Dynamic testing (eg, GnRH analogue test or 96-hour dexamethasone-suppression test) should be considered in selected patients to aid in localizing the source of androgen excess. Triptorelin should be administered at a dose of 3 mg via intramuscular injection, with measurement of gonadotropins and serum androgens at baseline and after 28 days. A prolonged dexamethasone-suppression test (0.5 mg QDS for 96 hours, due to the long half-life of DHEA-S) is recommended in the investigation of suspected adrenal androgen

excess, although it is not necessary in patients with a suspicious adrenal mass who are likely to have ACTH-independent (and therefore likely malignant) adrenal androgen generation.

Imaging

- If clinical indications suggest non-PCOS pathology, cross-sectional imaging of the ovaries and/or adrenal glands should be performed as appropriate.
- Pelvic MRI should be performed if an ovarian tumor is strongly suspected.
- Urgent cross-sectional imaging (CT or MRI) should be performed if adrenal pathology is suspected.

References

1. Elhassan YS, Idkowiak J, Smith K, et al. Causes, patterns, and severity of androgen excess in 1205 consecutively recruited women. *J Clin Endocrinol Metab.* 2018;103(3):1214-1223. PMID: 29342266

2. Escobar-Morreale HF, Carmina E, Dewailly D, et al. Epidemiology, diagnosis and management of hirsutism: a consensus statement by the Androgen Excess and Polycystic Ovary Syndrome Society. *Hum Reprod Update.* 2012;18(2):146-170. PMID: 22064667

3. Cussen L, McDonnell T, Bennett G, Thompson CJ, Sherlock M, O'Reilly MW. Approach to androgen excess in women: clinical and biochemical insights. *Clin Endocrinol (Oxf).* 2022;97(2):174-186. PMID: 35349173

4. Dennedy MC, Smith D, O'Shea D, McKenna TJ. Investigation of patients with atypical or severe hyperandrogenaemia including androgen-secreting ovarian teratoma. *Eur J Endocrinol.* 2010;162(2):213-220. PMID: 19906851

5. Poretsky L, Cataldo NA, Rosenwaks Z, Giudice LC. The insulin-related ovarian regulatory system in health and disease. *Endocr Rev.* 1999;20(4):535-582. PMID: 10453357

6. Hirschberg AL. Approach to investigation of hyperandrogenism in a postmenopausal woman. *J Clin Endocrinol Metab.* 2023;108(5):1243-1253. PMID: 36409990

7. Doyle LM, Cussen L, McDonnell T, O'Reilly MW. Clinical utility of GnRH analogues in female androgen excess: highlighting diagnostic and therapeutic applications. *JCEM Case Rep.* 2023;1(5):luad108. PMID: 37908205

8. Tng E-L, Tan JM-M. Dexamethasone suppression test versus selective ovarian and adrenal vein catheterization in identifying virilizing tumors in postmenopausal hyperandrogenism-a systematic review and meta-analysis. *Gynecol Endocrinol.* 2021;37(7):600-608. PMID: 33660585

9. Bancos I, Taylor AE, Chortis V, et al; ENSAT EURINE-ACT Investigators. Urine steroid metabolomics for the differential diagnosis of adrenal incidentalomas in the EURINE-ACT study: a prospective test validation study. *Lancet Diabetes Endocrinol.* 2020;8(9):773-781. PMID: 32711725

10. Yance VRV, Marcondes JAM, Rocha MP, et al. Discriminating between virilizing ovary tumors and ovary hyperthecosis in postmenopausal women: clinical data, hormonal profiles and image studies. *Eur J Endocrinol.* 2017;177(1):93.102. PMID: 28432270

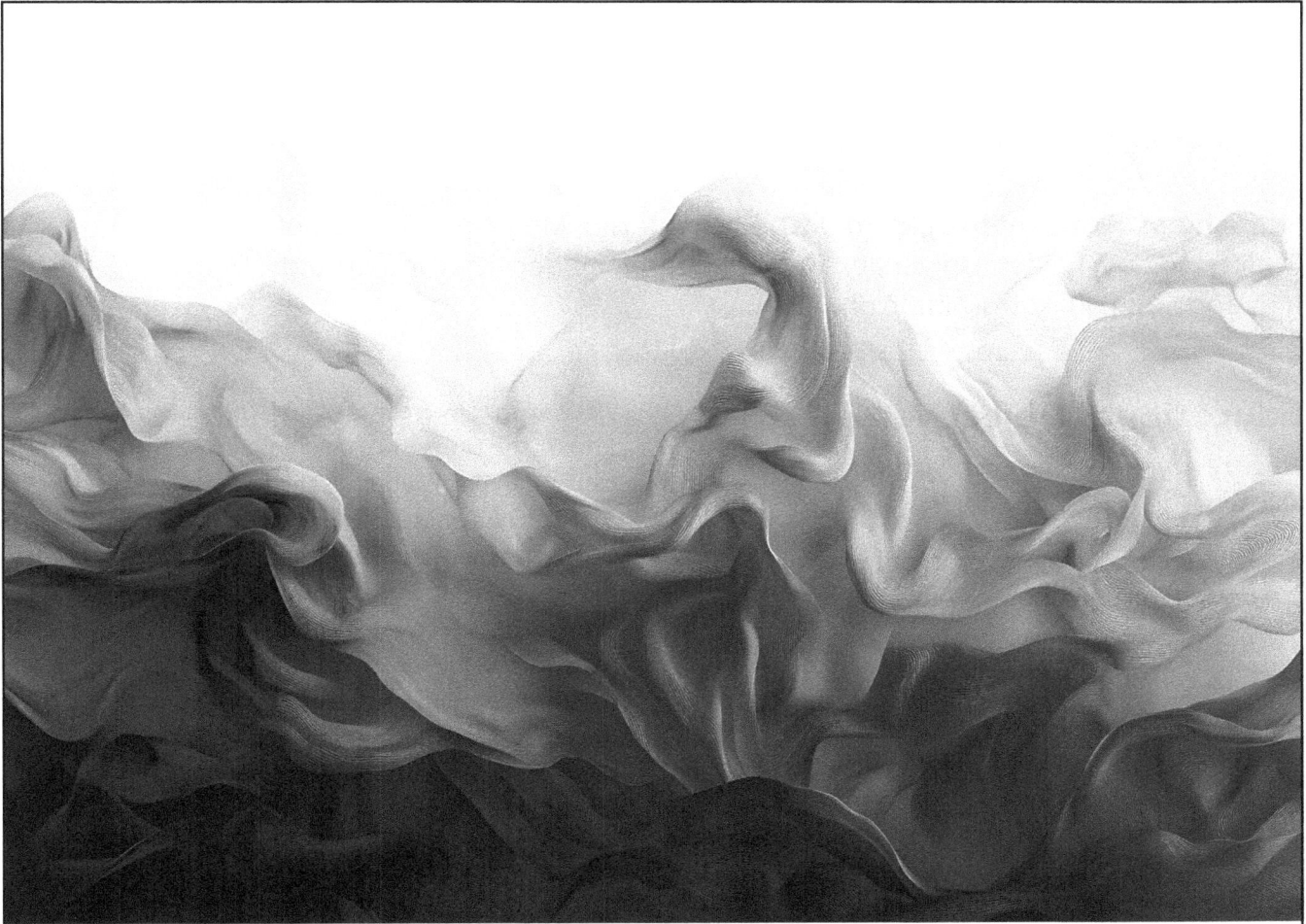

BONE AND MINERAL METABOLISM

Managing Calcium Disorders in Pregnancy

Natasha M. Appelman-Dijkstra, MD, PhD. Internal Medicine, Division of Endocrinology, Leiden University Medical Center, Leiden, the Netherlands; Email: n.m.appelman-dijkstra@lumc.nl

Educational Objectives

After reviewing this chapter, learners should be able to:

- Develop management plans tailored to the type of calcium disorder and gestational stage.

- Recognize and mitigate potential maternal and fetal complications of calcium disorders.

- Identify and diagnose calcium disorders in pregnant patients based on clinical and laboratory findings.

Significance of the Clinical Problem

Calcium disorders during pregnancy, including hypocalcemia and hypercalcemia, present unique challenges due to their profound implications for both maternal and fetal health. Maternal hypocalcemia can result in neuromuscular irritability, tetany, seizures, and cardiac arrhythmias, posing significant risks to the mother's well-being. In contrast, maternal hypercalcemia is associated with complications, such as nephrolithiasis, pancreatitis, and acute kidney injury, which can exacerbate pregnancy-related physiological stress. For the fetus, disruptions in maternal calcium homeostasis can affect the placenta, causing calcifications and subsequent negative consequences. In addition, maternal hypercalcemia can suppress fetal PTH secretion, potentially leading to neonatal hypocalcemia, tetany, and even seizures shortly after birth. Severe maternal hypocalcemia may impair the transfer of calcium across the placenta, causing hypocalcemia in the fetus.

Pregnancy induces physiological changes, including increased intestinal calcium absorption driven by elevated 1,25-dihydroxyvitamin D levels and altered PTHrP dynamics, which can obscure the presentation of calcium disorders. Mismanagement of these conditions can lead to adverse outcomes, including preterm delivery, fetal growth restriction, and long-term health effects for the neonate. Given these risks, proper identification and management of calcium disorders are important to minimize complications. This highlights the need for improved awareness, tailored diagnostic approaches, and management strategies to address these potentially life-threatening conditions effectively. Citations 1 through 5 provide additional background information and are used as references throughout the whole chapter.

Practice Gaps

- Limited awareness of physiological changes in calcium metabolism during pregnancy among clinicians.

- Variability in the diagnostic thresholds and management strategies for calcium disorders during pregnancy.

- Lack of consensus on the safety and timing of interventions, including the use of calcium supplements, vitamin D analogues, and other calcium-modifying information.

- Underrecognition of the risks and management of fetal and neonatal complications associated with maternal calcium imbalances.

Discussion

Pregnancy induces changes in calcium homeostasis to accommodate the growing fetal demand for calcium, particularly during the third trimester. These changes involve complex physiological adaptations that ensure adequate calcium availability while protecting maternal calcium stores.

One of the primary changes is an increase in intestinal calcium absorption, driven by a rise in circulating levels of 1,25-dihydroxyvitamin D (calcitriol), which may be 2 to 3 times higher than nonpregnant levels. This increase in calcitriol is facilitated by placental production of vitamin D-binding protein and enhanced renal conversion of 25-hydroxyvitamin D to 1,25-dihydroxyvitamin D, mediated by increased activity of the 1α-hydroxylase enzyme. The upregulation of calcitriol enhances calcium absorption in the maternal gastrointestinal tract, allowing the mother to meet the substantial calcium demands of the fetus without excessive reliance on bone resorption.

In addition to enhanced absorption, maternal skeletal calcium mobilization provides a secondary mechanism to supply calcium to the fetus. This is particularly evident in the later stages of pregnancy when fetal bone mineralization rates increase. The placental production of PTHrP plays a key role in this process, promoting bone resorption to release calcium into the maternal circulation. Unlike PTH, PTHrP can achieve this effect without significantly altering maternal serum calcium or phosphate levels, reflecting the finely tuned balance of maternal and fetal calcium needs. Although total serum calcium levels decrease during pregnancy, this is largely due to hemodilution caused by the 30% to 50% increase in maternal plasma volume. However, ionized calcium—the biologically active form of calcium—remains stable and should be measured to assess the calcium levels throughout pregnancy.

Hypocalcemia in Pregnancy

Hypocalcemia in pregnancy is mainly caused by hypoparathyroidism. The clinical presentation of hypocalcemia in pregnancy often includes muscle spasms and cramps or tetany. In more severe cases, patients may experience seizures due to increased neuronal excitability or arrhythmias resulting from altered cardiac conduction.

Management of hypocalcemia in pregnancy depends on its severity and underlying cause. Mild cases can often be addressed with oral calcium and vitamin D supplementation, while severe cases necessitate intravenous calcium replacement to rapidly restore serum calcium levels. Close monitoring of maternal calcium levels and fetal health is essential, as untreated hypocalcemia may lead to complications such as preterm labor, intrauterine growth restriction, or impaired neonatal skeletal development. Collaboration between endocrinologists, obstetricians, and other health care providers is crucial to optimize outcomes for both the mother and fetus.

Hypercalcemia in Pregnancy

Hypercalcemia during pregnancy is a rare but clinically significant condition that can arise from various etiologies, each with distinct implications for maternal and fetal health. The most common cause is primary hyperparathyroidism (PHPT), which is typically due to a parathyroid adenoma or, less commonly, parathyroid hyperplasia. Other potential causes of hypercalcemia include malignancy, such as metastases to bone or paraneoplastic syndromes associated with ectopic PTHrP production. Although rare in pregnancy, these malignancy-associated cases require prompt recognition and intervention. Additionally, excessive calcium or vitamin D supplementation can also result in hypercalcemia. This underscores the importance of cautious dosing and close monitoring of supplementation in pregnant patients.

Hypercalcemia can have serious maternal complications, such as nephrolithiasis, pancreatitis, peptic ulcer disease, hypertension, and fatigue, which can complicate pregnancy management. For the fetus, hypercalcemia poses significant risks, including fetal growth restriction, because altered calcium dynamics can impair normal placental function and nutrient delivery. Furthermore, maternal hypercalcemia suppresses fetal parathyroid gland function, potentially leading to neonatal hypocalcemia after delivery. Neonatal hypocalcemia can manifest as seizures, tetany, or other neuromuscular symptoms that may require urgent intervention.

Management of hypercalcemia during pregnancy depends on the underlying cause and the severity of the condition. Mild hypercalcemia can often be managed conservatively with adequate hydration and dietary adjustments, while severe cases or those due to PHPT may necessitate more aggressive interventions. Parathyroidectomy in the second trimester is considered safe and effective for treating PHPT in selected cases. Cinacalcet might be useful as well, but the safety of the drug during pregnancy is still to be debated. A multidisciplinary approach involving endocrinologists, obstetricians, and neonatologists is crucial in providing comprehensive care.

Diagnosis

Accurate diagnosis of calcium disorders in pregnancy requires careful consideration of physiological changes and a strategic approach to minimize risks to both mother and fetus. Pregnancy induces alterations in calcium metabolism, which must be accounted for when evaluating laboratory and clinical findings.

Due to the hemodilution and hypoalbuminemia commonly seen in pregnancy, total serum calcium levels may appear lower than normal even in the absence of a true calcium imbalance. However, ionized calcium levels are unaffected by changes in albumin and provide a more accurate assessment of calcium status in pregnant patients. If ionized calcium measurement is not available, corrected calcium can be calculated using the serum albumin level, although this is less precise.

Imaging Studies

Imaging may be necessary to evaluate potential causes of calcium imbalances, such as identifying parathyroid adenomas in primary hyperparathyroidism or assessing skeletal pathology. When imaging is required, special precautions should be taken to minimize fetal radiation exposure:

- *Ultrasonography* is the first-line imaging modality for evaluating parathyroid glands or kidneys given its demonstrated safety in pregnancy.

- *MRI* can be considered for more detailed anatomical assessments when necessary, as it does not use ionizing radiation.

- *CT or nuclear imaging* should generally be avoided during pregnancy unless absolutely critical, and radiation exposure should be minimized with appropriate shielding and dosing adjustments.

Additional Considerations

Diagnostic approaches must also include a thorough review of the patient's medical history, including prior diagnoses of calcium disorders, medication use (eg, calcium or vitamin D supplementation), and any symptoms suggestive of systemic conditions, such as malignancy or granulomatous disease. Family history of disorders, such as multiple endocrine neoplasia syndromes or other genetic conditions affecting calcium metabolism, should also be explored.

By using a careful and comprehensive diagnostic strategy, clinicians can accurately identify the etiology of calcium imbalances in pregnancy while ensuring maternal and fetal safety.

Management Principles for Calcium Disorders in Pregnancy

Effective management of calcium disorders during pregnancy requires a balance between maternal safety and fetal well-being. Management strategies should be tailored based on the severity of symptoms, underlying etiology, and gestational age. The following section discusses the key principles for addressing hypocalcemia and hypercalcemia in pregnant patients.

Management of Hypocalcemia

Acute Symptomatic Hypocalcemia

Acute hypocalcemia presenting with tetany, seizures, or cardiac arrhythmias necessitates urgent correction using intravenous calcium gluconate. Typical dosing is 1 to 2 g of calcium gluconate administered slowly over 10 to 20 minutes. Continuous cardiac monitoring is recommended to prevent arrhythmias during administration. The patient's regimen is transitioned to oral therapy once the acute episode is resolved.

Oral calcium supplementation is used as maintenance therapy. The mainstay of treatment is calcium carbonate (1-2 g elemental calcium daily) taken with food to enhance absorption. Active vitamin D analogues, such as calcitriol (0.25-1.0 mcg daily), are used to enhance intestinal calcium absorption and address deficiencies in 1,25-dihydroxyvitamin D production, especially in cases of hypoparathyroidism or kidney dysfunction. Regular assessment of serum calcium, phosphorus, and 24-hour urinary calcium levels is essential to balance effective treatment while avoiding complications, such as hypercalciuria or nephrocalcinosis.

Management of Hypercalcemia

Mild Hypercalcemia

Mild hypercalcemia (serum calcium <12 mg/dL [<3.0 mmol/L]) without significant symptoms can often be managed with hydration and dietary calcium restriction. Adequate hydration helps prevent nephrolithiasis and maintains renal calcium clearance.

Severe or Symptomatic Hypercalcemia

- Intravenous hydration: severe hypercalcemia (serum calcium >14 mg/dL [>3.5 mmol/L]) or symptomatic cases require aggressive hydration with normal saline to enhance renal calcium excretion.

  ○ Initial rate: 200-300 mL/h until rehydration is achieved; adjust to maintain adequate urine output.

- Pharmacological intervention:

  ○ Bisphosphonates: these agents are generally avoided in pregnancy due to potential fetal skeletal effects.

  ○ Cinacalcet: although not approved for the use during pregnancy, there have been reports of cinacalcet use during pregnancy, but the benefits should be considered on an individual basis.

Surgical Management

- If hypercalcemia is caused by a parathyroid adenoma, parathyroidectomy is typically deferred until the second trimester to minimize risks to the fetus. Second-trimester surgery has been shown to have lower rates of miscarriage and preterm labor.

- Maternal calcium levels should be optimized to ensure stable hydration status preoperatively.

General Management Considerations

- Serial measurements of ionized calcium, serum calcium, and relevant biomarkers are crucial during treatment.

- Fetal monitoring may be required in cases of severe maternal calcium imbalance, as both hypocalcemia and hypercalcemia can affect fetal bone mineralization and parathyroid function.

Fetal and Neonatal Considerations

Managing maternal calcium disorders during pregnancy requires careful attention to fetal and neonatal health, as disruptions in maternal calcium homeostasis can have profound effects on the developing fetus and newborn. Routine fetal ultrasonography is critical for assessing fetal growth and development, as maternal calcium imbalances—particularly hypercalcemia—are associated with intrauterine growth restriction.

Close monitoring of fetal skeletal formation is necessary, as both hypocalcemia and hypercalcemia can influence bone mineralization. Severe maternal hypercalcemia may lead to abnormal ossification or delayed bone growth.

Maternal calcium disorders can affect placental health, and close surveillance is warranted to ensure appropriate nutrient and calcium transfer to the fetus.

- Neonatal calcium levels

  - Newborns of mothers with hypercalcemia are at risk for neonatal hypocalcemia, a rebound effect caused by the suppression of fetal PTH production in utero.

  - Early and frequent monitoring of serum calcium levels in the first 48 to 72 hours post delivery is recommended to detect and address hypocalcemia promptly.

- Symptoms of neonatal hypocalcemia

  - Symptoms may include jitteriness, irritability, poor feeding, lethargy, and seizures.

  - Prompt recognition and treatment are critical to prevent complications, such as cardiac arrhythmias or long-term developmental delays.

Preventive Strategies
  - Optimizing maternal calcium and vitamin D status during pregnancy through adequate supplementation and careful monitoring can reduce the risk of neonatal complications.

  - Avoiding excessive maternal calcium or vitamin D supplementation during pregnancy is equally important to prevent fetal parathyroid suppression and subsequent neonatal hypocalcemia.

By addressing both maternal and fetal needs, clinicians can reduce the potential adverse outcomes of calcium disorders during pregnancy and the neonatal period. Coordination among obstetricians, endocrinologists, and neonatologists is essential for comprehensive care.

Clinical Case Vignettes
Case 1

A 35-year-old woman (G3, P1) at 20 weeks' gestation is referred for asymptomatic hypercalcemia detected on routine prenatal laboratory testing. She has no history of kidney stones, fractures, or gastrointestinal symptoms. She does not take calcium or vitamin D supplements. Her first pregnancy was uneventful.

Laboratory test results:

> Total calcium = 11.2 mg/dL (8.5-10.5 mg/dL) (SI: 2.8 mmol/L [2.1-2.6 mmol/L])
> Ionized calcium = 5.9 mg/dL (4.5-5.3 mg/dL) (SI: 1.48 mmol/L [1.12-1.32 mmol/L])
> PTH = 8 pg/mL (15-65 pg/mL) (SI: 0.85 pmol/L [1.59-6.90 pmol/L])
> 25-Hydroxyvitamin D = 42 ng/mL (20-50 ng/mL) (SI: 104.8 nmol/L [49.9-124.8 nmol/L])
> 1,25-Dihydroxyvitamin D = 80 pg/mL (30-80 pg/mL) (SI: 208 pmol/L [78-208 pmol/L])
> Creatinine = 0.7 mg/dL (SI: 61.9 μmol/L)
> Phosphorus = 2.6 mg/dL (2.5-4.5 mg/dL) (SI: 0.84 mmol/L [0.81-1.45 mmol/L])

Neck ultrasonography shows no parathyroid adenoma. A family history of hypercalcemia is noted, although no family member has had surgery to address it.

Which of the following is this patient's most likely diagnosis?

A. Primary hyperparathyroidism

B. Familial hypocalciuric hypercalcemia

C. Hypercalcemia of malignancy

D. Vitamin D intoxication

Answer: B) Familial hypocalciuric hypercalcemia

Hypercalcemia in pregnancy has a broad differential diagnosis, but misdiagnosis can lead to inappropriate management, such as unnecessary surgery. The key pitfall is assuming all hypercalcemia in pregnancy is due to PHPT, while familial hypocalciuric hypercalcemia (FHH) is an important alternative diagnosis. This pregnant patient has a low PTH concentration (not suppressed but inappropriately normal), a family history of hypercalcemia, and mild hypercalcemia with no classic PHPT symptoms. Pregnancy can unmask FHH due to increased calcium absorption. FHH is caused by pathogenic variants in the gene encoding the calcium-sensing receptor (*CASR*), leading to a higher set point for calcium homeostasis. The key test to distinguish FHH from PHPT is measuring calcium in a 24-hour urine collection. FHH shows low urinary calcium excretion (calcium-to-creatinine clearance ratio <0.01), whereas PHPT has normal or high urinary calcium excretion. However, these results can be blunted in pregnancy and in such cases genetic testing often holds the key to diagnosis.

Case 2

A 32-year-old woman (G2, P1) at 18 weeks' gestation is referred for evaluation of hypercalcemia. She reports fatigue, mild nausea, and intermittent constipation but has no polyuria or nephrolithiasis. There is no family history of endocrine disorders.

Laboratory test results:

Calcium = 11.5 mg/dL (8.5-10.5 mg/dL)
(SI: 2.9 mmol/L [2.1-2.6 mmol/L])
Ionized calcium = 6.0 mg/dL (4.5-5.3 mg/dL)
(SI: 1.5 mmol/L [1.12-1.32 mmol/L])
PTH = 95 pg/mL (15-65 pg/mL) (SI: 10.1 pmol/L
[1.6-6.9 pmol/L])
25-Hydroxyvitamin D = 30 ng/mL (20-50 ng/mL)
(SI: 74.9 nmol/L [49.9-124.8 nmol/L])
Creatinine = 0.7 mg/dL (SI: 61.9 μmol/L)

Neck ultrasonography identifies a 1.8-cm hypoechoic lesion posterior to the right thyroid lobe. A review of previous records shows persistent hypercalcemia for at least 2 years, although she was asymptomatic before pregnancy. The patient is concerned about maternal and fetal risks.

Which of the following is the most appropriate next step in this patient's management?

A. Encourage hydration and monitor calcium levels, deferring surgery until after delivery

B. Proceed with parathyroidectomy in the second trimester

C. Start cinacalcet to control hypercalcemia

D. Initiate bisphosphonate therapy to lower calcium

Answer: B) Proceed with parathyroidectomy in the second trimester

PHPT is the most common cause of hypercalcemia in pregnancy. Untreated maternal hypercalcemia increases the risk of complications, including nephrolithiasis, pancreatitis, hypertension, and preeclampsia, as well as neonatal hypocalcemia and tetany due to fetal suppression of parathyroid function. Parathyroidectomy (Answer B) is the only curative treatment for PHPT, and it eliminates the risks associated with prolonged maternal hypercalcemia. The second trimester is the safest period for surgery, minimizing risks of both fetal loss (higher in the first trimester) and preterm labor (higher in the third trimester). Studies show improved pregnancy outcomes with parathyroidectomy compared with outcomes associated with conservative management. Conservative management is considered if hypercalcemia is mild and asymptomatic, but given this patient's persistent hypercalcemia and symptoms, deferring surgery would increase maternal and fetal risks. Calcimimetics are not recommended in pregnancy due to insufficient safety data, and bisphosphonates are contraindicated in pregnancy because they cross the placenta and can impair fetal bone development. Thus, parathyroidectomy in the second trimester is the preferred treatment to optimize maternal and fetal outcomes.

Case 3

A 29-year-old woman (G1, P0) at 14 weeks' gestation presents for evaluation of muscle cramps, perioral tingling, and fatigue. She underwent total thyroidectomy for papillary thyroid carcinoma 2 years ago but was lost to follow-up. She is taking levothyroxine but no other medications.

Laboratory test results:

> Calcium = 7.1 mg/dL (8.5-10.5 mg/dL)
>   (SI: 1.8 mmol/L [2.1-2.6 mmol/L])
> Ionized calcium = 3.6 mg/dL (4.5-5.3 mg/dL)
>   (SI: 0.9 mmol/L [1.12-1.32 mmol/L])
> Phosphorus = 5.5 mg/dL (2.5-4.5 mg/dL)
>   (SI: 1.78 mmol/L [0.81-1.45 mmol/L])
> PTH = <5 pg/mL (15-65 pg/mL) (SI: <0.5 pmol/L
>   [1.6-6.9 pmol/L])
> 25-Hydroxyvitamin D = 32 ng/mL (20-50 ng/mL)
>   (SI: 79.9 nmol/L [49.9-124.8 nmol/L])
> Creatinine = 0.6 mg/dL (SI: 53.0 μmol/L)

The patient is diagnosed with postsurgical hypoparathyroidism with symptomatic hypocalcemia.

Which of the following is the most appropriate treatment approach for this patient during pregnancy?

A. Intravenous calcium gluconate and high-dosage vitamin D analogues

B. Calcium supplementation with calcitriol to maintain calcium in the lower normal range

C. Teriparatide (PTH analogue) for long-term management

D. No treatment is necessary, as pregnancy increases calcium absorption naturally

Answer: B) Calcium supplementation with calcitriol to maintain calcium in the lower normal range

Hypoparathyroidism during pregnancy requires careful calcium and vitamin D management to avoid maternal and fetal complications. Pregnancy increases intestinal calcium absorption due to placental production of 1,25-dihydroxyvitamin D, but PTH is still essential for calcium homeostasis. The goal is to maintain calcium in the low-normal range (8.0-8.5 mg/dL [2.0-2.1 mmol/L]) to avoid both maternal symptoms and fetal hypercalcemia, which can suppress neonatal parathyroid function. Drugs that can be initiated are active vitamin D metabolites and oral calcium supplements. Intravenous calcium and high-dosage vitamin D are used for severe or symptomatic hypocalcemia, but they are not needed for long-term management. PTH analogues are not approved for use in pregnancy due to unknown fetal effects. Thus, oral calcium and calcitriol are the standard treatment for hypoparathyroidism during pregnancy, ensuring both maternal and fetal safety.

Key Learning Points

- Pregnancy induces physiological adaptations in calcium metabolism that can mask or exacerbate underlying disorders.

- Maternal calcium disorders require a multidisciplinary approach, involving obstetrics, endocrinology, and neonatology.

- Tailored management based on gestational age and severity of the disorder is critical for optimizing outcomes.

- Close monitoring of fetal growth and neonatal calcium levels is essential to prevent long-term complications.

References

1. Kovacs CS. Maternal mineral and bone metabolism during pregnancy, lactation, and post-weaning recovery. *Physiol Rev.* 2016;96(2):449-547. PMID: 29053801

2. Kovacs CS, Ralston SH. Physiology and pathophysiology of bone turnover during pregnancy, lactation, and post-weaning recovery. *Endocr Rev.* 2023;44(1):1-34. PMID: 36546344

3. Eastell R, et al. Management of endocrine disease: bone and mineral metabolism in pregnancy and lactation. *Eur J Endocrinol.* 2022;186(1):R1-R13. PMID: 34863037

4. Appelman-Dijkstra NM, Pilz S. Approach to the patient: management of parathyroid diseases across pregnancy. *J Clin Endocrinol Metab.* 2023;108(6):1505-1513. PMID: 36546344

5. Bollerslev J, Rejnmark L, Zahn A, et al; 2021 PARAT Working Group. European expert consensus on practical management of specific aspects of parathyroid disorders in adults and in pregnancy: recommendations of the ESE Educational Program of Parathyroid Disorders. *Eur J Endocrinol.* 2022;186(2):R33-R63. PMID: 34863037

Long-Term Complications of Mild Asymptomatic Primary Hyperparathyroidism: To Treat or Not to Treat?

Ghada El-Hajj Fuleihan, MD, MPH. Calcium Metabolism and Osteoporosis Program, American University of Beirut, Beirut, Lebanon; Email: gf01@aub.edu.lb

Educational Objectives

After reviewing this chapter, learners should be able to:

- Define primary hyperparathyroidism (PHPT) and distinguish its phenotypes: symptomatic, asymptomatic (with end-organ damage), and normocalcemic.

- Describe the long-term complications of asymptomatic PHPT.

- Articulate a management plan for asymptomatic PHPT.

Significance of the Clinical Problem

This Meet the Professor session capitalizes on work and proceedings from the Fifth International Workshop on PHPT. The work was led by 4 task forces comprising 50 international experts and was published in a dedicated supplement in the *Journal of Bone and Mineral Research* in the November 2022 issue. The supplement provides a comprehensive update and clinical recommendations on the evaluation and management of this disease, based on GRADE methodology.[1,2] It consists of 7 manuscripts, including a summary statement, a manuscript describing methodology, several narrative reviews, systematic reviews, and meta-analyses that constitute the basis for the guidelines.[3-9]

PHPT is a common disease of mineral metabolism, only second in frequency to osteoporosis. It is most commonly a disease of postmenopausal women. Its prevalence and incidence vary widely globally.[5] In North America and Western Europe, PHPT mostly presents as an asymptomatic disease due to the wide availability of serum calcium measurement on automated chemistry analyzers. However, even asymptomatic PHPT can incur end-organ damage, manifesting as a decrease in bone density or quality, fractures, kidney stones, or nephrocalcinosis, in 20% to 50% of affected individuals.[6] In many countries of the developing world, PHPT is still mostly a symptomatic (>80%) and severe disease ("bones, stones and moans") due to a lack of routine serum biochemical screening.

Practice Gaps

The shift in the presentation of PHPT from a predominantly symptomatic condition to an asymptomatic and mild disease in western populations has presented several challenges. Subclinical nephrolithiasis and vertebral fractures are common in patients with mild and asymptomatic disease, but they can be missed unless searched for. Normocalcemic PHPT (NPHPT) is often diagnosed without the fulfillment of rigorous criteria. While observational and cross-sectional studies continue to show associations between PHPT and cardiovascular and neuropsychological abnormalities, their causal relationship is uncertain. Limited new data are available on the natural history of skeletal, renal, cardiovascular, neuropsychological, neuromuscular manifestations, and quality of life. Randomized controlled clinical trials have not demonstrated a consistent long-term benefit of parathyroidectomy vs observation on nonclassic manifestations. Knowledge and management gaps arise because of the heterogeneity of participants with PHPT reported in western cohort studies and in randomized clinical trials and the lack of clear phenotype identification in published series.

- The natural history of the various phenotypes of asymptomatic PHPT is unclear.
- The beneficial effects of interventions in the various subgroups of PHPT remain unclear.

Discussion
Definition of PHPT

Hypercalcemic PHPT: an elevated serum calcium level adjusted for albumin in the presence of an elevated or inappropriately normal intact PTH level (using either a second- or third-generation assay) on 2 occasions at least 2 weeks apart. Familial hypercalcemic hypocalciuria is the most common condition in the differential diagnosis of hypercalcemic PHPT.

NPHPT: normal adjusted total calcium and normal ionized calcium levels along with elevated intact PTH level (using either a second- or third-generation assay) on at least 2 occasions over 3 to 6 months after all alternative causes for secondary hyperparathyroidism have been ruled out. Secondary causes include a serum 25-hydroxyvitamin D value less than 30 ng/mL (<75 nmol/L), chronic kidney disease (eGFR <60 mL/min/1.73 m²), renal calcium loss (idiopathic hypercalciuria, and loop diuretics), and diseases of the gastrointestinal tract known to

affect calcium absorption, medications (denosumab, bisphosphonates, anticonvulsants, lithium, phosphorus).[5,6]

Clinical Phenotypes of PHPT

Symptomatic PHPT: associated with marked hypercalcemia (moderate or severe) or overt (clinically detected) skeletal and kidney complications that may include osteitis fibrosa cystica and/or fractures, chronic kidney disease, nephrolithiasis, and/or nephrocalcinosis.

Asymptomatic PHPT: no overt symptoms or signs on presentation; typically discovered by biochemical screening. Two forms of asymptomatic PHPT are defined after evaluation of the skeleton and kidneys:

- With target-organ involvement discovered upon performing the recommended radiologic procedures (eg, x-ray of the thoracolumbar spine [detecting asymptomatic fractures] or ultrasonography of the kidneys [detecting asymptomatic nephrolithiasis or nephrocalcinosis])
- Without target-organ involvement

NPHPT: may be symptomatic or asymptomatic, with/without target organ involvement.

Classic and Nonclassic Target Organs in PHPT and Disease Complications

Symptomatology may be related to disease chronicity and development of end-organ damage, severity of the serum calcium elevation, or the rapidity with which it is increased. Mild hypercalcemia usually implies an albumin-adjusted serum calcium value less than 1 mg/dL (<0.25 mmol/L) above upper normal limit (ie, <11.4 mg/dL [<2.85 mmol/L]) for most laboratories. Moderate hypercalcemia indicates an albumin-adjusted serum calcium value of 11.4 to 14.0 mg/dL (2.85-3.50 mmol/L), and severe hypercalcemia indicates an albumin-adjusted serum calcium value greater than 14 mg/dL (>3.5 mmol/L).

Disease causality has been clearly established only for biochemical abnormalities and for skeletal and kidney manifestations, namely manifestations that are reversible with parathyroidectomy (*Figure*).[6] The *Table* (*following page*) details PTH effects on cell targets, resulting pathophysiological changes, and clinical implications.

Management Plan for Asymptomatic PHPT, Including Surgical Indications

Unless surgery is contraindicated, parathyroidectomy is the recommended management for symptomatic patients, who by definition (for the most part) have end-organ involvement. The same approach applies to the clinical phenotype of asymptomatic patients with evidence of target-organ involvement. This is based on evidence of reversal of biochemical abnormalities, kidney, and bone complications (improvement in bone mineral density) after parathyroidectomy in both conditions.[4] The data become scarcer in asymptomatic patients with mild PHPT who have no evidence of target-organ involvement.

A thorough clinical evaluation of patients with confirmed PHPT is instrumental in guiding disease management. Evaluation includes a detailed family history of hypercalcemia, a careful clinical history to assess symptoms, review of laboratory findings (including multiple serum calcium levels over years before presentation and of intake of

Figure. Symptoms and Organ Involvement in Patients With PHPT

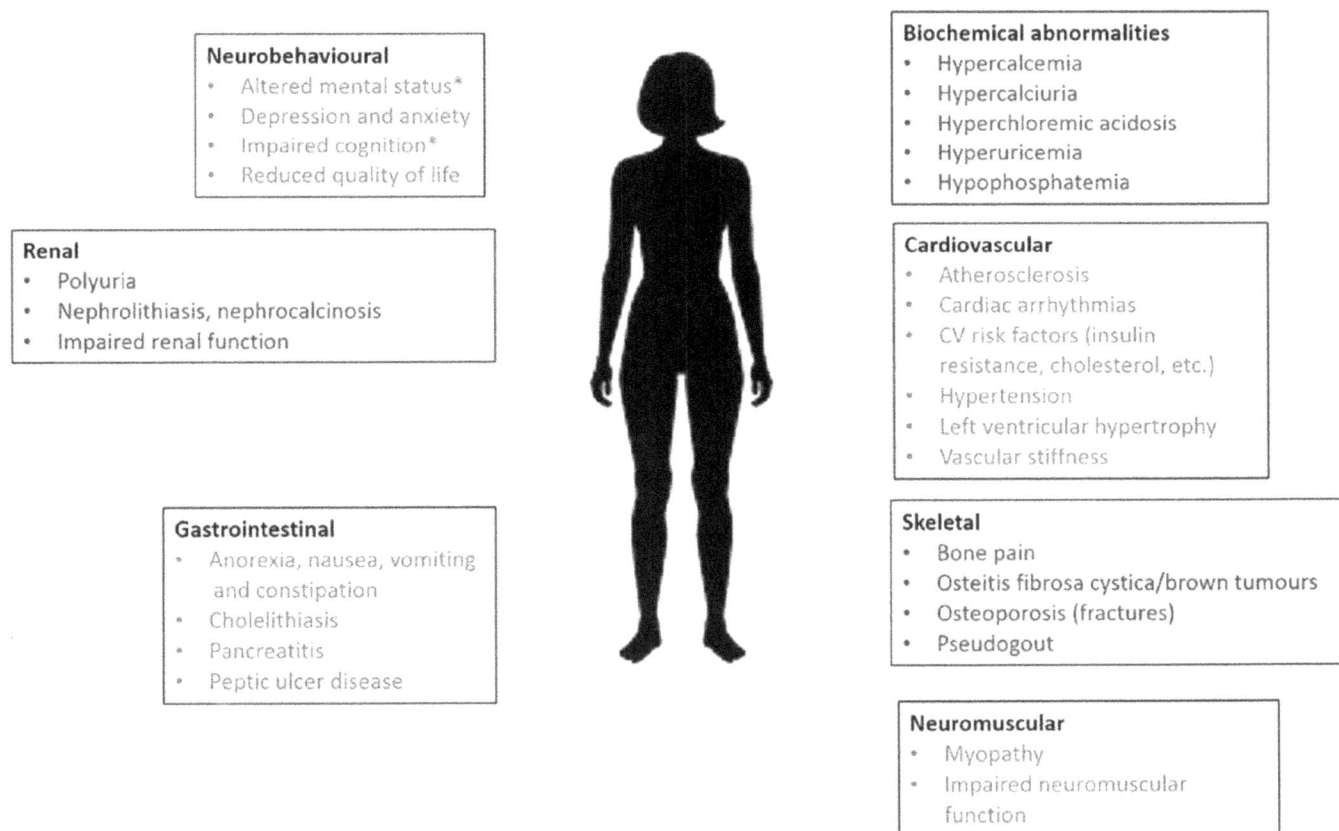

Neurobehavioural
- Altered mental status*
- Depression and anxiety
- Impaired cognition*
- Reduced quality of life

Renal
- Polyuria
- Nephrolithiasis, nephrocalcinosis
- Impaired renal function

Gastrointestinal
- Anorexia, nausea, vomiting and constipation
- Cholelithiasis
- Pancreatitis
- Peptic ulcer disease

Biochemical abnormalities
- Hypercalcemia
- Hypercalciuria
- Hyperchloremic acidosis
- Hyperuricemia
- Hypophosphatemia

Cardiovascular
- Atherosclerosis
- Cardiac arrhythmias
- CV risk factors (insulin resistance, cholesterol, etc.)
- Hypertension
- Left ventricular hypertrophy
- Vascular stiffness

Skeletal
- Bone pain
- Osteitis fibrosa cystica/brown tumours
- Osteoporosis (fractures)
- Pseudogout

Neuromuscular
- Myopathy
- Impaired neuromuscular function

Symptoms and complications depend on disease severity. Causality is implied from evidence by reversal with surgery or from mechanistic studies. Causal in is red, and association in green.

*Moderate to severe hypercalcemia may cause changes in mental status or cognitive function that are often reversible with correction of the serum calcium.

Reprinted from El-Hajj Fuleihan G et al. J Bone Miner Res, 2022; 37(11): 2330-2350. © The Authors. Published by Wiley Periodicals LLC on behalf of American Society for Bone and Mineral Research

[Color—Print (Color Gallery page CG8) or web & ePub editions]

medications that may affect PTH dynamics), thorough screening for target-organ involvement, and the request of additional laboratory studies (*Box, following page*).[4]

In patients with asymptomatic PHPT, the panel recommends surgery to cure the disease (strong recommendation/high-quality evidence, GRADE 1A). The panel states: "Although parathyroidectomy is an option for all patients, with concurrence of the patient and the physician and if there are no contraindications, the panel recommends surgery in all those in whom one or more of the following is present (including those who are asymptomatic, 4)." The conditions are listed in the right column of the *Box* (*following page*). Surgery cannot be recommended to improve neurocognitive function, quality of life, and/or cardiovascular indices because the evidence is inconclusive."[4] Because of limited data in NPHPT, the panel of experts could not recommend surgery.[4-6] In practice, parathyroidectomy is, however, performed in patients with NPHPT if evidence of end-organ damage is present. Preoperative localization is less successful in normocalcemic disease than in hypercalcemic disease due to hyperplasia. Surgery should always be performed by an experienced parathyroid surgeon.

Preoperative localization is not recommended for diagnostic purposes, but it is recommended for those who are going to have parathyroid surgery. Available modalities include ultrasonography, sestamibi scintigraphy, including SPECT-CT, parathyroid 4-dimensional CT, and MRI. PET-CT

Table. Effects of PTH on Classic and Nonclassic Target Organs and Ultimate Effects on Clinical Manifestations

Target organ	PTH cell target	PTH-regulated function	Pathophysiologic changes	Clinical implications
Kidney	Distal tubule Proximal and distal tubules Distal tubule Proximal tubule	Calcium reabsorption Phosphate reabsorption Bicarbonate reabsorption 1α-Hydroxylase	Hypercalcemia (with contributions from gut and bone) Hypophosphatemia Hyperchloremic acidosis Hypercalciuria (indirectly)	Hypercalcemic syndrome of increased mortality Fatigue/muscle weakness Nephrocalcinosis Kidney stones
Gut	Proximal and distal intestine	Indirect through 1,25-dihydroxyvitamin D-dependent increased calcium intestinal absorption	Hypercalciuria	Kidney stones
Bone	Osteoblast	Bone turnover	High bone turnover Bone loss	Fracture
Cardiovascular system	Cardiomyocyte Cardiac valves Smooth muscle cells	Hypercalcemia-dependent Interaction with RAAS Hypercalcemia-dependent vasodilatation Interaction with RAAS	Arrythmias Left ventricular hypertrophy Heart failure Soft-tissue calcification Decreased blood pressure Hypertension*	Possible increase in mortality Heart failure Decreased blood pressure Hypertension
Central nervous system	Axons	Hypercalcemia Cross-reactivity with PTH2R	Apoptosis* Stress response, anxiety*	
Skeletal/muscle	Myotube		Muscle weakness	
Dermis	Fibroblasts/hair follicles	Possible role in hair growth/differentiation	None known in nongenetic forms of PHPT	No known

* Possible PTH effect.

Reprinted from Minisola S et al. *J Bone Miner Res*, 2022; 37(11): 2315-29. © The Authors. Published by Wiley Periodicals LLC on behalf of American Society for Bone and Mineral Research.

Box. Evaluation of Patients With PHPT and Indications for Parathyroidectomy

How should patients with PHPT be evaluated?	For which patients is parathyroidectomy an option?
1. *Biochemical:* Measure adjusted total serum calcium (ionized if NPHPT is a consideration), phosphorus, intact PTH, 25-hydroxyvitamin D, creatinine; bone turnover may be added	1. *Serum calcium >1 mg/dL (>0.25 mmol/L) above the upper normal limit* **or**
2. *Skeletal:* Three-site DXA (lumbar spine, hip, distal one-third radius); imaging for vertebral fractures (vertebral fracture assessment or vertebral x-rays); trabecular bone score if available	2. *Skeletal involvement:* fracture by vertebral fracture assessment or vertebral x-ray or bone mineral density by T-score ≤ −2.5 at any site **or**
3. *Kidneys:* Estimated glomerular filtration rate or preferably, creatinine clearance, 24-hour urinary calcium and for biochemical risk factors for stones; imaging for nephrolithiasis/nephrocalcinosis	3. *Kidney involvement:* estimated glomerular filtration rate or creatinine clearance <60 mL/min; nephrocalcinosis or nephrolithiasis by x-ray, ultrasonography, or other imaging modality; hypercalciuria (eg, >250 mg/24 h in women; >300 mg/24 h in men) **or**
4. *Nonclassic manifestations* (neurocognitive, quality of life, cardiovascular): there are no data to support routine evaluation for these putative manifestations	4. *Age <50 years* (no other indications are necessary; age <50 years is a sufficient indication)
5. *Genetic:* genetic evaluation should be considered for patients younger than 30 years, those with multigland disease by history or imaging, and/or those with a family history of hypercalcemia and/or a syndromic disease	

Reprinted from Bilezikian JP et al. J Bone Miner Res, 2022; 37(11): 2293-314. © The Authors. Published by Wiley Periodicals LLC on behalf of American Society for Bone and Mineral Research.

with choline and methionine is used in Europe, but it is considered research methodology in the United States. There is no consensus on the best imaging protocol. It depends on institutional availability, radiologist expertise, the preference of the surgeon, and cost. The positive predictive values, on average, are lowest for ultrasonography (76%). Positive predictive values for sestamibi SPECT and 4-dimensional CT are 80% and 90%, respectively. For all modalities, localization is less accurate for multiglandular disease than for solitary adenomas: "The most important pre-op localization challenge in primary hyperparathyroidism is to localize the parathyroid surgeon," stated the late Dr. John Dopman, an interventional radiologist at the National Institutes of Health in 1975.

Medical Management and Monitoring

There may be instances where parathyroid surgery is not necessarily an option, such as when guidelines are not met, patients opt for nonsurgical management, there is a history of previous neck surgery (or surgeries), thus rendering surgery problematic, or there are coexisting medical issues.

The natural history of mild hyperparathyroidism over 15 years has been assessed in a cohort study.[10]

There was a very minimal increase in serum calcium over time, and PTH levels and urinary calcium levels remained stable, as did 25-hydroxyvitamin D and 1,25-dihydroxyvitamin D$_2$ levels. Bone density decreased in some patients after 10 years, especially at cortical sites. Thirty-seven percent of the cohort developed 1 or more indications for surgery during the 15 years of follow-up, including hypercalcemia, hypercalciuria, or reduced bone mineral density.[10] Despite the scare evidence at the time, parathyroidectomy was a valid consideration in view of the long-term complications of mild asymptomatic PHPT.[11]

In those who are not going to have parathyroid surgery, pharmacologic options can be considered to reduce serum calcium or to increase bone density (as a surrogate for fracture risk reduction in general). US FDA indications for a calcimimetic agent, such as cinacalcet, for PHPT include control of advanced disease, namely a serum calcium concentration greater than 1 mg/dL (>0.25 mmol/L) above the upper normal limit, in case parathyroidectomy is not indicated or the patient declines surgery.

The expert panel developed recommendations from systematic and narrative reviews regarding nutritional and pharmacologic interventions.[4]

- Calcium intake/supplementation: as per Institute of Medicine guidelines 1000 to 1200 mg of calcium daily

- Vitamin D supplementation: aim for a serum 25-hydroxyvitamin D concentration ≥30 ng/mL (≥75 nmol/L)

- Cinacalcet is useful to reduce the serum calcium level

- Effective options to increase bone density are alendronate or denosumab

- A combination of cinacalcet with a bisphosphonate or denosumab,[4] to reduce serum calcium and increase bone density

Monitoring for patients who do not undergo parathyroidectomy should include serum calcium and 25-hydroxyvitamin vitamin D measurement annually, skeletal visualization with 3-site DXA every 1 to 2 years, vertebral x-ray, vertebral fracture assessment or trabecular bone score if clinically indicated, creatinine clearance annually, abdominal imaging if clinically indicated, and 24-hour urinary calcium excretion if clinically indicated. In normocalcemic or hypercalcemic patients with PHPT monitored medically, parathyroid surgery should be recommended if the serum calcium concentration is consistently 1 mg/dL (>0.25 mmol/L) above the upper normal limit or if the patient develops a low-trauma fracture, a kidney stone, a significant reduction in bone mineral density exceeding the least significant change at any site, or a significant reduction in creatinine clearance (averaging more than 3 mL per minute over 1 to 2 years, if associated with other changes that indicate deterioration).

Clinical Case Vignettes

Case 1

A 52-year-old woman presents for evaluation of a high serum calcium concentration picked up on routine laboratory testing by her primary care physician. She is asymptomatic except for mild fatigue. She underwent menopause 2 years ago and has tolerable hot flashes. She has no polyuria,

no dry mouth, and no cognitive dysfunction. She has had no loss of height and no fractures or kidney stones. She has never been on lithium or thiazides. There is no known family history of hypercalcemia. Dietary calcium intake is approximately 500 mg elemental calcium daily. She exercises by walking twice weekly and swimming twice weekly. Her medical history is positive for essential hyperlipidemia that worsened slightly after menopause. She takes no medications except for calcium, 500 mg daily, and vitamin D, 800 IU daily (20 mcg daily).

Physical examination findings are normal, and there is no kyphosis.

Laboratory test results:

> Serum calcium = 10.8 mg/dL (8.5-10.2 mg/dL) (SI: 2.7 mmol/L [2.15-2.55 mmol/L])
> Phosphate = 3.8 mg/dL (SI: 1.2 mmol/L)
> Creatinine = 0.9 mg/dL (SI: 79.6 μmol/L)
> Albumin = 4.2 mg/dL (SI: 42 g/L)

Which of the following assessments are needed now?

A. Serum PTHrP and calcitriol measurement

B. Genetic testing for familial hypocalciuric hypercalcemia

C. Calcium/creatinine clearance ratio and PTH measurement

D. Review of documented calcium levels over the last few years

Answer: C) Calcium/creatinine clearance ratio and PTH measurement and D) Review of documented calcium levels over the last few years

This patient is unlikely to have a malignancy in view of her lack of symptoms and mild hypercalcemia. Vitamin D intoxication from active forms or from tumors secreting calcitriol (benign or malignant) are less likely. There is no suspicion for familial hypocalciuric hypercalcemia, as affected patients are usually younger. Genetic tests are expensive and are not warranted for this patient yet. The next step is confirmation of elevated serum calcium along with a concomitant measurement of PTH and 24-hour urinary calcium and creatinine excretion to calculate the calcium/creatinine clearance ratio. It is always helpful to review old laboratory values to assess the onset and duration of hypercalcemia. Calcium is expected to be slightly lower, on average, before menopause than after menopause, due to estrogen's masking of the bone resorptive effect of PTH.

Case 1, Continued

Laboratory test results:

> Repeated calcium =10.9 mg/dL (SI: 2.8 mmol/L)
> PTH = 76 pg/mL (15-76 pg/mL) (SI: 8.1 pmol/L [1.6-8.1 pmol/L])
> Creatinine = 0.9 mg/dL (SI: 79.6 μmol/L)
> Urinary calcium = 300 mg/24 h (SI: 7.5 mmol/d)
> Urinary creatinine = 900 mg/24 h

What are the indicated tests at this point?

A. Obtain labs on the patient's parents, siblings, and children

B. Determine bone mineral density of the spine, hip, and forearm and trabecular bone score and obtain vertebral fracture assessment or lateral spine films

C. Perform kidney ultrasonography

D. Order genetic testing for familial hypocalciuric hypercalcemia

E. A, B, and C

Answer: E) A, B, and C

PHPT is more common than familial hypocalciuric hypercalcemia, although the prevalence of the latter has been shown to be higher than expected as evidenced by examination of large repositories.[5] While PHPT can incur end-organ damage to the skeleton and kidney, familial hypocalciuric hypercalcemia is a benign condition, with no deleterious effects on these organ systems. It is inherited in an autosomal dominant pattern, and review of laboratory values of first-degree relatives is important. The calcium/creatinine clearance ratio may be useful to distinguish PHPT from familial hypocalciuric hypercalcemia. A ratio greater than 0.02 is more likely to be present in individuals with PHPT, while it is less than 0.01 in individuals with familial hypocalciuric hypercalcemia. However, values between 0.01 and 0.02 can be found in 30% to 40% of individuals with either condition.

This patient's calcium/creatinine clearance ratio is 0.027, and her family members (parents, 4 siblings, and 2 children) all have calcium concentrations below 10 mg/dL (<2.5 mmol/L). DXA shows osteopenia, spine T-score of −2.0, hip T-score of −1.2, and forearm T-score of −1.2. Her FRAX is below the country-specific threshold, and the trabecular bone score is 1.30. Vertebral fracture assessment is negative for compression fractures, and kidney ultrasonography is negative for nephrocalcinosis and kidney stones.

In summary, this patient has had elevated calcium on 2 occasions, inappropriately normal PTH (upper normal limit), high 24-hour urinary calcium excretion and calcium/creatinine clearance ratio, negative family history, and normal serum calcium levels in first-degree relatives. The patient has PHPT. The diagnosis can be further confirmed with genetic testing, but this is not needed at this point.

Case 1, Continued

After an informed discussion on benefits and risks of surgery and a discussion of alternative treatment options, the patient is referred for surgery.

Which criterion does the patient fulfill for consideration of surgical intervention?

A. Osteopenia

B. Elevated 24-hour urinary calcium excretion

C. Low trabecular bone score

D. None of the above

Answer: B) Elevated 24-hour urinary calcium excretion

The indications for parathyroidectomy are listed in the right column of the *Box*. The one that applies to the patient is high urinary calcium excretion (Answer B). Biological age matters more than chronological age, so the age cutoff is not absolute.

Case 2

A 30-year-old woman with bipolar disorder is self-referred for evaluation of hypercalcemia. She feels well and has no concerns or physical ailments. She has no gastrointestinal symptoms and no history of fractures or kidney stones. Review of systems is otherwise negative. Her family history is negative for hypercalcemia or endocrine disorders. She has taken lithium, 300 mg twice daily, for 10 years.

Laboratory test results:

> Serum calcium = 11 mg/dL (8.5-10.2 mg/dL) (SI: 2.75 mmol/L [2.15-2.55 mmol/L]) (review of her yearly labs reveals her serum calcium has been slowly rising over the last 10 years)
> Creatinine, normal
> Albumin, normal
> PTH = 120 pg/mL (15-76 pg/mL) (SI: 12.7 pmol/L [1.6-8.1 pmol/L])
> Serum calcium = 10.9 mg/dL (SI: 2.7 mmol/L)
> Albumin, normal

Review of laboratory studies of her family members reveals no hypercalcemia.

Which of the following is the most likely etiology of her hypercalcemia?

A. Familial hyperparathyroidism

B. Secondary hyperparathyroidism

C. Lithium-induced hypercalcemia and PHPT

D. Lithium-induced hypercalcemia independent of PTH

Answer: C) Lithium-induced hypercalcemia and PHPT

This patient may have sporadic or familial PHPT, although these scenarios are less likely in view of her young age (unlikely to be sporadic) and the negative family history PHPT (unlikely to be familial), and laboratory studies of family members did not detect hypercalcemia. Her rise in calcium is gradual and coincides with the start of lithium therapy. The patient may have thus developed de novo PHPT from long-term lithium intake, which decreased the sensitivity of the calcium-sensing receptor to calcium and gradually shifted the PTH-calcium set point to the right until parathyroid autonomy was clinically detectable through her biochemical abnormalities.

Case 2, Continued

At this point, what is the best advice for this patient?

A. Discontinue lithium now

B. Immediately consult a surgeon for parathyroidectomy

C. Consult her psychiatrist for tapering of lithium and switching to alternative therapy

D. Do nothing and monitor calcium and PTH every year

Answer: C) Consult her psychiatrist for tapering of lithium and switching to alternative therapy

Lithium increases serum total and ionized calcium and intact PTH levels within weeks, but these remain within the normal range in most individuals.[12] In a study of lithium-treated women (mean age, 40 years) followed up for 5 years, the mean baseline ionized calcium was lower and intact PTH levels were higher in the lithium-treated group than in the control group, although they were still within the normal range.[13] Lithium seems to affect the signal transduction pathway for calcium sensing by interfering with the calcium-sensing receptor at the level of parathyroid and kidney. Parathyroid autonomy, with both adenomas and 4-gland hyperplasia, has been described in this condition. It is therefore possible that lithium unmasks adenomas in patients with preexisting parathyroid lesions within a few years of starting therapy or induces parathyroid hyperplasia with more long-term therapy. If lithium therapy is short term and can be tapered and stopped without exacerbating the psychiatric condition, hypercalcemia may resolve. Long-term lithium therapy may have other adverse consequences, such as hypothyroidism, nephrogenic diabetes insipidus, and kidney failure. The effect on the skeleton is unclear. This patient was asked to see her psychiatrist to try to find an alternative treatment to lithium monitor calcium and PTH levels. In such a scenario, if normalization does not occur within a few months, consideration of parathyroidectomy with a neck exploration approach is reasonable considering the patient's age.

Case 3

A 60-year-old woman with dyslipidemia, hypertension, and osteoporosis is referred after her primary care physician felt a nodule in her thyroid gland. Neck ultrasonography performed at an outside hospital shows a 7 × 9 × 8-mm posteroinferior left thyroid lobe nodule, consistent with parathyroid adenoma. Menopause was at age 56 years, and she has never had a fracture. She has had no kidney stones. Her family history is negative for hypercalcemia.

Medications are candesartan, nebivolol, pravastatin, and magnesium.

On physical examination, her height is 65.0 in (165 cm) and weight is 143.3 lb (65 kg) (BMI = 23.8 kg/m²). Blood pressure is 120/80 mm Hg. Bone mineral density assessed (at an outside facility) September 2024 is as follows:

    Spine T-score = −2.0
    Hip T-score = −1.0
    Forearm T-score = −0.8

The patient has started alendronate, 70 mg once weekly, and vitamin D, 10,000 units once weekly. The patient's laboratory data are shown in the *Table*.

On sestamibi scan, subtraction images show abnormal focal uptake in the left neck projecting over the left lower thyroid pole, which is suspicious for an active left inferior parathyroid adenoma.

Which of the following is the most likely diagnosis?

A. PHPT

B. Secondary hyperparathyroidism

C. NPHPT

D. B and C

Answer: D) B and C

PHPT is a condition characterized by an elevated albumin-adjusted serum calcium level with an elevated PTH level (using second- or third-generation assays), documented on 2 occasions at least 2 weeks apart.[2] Secondary hyperparathyroidism is a condition characterized by an appropriate physiologic response of elevated PTH level to an initial hypocalcemic stimulus, such as what occurs in the setup of a malabsorptive syndrome, hypercalciuria, or kidney failure, in an

Analyte	Sept 2024 Outside lab	Sept 2024 Your lab	Jan 2025 Outside lab	Feb 2025 Your lab
Calcium (lab reference range: 8.5-10.5 mg/dL)	9.7 mg/dL		9.5 mg/dL	9.8 mg/dL
Phosphate	3.8 mg/dL		3.2 mg/dL	
PTH	73 pg/mL (lab reference range: 15-65 pg/mL)	40 pg/mL (second-generation) (lab reference range: 15-76 pg/mL)	80 pg/mL (lab reference range: 9-47 pg/mL)	40.7 pg/mL (second-generation) (lab reference range: 15-76 pg/mL)
25-Hydroxyvitamin D	35 ng/mL			42 ng/mL
Creatinine			0.7 mg/dL	
Other labs	TSH = 1.9 mIU/L Albumin, normal	24 hour Calcium = 408 mg Creatinine = 1.3 g Volume = 4.2 L		Ionized calcium = 1.4 mmol/L (lab reference range: 1.15-1.4 mmol/L) Albumin, normal

attempt to normalize serum calcium level. NPHPT is characterized by persistently normal albumin-adjusted total and ionized serum calcium levels on at least 2 consecutive measurements at least a week apart over a 3- to 6-month period, confirmed by elevated PTH levels. Other diseases and drugs that cause high PTH levels should be excluded.[5] Positive radiologic tests are not diagnostic of PHPT. False-positive sestamibi scans have been noted in patients with underlying thyroid disease at a rate reaching 15% to 20%.

Based the data in the vignette, this patient may have hypercalciuria with secondary hyperparathyroidism or NPHPT. Patients with NPHPT do not usually have elevated urinary calcium levels. They may have evidence of skeletal or kidney involvement (eg, osteoporosis, nephrolithiasis). The natural history of NPHPT is unclear in part because studies have not always used consistent terminology and the heterogenous nature of cohorts. In the latest guidelines, surgical intervention was not recommended for patients with NPHPT because of lack of evidence of any benefit on end-organs after parathyroidectomy. Furthermore, patients with NPHPT are more likely to have multiglandular disease and negative preoperative localizing studies, which complicates their surgical management.[14] This is a challenging, yet common, scenario that various experts may approach differently.

Key Learning Points

- A definite diagnosis of PHPT should be established using the accepted revised definitions.

- Patients with PHPT should be systematically assessed for silent end-organ involvement.

- If NPHPT is suspected, secondary causes of normal calcium and high PTH should be ruled out.

- Radiologic procedures are indicated to guide parathyroidectomy and not to diagnose PHPT.

- Parathyroidectomy is the only curative intervention for PHPT, but it is not recommended for individuals with NPHPT.

- Cinacalcet lowers serum calcium and PTH, but it does not improve bone mineral density or hypercalciuria. Bisphosphonates and denosumab maintain or modestly increase bone mineral density.

References

1. Civitelli R, Rosen C. Parathyroid disorders special sections. *J Bone Miner Res.* 2022;37(11):2288-2289. PMID: 36223904

2. Bilezikian JP, Khan AA, Clarke BL, Mannstadt M, Potts JT, Brandi ML. The fifth international workshop on the evaluation and management of primary hyperparathyroidism. *J Bone Miner Res.* 2022;37(11):2290-2292. PMID: 36245277

3. Yao L, Guyatt G, Ye Z, et al. Methodology for the guidelines on evaluation and management of hypoparathyroidism and primary hyperparathyroidism. *J Bone Miner Res.* 2022;37(11):2404-2410. PMID: 36053800

4. Bilezikian JP, Khan AA, Silverberg SJ, et al; International Workshop on Primary Hyperparathyroidism. Evaluation and management of primary hyperparathyroidism: summary statement and guidelines from the fifth international workshop. *J Bone Miner Res.* 2022;37(11):2293-2314. PMID: 36245251

5. Minisola S, Arnold A, Belaya Z, et al. Epidemiology, pathophysiology, and genetics of primary hyperparathyroidism. *J Bone Miner Res.* 2022;37(11):2315-2329. PMID: 36245271

6. El-Hajj Fuleihan G, Chakhtoura M, Cipriani C, et al. Classical and nonclassical manifestations of primary hyperparathyroidism. *J Bone Miner Res.* 2022;37(11):2330-2350. PMID: 36245249

7. Perrier N, Lang BH, Farias LCB, et al. Surgical aspects of primary hyperparathyroidism. *J Bone Miner Res.* 2022;37(11):2373-2390. PMID: 36054175

8. Ye Z, Silverberg SJ, Sreekanta A, et al. The efficacy and safety of medical and surgical therapy in patients with primary hyperparathyroidism: a systematic review and meta-analysis of randomized controlled trials. *Bone Miner Res.* 2022;37(11):2351-2372. PMID: 36054175

9. Bilezikian JP, Silverberg SJ, Bandeira F, et al. Management of primary hyperparathyroidism. *J Bone Miner Res.* 2022;37(11):2391-2403. PMID: 36054638

10. Rubin M, Bilezikian JP, McMahon DJ, et al. The natural history of primary hyperparathyroidism with or without parathyroid surgery after 15 years. *J Clin Endocrinol Metab.* 2008;93(9):3462-3470. PMID: 18544625

11. El-Hajj Fuleihan G. Hyperparathyroidism: time to reconsider current clinical decision paradigms? *J Clin Endocrinol Metab.* 2008;93(9):3302-3304. PMID: 18772461

12. El-Hajj Fuleihan G, Silverberg S. Pathogenesis and etiology of primary hyperparathyroidism. *UpToDate.* Wolters Kluwer.

13. Haden ST, Stoll AL, McCormick S, Scott J, El-Hajj Fuleihan G. Alterations in parathyroid dynamics in lithium-treated subjects. *J Clin Endocrinol Metab.* 1997;82(9):2844-2848. PMID: 9284708

14. Liu Y, Gregory NS, Andreopoulou P, Kashyap S, Cusano N. Approach to the patient: normocalcemic primary hyperparathyroidism. *J Clin Endocrinol Metab.* 2025;110(3):e868-e877. PMID: 39319404

*References 1 through 9 are part of the publications from the 5th International Workshop on Primary Hyperparathyroidism published in the *Journal of Bone and Mineral Research* in the 2022 Fall issue.

Addressing Bone Health in Underweight Individuals Across the Lifespan

Pouneh K. Fazeli, MD, MPH. Division of Endocrinology, Department of Medicine, UPMC Presbyterian Hospital, University of Pittsburgh, Pittsburgh, PA; Email: fazelipk@upmc.edu

Selma Feldman Witchel, MD. Division of Pediatric Endocrinology, Department of Pediatrics, UPMC Children's Hospital of Pittsburgh, University of Pittsburgh, Pittsburgh, PA; Email: selma.witchel@chp.edu

Educational Objectives

After reviewing this chapter, learners should be able to:

- Explain the relationship between bone health and nutrition.

- Describe the hormonal basis of low bone mineral density (BMD) in anorexia nervosa.

- Distinguish idiopathic hypogonadotropic hypogonadism from avoidant restrictive food disorder (ARFID) and anorexia nervosa.

Significance of the Clinical Problem

States of negative energy balance result in hormonal adaptations that help maintain a state of euglycemia and shunt energy expenditure away from processes that are unnecessary for survival. These adaptations lead to upregulation of counterregulatory hormones, including GH and cortisol, and redirect energy away from reproduction and IGF-1 dependent processes, neither of which is critical for survival.[1] Regardless of the cause of the state of negative energy balance, these adaptations are important for survival during periods of undernutrition.[1] Adaptations to prolonged caloric deprivation have long-term health consequences, including loss of bone mass and increased fracture risk.[2] Chronic conditions associated with undernutrition that affect bone health are listed in the *Box*. Herein, 3 situations representing different age groups are presented.

Box. Chronic Medical Conditions Associated With Increased Risk of Low BMD

Malabsorption/decreased caloric intake
- Crohn disease
- Ulcerative colitis
- Cystic fibrosis
- Systematic lupus erythematosus
- Ankylosing spondylitis
- Celiac disease
- Cancer and cancer treatments
- Solid organ transplant
- Anorexia nervosa
- Avoidant restrictive food disorder
- Chronic kidney disease
- Extreme prematurity and low birth weight

Endocrine dysfunction
- Hyperthyroidism
- Type 1 diabetes
- Adrenal insufficiency

Practice Gaps

- There is a lack of awareness of the role of hypophosphatemia in metabolic bone disease of prematurity.

- It is important for clinicians to understand potential causes of bone loss in states of undernutrition, as bone loss is rarely due to nutrient deficiency.

- Although hypoestrogenemia due to hypogonadotropic hypogonadism is a common finding in anorexia nervosa, combined oral contraceptives (COCs) are not effective in increasing BMD in this population.

Discussion

Fetal Skeletal Health

Skeletal health begins in utero. At approximately 8 to 12 weeks' gestation, the primary ossification centers appear in the vertebrae and long bones. Fetal bone mineral accretion is highly dependent on the active transport of calcium from the maternal to fetal circulation. The placenta also actively transports phosphorus and magnesium from the maternal circulation. Fetal intestinal mineral absorption is limited to the minerals excreted by the fetal kidney into amniotic fluid and swallowed by the fetus.

Typically, 30 g of calcium and 20 g of phosphate are deposited in the full-term fetal skeleton by term; most of this mineral accretion occurs during the third trimester. For the average fetus, calcium accretion increases from 60 mg per day at 24 weeks' gestation to 300 to 350 mg of calcium per day between 35 and 40 weeks' gestation. Phosphate accretion also increases from 40 mg per day at week 24 to 200 mg per day in the last 5 weeks of gestation.[3]

Total and ionized calcium concentrations, phosphorus, and magnesium concentrations are usually greater in the fetus than in the mother.[3] The higher fetal calcium concentrations suppress PTH secretion, resulting in lower fetal PTH concentrations compared with the mother's.

Calcitriol concentrations are also lower in the fetus than in the mother. Intact FGF-23 concentrations tend to be normal or slightly low.[3] The placenta and possibly the parathyroid glands produce PTHrP. Chronic placental insufficiency may be associated with intrauterine growth restriction and impaired phosphate transfer. Fetal skeletal mineralization is largely independent of maternal vitamin D status.[3]

Throughout pregnancy, the placenta is the major source of calcium. The cutting of the placenta is the switch that transforms regulation of mineral homeostasis in the newborn. Loss of placental calcium transport accompanied by the onset of breathing, respectively, decreases calcium transport and increases blood pH. This postnatal decline in serum calcium stimulates increased PTH secretion. Calcitriol concentrations also increase. The intestines then become the major calcium source. The kidneys start to reabsorb minerals and bone turnover contributes additional minerals to the circulation. FGF-23 becomes more active in the regulation of serum phosphorus, renal phosphorus excretion, and calcitriol synthesis and catabolism. Initially, intestinal calcium absorption is passive. The high lactose content of breast milk initially facilitates passive intestinal calcium absorption as the calcitriol-dependent active intestinal absorption pathways mature and become functional.[3]

Bone Health and Undernutrition Among Adolescents and Adults

Among adolescents and adults, the major causes of undernutrition can be classified into 2 etiologies: chronic medical conditions and psychiatric etiologies. Chronic medical conditions are often associated with malabsorption, undernutrition, or excessive energy demands. With appropriate diagnosis and ongoing treatment, weight generally improves. Psychiatric etiologies include anorexia nervosa and ARFID.

The psychiatric causes of undernutrition are more challenging to treat, with anorexia nervosa having a long-term remission rate of approximately 60% 2 decades after diagnosis.[4]

Anorexia nervosa is a chronic psychiatric disorder most commonly starting during adolescence.[5] The lifetime prevalence of anorexia nervosa is estimated to be 1.4% in women and 0.2% in men.[6] The *Diagnostic and Statistical Manual of Mental Disorders, 5th Edition*, criteria for anorexia nervosa include a low body weight in the setting of fear of weight gain. This results in self-induced inappropriate caloric intake. ARFID is a more recently described psychiatric condition in which there is food avoidance and a low-weight state, but not due to fear of gaining weight or due to a medical condition. Individuals with ARFID may avoid eating because of a fear of choking, for example, or may simply not eat due to lack of interest in food.

Clinical Case Vignettes

Case 1

A newborn boy is the 625 g product of a 26-week gestation (weight percentile, 3.4). He required mechanical ventilation for 7 days and now has chronic lung disease treated with furosemide and caffeine. He had 1 episode of medical necrotizing enterocolitis necessitating interruptions of enteral feeds. At 59 days of age, routine chest radiography identified rib fractures at various stages of healing. There is no family history of bone diseases or rickets.

Laboratory test results while on total parenteral nutrition:

Serum calcium = 9.9 mg/dL (9.0-11.0 mg/dL)
(SI: 2.5 mmol/L [2.3-2.8 mmol/L])
Serum phosphorus = 3.5 mg/dL (4.0-8.0 mg/dL)
(SI: 1.1 mmol/L [1.3-2.6 mmol/L])
Alkaline phosphatase = 1035 U/L (150-420 U/L)
(SI: 17.3 μkat/L [2.51-7.01 μkat/L])
25-Hydroxyvitamin D = 38 ng/mL (20-80 ng/mL)
(SI: 94.8 nmol/L [49.9-199.7 nmol/L])
Intact PTH = 63 pg/mL (15-65 pg/mL)
(SI: 6.7 mmol/L [1.6-6.9 mmol/L])
Tubular reabsorption of phosphate = 95% (78%-91%)

Which of the following is the most likely etiology of this infant's fractures?

A. Prematurity

B. Osteogenesis imperfecta

C. Metabolic bone disease of prematurity

D. X-linked hypophosphatemic rickets due to *PHEX* pathogenic variant

E. Vitamin D–dependent rickets due to *CYP27B1* pathogenic variant

Answer: C) Metabolic bone disease of prematurity

Although this baby is preterm, prematurity alone (Answer A) cannot explain his bone disease. Compared with term babies, preterm babies lack sufficient calcium and phosphorus storage because they are deprived of third-trimester calcium and phosphorus transport across the placenta. Extremely preterm and low–birth weight babies can develop metabolic bone disease of prematurity (MBDP) (Answer C), as is the case in this vignette. MBDP is characterized by decreased mineralization of the preterm infant skeleton due to insufficient calcium and phosphorus accretion. Peak MBDP occurrence is typically between 4 and 8 weeks of postnatal age.[7] Approximately 20% of very low–birth weight infants with gestational age younger than 32 weeks develop MBDP.[8] Rachitic changes and fractures may or may not be observed. MBDP sometimes goes undetected until marked demineralization is present with loss of 20% to 40% of bone mineral content.

The differential diagnosis of fractures in neonates include osteogenesis imperfecta, hypophosphatasia, X-linked hypophosphatemic rickets, and zinc deficiency. This baby's physical exam and x-ray findings are inconsistent with the features of osteogenesis imperfecta (Answer B).

Vitamin D–dependent rickets due to *CYP27B1* variants (Answer E) is unlikely because the infant has normal calcium and PTH values.

Although some biochemical findings are similar for MBDP and X-linked hypophosphatemic rickets (Answer D), the lack of a family history and this patient's clinical course suggest that MBDP is the most likely diagnosis. In addition, X-linked hypophosphatemic rickets, due to *PHEX* variants, is associated with low tubular reabsorption of phosphate, whereas MBDP is characterized by normal to elevated tubular reabsorption of phosphate.

The loss of the third trimester mineral bolus is exacerbated postnatally by impaired calcium and phosphorus supplementation/absorption, resulting in a suboptimally mineralized new and remodeled skeletal system. Human milk typically has a vitamin D concentration of 25 to 50 IU/L, which is insufficient to maintain serum 25-hydroxyvitamin D levels greater than 20 ng/mL (>50 nmol/L) in premature infants. In addition to insufficient vitamin D concentration, preterm human milk lacks sufficient calcium and phosphorous. Formulas designated for term infants, soy formulas, and lactose-free formulas should be avoided because their inadequate mineral and vitamin D concentrations may contribute to MBDP.

Vitamin D deficiency leads to hypocalcemia, secondary hyperparathyroidism, and phosphaturia. Appropriate supplementation is essential. The recommended vitamin D dosage is 400 IU daily (10 mcg daily) in healthy term and preterm infants.[9] For very low–birth weight infants, 200 IU daily (5 mcg daily) can be used and increased to 400 IU (10 mcg) when the infant weighs more than 1500 g and is tolerating enteral nutrition. Nevertheless, MBDP is generally not responsive to vitamin D or calcitriol treatment.[10]

The primary factor contributing to MBDP is phosphorus deficiency. Additional factors contributing to MBDP include chronic placental insufficiency, inadequate postnatal intestinal calcium and phosphorus absorption, parenteral nutrition, necrotizing enterocolitis, chronic lung disease, fluid restriction, and reduced physical activity. In necrotizing enterocolitis with bowel resection or other postsurgical short-gut complications, calcium absorption can be compromised, resulting in hypocalcemia. Medications, such as glucocorticoids, loop diuretics, methylxanthines, anticoagulants, and CYP450 3A4 inducers, may also contribute to the development of MBDP. Care of very low–birth weight babies involves titrating caloric intake, fluid balance, and mineral balance to enable extra-uterine maturation while minimizing long-term sequelae. In summary, numerous nutritional and biomechanical factors contribute to MBDP in low–birth weight and extremely low–birth weight preterm babies.

Currently, the optimal approach is prevention. Prevention involves diets containing appropriate calcium, phosphate, and vitamin D concentrations; screening; and fracture prevention. Formulas specially designed for preterm infants or human milk supplemented with fortifiers should be used for enteral feeds. While no optimal calcium to phosphorus ratio for intake has been validated, a 1.5 to 1.7:1 calcium to phosphorus ratio appears to be reasonable.[11]

Screening for MBDP should begin at 4 to 6 weeks of age for infants with risk factors (*Table, following page*). Monitoring should be repeated every 1 to 2 weeks.[12] Major risk factors include birth weight less than 1500 g, gestational age younger than 28 weeks, parenteral nutrition for longer than 4 weeks with insufficient enteral feeds, and use of medications with negative effects on bone. Screening should include serum calcium, phosphorus, and alkaline phosphatase. Low serum phosphorus values (<4 mg/dL [<1.3 mmol/L] for more than 1 to 2 weeks) and/or alkaline phosphatase values greater than 600 U/L (>193.8 μkat/L) warrant additional investigation for MBDP. Caveats regarding serum alkaline phosphatase include that it can be elevated in liver disease or decreased by zinc deficiency and use of glucocorticoids. Another potentially helpful screening test for MBDP is a tubular reabsorption of phosphate value greater than 95% accompanied by hypophosphatemia, which reflects complete renal phosphate reabsorption in an effort to compensate for inadequate phosphate intake.[12] However, samples for tubular reabsorption of phosphate calculations are best obtained in the fasting state, which might be difficult to collect from preterm infants who feed frequently or require continuous parenteral nutrition. PTH concentrations greater than 100 pg/mL (>10.6 pmol/L) suggest MBDP. With additional validation, low FGF-23 concentrations might prove to be another marker for MBDP.[13] To prevent fractures, bedside signage indicating the need for safe handling of high-risk infants can be displayed. Physical therapy can be used and taught to parents.

Table. Risk Factors Associated With Development of MBDP

Risk Factor	Mechanism
Prematurity (<28 weeks' gestation)	Deprivation of third trimester in utero transfer of calcium and phosphate
Low birth weight	Impaired placental mineral transfer in utero
Parenteral nutrition for >4 weeks' duration	Limited calcium and phosphate supplementation
Necrotizing enterocolitis	Disrupted enteral feeds, poor gut function, decreased calcium and phosphate absorption
Failure to tolerate formulas or human milk fortifiers with high mineral content	Decreased calcium and phosphate absorption
Chronic lung disease	Fluid restriction, need for loop diuretics and glucocorticoids, high energy needs
Decreased physical activity	Increased bone resorption, reduced bone formation
Glucocorticoid treatment	Increased bone resorption, reduced bone formation
Loop diuretics (eg, furosemide)	Hypercalciuria
CYP450 3A4 inducers (eg, phenobarbital)	Induce vitamin D metabolism
Methylxanthines (eg, caffeine and theophylline)	Increased bone resorption
Anticoagulants	Reduced bone formation
Aluminum in parenteral nutrition and other parental supplements	Reduced bone formation

Data regarding long-term outcome are heterogeneous. Most reports indicate that preterm children remain shorter than term peers and have decreased areal BMD.[14] Among young adults born preterm, even after accounting for height and weight, areal BMD at the femoral neck is significantly decreased, suggesting a role for additional influences, such as physical activity.[15] Currently adequate evidence-based data are unavailable regarding long-term outcomes for infants with MBDP and adult osteopenia/osteoporosis.

Case 2

A 30-year-old woman who has been running since high school, and currently runs 42 miles per week, experienced a tibial stress fracture. Her primary care physician performed DXA, which showed a T-score of –2.9 (Z-score, –2.9) at the L1-L4 spine. The left femoral neck T-score was –2.5 (Z-score, –2.5) and left total hip T- and Z-scores were both –2.3. She was referred to endocrinology for further evaluation. She reports no relevant medical or surgical history, and medications include a calcium citrate plus vitamin D supplement twice daily and a combined oral contraceptive pill. She underwent menarche at age 15.5 years and was started on a COC at the age of 17 years old for "irregular menses." Review of systems are negative for gastrointestinal symptoms; she has no abdominal pain or constipation. She follows a gluten-free and dairy-free diet and uses an app on her phone to count her caloric intake.

On physical examination, her blood pressure is 90/60 mm Hg and pulse rate is 45 beats/min. Her height is 65 in (165.1 cm), and weight is 100 lb (45.4 kg) (BMI = 16.6 kg/m²). She has lanugo hair on her arms.

Laboratory test results:

Calcium = 9.8 mg/dL (SI: 2.5 mmol/L)
Albumin, normal
25-Hydroxyvitamin D = 35 ng/mL (SI: 87.4 nmol/L)

Which of the following is the most likely cause of this patient's low BMD?

A. Vitamin D deficiency

B. Primary hyperparathyroidism

C. Low body weight resulting in low IGF-1, hypercortisolemia, and functional hypothalamic amenorrhea

D. All of the above

Answer: C) Low body weight resulting in low IGF-1, hypercortisolemia, and functional hypothalamic amenorrhea

In low-weight eating disorders, low BMD is very common, particularly in women with anorexia nervosa. Greater than 85% of women with anorexia nervosa have a BMD greater than one standard deviation below the mean of women at their peak BMD.[16] Although BMD is lower in both adolescents and adult women with anorexia nervosa compared with similarly aged normal-weight individuals, this low BMD is not associated with fracture history, despite the fact that girls and women with anorexia nervosa have a high prevalence of fractures. Therefore, although BMD should be followed to evaluate the trajectory of BMD loss, it may not be a predictor of fracture in this population. Importantly, low BMI, regardless of the cause (anorexia nervosa or ARFID), is associated with low BMD.[17] Although data on ARFID-associated low BMD are limited, it is possible that the same factors that affect BMD in anorexia nervosa may also result in low BMD in ARFID. Among the potential causes for low BMD, vitamin D deficiency can be excluded because she has a normal vitamin D concentration. Hyperparathyroidism is unlikely since her serum calcium concentration is normal. Thus, her low BMD is most likely attributed to anorexia nervosa accompanied by low IGF-1, hypercortisolemia, and functional hypothalamic amenorrhea (Answer C).

Although the patient does not present with a diagnosis of anorexia nervosa, the clinician should be highly suspicious of this diagnosis based on her BMI of less than 18.5 kg/m^2 and her restrictive dietary history, including counting her daily caloric intake. This patient has osteoporosis based on both the International Society for Clinical Densitometry definition, which defines premenopausal low BMD as a Z-score of −2 or less coupled with a secondary cause of low BMD (the patient is low weight and likely has anorexia nervosa), or the International Osteoporosis Foundation definition, which is based on a T-score of less than −2.5, in addition to a secondary cause of osteoporosis.[18,19] Many patients with anorexia nervosa present without a known diagnosis of anorexia nervosa and, therefore, it is important to remain vigilant about the possibility. Although

vitamin D deficiency (Answer A) should be screened for and treated in patients who have low BMD, vitamin D deficiency is an unlikely cause of low BMD in someone on a twice daily supplement. In a patient who is on vitamin D supplementation with a normal calcium level, primary hyperparathyroidism (Answer B) is also unlikely to be the explanation for low BMD.

Multiple hormonal adaptations that occur in states of undernutrition with resultant low body weight likely contribute to low BMD. Functional hypothalamic amenorrhea shunts energy away from the hypothalamic-pituitary-ovarian axis. Functional hypothalamic amenorrhea results in a low-estrogen state that is associated with increased bone resorption. Longer duration of amenorrhea is associated with lower BMD in anorexia nervosa. Long-term consequences may develop when the eating disorder begins before attainment of peak bone mass.[20] However, importantly, estradiol-containing COCs do not increase BMD relative to placebo in the setting of anorexia nervosa.[21] Lower, more physiologic doses of estradiol, predominantly in transdermal form, are beneficial for low BMD in adolescents.[22] Transdermal estradiol is also currently being studied in a randomized controlled study in adults after pilot data suggested benefit.

The lack of efficacy of COCs in improving BMD is due to suppression of hepatic IGF-1 secretion by oral estrogen. Transdermal estradiol may improve BMD because the transdermal route has minimal effects on IGF-1 concentrations.[23,24] In addition, GH resistance leads to decreased IGF-1 concentrations in underweight states.[25] In anorexia nervosa, low IGF-1 concentrations are associated with low BMD and, therefore, may be a cause of low BMD in low-weight states.[26] Recombinant human (rh) IGF-1 has been studied as a treatment for low BMD in anorexia nervosa. Nine months of rhIGF-1 combined with oral estrogen increases BMD in adults.[27] In contrast, in adolescents, 12 months of the combination of transdermal estradiol and rhIGF-1 does not increase BMD when compared with the effects of transdermal estradiol alone.[28]

Cortisol levels are increased in the setting of physiologic stress, such as the chronic undernutrition characteristic of anorexia nervosa.[29] High cortisol levels have been associated with low BMD in anorexia nervosa and therefore may also contribute to low BMD in this setting.[30] Importantly, because cortisol is a counterregulatory hormone and is critical for maintaining euglycemia during states of starvation, we would not consider treating hypercortisolemia in anorexia nervosa.

Case 3

A 26-year-old woman presents to an adult endocrine clinic with a history of idiopathic hypogonadotropic hypogonadism. She reports being diagnosed with primary amenorrhea at age 16 years at which time ARFID was also diagnosed. Her medical records from that time document a normal sense of smell and a reported weight loss of 60 lb (27.2 kg). Her lowest weight was noted to be 105 lb (47.6 kg), with a height of 67 in (170.2 cm) (BMI = 16.4 kg/m^2). The patient reported not eating at that time due to lack of hunger or interest in food. She had a full endocrine evaluation for primary amenorrhea, which included karyotype analysis (46,XX) and pelvic ultrasonography. Findings on pelvic ultrasonography were normal apart from a small uterus. There was no family history of infertility or anosmia. She was started on low-dose oral estradiol followed by cyclic progesterone. At age 19 years, her regimen was transitioned to a COC pill. Her lack of interest in eating diminished and she gained enough weight to achieve a normal BMI. She recently saw an adult endocrinologist who told her that she has idiopathic hypogonadotropic hypogonadism, would need to remain on COCs until menopause, and would likely need medical assistance to achieve pregnancy. She presents for a second opinion regarding this diagnosis. Her current BMI is 21 kg/m^2, and she reports stable weight for the last 5 years.

Which of the following is the best next step?

A. Continue COCs

B. Transition to a hormone replacement therapy dose of transdermal estradiol + progesterone

C. Stop COCs and reassess after 3 months

D. Encourage weight gain

Answer: C) Stop COCs and reassess after 3 months

This patient was diagnosed with idiopathic hypogonadotropic hypogonadism in the setting of significant weight loss and low body weight due to ARFID. Although it is possible that she has idiopathic hypogonadotropic hypogonadism, it is also possible that the low gonadotropins and low estradiol levels typical of idiopathic hypogonadotropic hypogonadism were due to hypogonadotropic hypogonadism in the setting of low body weight. Now that the patient has a normal body weight, the COCs can be discontinued to see if she is able to cycle without exogenous hormones and clarify the diagnosis (Answer C). If menstrual cycles do not resume in the absence of exogenous hormones, we would perform an amenorrhea evaluation that would include assessing thyroid function and measuring FSH, LH, estradiol, prolactin, and hCG. It is important to counsel the patient that she could become pregnant once she stops COCs. Additional weight gain does not need to be encouraged because she now has a normal BMI and her weight has been stable.

Individuals with ARFID are often significantly underweight. Substantial nutritional deficiencies may exist. Although ARFID was considered an eating disorder affecting primarily infants and children, individuals across the age spectrum can be affected. Some individuals are dependent on oral supplements or tube feeding. Psychiatric comorbidities, such as anxiety, obsessive-compulsive, and trauma-related disorders, are common among individuals with ARFID.

Key Learning Points

- Underweight states, regardless of the etiology, are a common cause of low BMD throughout the lifespan.

- Treating providers must be aware of the multiple effects of undernutrition on bone metabolism.

- In adolescents and adults, psychiatric causes of low body weight are a common cause of low BMD, but they are often underdiagnosed.

- Although hypoestrogenemia is a cause of low BMD in anorexia nervosa, combined COCs are not effective in increasing BMD in this population.

References

1. Amorim T, Khiyami A, Latif T, Fazeli PK. Neuroendocrine adaptations to starvation. *Psychoneuroendocrinology.* 2023;157:106365. PMID: 37573628

2. Fazeli PK, Klibanski A. Effects of anorexia nervosa on bone metabolism. *Endocr Rev.* 2018;39(6):895-910. PMID: 30165608

3. Ryan BA, Kovacs CS. Calciotropic and phosphotropic hormones in fetal and neonatal bone development. *Semin Fetal Neonatal Med.* 2020;25(1):101062. PMID: 31786156

4. Eddy KT, Tabri N, Thomas JJ, et al. Recovery from anorexia nervosa and bulimia nervosa at 22-year follow-up. *J Clin Psychiatry.* 2017;78(2):184-189. PMID: 28002660

5. Bulik CM, Reba L, Siega-Riz AM, Reichborn-Kjennerud T. Anorexia nervosa: definition, epidemiology, and cycle of risk. *Int J Eat Disord.* 2005;37(Suppl S2-S9). PMID: 15852310

6. Galmiche M, Déchelotte P, Lambert G, Tavolacci MP. Prevalence of eating disorders over the 2000-2018 period: a systematic literature review. *Am J Clin Nutr.* 2019;109(5):1402-1413. PMID: 31051507

7. Faienza MF, D'Amato E, Natale MP, et al. Metabolic bone disease of prematurity: diagnosis and management. *Front Pediatr.* 2019;7:143. PMID: 31032241

8. Perrone M, Casirati A, Stagi S, et al. Don't forget the bones: incidence and risk factors of metabolic bone disease in a cohort of preterm infants. *Int J Mol Sci.* 2022;23(18):10666. PMID: 36142579

9. Abrams SA; Committee on Nutrition. Calcium and vitamin d requirements of enterally fed preterm infants. *Pediatrics.* 2013;131(5):e1676-e1683. PMID: 23629620.

10. Venkataraman PS, Tsang RC, Steichen JJ, Grey I, Neylan M, Fleischman AR. Early neonatal hypocalcemia in extremely preterm infants. High incidence, early onset, and refractoriness to supraphysiologic doses of calcitriol. *Am J Dis Child.* 1986;140(10):1004-1008. PMID: 3755862

11. Rowe JC, Goetz CA, Carey DE, Horak E. Achievement of in utero retention of calcium and phosphorus accompanied by high calcium excretion in very low birth weight infants fed a fortified formula. *J Pediatr.* 1987;110(4):581-585. PMID: 3559809

12. Grover M, Ashraf AP, Bowden SA, et al. Invited mini review metabolic bone disease of prematurity: overview and practice recommendations. *Horm Res Paediatr.* 2025;98(1):40-50. PMID: 38211570

13. Llorente-Pelayo S, Docio P, Arriola S, et al. Role of fibroblast growth factor-23 as an early marker of metabolic bone disease of prematurity. *BMC Pediatr.* 2024;24(1):418. PMID: 38951759

14. Xie LF, Alos N, Cloutier A, Béland C, Dubois J, Nuyt AM, Luu TM. The long-term impact of very preterm birth on adult bone mineral density. *Bone Rep.* 2018;10:100189. PMID: 30627597

15. Balasuriya CND, Evensen KAI, Mosti MP, et al. Peak bone mass and bone microarchitecture in adults born with low birth weight preterm or at term: a cohort study. *J Clin Endocrinol Metab.* 2017;102(7):2491-2500. PMID: 28453635

16. Miller KK, Grinspoon SK, Ciampa J, Hier J, Herzog D, Klibanski A. *Medical findings in outpatients with anorexia nervosa. Arch Intern Med.* 2005;165(5):561-566. PMID: 15767533

17. Alberts Z, Fewtrell M, Nicholls DE, Biassoni L, Easty M, Hudson LD. Bone mineral density in Anorexia Nervosa versus Avoidant Restrictive Food Intake Disorder. *Bone.* 2020;134:115307. PMID: 32142910

18. Shuhart CR, Yeap SS, Anderson PA, Jankowski LG, Lewiecki EM, Morse LR, Rosen HN, Weber DR, Zemel BS, Shepherd JA. Executive summary of the 2019 ISCD position development conference on monitoring treatment, DXA cross-calibration and least significant change, spinal cord injury, peri-prosthetic and orthopedic bone health, transgender medicine, and pediatrics. *J Clin Densitom.* 2019;22(4):453-471. PMID: 31400968

19. Ferrari S, Bianchi ML, Eisman JA, et al; IOF Committee of Scientific Advisors Working Group on Osteoporosis Pathophysiology. Osteoporosis in young adults: pathophysiology, diagnosis, and management. Osteoporos Int. 2012;23(12):2735-2748. PMID: 22684497

20. Biller BM, Saxe V, Herzog DB, Rosenthal DI, Holzman S, Klibanski A. Mechanisms of osteoporosis in adult and adolescent women with anorexia nervosa. *J Clin Endocrinol Metab.* 1989;68(3):548-54. PMID: 2493036

21. Thavaraputta S, Fazeli PK. Estrogen for the treatment of low bone mineral density in anorexia nervosa. *J Psychiatr Brain Sci.* 2022;7(3):e220004. PMID: 35874115

22. Misra M, Katzman D, Miller KK, et al. Physiologic estrogen replacement increases bone density in adolescent girls with anorexia nervosa. *J Bone Miner Res.* 2011;26(10):2430-2438. PMID: 21698665

23. Weissberger AJ, Ho KK, Lazarus L. Contrasting effects of oral and transdermal routes of estrogen replacement therapy on 24-hour growth hormone (GH) secretion, insulin-like growth factor I, and GH-binding protein in postmenopausal women. *J Clin Endocrinol Metab.* 1991;72(2):374-381. PMID: 1991807

24. Kam GY, Leung KC, Baxter RC, Ho KK. Estrogens exert route- and dose-dependent effects on insulin-like growth factor (IGF)-binding protein-3 and the acid-labile subunit of the IGF ternary complex. *J Clin Endocrinol Metab.* 2000;85(5):1918-22. PMID: 10843175

25. Fazeli PK, Klibanski A. Determinants of GH resistance in malnutrition. *J Endocrinol.* 2014;220(3):R57-R65. PMID: 24363451

26. Grinspoon S, Miller K, Coyle C, et al. Severity of osteopenia in estrogen-deficient women with anorexia nervosa and hypothalamic amenorrhea. *J Clin Endocrinol Metab.* 1999;84(6):2049-2055. PMID: 10372709

27. Grinspoon S, Thomas L, Miller K, Herzog D, Klibanski A. Effects of recombinant human IGF-I and oral contraceptive administration on bone density in anorexia nervosa. *J Clin Endocrinol Metab.* 2002;87(6):2883-2891. PMID: 12050268

28. Singhal V, Bose A, Slattery M, et al. Effect of transdermal estradiol and insulin-like growth factor-1 on bone endpoints of young women with anorexia nervosa. *J Clin Endocrinol Metab.* 2021;106(7):2021-2035. PMID: 33693703

29. Thavaraputta S, Ungprasert P, Witchel SF, Fazeli PK. Anorexia nervosa and adrenal hormones: a systematic review and meta-analysis. *Eur J Endocrinol.* 2023;189(3):S64-S73. PMID: 37669399

30. Lawson EA, Donoho D, Miller KK, et al. Hypercortisolemia is associated with severity of bone loss and depression in hypothalamic amenorrhea and anorexia nervosa. *J Clin Endocrinol Metab.* 2009;94(12):4710-4716. PMID: 19837921

Complex Cases in Hypophosphatemia: Navigating Diagnostic and Treatment Challenges of Low Phosphate

Eva S. Liu, MD. Division of Endocrinology, Diabetes, and Hypertension, Brigham and Women's Hospital/Harvard Medical School, Boston, MA; Email: esliu@bwh.harvard.edu

Educational Objectives

After reviewing this chapter, learners should be able to:

- Illustrate the endocrine regulation of phosphate homeostasis.

- Identify and diagnose causes of hypophosphatemia in the clinic.

- Manage disorders of hypophosphatemia.

Significance of the Clinical Problem

Extracellular phosphate is a critical regulator of skeletal homeostasis, with 85% of phosphate localized to the skeleton/teeth and 15% in the soft tissue and extracellular fluid.[1] Phosphate plays an essential role in regulating growth plate maturation, with low serum phosphate leading to rickets in children.[2] Phosphate is also important for skeletal mineralization and structure, where in combination with calcium it forms the hydroxyapatite necessary for mineralization of skeletal tissues. Insufficient phosphate therefore results in osteomalacia. Dietary intake and hormones, including PTH, FGF-23, and 1,25-dihydroxyvitamin D_3, all regulate phosphate homeostasis. When one or multiple regulators of phosphate is abnormal, disorders of phosphate homeostasis may result. Causes of hypophosphatemia include inherited and acquired disorders and disorders of altered phosphate load and absorption. Symptoms of hypophosphatemia can be nonspecific, including myalgias, joint pain, and fatigue. Moreover, treatments of hypophosphatemia often lead to significant adverse effects, such as gastrointestinal distress or secondary/tertiary hyperparathyroidism. Therefore, it is important for health care providers to consider hypophosphatemic disorders in their patient workup and to be aware of the potential effects of medications used to treat these disorders.

Practice Gaps

- There is a lack of awareness among health care providers of the different causes of hypophosphatemia.

- There is a lack of awareness among health care providers regarding the treatment options and potential effects of medications used to treat disorders of hypophosphatemia.

Discussion

Diet, Intestine, and Kidney

Sixty to sixty-five percent of dietary phosphate is absorbed in the small intestine.[3] Circulating phosphate is filtered through the kidney, with 70%

of the filtered load being reabsorbed in the renal proximal tubules.[4] Sodium phosphate transporter 2b (NPT2b) is expressed in the intestine, while NPT2a/NPT2c are expressed in the proximal renal tubules to enable phosphate uptake in the intestine and kidney, respectively.[5,6] Renal reabsorption of phosphate increases until reaching a threshold termed the maximum tubular reabsorption rate for phosphate (TmP), which is normalized to glomerular filtration rate (GFR). TmP/GFR is a measure of renal tubular reabsorption.

PTH, 1,25-Dihydroxyvitamin D$_3$, and FGF-23

PTH promotes renal phosphate excretion by decreasing protein expression of sodium phosphate transporters NPT2a/c in the proximal renal tubules. In contrast, the active form of vitamin D, 1,25-dihydroxyvitamin D$_3$, enhances phosphate resorption in the small intestine by promoting the expression of NPT2b and enhances phosphate reabsorption in the proximal renal tubules. Dietary phosphate is also an important regulator of 1,25-dihydroxyvitamin D$_3$, with rodent and human studies demonstrating that phosphate deprivation leads to increased production of 1,25-dihydroxyvitamin D$_3$.

FGF-23 is predominantly synthesized by osteocytes and acts to decrease serum phosphate levels by (1) decreasing NPT2a/NPT2c expression in the kidney, leading to increased renal phosphate wasting and (2) inhibiting the expression of renal 1α-hydroxylase (CYP27B1) and increasing CYP24a1 expression, which together decreases 1,25-dihydroxyvitamin D$_3$ levels. *DMP1, PHEX, ENPP1,* and *FAM20C* all regulate FGF-23 levels. Inactivating pathogenic variants in these genes result in enhanced serum FGF-23 levels and thus hypophosphatemia (*Figure*).[7]

Figure. Regulation of Phosphate Homeostasis

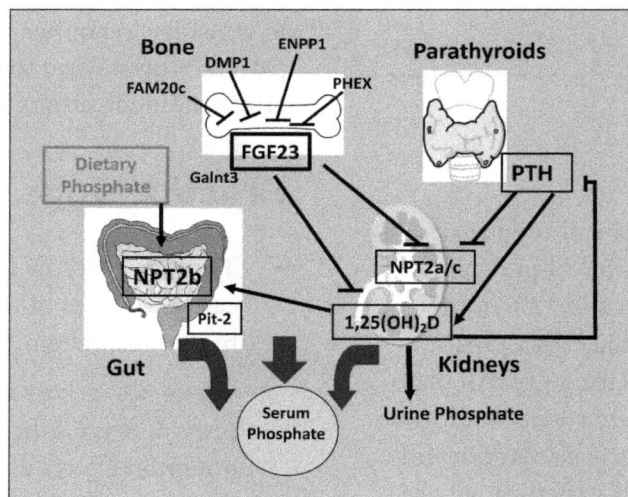

Dietary phosphate is absorbed in the gut by sodium phosphate transporter (NPT) 2b (NPT2b) and filtered by the kidneys. In the small intestine, phosphate transport is predominantly regulated by NPT2b. 1,25-dihydroxyvitamin D (1,25[OH]$_2$D) increases Pit-2 expression in the small intestine, which also leads to phosphate absorption. PTH binds to the PTHR1 to reduce NPT2a and NPT2c protein levels, resulting increased renal loss of phosphate. FGF-23 is predominantly expressed in bone and binds to the FGFR with α-Klotho (KL) as coreceptor in the kidneys. Urinary phosphate excretion increases with decreased renal proximal tubule expression of NPT2a and NPT2c. FGF-23 also stimulates 24-hydroxlase expression, and it reduces 1α-hydroxilase. The combined net effects of the actions of FGF-23 in the proximal renal tubules are decreased serum levels of phosphate and 1,25-(OH)$_2$D. FGF-23 expression is reduced by *PHEX, DMP1, ENPP1,* and *FAM20C*. Consequently, lack of these negative regulators leads to increased secretion of biologically active FGF-23, resulting in hypophosphatemia. GALNT3 glycosylates and thus stabilizes FGF-23; lack of this enzyme enhances FGF-23 degradation, thereby reducing urinary phosphate excretion.

Reprinted from Liu ES and Juppner H "Chapter 20: Disorders of Phosphate Homeostasis" in Radovich S and Misra M, Eds. *Pediatric Endocrinology*, 4th Edition: Springer 2024; 499-526.

[Color—Print (Color Gallery page CG9) or web & ePub editions]

Disorders of Hypophosphatemia

Many disorders of phosphate homeostasis lead to hypophosphatemia; the most common FGF-23–mediated and non–FGF-23–mediated disorders encountered in the clinic are discussed herein.

FGF-23–Mediated Disorders

X-Linked Hypophosphatemia

X-linked hypophosphatemia (XLH) is characterized by X-linked dominant pathogenic variants in the *PHEX* gene, and it is the most common form of inheritable rickets. *PHEX* pathogenic variants lead to high circulating levels of FGF-23, which in turn result in hypophosphatemia and impaired production of 1,25-dihydroxyvitamin D_3. Affected individuals present in childhood with impaired growth and rickets. Adults with XLH have osteomalacia and develop osteoarthritis and enthesopathy. All patients with XLH have impaired skeletal mineralization and are thus at risk for pseudofractures/fractures and dental caries/abscesses. Conventional treatment includes phosphate supplementation with calcitriol (*Table*). Due to the risk of secondary/tertiary hyperparathyroidism and nephrocalcinosis with phosphate supplements, the goal of conventional therapy is not to normalize serum phosphate levels.[8] Burosumab (*Table*), the humanized anti-FGF23 antibody, is FDA approved for treatment of children and adults with XLH. Burosumab maintains serum phosphate levels in the low-normal range without increasing urinary calcium and also improves quality of life, healing of pseudofractures, and bone mineralization.[9,10]

Table. Therapies for Disorders of Hypophosphatemia

Therapy	Administration	Effects
Burosumab	*Children* X-linked hypophosphatemia: 6 months-18 years old <10 kg: 1 mg/kg every 2 weeks ≥10 kg: 0.8 mg/kg every 2 weeks *Tumor-induced osteomalacia:* 2-18 years old 0.4 mg/kg every 2 weeks, up to 180 mg/dose *Adults* X-linked hypophosphatemia: 1 mg/kg subcutaneously, up to 90 mg every 4 weeks Tumor-induced osteomalacia: 0.5 mg/kg subcutaneously every 4 weeks, up to 2 mg/kg subcutaneously every 2 weeks (not to exceed 180 mg)	Decrease in vitamin D levels Rash Local site reaction Restless leg syndrome (in adults) Headache, cough, fever (in children)
Oral phosphate (sodium phosphate or potassium phosphate)	*Infants* Starting 40 mg elemental phosphorus/kg per day in divided doses *Children* >4 years old, adults: starting 250 mg daily (up to 250-500 mg 4 times daily)	Gastrointestinal symptoms (diarrhea, nausea, stomach pain) Muscle cramps/pain Hypocalcemia Secondary hyperparathyroidism
Active vitamin D	<u>Calcitriol</u> *Children* Starting 10-20 ng/kg per dose *Adults* Starting 0.25 mcg per dose <u>Alfacalcidol</u> (not available in United States) Starting 0.25 mcg per dose	Symptoms due to hypercalcemia (thirst, nausea, bone pain) or hyperphosphatemia (muscle cramps, joint pain)
Vitamin D	<u>Vitamin D_3 (cholecalciferol):</u> 400 IU, up to 50,000 IU per dose <u>Vitamin D (ergocalciferol):</u> 400 IU, up to 50,000 IU per dose	Can cause hypercalcemia at high dosages

Tumor-Induced Osteomalacia

Tumors can produce FGF-23, leading to tumor-induced osteomalacia (TIO). Such tumors are predominantly mesenchymal in origin and are often slow growing and located in obscure areas, making them difficult to localize on imaging. Imaging with ^{68}Ga-DOTATATE PET/CT has the highest sensitivity/specificity for localizing these tumors.[11] Surgical resection is curative, but if the tumor cannot be found or completely resected, therapy with calcitriol/phosphate supplementation or burosumab is initiated to improve mineral ion and hormone levels, prevent skeletal complications, and improve quality of life.[12]

Fibrous Dysplasia

In fibrous dysplasia (FD), normal bone is replaced by fibrous bone, leading to skeletal deformity, pain, and fracture. FD can manifest on its own or as part of McCune-Albright syndrome, characterized by postzygotic pathogenic variants in *GNAS*.[13] Patients with FD can have high serum FGF-23 levels, with the degree of resultant hypophosphatemia correlating with disease severity. Low phosphate is treated with phosphate/calcitriol, or potentially burosumab. Treatments that can be considered include bisphosphonates (may improve bone pain) and denosumab (decrease activity of bone lesions).

Non–FGF-23–Mediated Disorders

Fanconi Syndrome

Impaired proximal renal tubule function leads to proximal renal tubular acidosis and renal wasting of amino acids, bicarbonate, potassium, glucose, and phosphate. Since the urinary phosphate loss can result in rickets/osteomalacia, phosphate supplementation with calcitriol supplementation is used to treat the complications of hypophosphatemia. Fanconi syndrome can result from acquired secondary conditions, such as multiple myeloma or amyloidosis, or exposure to toxic metals or medications, such as tenofovir or cisplatin.[7]

Dietary Phosphate Deficiency

Hypophosphatemia due to very low dietary intake is rare, but it has been seen in children with kwashiorkor. Chronic ingestion of phosphate binders, including calcium acetate or sevelamer, or aluminum- or magnesium-containing antacids can present with low serum phosphate levels. Disorders that compromise the ability of the gastrointestinal tract to absorb phosphate, such as bariatric surgery, celiac disease, severe diarrhea, and small-bowel resection, also may lead to hypophosphatemia. In these disorders, vitamin D deficiency and/or malabsorption of calcium leads to increased PTH levels, which in turn increases urinary phosphate wasting.[7] Treatment includes replacement of calcium and phosphate by diet or supplement.

Clinical Case Vignettes

Case 1

A 50-year-old man has a history of XLH complicated by enthesopathy and osteoarthritis. For the past 10 years, he has been taking oral phosphate supplements up to a dosage of 750 mg 4 times daily and calcitriol up to 0.5 mcg twice daily, leading to the development of tertiary hyperparathyroidism for which he underwent parathyroidectomy. After surgery, he was treated with lower dosages of oral phosphate and optimized dosages of calcitriol to maintain normocalcemia and normal serum PTH levels. Due to the significant and worsening knee pain, he consulted with an orthopedist and has decided to purse bilateral osteotomies and knee replacements. He subsequently stopped conventional therapy and started burosumab and continues on cholecalciferol, 2000 international units daily (50 mcg daily). He has undergone 1 osteotomy and the contralateral osteotomy is scheduled in a few months.

Follow-up laboratory test results:

> Serum phosphate = 2.5 mg/dL (2.4-4.3 mg/dL)
> (SI: 0.8 mmol/L [0.8- 1.4 mmol/L])
> Serum calcium = 10.3 mg/dL (8.8-10.7 mg/dL)
> (SI: 2.6 mmol/L [2.2-2.7 mmol/L])

PTH = 71 pg/mL (SI: 7.53 pmol/L)
25-Hydroxyvitamin D = 39 ng/dL (97.3 nmol/L)

Which of the following is the most appropriate next step in this patient's management?

A. Stop burosumab and restart oral phosphate supplements

B. Refer for repeat parathyroidectomy

C. Continue burosumab and start cinacalcet

D. Change cholecalciferol to ergocalciferol, 50,000 international units weekly (1250 mcg weekly)

E. Increase the dosage of burosumab

Answer: C) Continue burosumab and start cinacalcet

Burosumab is the humanized FGF-23–blocking antibody that is FDA approved for the treatment of children and adults with XLH. Unlike conventional therapy, burosumab is able to sustain serum phosphate levels in the low-normal range without altering serum or urinary calcium levels. Burosumab therapy improves skeletal mineralization, fracture healing, and ambulatory function in treated patients with XLH.[9,14] Therefore, since this patient is going for additional orthopedic procedures, burosumab should not be stopped. Also, he has remnant tertiary hyperparathyroidism, so restarting oral phosphate supplements (Answer A), which can worsen hyperparathyroidism, would not be appropriate.

His 25-hydroxyvitamin D level is normal; therefore, changing cholecalciferol to ergocalciferol (Answer D) is not indicated.

The goal of burosumab is to maintain phosphate in the low-normal range, in part to prevent nephrocalcinosis. Burosumab is associated with increased PTH levels in treated patients with XLH with higher phosphate levels on prolonged therapy.[15] Therefore, increasing the burosumab dosage (Answer E) is not necessary.

This patient has remnant tertiary hyperparathyroidism. Discontinuing calcitriol and starting burosumab increased his serum PTH levels. Cinacalcet (Answer C), a calcimimetic

that acts as an allosteric activator of the calcium-sensing receptor, when administered with burosumab has been reported to help suppress serum PTH levels and decrease serum calcium levels in patients with XLH who have tertiary hyperparathyroidism.[16]

His PTH and calcium levels are mildly elevated; therefore, a repeat parathyroidectomy (Answer B) is not yet indicated.

Case 2

A 60-year-old woman has a history of osteopenia and T-cell large granular lymphocytic leukemia. Her clinical course has been complicated by development of stage 3 kidney insufficiency and Fanconi syndrome, thought to be secondary to interstitial infiltration of the renal proximal tubules by lymphoid. She was treated with oral cyclophosphamide, but this did not improve her urinary wasting of potassium, glucose, phosphate, and bicarbonate. For the hypophosphatemia, she is started on potassium phosphate, 250 mg tablets (3 tablets in the morning, 2 tablets at lunch, and 3 tablets at dinner).

Subsequent laboratory test results:

Serum phosphate, normal
Serum PTH = 62 pg/mL (15-65 pg/mL)
(SI: 6.6 pmol/L [1.6-6.9 pmol/L])

Her serum PTH concentration increases to 110 pg/mL (11.7 pmol/L) over the next year.

Which of the following would be most appropriate next step in managing this patient's hypophosphatemia?

A. Stop her phosphate supplements

B. Decrease phosphate supplements and add calcitriol

C. Refer for parathyroidectomy

D. Stop her phosphate supplements and start burosumab

E. No change in treatment, recommend yearly kidney ultrasonography

Answer: B) Decrease phosphate supplements and add calcitriol

Fanconi syndrome is a defect in the proximal renal tubules, leading to urinary wasting electrolytes, bicarbonate, glucose and phosphate. Treatment for this resultant hypophosphatemia includes a combination of oral phosphate supplements and calcitriol, with the goal of serum phosphate being in the low-normal range. It is not recommended that phosphate supplements be used increase serum phosphate levels to normal levels due to the risk of development of secondary hyperparathyroidism, which can eventually lead to tertiary hyperparathyroidism and nephrocalcinosis. In circulation, the reabsorbed phosphate binds to calcium, leading to a decrease in serum calcium and subsequent secondary hyperparathyroidism.[17] Therefore, it is recommended that daily phosphate supplements be administered along with calcitriol (Answer B), which can increase renal and intestinal absorption of phosphate and also suppress serum PTH levels.

Stopping the phosphate supplements (Answer A) would cause the patient to have persistent hypophosphatemia and is therefore not recommended.

She has secondary hyperparathyroidism from taking phosphate supplements alone; therefore, parathyroidectomy (Answer C) is not indicated.

Burosumab therapy (Answer D) is indicated for FGF-23–mediated hypophosphatemia, such as XLH and TIO, and therefore it is not recommended as treatment for this patient.

Since the serum PTH levels have begun to rise, it would not be advised to leave her on the high dosages of oral phosphate supplement alone (Answer E). While she is on oral phosphate and calcitriol, she should have intermittent kidney ultrasonography to monitor for nephrocalcinosis.

Case 3

A 47-year-old woman with osteopenia and history of vitamin D deficiency presents with intermittent low serum phosphate levels that range from 1.6 mg/dL (0.5 mmol/L) to 3.4 mg/dL (1.1 mmol/L) (reference range, 2.4-4.3 mg/dL [0.8-1.4 mmol/L]) over a few years. She does not consume dairy in her diet or take calcium/vitamin D supplements. On further workup, her kidney function is normal.

Laboratory test results:

> Serum calcium = 8.7 mg/dL (8.8-10.7 mg/dL)
>   (SI: 2.2 mmol/L [SI: 2.2-2.7 mmol/L])
> Serum PTH = 73 pg/mL (15-65 pg/mL)
>   (SI: 7.7 pmol/L [1.6-6.9 pmol/L])
> 25-Hydroxyvitamin D = 20 ng/dL (SI: 50 nmol/L)
> FGF-23 = 23 pg/mL (SI: >59 pg/mL)
> Serum phosphate = 3.1 mg/dL (2.4-4.3 mg/dL)
>   (SI: 1.0 mmol/L [0.8-1.4 mmol/L])
> Calcium-to-creatinine ratio = 0.004
> TmP/GFR = 2.8 mg/dL (2.6-3.8 mg/dL)
>   (SI: 0.9 mmol/L [0.8-1.2 mmol/L])

Which of the following is the most likely etiology of this patient's hypophosphatemia?

A. Inadequate calcium and phosphate intake

B. XLH

C. Primary hyperparathyroidism

D. Vitamin D deficiency

E. Fanconi syndrome

Answer: A) Inadequate calcium and phosphate intake

Patients with XLH (Answer B) can have inappropriately normal serum FGF-23 levels in the setting of hypophosphatemia. However, at the time of laboratory blood draw, this patient had normal serum FGF-23 and phosphate levels, making XLH an unlikely diagnosis.

This patient's laboratory workup shows a low-normal serum calcium level accompanied by a low renal calcium-to-creatinine ratio. In primary hyperparathyroidism, elevated PTH levels are accompanied by normal or elevated serum calcium levels and normal or increased urine calcium-to-creatinine ratio, thus ruling out the diagnosis of primary hyperparathyroidism (Answer C).

Impaired vitamin D action can lead to decreased renal resorption and intestinal reabsorption of calcium and phosphate, resulting in low serum calcium and phosphate levels and secondary hyperparathyroidism. However, this patient's serum vitamin D levels are normal per the Institute of Medicine guidelines. Therefore, she currently does not meet the criterion for vitamin D deficiency (Answer D).

Fanconi syndrome (Answer E) is characterized by renal phosphate wasting. This patient has a normal TmP/GFR, making Fanconi syndrome an unlikely diagnosis.

This patient has a history of vitamin D deficiency, low-normal serum calcium, and a low renal calcium-to-creatinine ratio, supporting a history of low dietary intake of calcium and phosphate. The serum PTH levels are likely elevated secondary to the decrease in serum calcium, where this elevation in PTH results in increased loss of urinary phosphate, which in combination with inadequate dietary dairy intake leads to low serum phosphate. The intermittent nature of the hypophosphatemia may be due to inconsistent dietary intake of calcium- and phosphate-rich foods (Answer A).

Case 3, Continued

Which of the following initial treatments for hypophosphatemia would be appropriate to offer this patient?

A. Start burosumab

B. Start cinacalet

C. Start ergocalciferol, 50,000 international units weekly (1250 mcg weekly)

D. Start oral phosphate supplements

E. Encourage dairy intake and start calcium and cholecalciferol supplements

Answer: E) Encourage dairy intake and start calcium and cholecalciferol supplements

Burosumab (Answer A) is a humanized FGF-23–blocking antibody that is FDA approved for the treatment of XLH and TIO. Since it unlikely that this patient has either diagnosis, there is no indication to start this therapy.

Cinacalcet (Answer B) is a calcimimetic that acts as an allosteric activator of the calcium-sensing receptor, leading to a decrease in serum PTH and calcium levels. It is often used as adjuvant therapy for patients with hypercalcemia mediated by high serum PTH levels. Since this patient has low serum calcium levels, cinacalcet would not be the appropriate therapy.

The 2024 Endocrine Society guidelines recommend that a generally heathy adult should adhere to the recommended daily allowance of vitamin D established by the Institute of Medicine. According to these guidelines, the recommended daily allowance of vitamin D_3 is 600 international units (15 mcg) for adults 70 years and younger and 800 international units (20 mcg) for adults older than 71 years.[18] Therefore, this patient should be encouraged to initiate vitamin D supplements to meet the daily intake recommendation (Answer E), but since she is not vitamin D deficient (per serum 25-hydroxyvitamin D levels), she does not need to be treated for vitamin D deficiency with ergocalciferol (Answer C).

The intermittent low serum phosphate levels may be secondary to low dairy intake and mild hyperparathyroidism in the setting of low calcium intake. Therefore, while oral phosphate supplements (Answer D) would improve serum phosphate levels, they would not address the primary issue of low dietary intake of calcium and phosphate. Also, oral phosphate supplements result in comorbidities, including worsening secondary hyperparathyroidism and nephrocalcinosis.

It is likely that this patient has inadequate dietary intake of calcium and phosphate. Since the Institute of Medicine recommends a daily dietary intake of 1000 mg calcium from diet or supplements for women younger than 50 years, this patient should be encouraged to take a balance of dairy and calcium supplements to meet the daily recommended calcium intake (Answer E).

Key Learning Points

- PTH, FGF-23, and 1,25-dihydroxyvitamin D_3 are key hormones that regulate phosphate homeostasis.

- Multiple causes for hypophosphatemia exist, which can be divided into FGF-23 and non–FGF-23–mediated disorders.

- Oral phosphate supplements should be accompanied by calcitriol to prevent secondary hyperparathyroidism.

- In patients with continued high PTH levels, burosumab may need to be accompanied by additional agents, such as cinacalcet, to decrease serum PTH and/or calcium levels.

References

1. Imel EA, Econs MJ. Approach to the hypophosphatemic patient. *J Clin Endocrinol Metab.* 2012;97(3):696-706. PMID: 22392950

2. Sabbagh Y, Carpenter TO, Demay MB. Hypophosphatemia leads to rickets by impairing caspase-mediated apoptosis of hypertrophic chondrocytes. *Proc Natl Acad Sci.* 2005;102(27):9637-9642. PMID: 15976027

3. Nordin BEC, ed. Calcium, *Phosphate, and Magnesium Metabolism: Clinical Physiology and Diagnostic Procedures.* Longman; 1976.

4. Tenenhouse HS. Cellular and molecular mechanisms of renal phosphate transport. J Bone Miner Res. 1997;12(2):159-164. PMID: 9041046

5. Sabbagh Y, Giral H, Caldas Y, Levi M, Schiavi SC. Intestinal phosphate transport. *Adv Chronic Kidney Dis.* 2011;18(2):85-90. PMID: 21406292

6. Murer H, Hernando N, Forster I, Biber J. Proximal tubular phosphate reabsorption: molecular mechanisms. *Physiol Rev.* 2000;80(4):1373-1409. PMID: 11015617

7. Hewison M, Bouillon R, Giovannucci E, Goltzman D, Meyer M, Welsh J. *Feldman and Pike's Vitamin D: Volume 2: Disease and Therapeutics.* Elsevier; 2024.

8. Carpenter TO, Imel EA, Holm IA, Jan de Beur SM, Insogna KL. A clinician's guide to X-linked hypophosphatemia. J Bone Miner Res. 2011;26(7):1381-1388. PMID: 21538511

9. Insogna KL, Rauch F, Kamenicky P, et al. Burosumab improved histomorphometric measures of osteomalacia in adults with X-linked hypophosphatemia: a phase 3, single-arm, international trial. J Bone Miner Res. 2019;34(12):2183-2191. PMID: 31369697

10. Insogna KL, Briot K, Imel EA, et al; AXLES 1 Investigators. A randomized, double-blind, placebo-controlled, phase 3 trial evaluating the efficacy of burosumab, an anti-FGF23 antibody, in adults with X-linked hypophosphatemia: week 24 primary analysis. *J Bone Miner Res.* 2018;33(8):1383-1393. PMID: 29947093

11. El-Maouche D, Sadowski SM, Papadakis GZ, et al. ^{68}Ga-DOTATATE for tumor localization in tumor-induced osteomalacia. *J Clin Endocrinol Metab.* 2016;101(10):3575-3581. PMID: 27533306

12. Jan de Beur SM, Miller PD, Weber TJ, et al. Burosumab for the treatment of tumor-induced osteomalacia. *J Bone Miner Res.* 2021;36(4):627-635. PMID: 33338281

13. Collins MT, Singer FR, Eugster E. McCune-Albright syndrome and the extraskeletal manifestations of fibrous dysplasia. *Orphanet J Rare Dis.* 2012;7(Suppl 1):S4. PMID: 22640971

14. Briot K, Portale AA, Brandi ML, et al. Burosumab treatment in adults with X-linked hypophosphataemia: 96-week patient-reported outcomes and ambulatory function from a randomised phase 3 trial and open-label extension. *RMD Open.* 2021;7(3):e001714. PMID: 34548383

15. Zhukouskaya VEA, Berkenou J, Audrain C, Bardet C, Chaussain C, Rothenbuhler A, Linglart A. Hyperparathyroidism after 3 years of burosumab in children affected with X-linked hypophosphatemia. *Annales d'Endocrinologie.* 2023;84(5):544.

16. Takashi, Y. et al. Combined treatment by burosumab and a calcimimetic can ameliorate hypophosphatemia due to excessive actions of FGF23 and PTH in adult XLH with tertiary hyperparathyroidism: a case report. *Front Endocrinol (Lausanne).* 2022;13:1004624. PMID: 36531500

17. Alon US, Levy-Olomucki R, Moore WV, Stubbs J, Liu S, Quarles D. Calcimimetics as an adjuvant treatment for familial hypophosphatemic rickets. *Clin J Am Soc Nephrol.* 2008;3(3):658-664. PMID: 18256372

18. Demay MB, Pittas AG, Bikle DD, et al. Vitamin D for the prevention of disease: an Endocrine Society clinical practice guideline. *J Clin Endocrinol.* 2014;109(8):1907-1947. PMID: 38828931

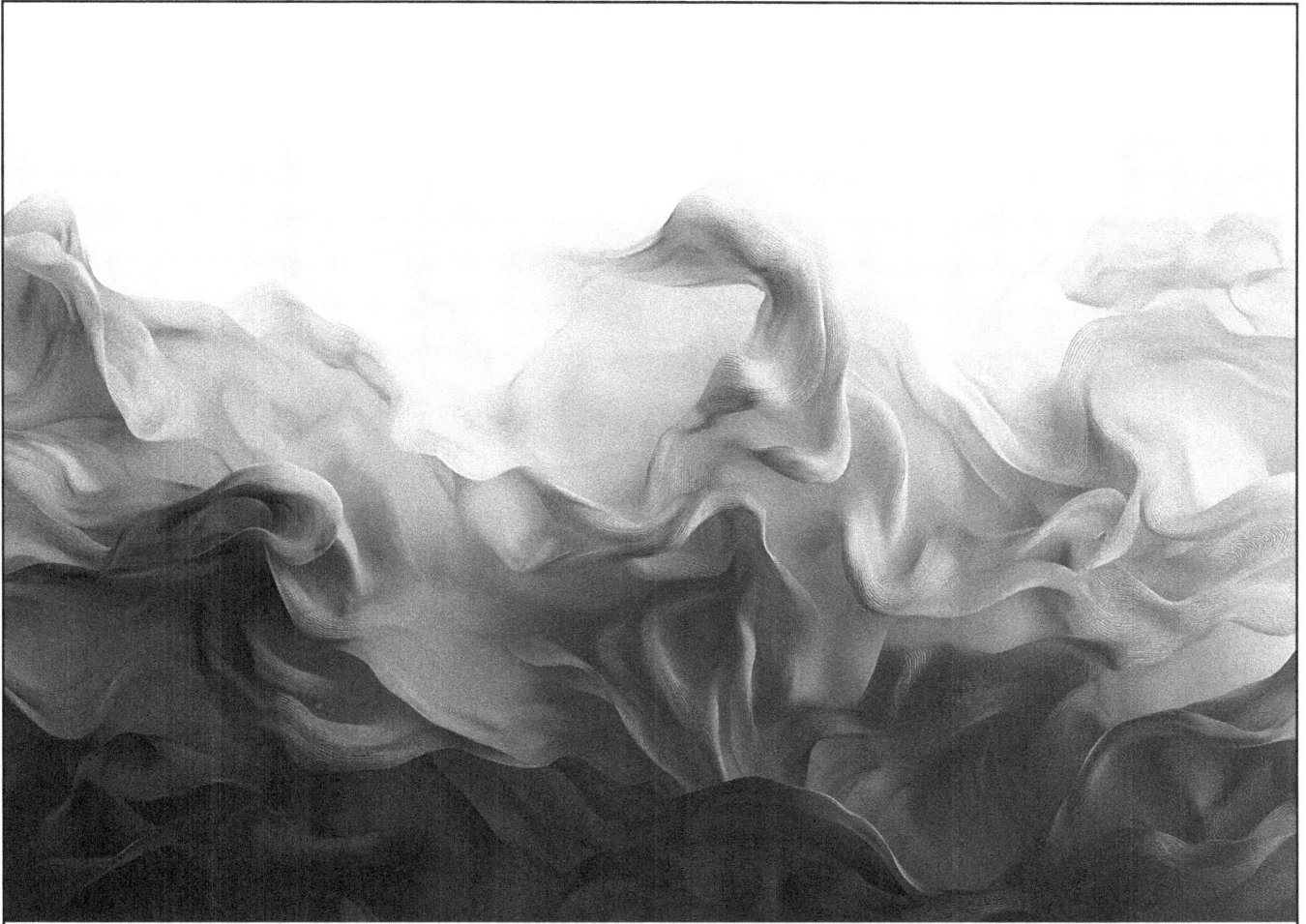

CARDIOVASCULAR
ENDOCRINOLOGY

Management of Patients With Elevated Lipoprotein(a)

David Saxon, MD, MSc. Division of Endocrinology, Metabolism, and Diabetes, University of Colorado School of Medicine, Rocky Mountain Regional VAMC, Aurora, CO; Email: david.saxon@cuanschutz.edu

Educational Objectives

After reviewing this chapter, learners should be able to:

- Identify the role of lipoprotein(a) (Lp[a]) as an independent cardiovascular risk factor and describe its pathophysiologic mechanisms.

- Explain current guideline recommendations for Lp(a) screening and identify practice gaps that contribute to its underuse in clinical practice.

- Evaluate available and emerging strategies for managing patients with elevated Lp(a), including risk factor modification, lipid apheresis, and investigational therapies in clinical trials.

Significance of the Clinical Problem

Cardiovascular disease (CVD) remains a leading cause of death worldwide.[1] Advancements in pharmacologic therapy and public health interventions have substantially reduced morbidity and mortality; however, even among aggressively treated patients in the setting of secondary prevention, residual risk persists for atherosclerotic cardiovascular disease (ASCVD). A unique target for addressing residual risk is Lp(a), a lipoprotein structurally similar to LDL but distinguished by the presence of apolipoprotein (a) (apo a), which is covalently bound to apolipoprotein B_{100} (apo B). Lp(a) is highly variable in size (300-800 kDa) due to more than 40 isoforms and 10 apo(a) subtypes, and it possesses proatherogenic, proinflammatory, and prothrombotic properties, the latter characteristic owing to apo(a) being homologous to plasminogen.[2]

Lp(a) levels above 30 mg/dL (>75 nmol/L) are associated with increased ASCVD risk and are thought to be elevated in more than 1.4 billion people worldwide.[3] Lp(a) levels of 50 mg/dL or higher (≥125 nmol/L) or higher are associated with very high risk of ASCVD and can increase the calculated 10-year ASCVD risk. Elevated levels are also a risk factor for stroke and calcific aortic stenosis. In a global population with established CVD, elevated Lp(a) levels were observed in the following proportions: 27.9% had levels greater than 50 mg/dL (>125 nmol/L), 20.7% had levels greater than 70 mg/dL (>175 nmol/L), 12.9% had levels greater than 90 mg/dL (>225 nmol/L), and 26.0% had levels greater than 150 mg/dL (>375 nmol/L).[4]

Lp(a) was first identified in 1963 by Kare Berg, and subsequent decades of research have provided a comprehensive understanding of its epidemiology, genetics, physiology, and pathophysiology. Its levels are largely genetically determined, driven by the codominant expression of 2 *LPA* alleles. However, nongenetic factors such as pregnancy, menopause, hypothyroidism, and kidney insufficiency or failure may increase Lp(a). Accurate measurement of Lp(a) is challenging due to the variable size of apo(a), and results can be confusing because 2 different measurement approaches are used—either mg/dL or nmol/L.

Clinicians may encounter both forms of measurement in practice, but the recommended gold standard ELISA method is calibrated in nmol/L, thus reflecting the number of Lp(a) particles.[2]

Practice Gaps

- Screening for Lp(a) remains underused, reflecting a lack of awareness about current guidelines and the importance of identifying this condition.

- There is a lack of clinical consensus on how to care for patients with elevated Lp(a), leaving many clinicians unsure about the optimal approach.

- While no medications specifically targeting elevated Lp(a) are FDA-approved, endocrinologists should be aware of several ongoing phase 3 clinical trials of such therapies.

Discussion

As previously mentioned, elevated Lp(a) levels are an independent risk factor for CVD, stroke, and calcific aortic stenosis. However, despite widespread acceptance of the health risks posed by elevated Lp(a), rates of Lp(a) screening are very low, perhaps because no proven targeted therapies to lower Lp(a) thus far exist. In one analysis of Lp(a) testing in individuals with various CVD conditions and individuals undergoing cardiac testing across 6 academic medical centers associated with the University of California from 2012 to 2021, only 0.3% of more than 5.5 million people had undergone Lp(a) testing.[5]

Now is a pivotal time for endocrinologists to deepen their understanding of Lp(a), as recent clinical guideline recommendations are shaping Lp(a) testing practices, strategies have emerged to guide the management of patients with elevated Lp(a), and promising therapies are advancing through clinical trials with the potential to transform care.

Clinical Guideline Recommendations Regarding Lp(a) Testing

Evolving societal guideline recommendations and statements highlight the growing role of Lp(a) measurement in CVD risk stratification and reinforce the need for broader clinical awareness of this condition. In the 2018 Multisociety Cholesterol Guidelines, Lp(a) was considered a risk enhancer, and testing was suggested in those with a family history of premature ASCVD or unexplained ASCVD who did not have major risk factors. However, universal Lp(a) screening was not recommended.[6] Subsequently, between 2019 and 2022, several guidelines and statements from Canada and Europe identified Lp(a) as a cardiovascular risk enhancer and went further by recommending testing at least once in all adults.[7-9] The 2020 Endocrine Society Clinical Practice Guideline on Lipid Management in Patients with Endocrine Disorders recommended Lp(a) measurement in adults with a family history of premature ASCVD or a personal history of ASCVD, or a family history of high Lp(a).[10] In 2024, the National Lipid Association published an Lp(a) Scientific Statement that advised testing all adults at least once for Lp(a) and recommended selective screening in high-risk youth (<18 years old) with suspected or confirmed familial hypercholesterolemia, ischemic stroke of unknown cause, a first-degree relative with premature ASCVD, or a first-degree relative with elevated Lp(a).[11]

Current Approach to Care of Patients With High Lp(a)

In patients without a history of ASCVD who have high Lp(a), cardiovascular risk factors should be evaluated, including LDL cholesterol (LDL-C), blood pressure, cigarette smoking history, and venous thrombosis, and management of these risk factors should be intensified. Imaging of coronary artery calcium (CAC) should be considered because CAC scores of 100 or greater in patients with the highest Lp(a) levels (upper quintile) are associated with increased ASCVD risk.[12] Since no targeted pharmacologic therapy indicated for Lp(a) lowering currently exists, current CVD risk reduction in the face of elevated Lp(a) should focus on aggressive management of modifiable traditional risk factors. Recently, reviews by Reyes-Soffer et al and Ellberg and Bhatia outlined strategies that can be used to manage patients with elevated Lp(a) based on current available evidence.[13,14] *Table 1* summarizes interventions for reducing LDL-C and Lp(a).

Therapies Under Investigation for Lp(a) Lowering

Now is an exciting time for targeted Lp(a) therapies, with at least 5 drugs currently in development that work through various mechanisms (*Table 2*). Among these, 3 therapies—pelacarsen, olpasiran, and lepodisiran—are either fully enrolled or actively enrolling in phase 3 cardiovascular outcome trials.[15-17] Approval of these medications will require evidence that they reduce Lp(a) and provide cardiovascular benefit.

Table 1. Approach to Treatment of Elevated Lp(a)

Treatment modality	Mechanism and rationale	Considerations
Statin therapy	Reduces overall CVD risk but does not lower—and may slightly increase—Lp(a) levels; residual risk can be mitigated by aggressive LDL-C or apo B lowering	Essential for overall risk reduction, but does not address Lp(a)-specific risk
PCSK9 inhibitors (evolocumab, alirocumab)	Lowers LDL-C and reduces Lp(a) levels by ~23%-27%	Not FDA-approved for Lp(a) lowering; potential role in residual risk management
Lipid apheresis	The only FDA-approved treatment for high Lp(a); removes apo B–containing lipoproteins, including Lp(a)	Reserved for patients at highest risk with Lp(a) >60 mg/dL (>150 nmol/L) and LDL-C >100 mg/dL (>2.59 mmol/L) with CVD
Aspirin in primary prevention	Potentially beneficial in patients at high risk with elevated Lp(a)	Not broadly recommended for primary prevention but may have selective benefit
Prolonged DAPT in secondary prevention	Extended DAPT (>1 year) may reduce CVD risk in patients with high Lp(a)	May benefit select secondary prevention patients with high Lp(a); further validation needed
Cascade screening of family members	Identifies individuals at risk through familial testing	Recommended by guidelines for family screening, particularly in familial hypercholesterolemia programs
Enrollment in clinical trials	Emerging Lp(a)-targeted therapies under investigation	Future Lp(a)-lowering therapies may transform treatment strategies

Abbreviations: CVD, cardiovascular disease; DAPT, dual antiplatelet therapy; LDL-C, low-density lipoprotein cholesterol; Lp(a), lipoprotein (a).

Table 2. Targeted Lp(a) Therapies in Development

Drug Name	Mechanism	Lp(a) lowering and administration frequency	Trial name and stage
Pelacarsen	Antisense oligonucleotide	~80%; once monthly injection	Phase 3: HORIZON (fully enrolled)
Olpasiran	Small interfering RNA	90%+; every 6 months injection	Phase 3: OCEAN(a) (fully enrolled)
Lepodisiran	Small interfering RNA	90%+; every 6 months injection	Phase 3: ACCLAIM-Lp(a) (enrolling)
Zerlasiran	Small interfering RNA	80%+; every 4- or 6-months injection in phase 2 trial	Phase 2: completed
Muvalaplin	Oral small molecule inhibitor	47.6%-85.8% reductions in phase 2 study using various daily oral doses	Phase 2: completed

These investigational treatments use different approaches, including antisense oligonucleotides, small interfering RNA molecules, and an oral small molecule inhibitor, some of which have demonstrated the ability to reduce Lp(a) levels between 80% and 99%. Additionally, these medications vary in their dosing schedules, with some administered as infrequently as every 6 months. The HORIZON trial, evaluating pelacarsen, is the furthest along, with an expected completion date in early 2026.

Clinical Case Vignettes

Case 1

A 45-year-old man with hypertension and a family history of premature coronary artery disease (father had a myocardial infarction at age 50 years) presents for a routine CVD risk assessment.

Lipid panel:

> LDL-C =110 mg/dL (SI: 2.85 mmol/L)
> HDL-C = 48 mg/dL (SI: 1.24 mmol/L)
> Triglycerides = 120 mg/dL (SI: 1.36 mmol/L)

He has never been tested for Lp(a).

According to the 2024 National Lipid Association Scientific Statement, which of the following is the most appropriate approach to Lp(a) testing in this patient?

A. No testing is needed unless he develops clinical ASCVD

B. Lp(a) testing is reasonable as part of routine adult screening

C. Lp(a) testing is only recommended in patients with LDL-C >190 mg/dL (>4.92 mmol/L)

D. Lp(a) testing should only be performed in the presence of familial hypercholesterolemia

E. Lp(a) testing is only indicated if the patient has a first-degree relative with Lp(a) >40 mg/dL (>100 nmol/L)

Answer: B) Lp(a) testing is reasonable as part of routine adult screening

The 2024 National Lipid Association Scientific Statement recommends that all adults have Lp(a) measured at least once (Answer B), as Lp(a) is largely genetically determined and remains stable over a lifetime. Testing can help identify individuals at increased risk for ASCVD, particularly those who may not have other traditional risk factors.

Lp(a) screening is recommended regardless of whether a person has already developed clinical ASCVD (thus, Answer A is incorrect). Waiting until ASCVD manifests may delay appropriate risk assessment and preventive strategies.

Lp(a) testing is not limited to individuals with an LDL-C value greater than 190 mg/dL (>4.92 mmol/L), although it is particularly relevant in this population (thus, Answer C is incorrect).

While individuals with familial hypercholesterolemia should be screened for Lp(a), testing is recommended for all adults, not just those with familial hypercholesterolemia (thus, Answer D is incorrect).

A first-degree relative with elevated Lp(a) is an indication for selective screening in youth, but this criterion does not apply to general adult screening, which is advised for everyone at least once in their lifetime (thus, Answer E is incorrect).

Case 2

A 58-year-old woman with a history of myocardial infarction at age 52 years, hypertension, and type 2 diabetes presents for CVD risk assessment. She is asymptomatic but is concerned about her long-term heart health. Her current medications include atorvastatin, 40 mg daily; ezetimibe, 10 mg daily; metformin, 1000 mg twice daily; and lisinopril, 10 mg daily.

Laboratory test results:

> Total cholesterol = 180 mg/dL (SI: 4.65 mmol/L)
> LDL-C = 78 mg/dL (SI: 2.02 mmol/L)
> High-density lipoprotein cholesterol (HDL-C) = 42 mg/dL (SI: 1.09 mmol/L)
> Triglycerides = 120 mg/dL (SI: 1.36 mmol/L)
> Apo B = 85 mg/dL (0.85 g/L)
> Lp(a) = 52 mg/dL (SI: 130 nmol/L)

Her blood pressure is well controlled at 118/72 mm Hg. She does not smoke cigarettes. She exercises regularly and has a healthy diet. Her father had a myocardial infarction at age 50, and her younger brother, age 55 years, recently underwent coronary artery bypass grafting.

She expresses concern about her elevated Lp(a) and asks about treatment options. You change the dosage of atorvastatin to 80 mg daily to further lower LDL-C.

Which of the following is the most appropriate next step in her lipid management?

A. Switch atorvastatin to simvastatin to lower Lp(a)

B. Initiate a PCSK9 inhibitor to lower both LDL-C and Lp(a)

C. Recommend lipid apheresis

D. Discontinue statin therapy, as it may increase Lp(a) levels

Answer: B) Initiate a PCSK9 inhibitor to lower both LDL-C and Lp(a)

PCSK9 inhibitors (evolocumab, alirocumab) lower LDL-C and have been shown in clinical trials to reduce Lp(a) levels by approximately 23% to 27%. This makes them an appropriate next step in patients at high risk who have elevated Lp(a) and residual ASCVD risk despite treatment with a high-intensity statin plus ezetimibe. This patient would benefit from the addition of a medication that targets PCSK9 (monoclonal antibodies to PCSK9 or a small interfering RNA) (Answer B). The PCSK9 inhibitor would reduce LDL-C further and may also reduce Lp(a) by 23% to 27% to mitigate some of the Lp(a)-associated risk. Another option for lowering LDL-C would be to switch atorvastatin to rosuvastatin, 20 or 40 mg daily. An LDL-C concentration of 78 mg/dL (2.02 mmol/L) is too high for a patient with a history of myocardial infarction.

Switching atorvastatin to simvastatin to lower Lp(a) (Answer A) is incorrect because while statins lower LDL-C effectively, they do not reduce Lp(a) levels and may even cause a slight increase. Also, simvastatin has less LDL-C–lowering potential than high-dosage atorvastatin. The 80 mg dosage of atorvastatin is the highest available. Increasing the statin dosage would reduce LDL-C and ASCVD risk, but it would not directly address the patient's Lp(a)-mediated risk.

Lipid apheresis (Answer C) is typically reserved for patients at very high risk of ASCVD who have both severely elevated Lp(a) and uncontrolled LDL-C (>100 mg/dL [>2.59 mmol/L]) despite maximal lipid-lowering therapy. This patient's LDL-C concentration was 78 mg/dL (2.02 mmol/L) on atorvastatin, 40 mg daily. Given the potential for additional medication adjustments to further lower LDL-C, lipid apheresis is not currently necessary.

Discontinuing statin therapy (Answer D) is incorrect because statins remain a cornerstone of CVD prevention and significantly reduce ASCVD risk. While statins do not lower Lp(a), stopping this therapy would remove a critical intervention for LDL-C reduction and overall CVD risk management.

Case 3

A 56-year-old man with a history of premature coronary artery disease, hypertension, and hyperlipidemia presents for lipid management. He underwent percutaneous coronary intervention at age 50 years and has since been on maximally tolerated statin therapy plus ezetimibe. His LDL-C remains well-controlled at 58 mg/dL (1.50 mmol/L), but his Lp(a) level is markedly elevated at 85 mg/dL (210 nmol/L). He has a strong family history of early myocardial infarction, with his father experiencing a myocardial infarction at age 48 years. The patient is concerned about his residual CVD risk and asks about emerging treatments for Lp(a) lowering.

Which of the following investigational therapies could the patient be informed about that are in phase 3 trials for Lp(a) lowering and reduction of CVD risk?

A. Inclisiran, evinacumab, and bempedoic acid

B. Niacin, colesevelam, and icosapent ethyl

C. Anacetrapib, lomitapide, and mipomersen

D. Pelacarsen, olpasiran, and lepodisiran

Answer: D) Pelacarsen, olpasiran, and lepodisiran

Pelacarsen, olpasiran, and lepodisiran (Answer D) are investigational therapies currently in phase 3 clinical outcome trials specifically targeting Lp(a) lowering and reduction in CVD risk. These agents are antisense oligonucleotides (pelacarsen) or small interfering RNAs (olpasiran and lepodisiran) designed to reduce hepatic *LPA* gene expression, thereby lowering Lp(a) levels, which have been implicated in residual CVD risk.

While inclisiran, evinacumab, and bempedoic acid (Answer A) are used in lipid management, they do not primarily target Lp(a). Inclisiran is a small interfering RNA that reduces PCSK9 levels, leading to LDL-C lowering, but it has minimal impact on Lp(a). Evinacumab is an ANGPTL3 inhibitor approved for LDL-C lowering in individuals with homozygous familial hypercholesterolemia, and it does not substantially affect Lp(a). Bempedoic acid inhibits ATP citrate lyase to reduce LDL-C, but it has no significant role in Lp(a) reduction.

Niacin, colesevelam, and icosapent ethyl (Answer B) are not in phase 3 trials for Lp(a) lowering. While niacin can modestly reduce Lp(a), it is no longer recommended for this purpose due to a lack of cardiovascular outcome benefit and poor tolerability. Colesevelam is a bile acid sequestrant that primarily lowers LDL-C and has no meaningful effect on Lp(a). Icosapent ethyl, an omega-3 fatty acid derivative, has demonstrated cardiovascular benefits in patients with moderate hypertriglyceridemia, but it does not lower Lp(a).

Anacetrapib, lomitapide, and mipomersen (Answer C) are lipid-altering drugs that are either not in phase 3 trials or are no longer clinically relevant. Anacetrapib is a CETP inhibitor that was shown to modestly lower Lp(a), but it is not available for clinical use. Lomitapide is used for homozygous familial hypercholesterolemia, and it does not significantly affect Lp(a). Mipomersen, an antisense oligonucleotide targeting apo B_{100}, was withdrawn from the market due to safety concerns and is not an Lp(a)-lowering therapy.

Key Learning Points

- Lp(a) is an independent risk factor for ASCVD, stroke, and calcific aortic stenosis. Genetics determines Lp(a) levels in 90% of people with high Lp(a). Its proatherogenic, proinflammatory, and prothrombotic properties contribute to residual CVD risk, even in patients with well-controlled LDL-C.

- Despite its recognized role in cardiovascular risk stratification, Lp(a) screening remains infrequent in clinical practice. The 2024 National Lipid Association Scientific Statement advises that all adults should have Lp(a) measured at least once in their lifetime.

- While no FDA-approved pharmacologic therapy exists for Lp(a) lowering, current management focuses on aggressive LDL-C and overall CVD risk reduction. Strategies include statins (despite their neutral or slight Lp[a]-raising effect), PCSK9 inhibitors (which modestly lower Lp[a] by ~25%), lipid apheresis for patients at high risk, and extended antiplatelet therapy in select patients.

- A new generation of targeted Lp(a)-lowering therapies, including pelacarsen, olpasiran, and lepodisiran, have shown promising reductions in Lp(a) levels of greater than 80%. These investigational drugs are in phase 3 clinical trials with CVD end points.

References

1. GBD 2017 Causes of Death Collaborators. Global, regional, and national age-sex-specific mortality for 282 causes of death in 195 countries and territories, 1980–2017: a systematic analysis for the Global Burden of Disease Study 2017. *Lancet.* 2018;392(10159):1736-1788. PMID: 30496103

2. Reyes-Soffer G, Ginsberg HN, Berglund L, et al. Lipoprotein(a): a genetically determined, causal, and prevalent risk factor for atherosclerotic cardiovascular disease: a scientific statement from the American Heart Association. *Arterioscler Thromb Vasc Biol.* 2022;42(1):e48-e60. PMID: 34647487

3. Tsimikas S, Fazio S, Ferdinand KC, et al. NHLBI Working Group recommendations to reduce risk of cardiovascular disease and aortic stenosis. *J Am Coll Cardiol.* 2018;71(2):177-192. PMID: 29325642

4. 4. Nissen SE, Wolski K, Cho L, et al. Lipoprotein(a) levels in a global population with established atherosclerotic cardiovascular disease. *Open Heart.* 2022;9(2):e002060. PMID: 36252994

5. Bhatia HS, Hurst S, Desai P, Zhu W, Yeang C. Lipoprotein(a) testing trends in a large academic health system in the United States. *J Am Heart Assoc.* 2023;12(18):e031255. PMID: 37702041

6. Grundy SM, Stone NJ, Bailey AL, et al. 2018 AHA/ACC/AACVPR/AAPA/ABC/ACPM/ADA/AGS/APhA/ASPC/NLA/PCNA Guideline on the Management of Blood Cholesterol: A Report of the American College of Cardiology/American Heart Association Task Force on Clinical Practice Guidelines. *J Am Coll Cardiol.* 2019;73(24):e285-e350. PMID: 30586774

7. Authors/Task Force Members, ESC Committee for Practice Guidelines (CPG), ESC National Cardiac Societies. 2019 ESC/EAS guidelines for the management of dyslipidaemias: lipid modification to reduce cardiovascular risk. *Atherosclerosis.* 2019;290:140-205. PMID: 31591002

8. 8. Pearson GJ, Thanassoulis G, Anderson TJ, et al. 2021 Canadian Cardiovascular Society guidelines for the management of dyslipidemia for the prevention of cardiovascular disease in adults. *Can J Cardiol.* 2021;37(8):1129-1150. PMID: 33781847

9. Kronenberg F, Mora S, Stroes ESG, et al. Lipoprotein(a) in atherosclerotic cardiovascular disease and aortic stenosis: a European Atherosclerosis Society consensus statement. *Eur Heart J.* 2022;43(39):3925-3946. PMID: 36036785

10. Newman CB, Blaha MJ, Boord JB, et al. Lipid management in patients with endocrine disorders: an Endocrine Society clinical practice guideline. *J Clin Endocrinol Metab.* 2020;105(12):dgaa674. PMID: 32951056

11. Koschinsky ML, Bajaj A, Boffa MB, et al. A focused update to the 2019 NLA scientific statement on use of lipoprotein(a) in clinical practice. *J Clin Lipidol.* 2024;18(3):e308-e319. PMID: 38565461

12. Mehta A, Vasquez N, Ayers CR, et al. Independent association of lipoprotein(a) and coronary artery calcification with atherosclerotic cardiovascular risk. *J Am Coll Cardiol.* 2022;79(8):757-768. PMID: 35210030

13. Reyes-Soffer G, Yeang C, Michos ED, Boatwright W, Ballantyne CM. High lipoprotein(a): Actionable strategies for risk assessment and mitigation. *Am J Prev Cardiol.* 2024;18:100651. PMID: 38646021

14. Ellberg CC, Bhatia HS. Strategies for management of patients with elevated lipoprotein(a). *Curr Opin Lipidol.* 2024;35(5):234-240. PMID: 39145610

15. Tsimikas S, Karwatowska-Prokopczuk E, Gouni-Berthold I, et al; AKCEA-APO(a)-LRx Study Investigators. Lipoprotein(a) reduction in persons with cardiovascular disease. *N Engl J Med.* 2020;382(3):244-255. PMID: 31893580

16. O'Donoghue ML, Rosenson RS, Gencer B, et al. Small interfering RNA to reduce lipoprotein(a) in cardiovascular disease. *N Engl J Med.* 2022;387(20):1855-1864. PMID: 36342163

17. Nissen SE, Linnebjerg H, Shen X, et al. Lepodisiran, an extended-duration short interfering RNA targeting lipoprotein(a): a randomized dose-ascending clinical trial. *JAMA.* 2023;330(21):2075-2083. PMID: 37952254

Interpreting Adrenal Vein Sampling

Michael Stowasser, MBBS, PhD. Endocrine Hypertension Research Centre, University of Queensland Frazer Institute, Princess Alexandra Hospital, Brisbane, Australia; Email: m.stowasser@uq.edu.au

Educational Objectives

After reviewing this chapter, learners should be able to:

- Describe implementation strategies that, when applied before and during adrenal vein sampling (AVS), can enhance procedure success and interpretability of results.

- Determine, based on AVS results, whether successful adrenal vein cannulation has been achieved and whether the patient has a bilateral or unilateral variety of primary aldosteronism (PA).

- Identify factors that can lead to inconclusive AVS results and steps that can be undertaken to overcome them.

Significance of the Clinical Problem

Accounting for at least 5% to 13% of patients with hypertension, PA is now recognized to be the most prevalent and specifically treatable (potentially curable) secondary endocrine form.[1,2] Detection is paramount, as these patients are at considerably higher risk of cardiovascular and kidney morbidity compared with blood pressure–matched patients with essential hypertension, and yet this increased morbidity is ameliorated and quality of life is improved by surgical intervention (unilateral adrenalectomy [ADX]) or medical treatment (most commonly mineralocorticoid receptor antagonist [MRA]) specifically directed toward addressing aldosterone excess.[3] Approximately 25% of patients with PA have unilateral forms (most commonly aldosterone-producing adenoma [APA]), for which ADX has the potential to cure or markedly improve control of hypertension and biochemical PA. In contrast, ADX is rarely undertaken in patients with bilateral PA (who make up most of the remainder of cases), as it is much less likely to provide such clinical and biochemical benefits. Instead, patients with bilateral PA are usually treated with MRAs. As a group, surgically treated patients demonstrate superior outcomes in terms of hypertension control, incidence of cardiovascular and kidney morbidities, and improved quality of life compared with patients with PA who are treated with MRAs.[4] Distinguishing unilateral from bilateral PA is therefore a critical step in the selection of optimal treatment options.

Because adrenal imaging by CT or MRI lacks reliability, and newer scintigraphic approaches, while promising, are still in development, AVS remains the favored approach for distinguishing unilateral from bilateral forms of PA. Guidelines suggest that AVS be performed in almost all patients diagnosed with PA who desire and are otherwise suitable candidates for ADX should they be found to have unilateral disease.[2] However, AVS is not widely available and requires considerable expertise to ensure acceptable rates of cannulation success, generation of reliable data, and correct result interpretation. In the wake of new clinical guidelines that currently recommend screening for PA among all patients with hypertension,[5] the demand for AVS is likely to increase markedly in coming years, making it timely and of vital importance to upscale availability of this important procedure and ensure it is performed correctly and results are interpreted accurately.

Practice Gaps

- There is an urgent need to expand AVS services to meet the demand among a rapidly growing number of patients being diagnosed with PA.

- There is a lack of awareness of optimal approaches to prepare patients for AVS, skillfully perform the procedure, and accurately interpret results.

- Disparity exists among institutions regarding how AVS is performed and how results are interpreted.

Discussion

AVS involves cannulation of both adrenal veins and measuring aldosterone and cortisol levels in adrenal vein (AV) and peripheral vein (PV) samples. There are numerous variations in AVS protocols related to patient preparation, performance of the procedure, and interpretation of results. Guidelines attempting to harmonize AVS approaches have thus recently been developed.[6,7]

Patient Preparation

Before performing AVS, potentially confounding factors should be controlled when possible. Lateralization on AVS depends on the gland contralateral to the source of aldosterone excess being suppressed in terms of aldosterone production. This, in turn, depends on the renin-angiotensin II system (RAS) also being suppressed. Certain factors (eg, medications) that stimulate the RAS may lead to inadequate suppression of the contralateral adrenal and loss of lateralization. In addition to measuring plasma potassium and plasma renin, an inventory of medications should be assessed 4 to 6 weeks before AVS. Hypokalemia (which can decrease adrenal aldosterone production) should be corrected, renin should be

suppressed, and, when feasible, medications that stimulate renin should be withdrawn before AVS (≥4 weeks for MRAs and diuretics; ≥2 weeks for ACE inhibitors, angiotensin II receptor blockers, and dihydropyridine calcium channel blockers).[6] Contrast-enhanced CT should be performed to localize the adrenal veins and thereby increase the chance of successful cannulation.[8]

Concomitant autonomous cortisol secretion, which may occur in as many as 5% to 18% of patients with PA,[9,10] can confound the interpretation of AVS results.[11,12] Cortisol production from an adrenal adenoma may be sufficient to cause ACTH suppression and contralateral suppression of cortisol secretion. As a result, cannulation may be incorrectly deemed unsuccessful on the contralateral side. In addition, increased cortisol production on the side of the adenoma may lower the aldosterone-to-cortisol ratio on that side and thereby mask lateralization. Because of these issues, some groups recommend performing a 1-mg overnight dexamethasone-suppression test before AVS.[6] While mild autonomous cortisol excess is unlikely to significantly alter cannulation or lateralization outcomes during AVS, in individuals with a cortisol value greater than 5 μg/dL (>137 nmol/L) after a 1-mg dexamethasone-suppression test, lower selectivity index values have been reported.[13] In such patients, it can be useful to measure an additional marker, such as plasma metanephrine, to assess for selectivity and lateralization of aldosterone production.

Performing AVS

In Brisbane hypertension units, AVS is performed in the morning (when endogenous ACTH levels are highest, ensuring maximal ACTH-induced stimulation of aldosterone and cortisol production) and following overnight recumbency (thereby avoiding confounding effects of postural changes on aldosterone levels).[14] Administration of sedatives, anesthetic agents, and narcotics are avoided for at least 24 hours before AVS because of their potential to suppress steroid production. A radiologist highly skilled in AVS collects samples from each of the adrenal veins and, simultaneously with each AV sample, from a PV (antecubital fossa vein, inferior vena cava well below the adrenal veins, or iliac vein). At least 2 samples are collected from each side to maximize the chances of successful sampling and as a safeguard should sample handling issues occur.

A learning curve has been well described in AVS.[15,16] Success rates by a single operator improved from 50% to 60% to 80% to 95% after 30 to 50 procedures were performed, with more than 15 to 25 procedures needed per year to maintain a success rate of approximately 95% over 8 years.[16] If fewer than 20 procedures at a site are performed annually, these should be performed by a single operator.[16]

Several groups use exogenous ACTH (cosyntropin) stimulation during AVS to (1) maximize AV/PV cortisol gradients, (2) reduce fluctuations in steroid secretion during nonsimultaneous AVS, and (3) stimulate aldosterone production by APAs and thus avoid sampling during a period of secretion "quiescence."[2,17,18] ACTH stimulation may, however, lead to loss of lateralization by stimulating the contralateral gland in patients with unilateral PA. ACTH stimulation can assist subtype differentiation in patients whose basal AVS results were inconclusive because of apparent quiescence in terms of aldosterone production (ie, AV aldosterone/cortisol levels lower than peripheral) on both sides at the time of AVS.[19,20] Administration of cosyntropin as an intravenous infusion (50 mcg/h) ensures adequate and stable concentrations at the time of sampling.

Should the 2 adrenal veins be cannulated sequentially or simultaneously? Simultaneous sampling avoids biological variations in steroid production over time, but it is more difficult to achieve. If sequential sampling is used, the right (which is harder to cannulate) should be cannulated first to minimize the time between sampling the 2 sides.[6,19-21]

Result Interpretation

Adequacy of AVS is assessed by examining the gradient between AV and PV cortisol levels (the selectivity index), with gradients of at least 2 to 3

(we prefer 3) for nonstimulated AVS and at least 5 for ACTH-stimulated AVS indicating adequate sampling.[6,19-21] In highly experienced units, success rates can reach 90% or higher.[8,18] Aids to successful cannulation include using CT to localize the adrenal veins before AVS,[8] restricting the number of AVS proceduralists at each center, and using point-of-care plasma cortisol measurement to permit semiquantitative comparison of AV and PV cortisol levels within minutes of collection.[22]

AV samples can differ considerably in the degree to which they are "diluted" with non-AV blood. Because of this, direct comparison of aldosterone concentrations in these samples frequently gives misleading results. Calculating the aldosterone-to-cortisol ratio for each AV and PV sample corrects for differences in dilution. In unstimulated AVS, if the average AV aldosterone-to-cortisol ratio on 1 side is at least 2 times higher than the simultaneous PV ratio, with a ratio no higher than peripheral on the other side (contralateral suppression), lateralization has been demonstrated, indicating that unilateral ADX should cure or improve the patient's hypertension.[3,23] Criteria for lateralization vary widely from one institution to another.[6,7,21] Many centers rely only on the comparison of aldosterone-to-cortisol ratios on 1 side vs the other (the lateralization index), with lateralization defined as the ratio on the higher side being at least 4 times greater than that on the lower side. It is possible that the presence of contralateral suppression is of particular importance for predicting hypertension cure or improvement in the subgroup whose lateralization indices fall between 2.0 and 4.0, and less so for those with indices greater than 4.0.

As stated above, in patients who demonstrate cortisol values greater than 5 μg/dL (>137 nmol/L) after a 1-mg dexamethasone suppression, it can be useful to measure an additional marker, such as plasma metanephrine, to assess for selectivity and lateralization of aldosterone production. Suggested thresholds using metadrenaline in place of cortisol include a selectivity index greater than 12 and a lateralization index greater than 4.[24]

Clinical Case Vignettes

Case 1

A 56-year-old woman with hypertension, unprovoked hypokalemia, a markedly elevated plasma aldosterone-to-renin ratio, a positive seated saline-suppression test (confirming PA), and an 8-mm nodule in the left adrenal gland on CT scanning undergoes AVS with cosyntropin stimulation several weeks after correction of hypokalemia and while receiving verapamil, hydralazine, and prazosin.

AVS results are shown in the *Table*.

Which of the following is the most accurate interpretation of the AVS results?

A. Bilateral adrenal aldosterone production

B. Left unilateral adrenal aldosterone production

C. Right unilateral adrenal aldosterone production

D. Neither adrenal producing significant amounts of aldosterone

E. Inconclusive; 1 or both adrenal veins not successfully cannulated

Answer: B) Left unilateral adrenal aldosterone production

In this AVS, successful cannulation of both adrenal veins is confirmed by the demonstration of AV-to-PV cortisol ratios (selectivity indices) of 5.0 or greater (in this case, 28 to 55) for all samples collected. The left AV aldosterone-to-cortisol ratios are more than twice PV values, and those on the right side are lower than the PV (contralateral suppression), consistent with left unilateral aldosterone production. Furthermore, the left AV aldosterone-to-cortisol ratios are more than 30 times those on the right, which well exceeds the cutoff lateralization index for unilateral PA of 4.0 or higher. Although the cortisol-corrected aldosterone levels on the right side are much lower than the PV values, the absolute aldosterone levels are higher than the PV values (which is often the case, even in unstimulated AVS), emphasizing the importance of comparing aldosterone-to-cortisol ratios rather than uncorrected aldosterone levels for the purpose of lateralization. As is usually the case, cortisol levels are higher on the right than on the left, probably because the left AV receives inflow from the phrenic vein, which dilutes steroid levels.

Table. Case 1

Time of collection	Site of collection	Aldosterone	Cortisol	Cortisol AV-to-PV ratio	Aldosterone-to-cortisol ratio
08:30	Right AV 1	306.2 ng/dL (SI: 8493 pmol/L)	1324.8 µg/dL (SI: 36,548 nmol/L)	49	0.2
08:30	PV	58.4 ng/dL (SI: 1621 pmol/L)	27.3 µg/dL (SI: 754 nmol/L)		2.1
08:36	Right AV 2	282.0 ng/dL (SI: 7823 pmol/L)	1489.9 µg/dL (SI: 41,103 nmol/L)	55	0.2
08:36	PV	59.6 ng/dL (SI: 1652 pmol/L)	27.2 µg/dL (SI: 751 nmol/L)		2.2
08:42	Left AV 1	5407.4 ng/dL (SI: 150,000 pmol/L)	741.2 µg/dL (SI: 20,447 nmol/L)	28	7.3
08:42	PV	62.4 ng/dL (SI: 1732 pmol/L)	26.5 µg/dL (SI: 731 nmol/L)		2.4
08:45	Left AV 2	576.7 ng/dL (SI: 15,999 pmol/L)	881.0 µg/dL (SI: 24,305 nmol/L)	33	6.2
08:45	PV	62.2 ng/dL (SI: 1726 pmol/L)	27.1 µg/dL (SI: 747 nmol/L)		2.4

Abbreviations: AV, adrenal vein; PV, peripheral vein.

Case 2

A 64-year-old hypertensive, normokalemic man has elevated aldosterone-to-renin ratios while off interfering medications. He has a positive result on a seated saline-suppression test, and a 12-mm nodule in the right adrenal gland is identified on CT. He undergoes AVS during cosyntropin infusion while receiving verapamil, prazosin, and moxonidine.

AVS results are shown in the *Table.*

Which of the following is the most accurate interpretation of the AVS results?

A. Bilateral adrenal aldosterone production

B. Left unilateral adrenal aldosterone production

C. Right unilateral adrenal aldosterone production

D. Neither adrenal producing significant amounts of aldosterone

E. Inconclusive; 1 or both adrenal veins not successfully cannulated

Answer: A) Bilateral adrenal aldosterone production

While the first sampling attempt of the right AV was unsuccessful based on the AV-to-PV cortisol gradient of only 1.0, adequate AV samples were obtained on the second attempt (gradient 37) and with both attempts when cannulating the left AV. If the unsuccessful sample is ignored, the demonstration of aldosterone-to-cortisol ratios being higher than peripheral on both sides, the lack of contralateral suppression (defined as a contralateral suppression index of <1.0) on the lower (left) side, and right/left aldosterone-to-cortisol ratios (lateralization indices) less than 2 to 4 all support bilateral adrenal aldosterone production. In this case, reliance on CT alone would to have led to an incorrect diagnosis of right unilateral PA and potentially inappropriate surgery.

Case 3

A 48-year-old man with hypertension, unprovoked hypokalemia, elevated plasma aldosterone-to-renin ratios, a positive result on a seated saline-suppression test, and a 6-mm nodule in the left adrenal gland on CT undergoes AVS without cosyntropin stimulation in the morning after overnight recumbency several weeks after correction of hypokalemia and while receiving verapamil SR and hydralazine.

Table. Case 2

Time of collection	Site of collection	Aldosterone	Cortisol	Cortisol AV-to-PV ratio	Aldosterone-to-cortisol ratio
09:23	Right AV 1	23.4 ng/dL (SI: 650 pmol/L)	34.1 µg/dL (SI: 940 nmol/L)	1.0	0.7
09:23	PV	22.5 ng/dL (SI: 623 pmol/L)	34.1 µg/dL (SI: 942 nmol/L)		0.7
09:26	Right AV 2	3721.5 ng/dL (SI: 103,235 pmol/L)	1343.8 µg/dL (SI: 37,074 nmol/L)	37	2.8
09:26	PV	21.1 ng/dL (SI: 586 pmol/L)	36.6 µg/dL (SI: 1009 nmol/L)		0.6
09:28	Left AV 1	1692.5 ng/dL (SI: 46,949 pmol/L)	904.9 µg/dL (SI: 24,965 nmol/L)	25	1.0
09:28	PV	23.2 ng/dL (SI: 643 pmol/L)	36.8 µg/dL (SI: 1014 nmol/L)		0.6
09:29	Left AV 2	1967.6 ng/dL (SI: 54,581 pmol/L)	1026.4 µg/dL (SI: 28,317 nmol/L)	29	1.9
09:29	PV	22.0 ng/dL (SI: 609 pmol/L)	35.1 µg/dL (SI: 967 nmol/L)		0.6

Abbreviations: AV, adrenal vein; PV, peripheral vein.

AVS results are shown in the *Table*.

Which of the following is the most accurate interpretation of the AVS results?

A. Bilateral adrenal aldosterone production

B. Left unilateral adrenal aldosterone production

C. Right unilateral adrenal aldosterone production

D. Neither adrenal producing significant amounts of aldosterone

E. Inconclusive; 1 one or both adrenal veins not successfully cannulated

Answer: D) Neither adrenal producing significant amounts of aldosterone

In this unstimulated AVS, although both AVs have been successfully cannulated based on the AV-to-PV cortisol gradients of 3.0 or higher, both left and right AV aldosterone-to-cortisol gradients are no higher than peripheral. This is usually because sampling has been undertaken during a quiescent phase of aldosterone production. We have observed this to occur after patients have received a sedating agent or narcotic in the hours before AVS and in very stressed patients in whom early stimulation of aldosterone by ACTH may have been followed by suppression. Much less likely explanations include an ectopic (extra-adrenal) source of aldosterone excess, aberrant venous draining of an APA, or placement of the catheter into a branch vein that is distal to, and not receiving blood from, the tumor. It is probable, however, that neither adrenal gland was producing much aldosterone at the time of sampling. In our experience, whereas unilateral disease comprises only 25% to 30% of patients with PA, approximately 50% of patients who demonstrate this pattern have lateralization on repeat AVS.[25] As a result, we routinely offer these patients repeat AVS, preferably with cosyntropin stimulation, which seems to lessen the chance of a similar pattern occurring.

Key Learning Points

- AVS is the most reliable method of distinguishing unilateral (surgically correctable) from bilateral (usually treated medically) forms of PA.

Table. Case 3

Time of collection	Site of collection	Aldosterone	Cortisol	Cortisol AV-to-PV ratio	Aldosterone-to-cortisol ratio
09:10	Right AV 1	97.3 ng/dL (SI: 2700 pmol/L)	244.7 µg/dL (SI: 6750 nmol/L)	21	0.4
09:10	PV	7.0 ng/dL (SI: 194 pmol/L)	11.7 µg/dL (SI: 324 nmol/L)		0.4
09:13	Right AV 2	126.5 ng/dL (SI: 3510 pmol/L)	254.5 µg/dL (SI: 7020 nmol/L)	20	0.5
09:13	PV	8.0 ng/dL (SI: 222 pmol/L)	12.7 µg/dL (SI: 351 nmol/L)		0.6
09:18	Left AV 1	116.8 ng/dL (SI: 3240 pmol/L)	195.7 µg/dL (SI: 5400 nmol/L)	17	0.7
09:18	PV	9.0 ng/dL (SI: 250 pmol/L)	11.7 µg/dL (SI: 324 nmol/L)		0.8
09:20	Left AV 2	122.6 ng/dL (SI: 3402 pmol/L)	205.5 µg/dL (SI: 5670 nmol/L)	16	0.6
09:20	PV	9.0 ng/dL (SI: 250 pmol/L)	12.7 µg/dL (SI: 351 nmol/L)		0.7

Abbreviations: AV, adrenal vein; PV, peripheral vein.

- Established criteria exist for assessing whether AVs have been successful cannulated and for distinguishing unilateral from bilateral forms of PA.

- Success rates for AV cannulation can be enhanced with experienced operators, maintaining a high throughput, performing contrast CT of the adrenal glands before AVS, use of ACTH stimulation, and point-of-care cortisol measurement during the procedure.

- Correct result interpretation is dependent on awareness of the importance of optimal patient preparation (including withdrawal of medications that affect renin and aldosterone levels); criteria for cannulation success and lateralization for both ACTH-stimulated and nonstimulated procedures; and the effects of time of day, postural changes, stress, and administration of sedating or narcotic agents leading up to the procedure.

References

1. Reincke M, Bancos I, Mulatero P, Scholl UI, Stowasser M, Williams TA. Diagnosis and treatment of primary aldosteronism. *Lancet Diabetes Endocrinol.* 2021;9(12):876-892. PMID: 34798068

2. Funder JW, Carey RM, Mantero F, et al. The management of primary aldosteronism: case detection, diagnosis, and treatment: an Endocrine Society clinical practice guideline. *J Clin Endocrinol Metab.* 2016;101(5):1889-1916. PMID: 26934393

3. Stowasser M, Gordon RD. Primary aldosteronism: changing definitions and new concepts of physiology and pathophysiology both inside and outside the kidney. *Physiol Rev.* 2016;96(4):1327-1384. PMID: 27535640

4. Samnani S, Cenzer I, Kline GA, et al. Time to benefit of surgery vs targeted medical therapy for patients with primary aldosteronism: a meta-analysis. *J Clin Endocrinol Metab.* 2024;109(3):e1280-e1289. PMID: 37946600

5. McEvoy JW, McCarthy CP, Bruno RM, et al. 2024 ESC guidelines for the management of elevated blood pressure and hypertension. *Eur Heart J.* 2024;45(38):3912-4018.

6. Yang J, Bell DA, Carroll R, et al. Adrenal vein sampling for primary aldosteronism: recommendations from the Australian and New Zealand Working Group. *Clin Endocrinol (Oxf).* 2025;102(1):31-43. PMID: 39360599

7. Monticone S, Viola A, Rossato D, et al. Adrenal vein sampling in primary aldosteronism: towards a standardised protocol. Lancet Diabetes Endocrinol. 2015;3(4):296-303. PMID: 24831990

8. Daunt N. Adrenal vein sampling: how to make it quick, easy, and successful. *Radiographics.* 2005;25(Suppl 1):S143-S158. PMID: 16227488

9. Buffolo F, Pieroni J, Ponzetto F, et al. Prevalence of cortisol cosecretion in patients with primary aldosteronism: role of metanephrine in adrenal vein sampling. *J Clin Endocrinol Metab.* 2023;108(9):e720-e725. PMID: 36974473

10. Fallo F, Bertello C, Tizzani D, et al. Concurrent primary aldosteronism and subclinical cortisol hypersecretion: a prospective study. *J Hypertens.* 2011;29(9):1773-1777. PMID: 21720261

11. Goupil R, Wolley M, Ahmed AH, Gordon RD, Stowasser M. Does concomitant autonomous adrenal cortisol overproduction have the potential to confound the interpretation of adrenal venous sampling in primary aldosteronism? *Clin Endocrinol (Oxf).* 2015;83(4):456-461. PMID: 25683582

12. Kline GA, So B, Campbell DJT, et al. Apparent failed and discordant adrenal vein sampling: a potential confounding role of cortisol cosecretion? *Clin Endocrinol (Oxf).* 2022;96(2):123-131. PMID: 34160833

13. Heinrich DA, Quinkler M, Adolf C, et al. Influence of cortisol cosecretion on non-ACTH-stimulated adrenal venous sampling in primary aldosteronism: a retrospective cohort study. *Eur J Endocrinol.* 2022;187(5):637-650. PMID: 36070424

14. Stowasser M, Gordon RD. Primary aldosteronism. *Best Pract Res Clin Endocrinol Metab.* 2003;17(4):591-605. PMID: 14687591

15. Vonend O, Ockenfels N, Gao X, et al. Adrenal venous sampling: evaluation of the German Conn's registry. *Hypertension.* 2011;57(5):990-995. PMID: 21383311

16. Jakobsson H, Farmaki K, Sakinis A, Ehn O, Johannsson G, Ragnarsson O. Adrenal venous sampling: the learning curve of a single interventionalist with 282 consecutive procedures. *Diagn Interv Radiol.* 2018;24(2):89-93. PMID: 29467114

17. Monticone S, Satoh F, Giacchetti G, et al. Effect of adrenocorticotropic hormone stimulation during adrenal vein sampling in primary aldosteronism. *Hypertension.* 2012;59(4):840-846. PMID: 22331382

18. Young WF, Stanson AW. What are the keys to successful adrenal venous sampling (AVS) in patients with primary aldosteronism? *Clin Endocrinol (Oxf).* 2009;70(1):14-17. PMID: 19128364

19. Wolley M, Thuzar M, Stowasser M. Controversies and advances in adrenal venous sampling in the diagnostic workup of primary aldosteronism. *Best Pract Res Clin Endocrinol Metab.* 2020;34(3):101400. PMID: 32115358

20. Wolley MJ, Ahmed AH, Gordon RD, Stowasser M. Does ACTH improve the diagnostic performance of adrenal vein sampling for subtyping primary aldosteronism? *Clin Endocrinol (Oxf).* 2016;85(5):703-709. PMID: 27213822

21. Rossi GP, Barisa M, Allolio B, et al. The Adrenal Vein Sampling International Study (AVIS) for identifying the major subtypes of primary aldosteronism. *J Clin Endocrinol Metab.* 2012;97(5):1606-1614. PMID: 22399502

22. Yoneda T, Karashima S, Kometani M, et al. Impact of new quick gold nanoparticle-based cortisol assay during adrenal vein sampling for primary aldosteronism. *J Clin Endocrinol Metab.* 2016;101(6):2554-2561. PMID: 27011114

23. Stowasser M, Gordon RD, Rutherford JC, Nikwan NZ, Daunt N, Slater GJ. Diagnosis and management of primary aldosteronism. *J Renin Angiotensin Aldosterone Syst.* 2001;2(3):156-169. PMID: 33234000

24. Carroll RW, Corley B, Feltham J, et al. The value of plasma metanephrine measurements during adrenal vein sampling. *Endocr Connect.* 2024;13(2):e230300. PMID: 38055778

25. Wolley M, Gordon RD, Pimenta E, et al. Repeating adrenal vein sampling when neither aldosterone/cortisol ratio exceeds peripheral yields a high incidence of aldosterone-producing adenoma. *J Hypertens.* 2013;31(10):2005-2009. PMID: 24107732

Managing Severe Hypertriglyceridemia: Best Practices and New Approaches

Lisa R. Tannock, MD. Dean, Faculty of Health Sciences, Queen's University, Kingston, Ontario, Canada; Email: deanfhs@queensu.ca

Educational Objectives

After reviewing this chapter, learners should be able to:

- Identify the patient population that should be treated.

- Describe the current evidence-based guidelines for treatment of hypertriglyceridemia.

- Discuss the risks and benefits of lipid-lowering therapy, including combination therapy.

- Discuss the use of lipid-lowering medications in pregnancy.

Significance of the Clinical Problem

Elevated triglyceride levels are a common occurrence in the setting of comorbidities, such as obesity, diabetes, metabolic syndrome, and chronic inflammatory diseases. While it has long been known that severe hypertriglyceridemia can cause acute pancreatitis, the role of elevated triglycerides in atherosclerotic cardiovascular disease (ASCVD) has remained controversial. However, current guidelines do indicate that elevated triglycerides are a contributing risk factor and should be addressed.[1] Given that most health care providers are focused on ASCVD risk reduction, the primary focus of lipid management has been on LDL-lowering therapies, and many health care providers are unsure what to do about elevated triglycerides.

Triglycerides have wide variability both within individuals and across populations. While there is not a standardized definition of "severe hypertriglyceridemia," in general it is stated to be triglyceride levels at which the risk of acute pancreatitis is high—often considered to be above 800 to 1000 mg/dL (9.04-11.30 mmol/L). However, triglycerides are a particularly labile lipid and can vary within an individual over time and be influenced by food intake, exercise, alcohol consumption, and medication use, among other factors. Thus, providers and patients may not necessarily recognize when the triglyceride levels become "severe," and this can cause missed opportunities to treat and prevent an episode of acute pancreatitis.

Further compounding the situation is a common misperception that combination lipid-lowering therapy with agents targeting LDL cholesterol (eg, statins) and agents targeting triglycerides (eg, fibrates) can be dangerous. This can lead to provider hesitancy to provide prescription therapy for patients with or at risk of severe hypertriglyceridemia. Another challenge is that hesitancy around combination therapy can lead to missed opportunities to provide ASCVD-reducing LDL cholesterol–targeted therapies in patients with a history of triglyceride-induced pancreatitis.

Practice Gaps

- Lack of awareness of how to identify patients at risk of severe hypertriglyceridemia.

- Hesitancy to prescribe combination lipid-lowering therapy for patients with or at risk of severe hypertriglyceridemia and/or for patients with a history of severe hypertriglyceridemia and acute pancreatitis who also have increased ASCVD risk.

- Lack of comfort in treating pregnant women with hypertriglyceridemia.

Discussion

Triglyceride Metabolism

Triglycerides are a lipid molecule found on chylomicrons (produced by the gut) and VLDL particles (produced by the liver) and their respective remnant particles. Collectively, these particles are termed triglyceride-rich lipoproteins (TRL). Dietary triglycerides consumed in a fatty meal are hydrolyzed in the intestine to free fatty acids and monoglycerides; these are then absorbed by enterocytes and resynthesized to form triglycerides. The intestinal enterocytes reassemble triglycerides into chylomicrons containing apolipoprotein (apo) B_{48}. The chylomicrons are released from the cells into the lymphatic system, move into the thoracic duct, and then enter plasma. Chylomicrons are metabolized by lipoprotein lipase (LPL) to yield smaller particles termed chylomicron remnants. Chylomicrons and chylomicron remnants are taken up by the liver. Both lipids derived from chylomicron remnants and those synthesized de novo are reassembled in the liver as VLDL particles containing apo B_{100} and are secreted into the plasma. VLDL particles are also metabolized by LPL, which generates atherogenic remnant particles. Free fatty acids liberated by the action of LPL on TRLs can be directed to adipose tissue for storage or used by other tissues (eg, skeletal muscle, heart) as energy substrates. For more details, see the chapter by Boren and Taskinen.[2]

Classification of Hypertriglyceridemia

Various guidelines and committees have slightly different classification of triglyceride levels. *Table 1* reflects the Endocrine Society classification.[3]

Table 1. Classification of Triglyceride Levels

Classification	Triglyceride concentration
Normal	<150 mg/dL (SI: <1.70 mmol/L)
Mild hypertriglyceridemia	150-199 mg/dL (SI: 1.70-2.25 mmol/L)
Moderate hypertriglyceridemia	200-999 mg/dL (SI: 2.26-11.29 mmol/L)
Severe hypertriglyceridemia	1000-1999 mg/dL (SI: 11.30-22.59 mmol/L)
Very severe hypertriglyceridemia	>2000 mg/dL (SI: >22.60 mmol/L)

Reprinted from Berglund L et al. *J Clin Endocrinol Metab*, 2012; 97(9): 2969-2989. © by The Endocrine Society.

The plasma composition of lipid particles varies among individuals, but when fasting triglycerides are greater than 1000 mg/dL (>11.30 mmol/L), chylomicrons are present in addition to VLDL. Individuals with triglyceride levels greater than 1000 mg/dL (>11.30 mmol/L), and especially greater than 2000 mg/dL (>22.60 mmol/L), are considered to be at high risk for acute pancreatitis.

Genetic Causes of High Triglycerides

There are a number of genetic causes of hypertriglyceridemia (*Table 2, following page*). Patients with severe hypertriglyceridemia often have genetic causes or predispositions to high triglycerides, although environmental factors also have a role. For a review, see the article by Dron and Hegele.[4]

Individuals with monogenic hypertriglyceridemia often have elevated triglycerides throughout the lifespan and may present in infancy. Polygenic causes of hypertriglyceridemia have variable ages of presentation.

Table 2. Genetic Causes of Hypertriglyceridemia

Syndrome	Genetic cause	Typical triglyceride levels
Monogenic familial chylomicronemia	LPL deficiency Apolipoprotein C-II deficiency Apolipoprotein A-V pathogenic variants *LMF1* pathogenic variants GPIHP1 deficiency	>1000 mg/dL (SI: >11.30 mmol/L)
Polygenic chylomicronemia	Unknown	>1000 mg/dL (SI: >11.30 mmol/L)
Familial hypertriglyceridemia	Unknown, likely polygenic	200-1000 mg/dL (SI: 2.26-11.30 mmol/L)
Dysbetalipoproteinemia or type 3 hyperlipoproteinemia	Apolipoprotein E2/E2 and other polygenic susceptibility	200-1000 mg/dL (SI: 2.26-11.30 mmol/L)
Familial combined hyperlipidemia	Polygenic	200-1000 mg/dL (SI: 2.26-11.30 mmol/L)

Causes of Acute Elevations in Triglycerides

Environmental factors can affect triglyceride metabolism, particularly but not exclusively in patients with underlying genetic predisposition to hypertriglyceridemia (also termed the "second hit"). Factors can affect triglyceride production and/or triglyceride metabolism. Common acquired and environmental factors include:

- Alcohol
- High-calorie diet (fat, glucose, and fructose)
- Hypothyroidism
- Insulin resistance (associated with obesity, metabolic syndrome, type 2 diabetes, pregnancy, chronic kidney failure, chronic inflammatory conditions, etc)
- Multiple myeloma
- Pregnancy
- Kidney diseases (nephrotic syndrome, glomerulonephritis)

In addition, although less common than the factors listed above, additional endocrine disorders associated with elevated triglycerides are type 1 diabetes, Cushing syndrome, acromegaly, polycystic ovarian syndrome, and male hypogonadism.[5]

Many medications can also trigger elevations in triglycerides:

- Antipsychotic medications (clozapine, olanzapine)
- β-Adrenergic blockers
- Bile acid–binding agents (due to the risk of increasing triglycerides, these agents are generally contraindicated in patients with triglycerides >400 mg/dL [>4.52 mmol/L])
- Estrogens (especially oral estrogens) and the selective estrogen receptor modulators tamoxifen, raloxifene, clomiphene
- Glucocorticoids
- HIV antiretroviral medications
- Immunosuppressants (cyclosporine, everolimus, sirolimus)
- Retinoic acids
- Thiazide diuretics

Lability of Triglycerides

Humans spend a significant amount of time in a postprandial state, and some individuals have dramatic postprandial elevations of TRLs. These patients tend to have saturation of the LPL removal system and can experience a rapid increase of triglyceride levels after consumption of high-fat meals; this can be exacerbated by consumption of simple sugars, fructose, and alcohol in susceptible individuals. However, most guidelines are based on measurements of fasting triglycerides, which can lead to providers missing patients at risk of severe hypertriglyceridemia and associated complications.

High Triglycerides and Risk of Pancreatitis

Hypertriglyceridemia-induced pancreatitis is a common cause of acute pancreatitis (gallstone-induced and alcohol-induced pancreatitis are the leading causes). The incidence of acute pancreatitis is estimated to be up to 5% in patients with triglyceride concentrations greater than 1000 mg/dL (>11.30 mmol/L) and up to 20% in patients with triglycerides greater than 2000 mg/dL (>22.60 mmol/L).[6] While the mechanism(s) underlying hypertriglyceridemia-induced acute pancreatitis are not fully understood, theories include toxicity induced by triglyceride lipolysis and high levels of free fatty acids, as well as hyperviscosity leading to decreased microcirculation and pancreatic ischemia.[7]

Triglycerides in ASCVD

In addition to being a risk factor for acute pancreatitis, guidelines consider chronic hypertriglyceridemia to be a risk-enhancing factor for ASCVD, related to the atherogenic potential of TRLs, particularly remnant particles. The American College of Cardiology recommends lifestyle interventions (low-fat/calorie diet and avoidance of alcohol) and consideration of addition of triglyceride-reducing medications (icosapent ethyl or fibrates) to maximally tolerated statin therapy in patients with triglyceride concentrations greater than 500 mg/dL (>5.65 mmol/L).[1]

Triglyceride Lowering and Combination Therapy

Due to the significant impact of diet on triglycerides, a low-fat/low-sugar diet and weight loss, especially when combined with increased physical activity, can induce triglyceride reductions of 10% to 70%. In patients with severe hypertriglyceridemia, intermittent fasting or consumption of a diet with total fat less than 15% of daily calories can reduce triglycerides. The Endocrine Society's Lipid Management in Patients with Endocrine Disorders Clinical Practice Guideline recommends the use of pharmacologic treatment as adjunct to diet and exercise to prevent pancreatitis in adults with fasting triglyceride levels above 500 mg/dL (>5.65 mmol/L).[5] *Table 3* indicates the expected triglyceride lowering of common lipid-lowering agents.

Table 3. Expected Triglyceride Lowering With Common Lipid-Lowering Agents

Agent	Expected triglyceride reduction
Statins	10%-30%
Ezetimibe	Up to 10%
Niacin	35%-50%
PCSK9 inhibitors	Up to 25%
Bile acid binders	No change or increase
Bempedoic acid	No change
Icosapent ethyl	20%-45%
Fibrates	35%-50%

Although there have been warnings of increased risks of adverse effects with statin and fibrate combinations, randomized controlled trials and meta-analyses have demonstrated the safety and efficacy of using these drugs in combination, particularly when fenofibrate is the triglyceride-reducing agent used.[8,9] However, due to longstanding concerns about increased toxicity, many providers are reluctant to use these medications in combination, thus potentially depriving patients of benefit.

New and Potential Therapies

Since patients with familial chylomicronemia syndrome are often minimally responsive or nonresponsive to currently available triglyceride-lowering agents due to a lack of LPL activity, new therapies are urgently needed. Approaches to antagonize apo CIII are the most promising. Apo CIII increases triglyceride levels via inhibiting LPL and decreasing hepatic clearance of TRLs. Thus, targeting apo CIII has emerged as a therapeutic approach. In Europe, volanesorsen, an unconjugated antisense oligonucleotide against APOC3 mRNA, has been shown to reduce triglyceride levels and reduce the risk of acute pancreatitis. However, volanesorsen has not been approved in the United States. Olezarsen is a conjugated antisense oligonucleotide against APOC3 mRNA that was recently approved in the United States based on its ability to decrease triglyceride levels by approximately 50% with no major adverse effects.[10]

Triglycerides in Pregnancy

Estrogens increase triglyceride levels by stimulating hepatic triglyceride production. In women with a genetic predisposition to hypertriglyceridemia, pregnancy can impose significant increased risk for the development of severe hypertriglyceridemia and acute pancreatitis. In pregnant patients at high risk, omega-3 fatty acids and fibrates have been used with no apparent adverse outcomes. Fibrates were considered category C in pregnancy until 2015 when these categories were eliminated by the US FDA. The 2018 FDA label for the fenofibrate Tricor states that data in pregnant women are insufficient to determine the risk of major birth defects, miscarriage, or adverse maternal or fetal outcomes and that this drug should be used during pregnancy only if the potential benefit justifies the potential risk to the fetus. For patients at high risk of triglyceride-induced complications (triglyceride >500 mg/dL [>5.65 mmol/L]) during pregnancy, the National Lipid Association recommends use of dietary interventions, omega-3 fatty acids, or

fibrates in the second trimester.[11] Pancreatitis in pregnancy confers a high risk for fetal loss, particularly in the first trimester.

Clinical Case Vignettes

Case 1

A 48-year-old woman with a history of hypertriglyceridemia-induced pancreatitis presents for routine follow-up. She reports that she has followed management advice and is now consuming a very low-fat diet. She continues to take icosapent ethyl, 2 g twice daily; fenofibrate, 137 mg daily; and atorvastatin, 20 mg daily. The table shows her current and previous (6 months ago) lipid panels, on the same lipid-lowering medications. She has ongoing fatigue, some puffiness in her hands and feet, and hot flashes, for which she recently started estrogen and progesterone therapy.

Parameter	Current	6 months ago
Total cholesterol	238 mg/dL (SI: 6.16 mmol/L)	160 mg/dL (SI: 4.14 mmol/L)
Triglycerides	1548 mg/dL (SI: 17.49 mmol/L)	660 mg/dL (SI: 7.46 mmol/L)
HDL cholesterol	24 mg/dL (SI: 0.62 mmol/L)	32 mg/dL (SI: 0.83 mmol/L)

Which of the following is the first priority in this patient's management?

A. Advise a lower-carbohydrate diet

B. Assess alcohol intake

C. Discontinue estrogen and progesterone therapy

D. Measure kidney function

E. Measure TSH

Answer: C) Discontinue estrogen therapy

The patient in this vignette has known hypertriglyceridemia and a history of acute pancreatitis. However, on her current medications, her triglyceride levels have been relatively well controlled. She now presents with a significant increase in triglycerides, but fortunately she has no symptoms of acute pancreatitis. Numerous environmental and dietary factors affect triglyceride metabolism, including hypothyroidism, high-carbohydrate diet, kidney dysfunction (in particular, nephrotic syndrome), medications (eg, estrogen), alcohol intake, and others. However, in patients with genetic hypertriglyceridemia, such as the patient in this vignette, estrogen therapy is a relative contraindication and is the most likely contributor to the dramatic increase in her triglyceride levels. Discontinuing estrogen (Answer C) is the best next step.

While hypothyroidism can lead to slower lipid metabolism, the relative change in triglyceride levels tends to be minimal,[12] and measuring TSH (Answer E) is not the highest priority.

When patients consume a low-fat diet, the relative consumption of carbohydrates increases, and these carbohydrates can lead to increased fatty acid synthesis and increased triglyceride levels.[13,14] However, this would be unlikely to cause such a degree of triglyceride elevation, and advising a lower-carbohydrate diet (Answer B) is not the best next step.

Kidney dysfunction and nephrotic syndrome can cause significant changes in lipid metabolism; however, there are no indications in the vignette that this patient has nephrotic syndrome. While measuring kidney function (Answer D) would be prudent, it is not the most important next step.

Finally, while alcohol consumption can raise triglycerides, especially in the postprandial stage,[15] and assessing alcohol consumption (Answer B) is prudent, there is no information suggesting an increase in alcohol consumption.

Case 2

A 27-year-old woman is referred by her obstetrician who noticed that her blood looked like a strawberry milkshake after a blood draw for recent labs. She is 14 weeks pregnant, takes no medications other than a prenatal multivitamin, and has no concerns on review of systems.

Fasting lipid panel:

> Total cholesterol = 238 mg/dL (<200 mg/dL [optimal]) (SI: 6.16 mmol/L [<5.18 mmol/L])
> Triglycerides = >1400 mg/dL (<150 mg/dL [optimal]) (SI: >15.82 mmol/L [<1.70 mmol/L])
> HDL cholesterol = 22 mg/dL (>60 mg/dL [optimal]) (SI: 0.57 mmol/L [>1.55 mmol/L])
> Fasting glucose = 136 mg/dL (70-99 mg/dL) (SI: 7.5 mmol/L [3.9-5.5 mmol/L])

Which of the following is the best next step?

A. Admit to the hospital and initiate intravenous insulin therapy

B. Admit to the hospital and initiate plasmapheresis

C. Initiate a very low-fat diet

D. Initiate statin therapy

E. Initiate omega-3 fatty acids and fenofibrate

Answer: E) Initiate omega-3 fatty acids and fenofibrate

This asymptomatic pregnant patient has incidentally discovered severe hypertriglyceridemia. While her triglycerides are significantly elevated, she has no symptoms suggesting acute pancreatitis. Thus, while treatment should be initiated, it is not an emergency, and she does not require hospital admission (Answers A and B). If she had symptoms suggestive of pancreatitis, then plasmapheresis could be considered; however, plasmapheresis should not be initiated unless a trial of medical management has failed. Her fasting glucose is elevated, indicating she likely has diabetes, which is another risk factor possibly contributing to her hypertriglyceridemia. Unless her glucose level was much higher and she had acute pancreatitis, there is no indication for intravenous insulin therapy now.

While omega-3 fatty acids and fibrates (Answer E) are considered pregnancy category C (risk in pregnancy cannot be ruled out), she is at high risk for pancreatitis due to her elevated triglycerides, which confers both fetal and maternal risks. Thus, initiation of triglyceride-lowering therapy is the best next step.[16,17]

Although statin therapy (Answer D) could be considered in pregnancy for severe hypercholesterolemia, statins have weak triglyceride-lowering effects and are not the best next step.

Providing dietary advice for a low-fat diet (Answer C) is appropriate for both her lipid disorder and presumptive diabetes, but it is insufficient to address her risk and pharmacotherapy should be initiated.

Case 3

A 52-year-old man is referred for assessment of cardiovascular risk reduction. He has never had an atherosclerotic cardiac event and has no cardiac symptoms. However, 5 years ago he had acute pancreatitis thought to be due to hypertriglyceridemia. He has a history of type 2 diabetes diagnosed 5 years ago, which is currently treated with metformin and glargine insulin once daily. He is a former cigarette smoker but quit 5 years ago at the time of diabetes diagnosis. He tries to eat a healthy diet but struggles, and he acknowledges that he consumes alcohol most days of the week. He takes atorvastatin, 40 mg daily, and has been hesitant to increase the dosage. He also takes metoprolol, gabapentin, and sertraline.

The consultation information includes a fasting lipid panel from 3 months ago:

> Total cholesterol = 183 mg/dL (<200 mg/dL [optimal]) (SI: 4.74 mmol/L [<5.18 mmol/L])
> Triglycerides = 602 mg/dL (<150 mg/dL [optimal]) (SI: 6.80 mmol/L [<1.70 mmol/L])
> HDL cholesterol = 31 mg/dL (>60 mg/dL [optimal]) (SI: 0.80 mmol/L [>1.55 mmol/L])
> Direct LDL cholesterol = 72 mg/dL (<100 mg/dL [optimal]) (SI: 1.86 mmol/L [<2.59 mmol/L])
> Hemoglobin A_{1c} = 7.8% (4.0%-5.6%) (62 mmol/mol [20-38 mmol/mol])

You decide to repeat the lipid panel even though he ate breakfast 2 hours ago (he reports stopping at a fast-food restaurant on his way to clinic).

> Total cholesterol = 262 mg/dL (SI: 6.79 mmol/L)
> Triglycerides = 1368 mg/dL (SI: 15.46 mmol/L)
> HDL cholesterol = 22 mg/dL (SI: 0.57 mmol/L)
> LDL cholesterol, cannot be calculated
> Hemoglobin A_{1c} = 8.2% (66 mmol/mol)

Which of the following changes to his lipid-lowering therapy should be recommended?

A. Add ezetimibe

B. Add fenofibrate

C. Add niacin

D. Change atorvastatin to rosuvastatin, 40 mg daily

E. Recommend no changes

Answer: B) Add fenofibrate

The patient in this vignette was sent for consultation for cardiovascular risk but is actually at high risk of severe hypertriglyceridemia. He is on appropriate statin therapy for cardiovascular risk. Three months ago, his fasting triglyceride concentration was elevated, but his direct LDL-cholesterol concentration was almost at goal (his LDL-cholesterol goal would be <70 mg/dL [<1.81 mmol/L] given his diabetes). However, a nonfasting lipid panel today demonstrates very high triglyceride levels, conferring increased risk for acute pancreatitis. His glycemic control has worsened, likely contributing to the triglyceride elevation. Given his previous episode of acute pancreatitis and his elevated triglycerides, the acute risk of pancreatitis is the top priority, and a triglyceride-lowering drug (fenofibrate [Answer B]) should be added to his regimen.

Changing atorvastatin to rosuvastatin (Answer D) or adding ezetimibe (Answer A) would help reduce his cardiovascular risk but would not lower his triglycerides very much.

Adding niacin (Answer C) could lower triglycerides, but niacin is poorly tolerated and could lead to further deterioration in glycemic control.

Doing nothing (Answer E) is not appropriate given his acute pancreatitis risk and cardiovascular risk. Using combination statin plus fibrate therapy is indicated to address both his cardiovascular and hypertriglyceridemia risk.

Key Learning Points

- Severe hypertriglyceridemia conveys risk for acute pancreatitis; providers should consider both cardiovascular risk reduction and prevention of acute pancreatitis in patients with high triglycerides.

- Environmental, medical, and lifestyle factors can significantly raise triglycerides in susceptible individuals; providers should screen and remove or treat contributing factors.

- Severe hypertriglyceridemia in pregnancy confers high risk for fetal loss due to pancreatitis. Neither fibrates nor statins are contraindicated in pregnancy. Fenofibrate may be used cautiously in women at high risk who have severe hypertriglyceridemia. The use of statins in pregnancy is discouraged except in women with familial hypercholesterolemia, other severe LDL increases, or ASCVD when the benefits outweigh the risks.

- Nonfasting triglyceride levels may be a better indicator of risk than fasting triglyceride levels.

References

1. Grundy SM, Stone NJ, Bailey AL, et al. 2018 AHA/ACC/AACVPR/AAPA/ABC/ACPM/ADA/AGS/APhA/ASPC/NLA/PCNA Guideline on the Management of Blood Cholesterol: A Report of the American College of Cardiology/American Heart Association Task Force on Clinical Practice Guidelines. *J Am Coll Cardiol.* 2019;73(24):e285-e350. PMID: 30423391

2. Boren J and Taskinen MR. Metabolism of triglyceride-rich lipoproteins. In: von Eckardstein A, Binder CJ, eds. *Prevention and Treatment of Atherosclerosis: Improving State-of-the-Art Management and Search for Novel Targets.* Cham (CH): Springer; 2022:133-156.

3. Berglund L, Brunzell AC, Goldberg IJ, et al; Endocrine Society. Evaluation and treatment of hypertriglyceridemia: an Endocrine Society clinical practice guideline. *J Clin Endocrinol Metab.* 2012;97(9):2969-2989. PMID: 22962670

4. Dron JS, Hegele RA. Genetics of hypertriglyceridemia. *Front Endocrinol (Lausanne).* 2020;11:455. PMID: 32793115

5. Newman CB, Blaha MJ, Boord JB, et al. Lipid management in patients with endocrine disorders: an Endocrine Society clinical practice guideline. *J Clin Endocrinol Metab.* 2020;105(12):dgaa674. PMID: 32951056

6. Rawla PT, Sunkara KC, Thandra KC, Gaduputi V. Hypertriglyceridemia-induced pancreatitis: updated review of current treatment and preventive strategies. *Clin J Gastroenterol.* 2018;11(6):441-448. PMID: 29923163

7. Meng Y, Han P, Ma X, He Y, Chen H, Ren H. Research progress on the mechanism of acute hypertriglyceridemic pancreatitis. *Pancreas.* 2024;53(8):e700-e709. PMID: 38696438

8. Keech A, Simes RJ, Barter P, et al; FIELD Study Investigators. Effects of long-term fenofibrate therapy on cardiovascular events in 9795 people with type 2 diabetes mellitus (the FIELD study): randomised controlled trial. *Lancet.* 2005;366(9500):1849-1861. PMID: 16310551

9. Guo J, Meng F, Ma N, et al. Meta-analysis of safety of the coadministration of statin with fenofibrate in patients with combined hyperlipidemia. *Am J Cardiol.* 2012;110(9):1296-1301. PMID: 22840347

10. Bergmark BA, Marston NA, Prohaska TA, et al; Bridge-TIMI 73a Investigators. Olezarsen for hypertriglyceridemia in patients at high cardiovascular risk. *N Engl J Med.* 2024;390(19):1770-1780. PMID: 38587249

11. Jacobson TA, Maki KC, Orringer CE, et al; NLA Expert Panel. National Lipid Association recommendations for patient-centered management of dyslipidemia: part 2. *J Clin Lipidol.* 2015;9(Suppl 6)S1-122.e1. PMID: 26699442

12. Kotwal A, Cortes T, Genere N, et al. Treatment of thyroid dysfunction and serum lipids: a systematic review and meta-analysis. *J Clin Endocrinol Metab.* 2020;105(12):dgaa672. PMID: 32954428

13. Hudgins, L. C. 2000. Effect of high-carbohydrate feeding on triglyceride and saturated fatty acid synthesis. *Proc Soc Exp Biol Med* 225: 178-183.

14. Schwarz, J. M., P. Linfoot, D. Dare, and K. Aghajanian. 2003. Hepatic de novo lipogenesis in normoinsulinemic and hyperinsulinemic subjects consuming high-fat, low-carbohydrate and low-fat, high-carbohydrate isoenergetic diets. *Am J Clin Nutr* 77: 43-50.

15. Van de Wiel, A. 2012. The effect of alcohol on postprandial and fasting triglycerides. *Int J Vasc Med* 2012: 862504.

16. Gupta, M., B. Liti, C. Barrett, P. D. Thompson, and A. B. Fernandez. 2022. Prevention and Management of Hypertriglyceridemia-Induced Acute Pancreatitis During Pregnancy: A Systematic Review. *Am J Med* 135: 709-714.

17. Schatoff, D., I. Y. Jung, and I. J. Goldberg. 2024. Lipid Disorders and Pregnancy. *Endocrinol Metab Clin North Am* 53: 483-495.

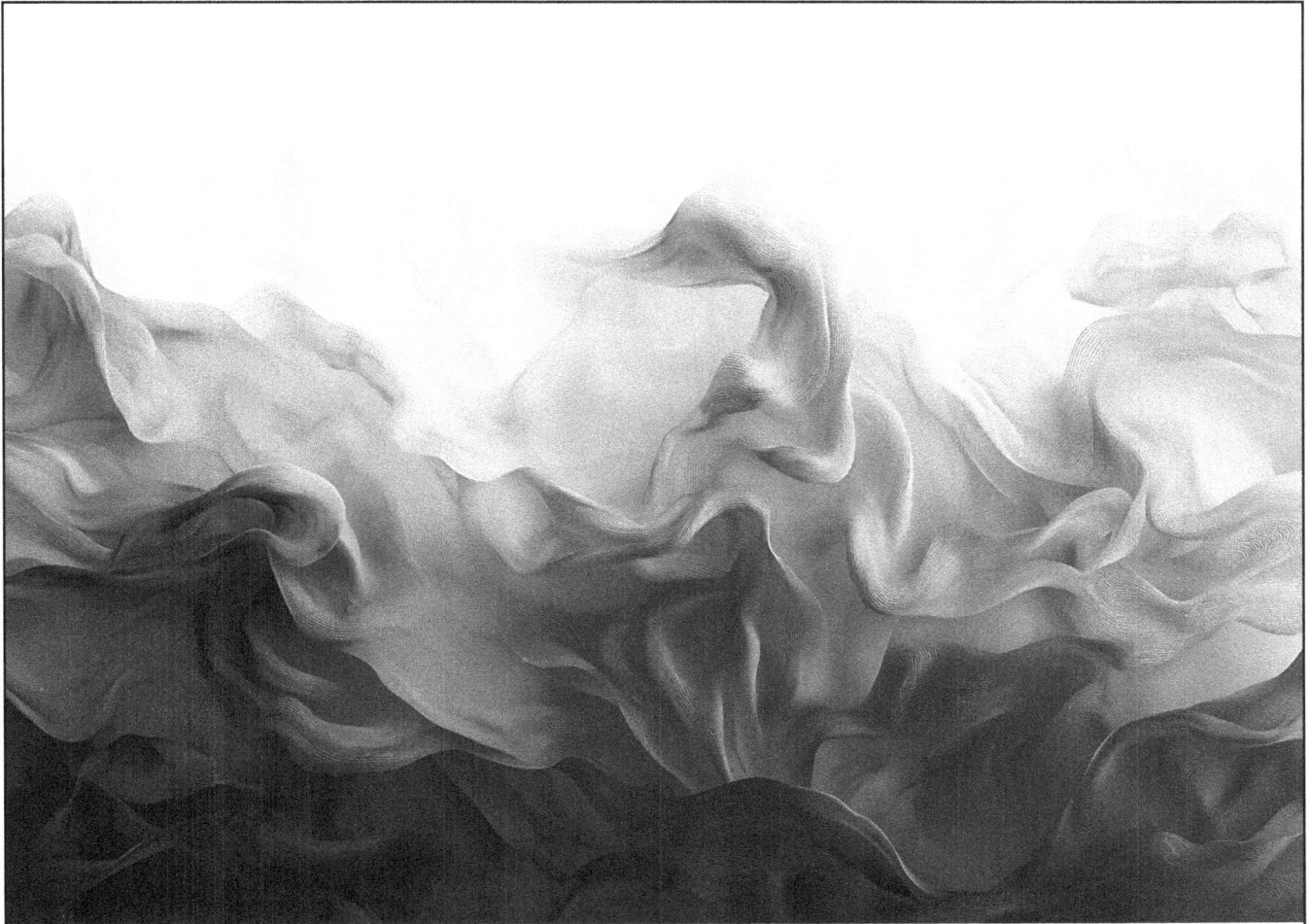

DIABETES AND VASCULAR DISEASE

Monitoring Diabetes Control Using Hemoglobin A$_{1c}$ and Continuous Glucose Monitoring: Advantages and Pitfalls

Shichun Bao, MD, PhD. Division of Diabetes, Endocrinology, and Metabolism, Department of Medicine, Vanderbilt University Medical Center, Nashville, TN; Email: shichun.bao@vumc.org

Educational Objectives

After reviewing this chapter, learners should be able to:

- Explain the advantages and pitfalls of hemoglobin A$_{1c}$ (HbA$_{1c}$) and continuous glucose monitoring (CGM).

- Identify potential causes of glucose monitoring discrepancies.

- Manage CGM therapy using a personalized approach.

Significance of the Clinical Problem

Monitoring glycemic control using HbA$_{1c}$ and CGM each has advantages and pitfalls. HbA$_{1c}$ is a useful tool for the diagnosis and management of diabetes and is generally an excellent marker of overall glycemic control for the preceding 8 to 12 weeks.[1] However, HbA$_{1c}$ does not capture short-term glucose fluctuations or hypoglycemic episodes. It may not reflect recent improvements or deteriorations in glycemic control. HbA$_{1c}$ accuracy can be affected by many conditions.[2] CGM provides real-time glucose readings, allowing users to see immediate changes in glucose levels all the time and track glucose trends, which can help them understand how food, exercise, stress, or medications affect their glucose levels and how to prevent hypoglycemia[3]; however, many factors can affect the accuracy of CGM.[4] Cost and accessibility, sensor calibration, skin sensitivity, and user overload can be problems. Health care providers must be able to identify problems with glucose monitoring, investigate potential causes, provide better education, and deliver high-quality care to patients using personalized approaches.

Practice Gaps

- Lack of awareness of the conditions that can affect HbA$_{1c}$ and CGM accuracy.

- Insufficient knowledge about different features of various CGMs and skills related to CGM problem-solving.

- Lack of extensive training on CGM ordering for different patient populations, data analysis, and management.

Discussion

Monitoring glycemic control using HbA$_{1c}$ and CGM has advantages and pitfalls. HbA$_{1c}$ is formed by the concentration-dependent nonenzymatic linkage of glucose to the N-terminal valine of the hemoglobin β chain.[5] It is an excellent marker of overall glycemic control during the time frame of the 120-day lifespan of a normal erythrocyte and is routinely used for both management and diagnosis of diabetes.[2] Four basic methodologies are used for HbA_{1c} measurement, as standardized by the National Glycohemoglobin Standardization Program (NGSP): immunoassay, ion-exchange high-performance liquid chromatography (HPLC), boronate affinity HPLC, and enzymatic assays.[6] Point-of-care (POC) HbA_{1c} measurements are generally immunoassay-based. POC HbA_{1c} is commonly used in the provider's office to obtain immediate results and provide feedback for timely adjustment in the treatment regimen. POC values can have small variations from values obtained in the central laboratory, and this is attributed to different methodologies.[7]

The main pitfalls of HbA_{1c}:

1. HbA_{1c} does not capture short-term glucose fluctuations and hypoglycemic episodes. It may not reflect recent improvements or deteriorations in glycemic control.

2. Multiple conditions can interfere with HbA_{1c} results in 2 basic ways: direct interference with the assay's ability to accurately detect glycated hemoglobin molecules, and physiologic factors that alter the concentration of HbA_{1c} in the patient's blood in such a way that it no longer accurately reflects glycemic control. Hemoglobin variants can directly interfere with some assays' detection of glycated hemoglobin. The degree of interference depends on the assay used, leading to artificially increased or decreased results.[6] Conversely, any condition that prolongs erythrocyte survival, such as asplenia, or that decreases erythrocyte turnover, such as iron deficiency anemia, B_{12} deficiency, or folate deficiency anemia, can cause falsely elevated HbA_{1c}. Uremia and chronic ingestion of alcohol, salicylates, opioids, or lead poisoning have also been associated with falsely elevated HbA_{1c}.[2] Similarly, any condition that shortens the life of erythrocytes or is associated with increased erythrocyte turnover, such as splenomegaly, hemolytic anemia, or acute or chronic blood loss, can cause falsely lowered HbA_{1c} results. Patients with end-stage kidney disease generally have falsely low HbA_{1c} values, primarily due to the associated chronic anemia with increased erythrocyte turnover.

CGM is widely used, especially in the last few years, as part of diabetes management, and should be recommended to every person with diabetes who is on insulin treatment.[8] CGM provides real-time glucose readings, allowing users to see immediate changes in glucose levels all the time and track glucose trends, which helps users understand how food, exercise, stress, and medications affect their glucose levels and how to prevent hypoglycemia.[3] Over-the-counter CGM has been increasingly used by people without diabetes who are seeking personalized insight into metabolic health, behavioral motivation, enhanced athletic performance, and early detection of glucose dysregulation.[9]

The main pitfalls of CGM:

1. Many factors affect the accuracy of CGM systems
   - *Physiological factors*: lag time (typically 5- to 15-minute delay in blood glucose changes and CGM readings), hydration levels, body temperature, and sweat can affect CGM readings.
   - *Device-related factors*: sensor placement, sensor calibration, sensor age, and insertion site issues can affect CGM readings.
   - *Environmental factors*: compression artifacts, altitude, and electromagnetic interference can affect CGM performance.
   - *Medication and substance interference*: acetaminophen, hydroxyurea, vitamin C, salicylic acid, tetracycline, mannitol, etc, can affect certain CGM readings.
   - *Calibration time errors*: calibration should be done during stable glucose periods, not during times of rapid blood glucose changes.

- *Sensor adhesion and movement:* Loose or poor adhesion, movement, or improper attachment can affect the sensor's ability to provide accurate readings.
  - *Individual variability:* skin composition (differences in skin thickness, body fat distribution and immune response (in some cases, the body may mount an immune response against the sensor, causing inflammation or irritation of surrounding skin) can cause inaccurate CGM readings.

2. Cost and accessibility: CGM can be expensive and may not be accessible for everyone due to insurance coverage or out-of-pocket costs. Coverage and the ordering process vary for different patient populations (via formulary prescription plan vs Duel Medical Equipment coverage).

3. User overload: The constant flow of data and glucose alerts can be overwhelming for some individuals. Insufficient training on how to properly use CGM can cause data misinterpretation, anxiety, and frustration for both patients and providers.

Clinical Case Vignettes

Case 1

A 54-year-old African American woman with type 2 diabetes is treated with dapagliflozin, 10 mg daily; metformin, 1000 mg twice daily; and liraglutide subcutaneous injection, 1.8 mg daily. The only other medication she takes is irbesartan/hydrochlorothiazide, 300/25 mg daily, for hypertension, and she takes no supplements. She needs a knee replacement for severe arthritis and was told she could not have surgery until her HbA_{1c} is below 8.0% (<64 mmol/mol). Her recent HbA_{1c} measurement was 9.5% (80 mmol/mol), and she needs help to decrease this value. Her POC HbA_{1c} value in the clinic today is 10.8% (95 mmol/mol). Review of her home glucose

meter data shows that she is checking fingerstick blood glucose on average 0.5 times a day, usually fasting in the morning or before dinner, with a 3-month average glucose concentration of 138 mg/dL (7.7 mmol/L) (range, 110-164 mg/dL [6.1-9.1 mmol/L]), A repeat HbA_{1c} measurement by a central laboratory is 9.2% (77 mmol/mol). Her fructosamine concentration is 340 µmol/L (reference range, 170-285 µmol/L).

Which of the following is the best next step given this patient's goal?

A. Add glimepiride

B. Add long-acting insulin

C. Add short-acting insulin

D. Instruct her to measure fingerstick blood glucose 3 to 4 times a day, before meals and at bedtime, and return in 3 months to measure HbA_{1c}

E. Instruct her to measure fingerstick blood glucose 3 to 4 times a day, before meals and at bedtime, initiate a blinded professional CGM, and reassess in 2 weeks

Answer: E) Instruct her to measure fingerstick blood glucose 3 to 4 times a day, before meals and at bedtime, initiate a blinded professional CGM, and reassess in 2 weeks

HbA_{1c} has been routinely used for management and diagnosis of diabetes. HbA_{1c} is generally an excellent marker of overall glycemic control for the preceding 8 to 12 weeks; however, it does not capture short-term glucose fluctuations or hypoglycemic episodes. It may also not reflect recent improvements or deteriorations in glycemic control. POC HbA_{1c} values can have small variations from central laboratory measurements of HbA_{1c}, which is attributed to the different methodologies. HbA_{1c} accuracy can be affected by many conditions; therefore, the result should be interpreted with caution. This patient's HbA_{1c} did not correlate with her fingerstick blood glucose values, with much lower-than-expected fingerstick blood glucose readings based on her high HbA_{1c} measurement, which could be due to her infrequent fingerstick blood glucose sampling and missed high readings. While more frequent measurement of blood glucose should be recommended, inaccurate HbA_{1c} should also be suspected.

Fructosamine can be used as an alternative analyte to monitor glycemic control in patients with known or suspected inaccurate HbA_{1c}. Fructosamine refers to the product formed by nonenzymatic reaction of glucose and albumin and reflects a much shorter period of glycemic control than HbA_{1c} (about 20 days vs 120 days), due to the shorter half-life of albumin.[5] Unfortunately, conditions such as nephrotic syndrome and cirrhosis can interfere with fructosamine measurement,[10] and these values must be interpreted with the clinical context in mind. This patient's fructosamine concentration was slightly elevated at 340 μmol/L (reference range, 170-285 μmol/L), which should correlate to an estimated HbA_{1c} value of 8.0% (64 mmol/mol) and an average glucose concentration of 180 mg/dL (9.9 mmol/L),[5] suggesting her HbA_{1c} could be falsely elevated.

In the meantime, an alternative method of glucose monitoring, such as a professional CGM (Answer E), should be considered to investigate the big discrepancy between this patient's HbA_{1c} and fingerstick blood glucose values. In this case, a blinded CGM trial would be a good option, so the patient would not see her CGM readings and subsequently change her lifestyle, which could affect readings during the CGM trial period. This patient was placed on a 14-day blinded professional CGM and was told to come back in 2 weeks for reevaluation. Simply measuring fingerstick blood glucose more frequently and coming back in 3 months to measure HbA_{1c} (Answer D) would delay her surgery unnecessarily.

Medications that could cause hypoglycemia (Answers A, B, and C) should not be added before confirming the accuracy of her high HbA_{1c}.

Case 1, Continued

Her CGM and glucose meter data are downloaded at her 2-week follow-up visit. Her CGM ambulatory glucose profile shows an average glucose concentration of 165 mg/dL (9.1 mmol/L), 73% of readings in the target range of 70 to 180 mg/dL (3.9-10.0 mmol/L), and an estimated HbA_{1c} of 7.4% (57 mmol/mol) (*Figure*),[10]

Figure.

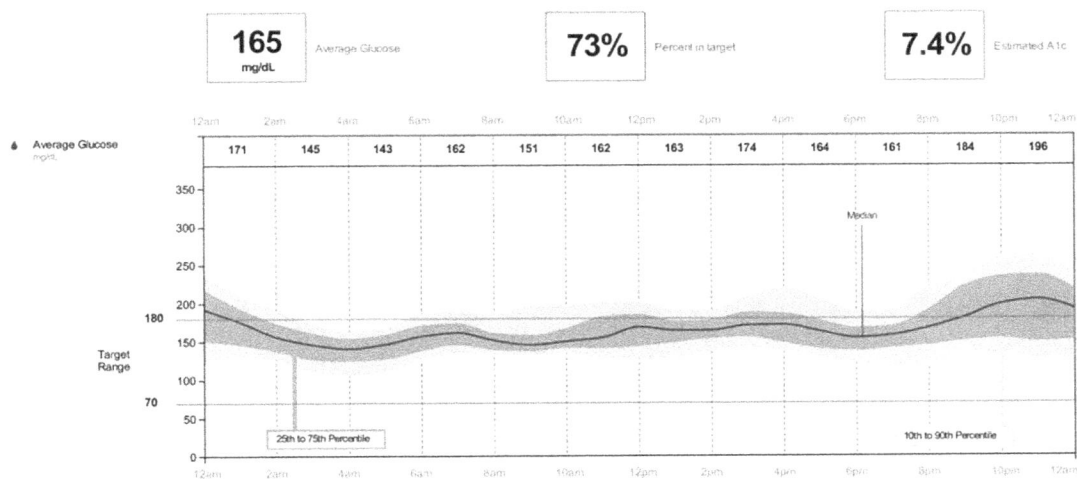

LibreView daily patterns report shows ambulatory glucose profile with average sensor glucose of 165 mg/dL (9.2 mmol/L), 73% readings within the target range of 70 to 180 mg/dL (3.9-10.0 mmol/L), and an estimated HbA_{1c} of 7.4% (57 mmol/mol). Dark and light shading shows 25th-75th and 10th-90th percentiles, respectively.

[Color—Print (Color Gallery page CG9) or web & ePub editions]

correlating reasonably well with her fingerstick blood glucose data (average 3.4 readings per day, mean glucose concentration of 142 mg/dL (7.9 mmol/L) (range 108-181 mg/dL [6.0-10.0 mmol/L]). You tell her that her HbA$_{1c}$ was falsely higher and that you will explain this to her surgeon, so her surgery does not need to be delayed. She asks why her HbA$_{1c}$ is falsely high and wonders what additional tests could be done to evaluate the possible cause. She does not use alcohol, salicylate, vitamin C, or opioids and has no history of asplenia.

Which of the following should be ordered next?

A. Hematocrit and lactate dehydrogenase measurement

B. Bone marrow biopsy

C. Hematocrit, iron, folic acid, and vitamin B$_{12}$ measurement and hemoglobin electrophoresis

D. Blood alcohol measurement

E. Blood lead measurement

Answer: C) Hematocrit, iron, folic acid, and vitamin B$_{12}$ measurement and hemoglobin electrophoresis

Conditions that prolong erythrocyte survival, such as asplenia, or that decreases erythrocyte turnover, such as iron deficiency anemia, vitamin B$_{12}$ deficiency, or folate deficiency anemia can cause falsely elevated HbA$_{1c}$. Uremia and chronic ingestion of alcohol, salicylates, opioids, or lead poisoning have also been associated with falsely elevated HbA$_{1c}$.[2] The patient's hematocrit, creatinine, iron, folic acid, and vitamin B$_{12}$ levels were all within reference range.

Hemoglobin (Hb) variants, including HbS, HbC, or HbF, are found in approximately 7% of the world's population and in about 10% of the African American population,[10] and they can directly interfere with some assays' detection of glycated hemoglobin. The degree of interference depends on the assay used.[2] The best next step in this patient's care is to measure hematocrit, iron, folic acid, and vitamin B$_{12}$ and perform hemoglobin electrophoresis (Answer C). Her Hb

variant analysis revealed an HbC percentage of 31%, consistent with HbC trait. HbC trait has been reported to be a cause of inappropriately elevated HbA$_{1c}$.[12] Hemolytic anemia and acute or chronic blood loss can cause falsely low, not high, HbA$_{1c}$ results. Therefore, studies to evaluate hemolytic anemia and its causes (Answers A and B) are not indicated. This patient did not have a history of chronic alcohol ingestion or lead poisoning (Answers D and E).

In conclusion, CGM is a valuable tool to assess discordance between HbA$_{1c}$ and fingerstick blood glucose values and to guide subsequent diabetes management. HbA$_{1c}$ values are useful in most cases, but they can also be subject to elevations or depressions that are not indicative of the patient's clinical picture and must be interpreted with the clinical context in mind. An alternative assay or analyte can also be used to investigate the discrepancy. With the availability of relatively easier-to-use, lower-cost, and longer-duration CGM, clinicians should consider using CGM to investigate the accuracy of HbA$_{1c}$ and the reliability of fingerstick blood glucose and to explore the causality of discrepancy with HbA$_{1c}$.

Case 2

A 72-year-old woman with type 1 diabetes uses a Medtronic insulin pump. She has a history of mini stroke with some weakness in her left hand. She also has thrombocythemia treated with hydroxyurea and clopidogrel. She does not take high-dosage vitamin C. Her POC HbA$_{1c}$ in the clinic office is 8.1% (65 mmol/mol). She has been using a glucose meter to monitor her blood glucose 3 to 4 times per day. Her meter download reveals frequent hyperglycemia but also frequent hypoglycemia with glucose readings in the range of 50 to 60 mg/dL (2.8-3.3 mmol/L). CGM is recommended.

Which CGM should be considered as the first choice for this patient?

A. Disposable CGM not interfered by platelet count

B. Disposable CGM not interfered by hydroxyurea

C. Disposable CGM not interfered by clopidogrel

D. Implantable CGM not interfered by hydroxyurea

E. Blinded professional CGM

Answer: B) Disposable CGM not interfered by hydroxyurea

Managing type 1 diabetes in elderly patients presents unique challenges. Age-related factors, such as cognitive decline, physical limitations, and coexisting medical conditions, can complicate glycemic control and increase risks of both hyperglycemia and hypoglycemia. Hypoglycemia can be particularly dangerous for elderly patients due to their increased vulnerability and the more severe consequences it can have on their health. Studies have shown that CGM improves glycemic outcomes in older patients with type 1 diabetes.[13] This patient has hypoglycemia unawareness. She would benefit from using a CGM with glucose alerts to reduce the risk of severe hypoglycemia. Choosing the right CGM for a particular patient requires an individualized approach, balancing ease of use, accuracy, and compatibility with an individual's lifestyle and health care needs.

Hydroxyurea is known to interfere with Medtronic's disposable CGM and Dexcom CGM sensors, can cause falsely higher CGM glucose readings, which could result in missed hypoglycemia alerts or errors in diabetes management, such as administering too much insulin due to falsely high sensor glucose values.[14] Therefore, this patient should not use those CGMs, although she would benefit from using a Medtronic automatic insulin delivery system integrated with Medtronic CGM if she were not on hydroxyurea. A very high platelet count might contribute to local clotting or inflammation at the sensor site, potentially leading to inaccurate readings or sensor failures. Clopidogrel reduces platelet function, which may increase the risk of bruising or minor bleeding when inserting a CGM sensor, but platelet count (Answer A) and clopidogrel (Answer C) generally do not directly interfere with CGM accuracy. A disposable CGM not interfered by hydroxyurea (Answer B), such as Abbott's CGM, is easy to use and could be considered as the first choice for this patient. Abbott's CGM can be affected by high levels of vitamin C.[15] Taking more than 500 mg of vitamin C a day may lead to falsely higher sensor glucose readings. This patient is not on high-dosage vitamin C. An implantable CGM not interfered by hydroxyurea (Answer D) such as Eversense CGM, could also be an option. It is not interfered by hydroxyurea, although could be affected by tetracycline and mannitol, causing falsely lower and higher sensor readings, respectively.[16] Eversense CGM requires a small surgical procedure for sensor implantation and removal, wearing a transmitter on top of the sensor, and sensor calibration with fingerstick blood glucose measurement. Therefore, it would be considered as the second choice for this patient. A blinded professional CGM (Answer E) would not provide immediate glucose feedback and low glucose alerts.

Case 3

A 45-year-old man with type 1 diabetes is scheduled to have a brain MRI for evaluation of frequent headache. He has been using Abbott's CGM. He asks whether he should remove his CGM sensor before the MRI or continue to wear it throughout the procedure.

Which of the following is the best recommendation?

A. Remove it before MRI, replace with a new sensor right after the procedure is completed, and call the sensor company to ask for free sensor replacement

B. Remove it before MRI, but do not replace it with a new sensor until the scheduled time for a new sensor, as her insurance might not cover replacement of the one removed for MRI

C. Remove it before MRI, self-pay for a new sensor, and start the new sensor right after the procedure is completed

D. Continue wearing it throughout the procedure, but monitor blood glucose closely with a glucose meter during and until at least 1 hour after the procedure to confirm the sensor is still providing proper readings

E. Continue wearing it throughout the procedure; no additional steps are required

Answer: D) Continue wearing it throughout the procedure, but monitor blood glucose closely with a glucose meter during and until at least 1 hour after the procedure to confirm the sensor is still providing proper readings

Electromagnetic interference can affect CGM performance. Some sensors contain metal components that can interfere with MRI. In November 2024, Abbott's CGM systems were cleared by the FDA to stay on during MRI, CT, and x-ray procedures. Medtronic's and Dexcom's current guidance still state their sensors should be removed for MRI and CT. For Eversense CGM, the sensor that is implanted under the skin is safe, but the transmitter should be removed for MRI, CT, and x-rays and reapplied after the procedure. Glucose data return within 10 minutes of reconnecting the transmitter.

Abbott states their Libre CGM readings may not be accurate during MRI, although "uncompromised" readings will usually return after 1 hour. Users are advised to have their glucose monitored closely during and after MRI using a glucose meter, until it is confirmed that the sensor is still providing proper readings after MRI (thus, Answer D is correct and Answer E is incorrect). The sensor does not need to be removed in advance of MRI (Answers A, B, and C).

Key Learning Points

- HbA$_{1c}$ and CGM monitoring have advantages and pitfalls. Clinicians must be aware of the conditions that can affect HbA$_{1c}$ and CGM accuracy and interpret the results with the clinical context in mind.

- CGM can be a valuable tool to evaluate discordance of HbA$_{1c}$ and fingerstick blood glucose values, and to guide subsequent diabetes management. Clinicians should consider using CGM to investigate the accuracy of HbA$_{1c}$ and the reliability of fingerstick blood glucose, and to identify potential causes of glucose monitoring discrepancies.

- Managing CGM requires a personalized approach; sufficient knowledge of different features of various CGMs; skills on CGM problem-solving; and extensive training on CGM ordering for different patient populations, data analysis, and management.

References

1. Nathan DM, Kuenen J, Borg R, et al. Translating the A1C assay into estimated average glucose values. *Diabetes Care.* 2008;31(8):1473-1478. PMID: 18540046

2. Radin MS. Pitfalls in hemoglobin A1c measurement: when results may be misleading. *J Gen Intern Med.* 2014;29(2):388-394. PMID: 24002631

3. Rodbard D. Continuous glucose monitoring: a review of recent studies demonstrating improved glycemic outcomes. *Diabetes Technol Ther.* 2017;19(Suppl 3):S25-S37. PMID: 28585879

4. Bellido V, Freckman G, Perez A, et al. Accuracy and potential interferences of continuous glucose monitoring sensors in the hospital. *Endocr Pract.* 2023;29(11):919-927. PMID: 37369291

5. Wright LA-C, Hirsch IB. The challenge of the use of glycemic biomarkers in diabetes: reflecting on hemoglobin A1C, 1, 5-anhydroglucitol, and the glycated proteins fructosamine and glycated albumin. *Diabetes spectrum*. 2012; 25(3):141-148.

6. Little RR, Roberts WL. A review of variant hemoglobins interfering with hemoglobin A1c measurement. *J Diabetes Sci Technol*. 2009;3(3):446-451. PMID: 20144281

7. Lenters-Westra E, Slingerland RJ. Three of 7 hemoglobin A1c point-of-care instruments do not meet generally accepted analytical performance criteria. *Clin Chem*. 2014;60(8):1062-1072. PMID: 24865164

8. American Diabetes Association Professional Practice Committee. Summary of revisions: standards of care in diabetes-2025. *Diabetes Care*. 2025;48(Suppl 1). PMID: 39651984

9. Klonoff DC, Nguyen KT, Xu NY, et al. Use of continuous glucose monitors by people without diabetes: an idea whose time has come? *J Diabetes Sci Technol*. 2023;17(6):1686-1697. PMID: 35856435

10. Sundaram RC, Selvaraj N, Vijayan G, Bobby Z, Hamide A, Dasse NR. Increased plasma malondialdehyde and fructosamine in iron deficiency anemia: effect of treatment. *Biomed Pharmacother*. 2007;61(10):682-685. PMID: 17698317

11. Wright JJ, Hu IR, Shajani-Yi Z, Bao S. Use of continuous glucose monitoring leads to diagnosis of hemoglobin C trait in a patient with discrepant hemoglobin A1C and self-monitored blood glucose. *AACE Clin Case Rep*. 2019;5(1):e31-e34. PMID: 31966996

12. Lorenzo-Medina M, De-La-Iglesia S, Ropero P, Nogueira-Salgueiro P, Santana-Benitez J. Effects of hemoglobin variants on hemoglobin a1c values measured using a high-performance liquid chromatography method. *J Diabetes Sci Technol*. 2014;8(6):1168-1176. PMID: 25355712

13. Pratley RE, Kanapka LG, Rickels MR, et al; Wireless Innovation for Seniors with Diabetes Mellitus (WISDM) Study Group. Effect of continuous glucose monitoring on hypoglycemia in older adults with type 1 diabetes: a randomized clinical trial. *JAMA*. 2020;323(23):2397-2406. PMID: 32543682

14. Szmullowicz ED, Aleppo G. Interferent effect of hydroxyurea on continuous glucose monitoring. *Diabetes Care*. 2021;44(5):e89-e90. PMID: 33653823

15. Heinemann L. Interference with CGM systems: practical relevance? *J Diabetes Sci Technol*. 2021;16(2):271-274. PMID: 34911382

16. Lorenz C, Sandoval W, Mortllaro M. Interference assessment of various endogenous and exogenous substances on the performance of the Eversense long-term implantable continuous glucose monitoring system. *Diabetes Technol Ther*. 2018;20(5):344-352. PMID: 29600877

SGLT-2 Inhibitor Therapy in Type 2 Diabetes: Advantages and Pitfalls

Aidar R. Gosmanov, MD, DMSc. Division of Endocrinology, Albany Medical College and Section of Endocrinology, Stratton VAMC, Albany, NY; Email: agosmanov@gmail.com

Educational Objectives

After reviewing this chapter, learners should be able to:

- Identify the clinical benefits and most frequently observed adverse effects that occur in people with type 2 diabetes (T2D) after initiation of SGLT-2 inhibitors.

- Identify approaches to effectively diagnose and manage adverse effects of SGLT-2 inhibitors.

- Develop patient-centric strategies to reduce the risk of SGLT-2 inhibitor–associated adverse effects.

Significance of the Clinical Problem

The landscape of diabetes pharmacotherapy has been revolutionized following FDA approval in 2013 of the first SGLT-2 inhibitor, canagliflozin, for glycemic management in people with T2D. In general, SGLT-2 inhibitors lead to modest hemoglobin A_{1c} reduction by 0.5% to 1.0% depending on whether they were initiated in drug-naïve patients or in patients already taking metformin.[1] The subsequent increase of SGLT-2 inhibitor use in clinical practice was, however, driven not by their glycemic effects but rather by clear evidence of cardiovascular (CV) and kidney benefits that occur independent of their impact on glycemic control. In prospective, randomized placebo-controlled trials, canagliflozin, dapagliflozin, and empagliflozin—but not ertugliflozin—were shown to significantly reduce CV death, heart failure hospitalizations, and kidney end points.[2-5] A recent meta-analysis of SGLT-2 inhibitor effects on major adverse CV events clearly demonstrates that the therapeutic effects are driven by a reduction in CV death, which in turn is explained by reductions in heart failure death and sudden cardiac death.[6] In the T2D trials with prespecified primary kidney end points, SGLT-2 inhibitors consistently and significantly reduced the risk of kidney disease progression in patients, regardless of baseline estimated glomerular filtration rate.[7]

Despite the initial enthusiasm in the field, prescription of SGLT-2 inhibitors in clinical practice remains lower than expected, placing a large number of patients who could have benefitted from this class of medication at a disadvantage.[8] While therapeutic inertia can frequently explain delay in implementation of novel treatment modalities in the management of chronic diseases, this notion by itself is unlikely to explain the persistently low prescription rate more than 10 years since approval of the first SGLT-2 inhibitor. We believe that unique and sometimes serious, yet poorly predictable, adverse effects associated with the use of gliflozins make some providers cautious to initiate these agents. In this chapter, the most frequently observed adverse effects associated with SGLT-2 inhibitors are discussed, as well as current knowledge in their evaluation and management and challenges in predicting patient populations prone to develop these adverse effects.

Practice Gaps

- The possibility of SGLT-2 inhibitor–induced adverse effects in clinical practice is overshadowed by the default assumption that the risk–benefit profile favors therapeutic efficacy over the risk of adverse effects.

- Providers may not be fully aware of the previous and evolving body of evidence demonstrating that prescription of SGLT-2 inhibitors can first lead to the development of serious adverse effects that can negatively affect patients' health in the short-term before expected clinical benefits are attained.

- While there is clear agreement on when and how to prescribe SGLT-2 inhibitors for optimization of T2D management, there is less agreement on how to predict, diagnose, and manage on-treatment adverse effects following the initiation of SGLT-2 inhibitors.

Discussion

The very first landmark trials that demonstrated cardiovascular and kidney benefits of different SGLT-2 inhibitors in T2D have consistently reported clinically important safety events (*Table*). Use of SGLT-2 inhibitors increases risk of genital mycotic infections (GMIs) but not urinary tract infections (UTIs). The most serious yet rare adverse effect reported in these trials was the development of diabetic ketoacidosis (DKA). Finally, with the landmark trials demonstrating consistent placebo-adjusted increases in hematocrit in those treated with SGLT-2 inhibitors,[9] recent postmarketing observations revealed that some patients with T2D who are treated with SGLT-2 inhibitors develop new-onset erythrocytosis.[10,11]

Genitourinary Infections

There was no meaningful excess in UTI risk with SGLT-2 inhibitor exposure compared with risk in the placebo arm.[12] Nevertheless, in 2015, the FDA issued a black box warning to the labels of all SGLT-2 inhibitors regarding the risk for severe UTIs following reports of severe sepsis and pyelonephritis in patients treated with gliflozins.[13] This was downgraded to a warning in 2023. Glycosuria from uncontrolled diabetes or SGLT-2 inhibition can create a favorable environment for the growth of *Candida* species in the lower genitourinary tract. *Candida* organisms can adhere to genitalia more extensively in the presence of glycosuria and via attachment to the host cells, which in turn can result in local yeast infection signs and symptoms, such as pain, redness, swelling, and/or pruritis. Therefore, it is not surprising to see a 3-fold higher risk of GMIs in large SGLT-2 inhibitor trials (*Table*), as well as in real-world practice.[14] The clinical presentation can range from balanitis in males and vulvovaginal

Table. Adverse Events and Off-Target Biological Effects Observed in Landmark Randomized Placebo-Controlled SGLT-2 Inhibitor Trials

| Type 2 diabetes trial / SGLT-2 inhibitor | Genitourinary infections SGLT-2 inhibitor vs placebo, % incidence | | DKA SGLT-2 inhibitor vs placebo, new cases/total participants | Hematocrit Placebo-adjusted absolute change, % |
	GMI	UTI		
EMPA-REG OUTCOME / empagliflozin[5]	6.4 vs 1.8	18.1 vs 18.0	4/4687 vs 1/2333	+ 2.6%
DECLARE-TIMI 58 / dapagliflozin[4]	0.9 vs 0.1	1.5 vs 1.6	27/8574 vs 12/8569	+ 2.6%
CREDENCE / canagliflozin[3]	2.3 vs 0.6	11.1 vs 10.1	11/2200 vs 1/2197	+ 2.4%
VERTIS CV / ertugliflozin[2]	5.4 vs 1.5	12 vs 10	19/5493 vs 2/2745	+ 2.1%

candidiasis in females to Fournier gangrene in advanced cases. GMIs usually occur within the first 6 months after SGLT-2 inhibitor initiation. Other risk factors for GMIs in T2D include female sex, uncircumcised males, obesity, and history of recurrent GMIs.

Diabetic Ketoacidosis

The initial warning that SGLT-2 inhibitors can cause DKA in people with diabetes came within first 2 years following the approval of the first-in-class agent, canagliflozin.[15] Since then, DKA risk has become a theme of multiple publications.[16] The absolute risk of DKA is less than 0.1%, and relative risk is about 2-fold higher than that of people with T2D treated with other hypoglycemic agents. These risks collectively translate to 1 to 2 additional cases of DKA per 1000 patients with T2D who are treated with an SGLT-2 inhibitor over 1 year.[7] The mechanisms that predispose to SGLT-2 inhibitor–induced DKA include a decrease in insulin and an increase in glucagon production and an increase in blood concentration of ketone bodies, which, in settings of volume depletion, caloric deprivation, reduction or discontinuation of insulin therapy, alcohol intake, and/or infection, can lead to ketoacidosis.[15,16] SGLT-2 inhibitor–induced DKA can present initially without hyperglycemia (ie, euglycemic DKA) or classically with hyperglycemia.[16,17] It should be highlighted that in the landmark T2D trials, patients with a hemoglobin A_{1c} value above 10.0% (>86 mmol/mol)[2,5] or 12.0% (>108 mmol/mol)[3,4] were excluded from study participation. Indeed, severe hyperglycemia in people with non–insulin-treated T2D already results in β-cell dysfunction and insulinopenia.[18] This clearly argues against initiation of SGLT-2 inhibitors in patients who have a hemoglobin A_{1c} value greater than 10% to 12% (86-108 mmol/mol).

Erythrocytosis

As SGLT-2 inhibitors can lead to hematocrit elevation (*Table*), of particular interest are recent studies that demonstrate an increased risk of SGLT-2 inhibitor–triggered erythrocytosis, including studies in men receiving testosterone replacement therapy. The absolute erythrocytosis incidence can reach up to 10%.[10,11] It was shown that SGLT-2 inhibitors increase erythropoiesis via stimulation of erythropoietin production and inhibition of hepcidin synthesis.[19,20] SGLT-2 inhibitor–induced erythrocytosis is a clinically relevant finding, as a more pronounced rise in hematocrit could potentially increase blood viscosity and, hence, reduce blood flow, resulting in tissue ischemia. It is unclear why only a small fraction of patients develop de novo erythrocytosis following the initiation of SGLT-2 inhibitors. It could be that some patients have a genetic predisposition to excessive red blood cell production and initiation of an SGLT-2 inhibitor unmasks propensity towards unregulated erythropoiesis.[21] Until more information becomes available, prescribers should consider following hematocrit trends in people with T2D treated with SGLT-2 inhibitors regardless of the presence of background testosterone replacement. In those who develop marked rise in hematocrit meeting criteria for erythrocytosis, blood donation should be strongly considered pending results of ancillary laboratory assessments for other causes of new-onset erythrocytosis following initiation of SGLT-2 inhibitor therapy.

Clinical Case Vignettes

Case 1

A 69-year-old woman with a 15-year history of T2D returns to clinic for regular follow-up. The patient also has osteoporosis, dyslipidemia, nephrolithiasis, history of total hysterectomy, and diabetic kidney disease. She is intolerant of metformin and alogliptin due to abdominal discomfort. Her T2D is currently diet-controlled.

On physical examination, her BMI is 27.8 kg/m² and blood pressure is normal.

Her hemoglobin A_{1c} level has increased from 6.9% (52 mmol/mol) at the last visit to 7.5% (58 mmol/mol) today. Other laboratory studies are significant for an estimated glomerular filtration rate of 70 mL/min per m² and spot urine albumin-to-creatinine ratio of 200 mg/g (normal <30 mg/g).

Based on the above data, dapagliflozin, 10 mg daily, is initiated. One month later, she calls the clinic and describes a 1-week history of itching in her labia and vagina. She has no fever/chills and no urinary symptoms. She had a similar episode about 10 years ago.

Which of the following is the best next step in this patient's management?

A. Initiate nitrofurantoin

B. Hold dapagliflozin and start fluconazole, 150 mg daily × 3 days

C. Recommend no changes

D. Continue dapagliflozin and start fluconazole, 150 mg daily × 3 days

E. Obtain urinalysis

Answer: B) Hold dapagliflozin and start fluconazole, 150 mg daily × 3 days

This patient likely has vulvovaginal candidiasis without systemic manifestations and is unlikely to have a bacterial infection. Thus, initiating nitrofurantoin (Answer A) or obtaining urinalysis (Answer E) is not the best next step. There are no outcome studies to guide whether to advise holding or continuing an SGLT-2 inhibitor in this situation. As patient safety is the utmost concern and her glycemic control is near-optimal, her metabolic health would not be compromised by holding dapagliflozin to reduce glucosuria for several days (thus, Answers C and D are incorrect). Holding dapagliflozin for several days and administering topical or oral antifungal agents (Answer B) should address her GMI. In discussing long-term plans regarding whether an SGLT-2 inhibitor could be safely continued after an initial episode of GMI, preventive strategies should be discussed, including advice on adequate hydration, maintenance of personal hygiene, emptying the bladder regularly, and wearing loose-fitting cotton underwear. In patients with an initial episode of successfully treated, uncomplicated GMI, SGLT-2

inhibitor therapy can be resumed after providing appropriate counseling.

Case 1, Continued

The patient returns for regular follow-up 3 months later. The GMI episode reported at the last encounter resolved following a short course of fluconazole. Her hemoglobin A_{1c} level has improved to 7.1% (54 mmol/mol) while on dapagliflozin. Today, she reports that for the last 2 weeks she has had new-onset intermittent urinary frequency and hesitancy, which she attributes to possible recurrent kidney stones. She does not report passing any stones. She has no fever/chills, back pain, vaginal itching, or hematuria. Preclinic blood work shows no abnormalities of serum biochemical parameters, and preclinic urinalysis performed 3 days ago demonstrates following:

> Glucose = >1000 mg/dL (SI: >55.5 mmol/L)
> Ketones, negative
> Small blood
> Trace protein
> Nitrite, negative
> Leukocyte esterase, moderate
> White blood cell count = 11-25 per high-power field (normal, 0-2)
> Red blood cell count = 3-5 per high-power field (normal, 0-2)
> Squamous epithelial cells = 11-25 (normal, 0-5)
> Trace bacteria

During the clinic visit, the patient asks for advice to help manage her urinary symptoms.

Which of the following is the best next step in this patient's management?

A. Repeat urinalysis in 1 week

B. Discontinue dapagliflozin

C. Obtain urine culture

D. Discontinue dapagliflozin and start nitrofurantoin, 100 mg twice daily × 7 days

E. Refer to urology clinic

Answer: D) Discontinue dapagliflozin and start nitrofurantoin, 100 mg twice daily × 7 days

She has likely developed cystitis in the background of SGLT-2 inhibitor therapy and history of kidney stones. Interestingly, recent reports suggested that dapagliflozin increases UTI risk in a dose-dependent manner. Given the risk of complicated UTI, she should be started on an antibacterial regimen. Experts advise a 3- to 5-day course of cotrimoxazole or nitrofurantoin for treatment of the first episode of bacterial cystitis.[22] Therefore, stopping the SGLT-2 inhibitor as the only strategy (Answer B) may not be sufficient, while holding the SGLT-2 inhibitor and starting an antibacterial agent (Answer D) that can attain high concentrations in the urine is most appropriate.

Obtaining urine culture (Answer C), repeating urinalysis later (Answer A), or referring to urology clinic (Answer E) could be suggested, but none of these options addresses the core problem, which is high suspicion for urinary bacterial infection in a person with complicated genitourinary history. If left untreated, a bacterial infection in this setting could lead to more severe UTI. Previous uncomplicated UTI is currently not a contraindication to SGLT-2 inhibitor therapy. There are no clear clinical guidelines on whether SGLT-2 inhibitors can be resumed in patients after an initial UTI. Until then, it might be a safe practice not to continue SGLT-2 inhibitors in patients whose first UTI was severe or if there is known accompanying genitourinary history, including structural abnormalities, benign prostate hyperplasia, presence of indwelling Foley catheter, nephrolithiasis, and/or kidney cysts.

Case 2

A 76-year-old man with a 20-year history of T2D is evaluated in the emergency department for confusion. He also has obesity (BMI = 38 kg/m^2), atrial fibrillation, hypertension, depression, and frailty. His home-based primary care provider was repeatedly unable to contact the patient who lives alone. The provider requested a wellness check by local police who found the patient to be confused. In the emergency department, he was afebrile and hemodynamically stable and had generalized nonfocal weakness.

He takes 15 prescription medications. T2D is treated with metformin, 1 g twice daily; empagliflozin, 25 mg daily; semaglutide, 2 mg subcutaneously weekly; and insulin glargine, 40 units daily. Brief medical record review reveals his hemoglobin A$_{1c}$ level 2 months ago was 7.8% (62 mmol/mol). Insulin was added to his treatment regimen about 2 years ago, and empagliflozin was started 6 months ago.

Laboratory test results:

> Sodium = 137 mEq/L (SI: 137 mmol/L)
> Chloride = 102 mEq/L (SI: 102 mmol/L)
> Bicarbonate = 16 mEq/L (22-32 mEq/L)
>   (SI: 16 mmol/L [22-32 mmol/L])
> Potassium = 4.5 mEq/L (4.5 mmol/L)
> Glucose = 141 mg/dL (SI: 7.8 mmol/L)
> Lactic acid, normal
> White blood cell count, normal
> Troponin, normal
> Kidney function, normal
> Chest x-ray, normal

Urinalysis:

> Glucose = >1000 mg/dL (>55.5 mmol/L)
> Ketones = >150 mg/dL
> Large leukocyte esterase
> White blood cell count = >50 per high-power field
> Few bacteria
> Few yeasts

The emergency department provider consults endocrinology in light of recent reports of SGLT-2 inhibitor–induced euglycemic DKA.

Which of the following is the best next step in this patient's management?

A. Measure β-hydroxybutyrate in blood

B. Obtain arterial blood gases

C. Repeat biochemistries, as the blood glucose value of 141 mg/dL is likely an error

D. Begin intravenous infusion of insulin and dextrose-containing fluids

E. Start fluconazole

Answer: D) Begin intravenous infusion of insulin and dextrose-containing fluids

This patient has euglycemic DKA. Following recent recommendations on the evaluation of patients with suspected DKA,[18] the diagnosis here is made based on history of T2D, significant ketonuria, and bicarbonate value less than 18 mEq/L (<18 mmol/L). Therefore, additional studies to prove he has ketosis (Answer A) or acidosis (Answer B) are only confirmatory and they would only delay initiation of DKA therapy. Nevertheless, the admitting team measured serum ketones before insulin was initiated (β-hydroxybutyrate assay was not available), which later was reported as "moderately" positive (equivalent to 2+ grade [~ 30-40 mg/dL] ketonemia). The patient is clearly adherent to SGLT-2 inhibitor therapy given significant glucosuria in the setting of euglycemia. Therefore, there is no indication to repeat biochemistries (Answer C). Although the urinalysis results may suggest he has UTI or GMI (Answer E), the priority at this time is to commence comprehensive therapy of DKA consisting of intravenous infusion of insulin and fluids (Answer D). The fact that he is euglycemic necessitates use of dextrose-containing fluids to prevent hypoglycemia in the background of insulin infusion. A recent report highlighted that resolution of SGLT-2 inhibitor–induced DKA can, in some cases, take up to 20 days, and this is likely commensurate with the degree of acidosis on presentation and/or prolonged elimination of SGLT-2 inhibitors from the circulation.[23]

Case 2, Continued

Follow-up conversation with the patient revealed that 1 to 2 weeks before this admission, he self-discontinued insulin because he was tired of taking multiple medications. Four days after admission, the primary team informs the endocrinology consulting team that the patient will be discharged home soon.

In preparation for discharge, which of the following is the best next step in this patient's management?

A. Measure serum fasting C-peptide

B. Stop empagliflozin and emphasize that insulin glargine should be administered daily as prescribed

C. Measure glutamic acid decarboxylase 65 antibody titer

D. Resume all home medications

E. Resume all home medications and advise use of fluconazole if he develops genitourinary symptoms

Answer: B) Stop empagliflozin and emphasize that insulin glargine should be administered daily as prescribed

The main task in this case is to reduce risk of recurrent DKA. The factor that likely precipitated euglycemic DKA is omission of insulin in the setting of concomitant SGLT-2 inhibitor use in a person with longstanding T2D who already has significantly diminished capacity for endogenous insulin production. Immediately following the DKA episode, endogenous insulin production, judged by C-peptide level (Answer A), will be low.

A subset of patients with T2D may have latent autoimmune diabetes in adults (LADA), which is characterized by progressive loss of β-cell function requiring early introduction of insulin therapy to aid glycemic control. In this case, the presence of longstanding diabetes and only recent initiation of basal insulin would suggest testing for glutamic acid decarboxylase 65 antibodies (Answer C) is unnecessary.

Reassurance that resuming home medications (Answer D), including empagliflozin, will not put him at risk for another DKA episode is not substantiated by systematic evidence. In addition, there are no studies to suggest that empiric treatment for suspected GUI (Answer E) while being treated with SGLT-2 inhibitors in the outpatient setting can reduce DKA risk.

Therefore, at this time, the safest approach would be discontinuation of empagliflozin and patient reeducation on the importance of adherence to a diabetes treatment regimen, including basal insulin (Answer B).

Case 3

A 67-year-old White man with a history of T2D, ischemic stroke, hypertension, and dyslipidemia comes for a 6-month follow-up appointment for hypogonadism management. He is clinically and biochemically eugonadal while on testosterone cypionate, 200 mg intramuscularly every 10 days for past the 7 years. He has no history of tobacco use or sleep apnea. His BMI is 33.1 kg/m². Four months ago, his primary provider added empagliflozin, 10 mg daily, to his regimen of metformin and sitagliptin. One month ago, he was in the emergency department for evaluation of progressive headaches. At that time, extensive clinical, biochemical, and radiological evaluation revealed presence of hypertensive urgency and elevated hematocrit of 53.5% (normal, 32%-50%). An antihypertensive medication, amlodipine, was added. His hematocrit and hemoglobin A_{1c} values before empagliflozin initiation were 49.2% and 7.0% (53 mmol/mol), respectively.

In clinic, his blood pressure is 145/90 mm Hg while on lisinopril, 20 mg daily, and amlodipine, 5 mg daily. He reports a 10-lb (4.5-kg) weight loss since starting the SGLT-2 inhibitor. His current hemoglobin A_{1c} value is 6.4% (46 mmol/mol), and repeat hematocrit remains elevated at 56%.

Which of the following is the best next step in this patient's management?

A. Hold testosterone replacement therapy

B. Refer to a hematologist

C. Discontinue the SGLT-2 inhibitor

D. Begin low-dosage aspirin

E. Increase the lisinopril dosage to 40 mg daily

Answer: A) Hold testosterone replacement therapy

This patient developed secondary erythrocytosis defined as a hematocrit value greater than 50% following the initiation of empagliflozin. Recent

cohort studies provided early evidence that men with T2D commencing SGLT-2 inhibitors have a higher risk of developing erythrocytosis.[10,11] Such risk is particularly evident in hypogonadal men receiving concurrent testosterone replacement therapy.[24] In this case, the patient has experienced erythrocytosis, which likely led to blood pressure elevation; thus, prompt action to correct erythrocytosis is indicated.

Referring to a hematologist (Answer B), commencing aspirin (Answer D), or increasing the lisinopril dosage (Answer E) could be considered, but they do not address the core of his present problem.

He successfully lost weight and reduced his hemoglobin A_{1c} level after empagliflozin initiation. Therefore, discontinuing the SGLT-2 inhibitor (Answer C) is not warranted.

Although his current testosterone regimen resulted in optimal management of his hypogonadism over years, holding it (Answer A) would offer the fastest short-term solution to lower his hematocrit and prothrombotic risk and improve blood pressure.

Case 3, Continued

Four weeks later, the patient returns because he is experiencing hypogonadal symptoms while off testosterone injections and asks to resume treatment. He is willing to continue empagliflozin given its proven health benefits in patients with T2D. His hematocrit is now normal at 45%. Testosterone is resumed at a lower dosage.

Which of the following assessments would help determine whether the patient remains at risk for erythrocytosis?

A. *HFE* (human iron homeostatic protein) genetic testing

B. *JAK2* genetic testing

C. Polysomnography

D. Iron measurement

E. Bone marrow biopsy

Answer: A) HFE (human iron homeostatic protein) genetic testing

When screening for hemochromatosis, iron measurement by itself (Answer D) has no value. Also, SGLT-2 inhibitors increase erythropoiesis and inhibit the hepcidin pathway[19]; thus, interpretation of iron metabolism in this patient may be challenging.

The prevalence of *JAK2* pathogenic variants (Answer B) that predispose to polycythemia vera in the general population and in patients with secondary erythrocytosis, as in this case, is very low.

The patient did not report snoring, and he experienced weight loss after initiation of SGLT-2 inhibitor therapy, so screening for sleep apnea (Answer C) is not warranted.

Knowing that up to 20% of US non-Hispanic White persons may be asymptomatic carriers of a hemochromatosis gene allele,[25] we requested *HFE* genetic analysis (Answer A), which revealed that the patient's genotype was C282Y –/– (he was heterozygous for the H63D pathogenic variant). In one case series describing White men who developed erythrocytosis while on combined testosterone and SGLT-2 inhibitor therapy, there was high prevalence of newly diagnosed heterozygosity in one *HFE* allele.[21]

Finally, bone marrow biopsy (Answer E) is an invasive procedure and is unlikely to help in the evaluation of secondary erythrocytosis.

The patient`s sexual symptoms improved while on a less-intense testosterone regimen of 150 mg every 2 weeks. Repeat hematocrit measurements were consistently below 50%, which allowed for safe continuation of his endocrine treatments with plans to closely monitor hematocrit trends.

Key Learning Points

- SGLT-2 inhibitors offer numerous health benefits to people with T2D.

- Initiation of SGLT-2 inhibitors may, however, increase risk of GUI, DKA, and new-onset erythrocytosis.

- Timely identification of patients who are at risk for serious adverse effects is critical before initiation of SGLT-2 inhibitor therapy.

- Although early reports can help to shape initial approaches to enhance safety of SGLT-2 inhibitor prescription, prediction, diagnosis, and management of adverse effects can be challenging due to lack of systematic postmarketing data reporting and consensus among content experts.

- As SGLT-2 inhibitors are frequently prescribed by nonendocrinology providers, the role of endocrinologists and diabetologists in educating trainees and primary care, cardiology, and nephrology specialists on avoiding these adverse effects must be revitalized, which, in turn, should enhance confidence of practitioners in initiating SGLT-2 inhibitor therapy.

- When initiating SGLT-2 inhibitors to improve care for people with diabetes, providers should always discuss the spectrum of adverse effects, reassess clinical and laboratory parameters at each follow-up visit, and advise the patient to contact the clinic any time an adverse reaction develops.

References

1. Tsapas A, Avgerinos I, Karagiannis T, et al. Comparative effectiveness of glucose-lowering drugs for type 2 diabetes: a systematic review and network meta-analysis. *Ann Intern Med.* 2020;173(4):278-286. PMID: 32598218

2. Cannon CP, Pratley R, Dagogo-Jack S, et al; VERTIS CV Investigators. Cardiovascular outcomes with ertugliflozin in type 2 diabetes. *N Engl J Med.* 2020;383(15):1425-1435. PMID: 32966714

3. Perkovic V, Jardine MJ, Neal B, et al; CREDENCE Trial Investigators. Canagliflozin and renal outcomes in type 2 diabetes and nephropathy. *N Engl J Med.* 2019;380(24):2295-2306. PMID: 30990260

4. Wiviott SD, Raz I, Bonaca MP, et al; DECLARE-TIMI 58 Investigators. Dapagliflozin and cardiovascular outcomes in type 2 diabetes. *N Engl J Med.* 2019;380(4):347-357. PMID: 30415602

5. Zinman B, Wanner C, Lachin JM, et al. Empagliflozin, cardiovascular outcomes, and mortality in type 2 diabetes. *N Engl J Med*. 2015;373(22):2117-2128. PMID: 26378978

6. Patel SM, Kang YM, Im K, et al. Sodium-glucose cotransporter-2 inhibitors and major adverse cardiovascular outcomes: a SMART-C collaborative meta-analysis. *Circulation*. 2024;149(23):1789-1801. PMID: 38583093

7. Nuffield Department of Population Health Renal Studies G, Consortium SiM-AC-RT. Impact of diabetes on the effects of sodium glucose co-transporter-2 inhibitors on kidney outcomes: collaborative meta-analysis of large placebo-controlled trials. *Lancet*. 2022;400(10365):1788-1801. PMID: 36351458

8. Mahtta D, Ramsey DJ, Lee MT, et al. Utilization rates of SGLT2 inhibitors and GLP-1 receptor agonists and their facility-level variation among patients with atherosclerotic cardiovascular disease and type 2 diabetes: insights from the Department of Veterans Affairs. *Diabetes Care*. 2022;45(2):372-380. PMID: 35015080

9. Inzucchi SE, Zinman B, Fitchett D, et al. How does empagliflozin reduce cardiovascular mortality? Insights from a mediation analysis of the EMPA-REG OUTCOME trial. *Diabetes Care*. 2018;41(2):356-363. PMID: 29203583

10. Schwarz Y, Klein P, Lev-Shalem L. Masked anemia and hematocrit elevation under sodium glucose transporter inhibitors: findings from a large real-world study. *Acta Diabetol*. 2024;61(1):99-105. PMID: 37698758

11. Gosmanov AR. Haematocrit trends and risk of erythrocytosis in persons with type 2 diabetes treated with sodium-glucose cotransporter-2 inhibitors in real world clinical practice. Diabetologia. 2024;67:S347.

12. Gorgojo-Martinez JJ, Gorriz JL, Cebrian-Cuenca A, Castro Conde A, Velasco Arribas M. Clinical recommendations for managing genitourinary adverse effects in patients treated with SGLT-2 inhibitors: a multidisciplinary expert consensus. *J Clin Med*. 2024;13(21):6509. PMID: 39518647

13. Dave CV, Schneeweiss S, Kim D, Fralick M, Tong A, Patorno E. Sodium-glucose cotransporter-2 inhibitors and the risk for severe urinary tract infections: a population-based cohort study. *Ann Intern Med*. 2019;171(4):248-256. PMID: 31357213

14. Fralick M, MacFadden DR. A hypothesis for why sodium glucose co-transporter 2 inhibitors have been found to cause genital infection, but not urinary tract infection. *Diabetes Obes Metab*. 2020;22(5):755-758. PMID: 31943733

15. Peters AL, Henry RR, Thakkar P, Tong C, Alba M. Diabetic ketoacidosis with canagliflozin, a sodium-glucose cotransporter 2 inhibitor, in patients with type 1 diabetes. *Diabetes Care*. 2016;39(4):532-538. PMID: 26989182

16. Chow E, Clement S, Garg R. Euglycemic diabetic ketoacidosis in the era of SGLT-2 inhibitors. *BMJ Open Diabetes Res Care*. 2023;11(5):e003666. PMID: 37797963

17. Kum-Nji JS, Gosmanov AR, Steinberg H, Dagogo-Jack S. Hyperglycemic, high anion-gap metabolic acidosis in patients receiving SGLT-2 inhibitors for diabetes management. *J Diabetes Complications*. 2017;31(3):611-614. PMID: 27913012

18. Umpierrez GE, Davis GM, ElSayed NA, et al. Hyperglycemic crises in adults with diabetes: a consensus report. *Diabetes Care*. 2024;47(8):1257-1275. PMID: 39052901

19. Ghanim H, Abuaysheh S, Hejna J, et al. Dapagliflozin suppresses hepcidin and increases erythropoiesis. *J Clin Endocrinol Metab*. 2020;105(4):dgaa057. PMID: 32044999

20. Sano M, Goto S. Possible mechanism of hematocrit elevation by sodium glucose cotransporter 2 inhibitors and associated beneficial renal and cardiovascular effects. *Circulation*. 2019;139(17):1985-1987. PMID: 31009585

21. Schumacher KA, Gosmanov AR. Hemochromatosis gene mutation in persons developing erythrocytosis on combined testosterone and SGLT-2 inhibitor therapy. *J Investig Med High Impact Case Rep*. 2022;10:23247096221111774. PMID: 35848311

22. Grigoryan L, Trautner BW, Gupta K. Diagnosis and management of urinary tract infections in the outpatient setting: a review. *JAMA*. 2014;312(16):1677-1684. PMID: 25335150

23. Woronow D, Chamberlain C, Houstoun M, Munoz M. Prolonged diabetic ketoacidosis associated with sodium-glucose cotransporter-2 inhibitors: a review of postmarketing cases. *Endocr Pract*. 2024;30(7):603-609. PMID: 38692489

24. Gosmanov AR, Gemoets DE, Schumacher KA. Increased risk of erythrocytosis in men with type 2 diabetes treated with combined sodium-glucose cotransporter-2 inhibitor and testosterone replacement therapy. *J Endocrinol Invest*. 2024;47(10):2615-2621. PMID: 38536657

25. Steinberg KK, Cogswell ME, Chang JC, et al. Prevalence of C282Y and H63D mutations in the hemochromatosis (HFE) gene in the United States. *JAMA*. 2001;285(17):2216-2222. PMID: 11325323

Recommended Reading

- Nanna MG, Kolkailah AA, Page C, Peterson ED, Navar AM. Use of sodium-glucose cotransporter 2 inhibitors and glucagonlike peptide-1 receptor agonists in patients with diabetes and cardiovascular disease in community practice. *JAMA Cardiol*. 2023;8(1):89-95. PMID: 36322056

- Dawwas GK, Flory JH, Hennessy S, Leonard CE, Lewis JD. Comparative safety of sodium-glucose cotransporter 2 inhibitors versus dipeptidyl peptidase 4 inhibitors and sulfonylureas on the risk of diabetic ketoacidosis. *Diabetes Care*. 2022;45(4):919-927. PMID: 35147696

- Gagnon DR, Zhang TJ, Brand FN, Kannel WB. Hematocrit and the risk of cardiovascular disease--the Framingham study: a 34-year follow-up. *Am Heart J*. 1994;127(3):674-682. PMID: 8122618

- Liew A, Lydia A, Matawaran BJ, Susantitaphong P, Tran HTB, Lim LL. Practical considerations for the use of SGLT-2 inhibitors in the Asia-Pacific countries-An expert consensus statement. *Nephrology (Carlton)*. 2023;28(8):415-424. PMID: 37153973

- Chandrashekar M, Philip S, Nesbitt A, Joshi A, Perera M. Sodium glucose-linked transport protein 2 inhibitors: an overview of genitourinary and perioperative implications. *Int J Urol*. 2021;28(10):984-990. PMID: 34155680

- Taylor SI, Blau JE, Rother KI. SGLT2 inhibitors may predispose to ketoacidosis. *J Clin Endocrinol Metab*. 2015;100(8):2849-2852. PMID: 26086329

- Mazer CD, Hare GMT, Connelly PW, et al. Effect of empagliflozin on erythropoietin levels, iron stores, and red blood cell morphology in patients with type 2 diabetes mellitus and coronary artery disease. *Circulation*. 2020;141(8):704-707. PMID: 31707794

- Gangat N, Szuber N, Alkhateeb H, Al-Kali A, Pardanani A, Tefferi A. JAK2 wild-type erythrocytosis associated with sodium-glucose cotransporter 2 inhibitor therapy. *Blood*. 2021;138(26):2886-2889. PMID: 34653249

- Pishdad R, Auwaerter PG, Kalyani RR. Diabetes, SGLT-2 inhibitors, and urinary tract infection: a review. Curr Diab Rep. 2024;24(5):108-117. PMID: 38427314

- Poitout V, Robertson RP. Glucolipotoxicity: fuel excess and beta-cell dysfunction. *Endocr Rev*. 2008;29(3):351-366. PMID: 18048763

Optimal Use of Diabetes Technology in the Clinical Management of Diabetes

Rayhan Lal, MD. Divisions of Endocrinology, Departments of Medicine and Pediatrics, Stanford University, Stanford, CA; Email: inforay@stanford.edu

Educational Objectives

After reviewing this chapter, learners should be able to:

- Describe components of an automated insulin dosing (AID) system and the current regulatory framework.

- Explain who can benefit from an AID system.

- Provide optimizations for people using an AID system.

Significance of the Clinical Problem

More than 2 million Americans with absolute insulinopenia require insulin replacement therapy. Network meta-analysis demonstrates that among studied diabetes technologies, AID results in the most significant improvements in time-in-range, hemoglobin A_{1c}, and severe hypoglycemia.[1,2] The 2025 American Diabetes Association Standards of Care now recommend continuous glucose monitors (CGMs) for all people with diabetes and AID for people requiring insulin when it can be used safely.[3] Keeping up-to-date with the latest technology, understanding how it works, ensuring access, and integrating this technology into life can pose barriers for people with diabetes and the providers caring for them.[4]

Practice Gaps

- Keeping up-to-date with new diabetes technology.

- Ensuring access to all available tools.

- Being provided full details of algorithm operation.

- Understanding what, if any, effect adjustments have on system operation.

Discussion

Every commercial insulin pump manufacturer in the United States offers an AID system. The US FDA has cleared 5 such systems (Tandem Control-IQ, iLet Bionic Pancreas, OmniPod 5, twiist with Tidepool Loop, CamAPS) as class II medical devices and approved the MiniMed 780G as a class III medical device. Under the class II designations are 3 components: the glucose sensor or integrated continuous glucose monitor (iCGM), alternate controller enabled (ACE) insulin pump, and algorithm dubbed iAGC (interoperable automated glycemic controller). While it may appear that these regulatory precedents guarantee interoperability (plug-and-play operation of any pump, CGM, and algorithm), pairing components requires commercial business agreements between manufacturers. In addition, these commercial options require announcement of meals and exercise to achieve optimal glycemic outcomes.

Many commercial AID options do not have full descriptions of how they automate glucose control (also known as closed source), as these mechanisms are held as trade secrets by manufacturers. There are 2 popular open-source AID (OS-AID) algorithms: the FDA-cleared Loop algorithm and the randomized controlled trial–validated OpenAPS algorithm.[5] The Loop algorithm is implemented in the iOS Loop app, while the OpenAPS algorithm can run on iOS (iAPS, Trio), Android (AndroidAPS), or Linux (OpenAPS). These algorithms are compatible with multiple sensors and pumps. The OpenAPS algorithm is the only current control software designed and tested for unannounced meals.[6] The 2025 American Diabetes Association Standards of Care encourage providers to support people with diabetes using OS-AID.[3]

With all the available options, it is theoretically possible for most people with type 1 diabetes to achieve glycemic targets even with unannounced meals. Unfortunately, access to diabetes technology is not equitable[7] and is driven by profit-based motives. As providers, it is critical to remain up-to-date and consistently offer diabetes technology to any person with type 1 diabetes.

Clinical Case Vignettes

Case 1

A 17-year-old girl with 12-year history of type 1 diabetes recently started using an AID system and reports that 1 night ago when her sensor expired, she woke up 8 hours after her last meal feeling hungry, shaky, and tired. The glucose value before the sensor cut off at 9 PM was recorded as 100 mg/dL (5.6 mmol/L), and a fingerstick value when she woke up at 2 AM was 45 mg/dL (2.5 mmol/L). She consumed carbohydrates appropriately to treat the hypoglycemia, replaced her sensor, and returned to sleep. Her estimated total daily dose over the last 2 weeks was 50 units. Her current therapy settings include a basal rate of 1.5 units/h, insulin-to-carbohydrate ratio of 8 g, and insulin sensitivity factor of 40 mg/dL (2.2 mmol/L).

Which of the following is the best advice for this patient?

A. Weaken the carbohydrate-to-insulin ratio

B. Weaken basal insulin and instruct her on basal insulin titration and timely CGM replacement

C. Weaken the insulin sensitivity factor

D. Instruct her to always have a bedtime snack

E. Counsel on the risk of dead-in-bed syndrome

Answer: B) Weaken basal insulin and instruct her on basal insulin titration and timely CGM replacement

In general, AID systems reduce basal insulin delivery in anticipation of hypoglycemia. This may make providers feel that basal rates do not really matter. However, in this case, without CGM input, the system fell back to the scheduled basal rate, resulting in hypoglycemia. The young woman had an overly aggressive basal rate relative to her other therapy settings. After reducing the basal insulin dosage, it may be useful for her to titrate basal insulin (potentially even with closed loop turned off) (Answer B).

Based on the timeline, her last meal was around 6 PM and most of her prandial insulin effect would have dissipated. In addition, her 9 PM glucose value was 100 mg/dL (5.6 mmol/L), so it is unlikely that any corrective insulin doses would have been at play. Therefore, weakening the carbohydrate-to-insulin ratio (Answer A) or insulin sensitivity factor (Answer C) would be unlikely to affect this overnight hypoglycemia.

Consuming extra calories from carbohydrates (Answer D) to counter nonphysiologic settings would not be appropriate.

It is important to reassure this young woman that while she did have a low glucose value, she woke up and treated hypoglycemia appropriately. Instilling fear of fatal overnight hypoglycemia (Answer E) is unlikely to result in any positive behavioral changes and could result in maladaptive behaviors.

Case 2

A 22-year-old man with a 10-year history of type 1 diabetes on a commercial AID seeks help to better control his postprandial blood glucose. He reports diminished satiety and substantial weight gain over the years, culminating in class 1 obesity (height, 71 in [180 cm]; weight, 216 lb [98 kg] [BMI = 30.1 kg/m^2]) and an increase in insulin needs to 120 units daily.

Physical examination findings are notable for hypertension and acanthosis nigricans on the neck and axillae.

A point-of-care hemoglobin A_{1c} value is 6.9% (52 mmol/mol).

Which of the following is the best next step to improve this patient's overall health?

A. Start a GLP-1 receptor agonist

B. Strengthen the carbohydrate-to-insulin ratio

C. Strengthen basal insulin

D. Strengthen the insulin sensitivity factor

E. Discontinue AID

Answer: A) Start a GLP-1 receptor agonist

This man has reasonable glycemic control but is dealing with obesity and type 2 diabetes on top of his known type 1 diabetes. It is important to realize that in this scenario, GLP-1 receptor agonist therapy (Answer A) is entirely on label (both for obesity and type 2 diabetes). Presently, obesity and insulin resistance are his primary health problems.

Increasing the aggressiveness of his therapy settings (Answers B, C, and D) would only lead to further weight gain and would not substantially improve health outcomes, even if there is a further hemoglobin A_{1c} reduction.

Discontinuing AID (Answer E) would likely increase the workload of diabetes and would not be appropriate at this time. Indeed, following the initiation of a GLP-1 receptor agonist, and especially as weight loss progresses, insulin modulation will be important to reduce the risk of hypoglycemia.

Case 3

A 39-year-old woman with a 14-year history of type 1 diabetes (using Loop) seeks assistance with insulin resistance occurring 1 week per menstrual cycle. During these weeks, her time-in-range drops to around 60%, but it is 80% at other times without significant time-below-range.

Which of the following is the best recommendation?

A. Make all therapy settings uniformly more aggressive

B. Change the glucose target

C. Make all therapy settings uniformly weaker

D. Set up a custom preset to manage periods of insulin resistance or offer a monophasic oral contraceptive pill

E. Change the glucose safety limit

Answer: D) Set up a custom preset to manage periods of insulin resistance or offer a monophasic oral contraceptive pill

Altered hormone levels during the menstrual cycle can affect insulin sensitivity. For example, elevated progesterone levels in the luteal phase (10-14 days before a period) may induce insulin resistance. This can make type 1 diabetes more difficult to manage in those with menstrual periods. Loop offers override presets that can uniformly intensify therapy settings by a fixed percentage for a duration of the user's choosing. It may, for example, be useful to set up a 110% preset for when this woman is experiencing insulin resistance (Answer D). This preset can be activated and deactivated when she feels it is appropriate. Alternatively, a monophasic oral contraceptive pill could eliminate the hormonal fluctuations and reduce these changes over the course of a cycle.

Changing the glucose target (Answer B) or uniformly strengthening or weakening the settings at all times (Answers A and C) would be a nuisance given that she is maintaining target time-in-range most of the time.

The glucose safety limit is a feature of Loop; in the case of an actual or predicted glucose value below the glucose safety limit, Loop will suspend all insulin delivery. Changing the value (Answer E) would not increase insulin delivery during times of resistance.

References

1. Pease A, Clement L, Earnest, Kiriakova V, Liew D, Zoungas S. Time in range for multiple technologies in type 1 diabetes: a systematic review and network meta-analysis. *Diabetes Care.* 2020;43(8):1967-1975. PMID: 32669412

2. Pease A, Clement L, Earnest A, Kiriakova, Liew D, Zoungas S. The efficacy of technology in type 1 diabetes: a systematic review, network meta-analysis, and narrative Synthesis. *Diabetes Technol Ther.* 2020;22(5):411-421. PMID: 31904262

3. American Diabetes Association Professional Practice Committee. 7. Diabetes technology: standards of care in diabetes-2025. *Diabetes Care.* 2025;48(Suppl_1):S146-S166. PMID: 39651978

4. Tanenbaum ML, Commissariat PV, Wilmot EG, Lange K. Navigating the unique challenges of automated insulin delivery systems to facilitate effective uptake, onboarding, and continued use. *J Diabetes Sci Technol.* 2025;19(1):47-53. PMID: 39212371

5. Braune K, Hussain S, Lal R. The first regulatory clearance of an open-source automated insulin delivery algorithm. *J Diabetes Sci Technol.* 2023;17(5):1139-1141. PMID: 37051947

6. Petruzelkova L, Neuman V, Plachy L, et al. First use of open-source automated insulin delivery AndroidAPS in full closed-loop scenario: Pancreas4ALL Randomized Pilot Study. *Diabetes Technol Ther.* 2023;25(5):315-323. PMID: 36826996

7. Burckhardt M-A. Addala A, and de Bock M. Editorial: equity in type 1 diabetes technology and beyond: where are we in 2022? *Front Endocrinol (Lausanne).* 2024;15:1400240. PMID: 38596223

Addressing Racial Health and Health Care Inequities in Diabetes

Alyson K. Myers, MD. Department of Medicine, Montefiore Einstein, Bronx, NY; Email: alymyers@montefiore.org

Educational Objectives

After reviewing this chapter, learners should be able to:

- Describe the role of systemic racism and bias in health outcomes.

- Identify racial/ethnic disparities in diabetes diagnosis, complications, and management.

- Illustrate methods for improving gaps in diabetes care.

Significance of the Clinical Problem

Race is social construct that has been used to categorize people by phenotype and ancestry. Unfortunately, race has also been used as a tool to discriminate against certain groups of people—racism. In a study of medical students at the University of Virginia, those who held a greater number of false beliefs about the differences between White and Black patients (eg, Black people have thicker skin than White people) were more likely to incorrectly assess or treat the pain of Black patients.[1]

Such discriminatory theories have also extended to diabetes, which was known in the late 1800s as *Judenkrankheit*—the Jewish malady—because doctors found that those who were Jewish were 2 to 6 times more likely to die of diabetes than those who were not Jewish.[2] During the 1930s, when involuntary sterilization was being imposed in Germany to prevent continuation of conditions such as epilepsy or manic depression, diabetes was considered but not selected.[2] In current times, diabetes disproportionately affects persons who identify as non-Hispanic Black, Hispanic/Latino, American Indian Alaskan Native, or Pacific Islander compared with non-Hispanic White persons.

Disparities in both diagnosis and management have led to increased rates of diabetes complications, such as end-stage kidney disease, blindness, or amputations, among people from these communities. Identifying the root causes of these disparities—discrimination, racism, bias, social determinants of health—is necessary to close these disparity gaps.[3]

Practice Gaps

- There is a lack of provider awareness about the need to consider the unique needs of racial and ethnic minorities who are living with diabetes.

- It is imperative for providers to consider how implicit bias, discrimination, and social determinants of health can affect patient care.

- There is a gap in understanding how individuals, health systems, and insurance organizations can improve health outcomes for people with diabetes from marginalized populations.

Discussion

Diabetes affects 38.4 million people or roughly 12% of the population, but the rates and complications are more prevalent in communities of color. People from racial and ethnic minoritized groups bear the extra burden of patient-provider discordance, discrimination, and the downstream effects of historical injustice (ie, slavery, redlining, Jim Crow laws). Such factors affect trust and access to care and ultimately create a system of inequitable care.

Diabetes Screening and Diagnosis

Diabetes screening should be done in people older than 40 years, as well as in people who are sedentary and/or have overweight or obesity. For persons of Asian descent, different BMI cutoffs are used to diagnose both overweight and obesity ($23 kg/m^2$ vs $25 kg/m^2$ and $28 kg/m^2$ vs $30 kg/m^2$, respectively).[4] In several studies, those who identify as Japanese American were diagnosed with diabetes at a BMI as low as $22 kg/m^2$.[4] As a result, it has been suggested that waist-to-height ratio of 0.5 or greater may be a better predictor than BMI for Chinese patients.[5]

Diabetes can be diagnosed with a fasting serum glucose measurement (or random glucose concentration >200 mg/dL [>10.0 mmol/L]), hemoglobin A_{1c} (HbA_{1c}) measurement, or oral glucose tolerance test (OGTT). HbA_{1c} can be falsely elevated or lowered in some populations due to the presence of anemia or hemoglobinopathies (eg, thalassemia, sickle cell anemia).[6] In addition, in some racial/ethnic groups, postprandial hyperglycemia is the problem as opposed to impaired fasting glucose, so using fasting glucose alone could potentially lead to an incorrect diagnosis. The Diabetes Epidemiology Collaborative Analysis of Diagnostic Criteria in Asia (DECODA) Study Group found that using both fasting glucose and OGTT identified more persons with diabetes than simply using fasting serum glucose alone.[7]

Diabetes Management

Diabetes is best managed with a patient-centered approach. It is important to consider medication cost, insurance status, comorbidities, lifestyle, housing and food security/insecurity when devising a treatment plan for a patient. For example, a patient who is undomiciled may not be able to store their unused insulin in the refrigerator. Alternatively, a patient with blindness from retinopathy may need help in organizing their pills or giving injections. Also, patients with a high deductible may not be able to afford newer diabetes medications until the middle or end of the year when that deductible has been reached.

Disparities in health insurance also can interfere with screening for diabetes complications. The National Health Interview Survey of persons recently diagnosed with diabetes found that Hispanic patients were less likely to be insured when compared with Black or White participants.[8] As a result, Hispanic participants were less likely to have lipid, blood pressure, or retinal screening.[8]

Insurance is not the sole barrier for screenings. In a review of the barriers of retinal screening for racial/ethnic minoritized populations, there were numerous social determinants of health that were highlighted as impeding care, including transportation issues, language barriers, cost, and low level of education.[9]

Unfortunately, provider bias may also impede a successful treatment plan. Studies in both the pediatric and adult literature have shown increased awareness and use of diabetes technology in White patients when compared with those who identify as Black or Hispanic.[10-12] Another study found that there was also favoritism when prescribing diabetes technology to those with English names or private insurance.[13]

Diabetes Complications

Racial and ethnic minority patients are also more likely to have diabetes complications, including blindness, end-stage kidney disease, peripheral arterial disease, and skin infections.[6] Persons with diabetes have a 25% lifetime chance of developing a diabetic foot ulcer, and nearly 20% of those with a diabetic foot ulcer will need a lower-extremity amputation.[14] Lower-extremity amputations are associated with a 5-year mortality of 50%, which is greater than the 5-year mortality of either colon or breast cancer.[15] Risk factors for amputation include male sex, age younger than 70 years, Black/Hispanic/Native American race/ethnicity, living in a rural area, depression, and tobacco use. Comorbid neuropathy and peripheral arterial disease in the setting of poor glycemic control can also increase the risk of lower-extremity amputation.[14] The use of the SGLT-2 inhibitor canagliflozin has not been consistently shown to lead to lower-extremity amputation. As a result, it is important to counsel patients on daily foot exams, proper footwear, and cigarette smoking cessation. Studies have shown that Hispanic patients are less likely than White patients to receive smoking cessation advice. Factors that contribute to these disparities include language, insurance status, frequency of doctor's visits, provider bias, and access to care.[16] Counseling and medication can be used together to most effectively help a patient quit smoking.[17]

Closing Disparity Gaps

To close the disparity gaps that exist for racial/ethnic minoritized groups, it is important to first start at the level of the provider. Providers must stay up-to-date with diabetes diagnosis and management. In addition, we need to transition from the paternalistic approach to care to that of a patient-centered model. This requires a discussion with patients about their goals for care and difficulties and ensuring that they understand their treatment plan. Using the teach-back method at the end of the visit is a great way to assess whether patients understand what was communicated.

We also must acknowledge and explore our biases to ensure that we are providing patients with the best care. In doing so, we must validate the feelings of discrimination and racism that our patients have endured. By ignoring such feelings,

the patient-provider relationship becomes one of mistrust and can lead to nonadherence. Lastly, we must continue to support research efforts to further close these diabetes disparity gaps and make diabetes care equitable.

Clinical Case Vignettes

Case 1

A 78-year-old Chinese woman with stage 3 chronic kidney disease, hearing loss, and polyneuropathy of the feet has been living with type 2 diabetes for the past 10 years. She also has hepatic steatosis, hypertension, and hyperlipidemia. She lives with her husband who is a retired maintenance worker at a bank. Her HbA$_{1c}$ is 6.8% (51 mmol/mol) on basal insulin, 14 units subcutaneously once daily at bedtime; metformin, 1000 mg twice daily; and an GLP-1 receptor agonist delivered subcutaneously at maximal dosage weekly. On review of her continuous glucose monitoring report, her time in range is 75%, with a coefficient of variation of 28%, and there is no hypoglycemia.

At today's visit, she laments that her son has been helping her pay for her GLP-1 receptor agonist therapy, as it costs $400 per month. On review of her insurance, she has a high deductible that she will not meet until the end of the year.

Which of the following is the best strategy in this patient's diabetes care?

A. Continue current therapy

A. Switch from subcutaneous to oral GLP-1 receptor agonist

B. Increase the metformin dosage

C. Add bolus insulin

D. Discontinue the GLP-1 receptor agonist and start pioglitazone

Answer: E) Discontinue the GLP-1 receptor agonist and start pioglitazone

GLP-1 receptor agonists and thiazolidinediones both can improve steatohepatitis and potentially prevent worsening of fibrosis.[18] If the cost of the GLP-1 receptor agonist is too high, then switching to a less expensive agent would be best (Answer E). Oral GLP-1 receptor agonists (Answer B) are also costly, so that would not help her financial issue. Her metformin is at maximal dosage, so increasing it (Answer C) would not be recommended. Her HbA$_{1c}$ goal is less than 7.5% (<58 mmol/mol) based on her age, so adding bolus insulin (Answer D) is not needed now.

Case 1, Continued

The patient is bilingual in English and Cantonese.

After adjusting her medications, what would be the best way to decide whether she understands her medication changes?

A. Give her a paper handout with her medication list in her preferred language

B. Read her the medication list

C. Perform a teach-back

D. Call her pharmacy

E. Schedule an appointment with the certified diabetes care and education specialist

Answer: C) Perform a teach-back

This patient's hearing loss may compromise what she processes through listening, so the only way to know if she heard what was said is to use the teach-back method (Answer C), as it would require her to explain what she was taught in her own words.[19] Paper handouts (Answer A), reading her the medication list (Answer B), and calling the pharmacy (Answer D) would not help the provider to determine if the patient understands the information. Although working with a certified diabetes care and education specialist (Answer D) has been shown to improve health outcomes,[17] it is important for the patient to adjust her medications at the time of her appointment, not at a future date.

Case 2

Patient 1

A 64-year-old retired city transit worker who immigrated from the Dominican Republic 30 years ago presents for a well visit. She lives with her husband of 40 years and her 2 adult sons in a community where the median annual income is $48,700.[20] She has hypertension, type 2 diabetes, dyslipidemia, and kidney stones. Her HbA$_{1c}$ level is 8.5% (69 mmol/mol). She is currently on metformin, 1000 mg twice daily, and glipizide, 10 mg daily. She has been minimally active since retiring 3 years ago.

Patient 2

A 60-year-old public school high school principal lives with his 2 dogs in a community where the median annual income is $79,190.[20] Three months ago, during an annual exam, he was diagnosed with type 2 diabetes (HbA$_{1c}$ = 9.0% [75 mmol/mol]). Semaglutide and metformin were initiated. At his follow-up visit today, he has lost 8 lb (3.6 kg), and his HbA$_{1c}$ level has decreased to 6.9% (52 mmol/mol). He works out at the gym at his job 3 to 4 times per week.

The 2 patients are treated by the same physician but are managed differently. What could be the reason?

A. Ageism

B. Implicit bias

C. Imposter syndrome

D. Intersectionality

E. Stereotype threat

Answer: B) Implicit bias

Implicit bias (Answer B) is an unconscious bias that we all have as human beings, which can lead to prescribing differences between patients. These 2 patients are similar in age, so ageism (Answer A) is not an issue. Intersectionality (Answer D) is a term used to recognize a person's multiple identities, such as race, ethnicity, gender, sexual orientation, and immigrant status as opposed to focusing on only one. The imposter syndrome (Answer C) occurs when one undervalues their own work while praising the work of others. Stereotype threat (Answer E) occurs when an individual purposely avoids behaving in a manner that is stereotypical of the group to which they belong.[21]

Case 2, Continued

On review of his medical records, the 60-year-old male patient in part 1 of this vignette has a mean corpuscular volume of 78 μm^3 (78 fL) with normal measurements of ferritin, transferrin, and reticulocyte count.

How does this finding affect his glycemic control measurements?

A. His HbA_{1c} is unaffected

B. His HbA_{1c} may be falsely elevated

C. His HbA_{1c} may be falsely low

D. His fructosamine may be falsely elevated

E. His fructosamine may be falsely low

Answer: C) His HbA$_{1c}$ may be falsely low

This patient's laboratory findings suggest a presence of a hemoglobinopathy, such as thalassemia trait, which can falsely lower HbA_{1c} (Answer C). Glycation of red blood cells occurs with mature cells, so conditions with high red blood cell turnover lead to a lower HbA_{1c} level.[6] Fructosamine involves glycation of albumin, so a hemoglobinopathy would not be an issue.

Case 3

A 28-year-old unemployed Hispanic/Latino man with uncontrolled type 1 diabetes (HbA_{1c} = 12.0% [108 mmol/mol]) presents to diabetes clinic for follow-up care. He was hospitalized 2 months ago with a right fifth metatarsal ulcer and was told to follow-up with podiatry in 2 weeks, but no appointment was made.

He has been living with type 1 diabetes for 12 years and has associated neuropathy. He also has a history of depression, anxiety, and polysubstance use (tobacco, marijuana, and cocaine). At home, he takes insulin glargine, 20 units subcutaneously daily at bedtime, and insulin lispro, 8 units subcutaneously 3 times a day before meals.

His vital signs are stable, and his glucose sensor shows a sideways arrow with a blood glucose value of 150 mg/dL (8.3 mmol/L).

On physical examination, he has an ulcer with an overlying callus. There is neither erythema nor pus expressed, but there is concern for an infection underneath the callus. His monofilament testing shows decreased sensation in the first metatarsal, and his pulses are 2+ in both the dorsal pedis and posterior tibialis pulses.

Which of the following factors increases risk for having an amputation in patients with diabetic foot ulcers?

A. Female sex

B. Age >70 years

C. Tobacco use

D. 20/20 vision

E. Type 1 diabetes

Answer: C) Tobacco use

Male sex, age younger than 70 years, and poor vision are all associated with increased risk of amputation (thus, Answers A, B, and D are incorrect).[22,23] There are more people with type 2 diabetes than type 1 diabetes, so the rate of diabetic foot ulcer in those with type 2 diabetes is greater than that of type 1 diabetes (thus, Answer E is incorrect).[14] Tobacco use (Answer C) increases risk for amputation in patients with diabetic foot ulcers.

Case 3, Continued

The patient has been smoking 1 pack of cigarettes per day for about 10 years. He wants to quit smoking cold turkey, starting today. He has tried several times in the past but has not been able to quit for more than a couple of weeks, as he develops problems with sleep, anxiety, worsening depression, and poor concentration. He does not have headaches or dizziness.

Which of the following is his diagnosis as it relates to tobacco use?

A. Tobacco use disorder

B. Tobacco dependence disorder

C. Tobacco abuse

D. Tobacco overuse disorder

E. Tobacco withdrawal

Answer: B) Tobacco dependence disorder

The diagnosis of tobacco dependence (Answer B) is based on his withdrawal symptoms (tolerance), his multiple attempts to quit, and his continued use of nicotine despite worsening depression.[24]

Case 3, Continued

Which of the following is the best management for his tobacco diagnosis?

A. Varenicline

B. Bupropion

C. Nicotine patch

D. E-cigarettes

E. Nicotine patch and counseling

Answer: E) Nicotine patch and counseling

In patients with diabetes who are trying to quit smoking, medical therapy with counseling is the best choice, so the nicotine patch paired with counseling (Answer E) would be a better option than the nicotine patch (Answer C), varenicline (Answer A), or bupropion (Answer B) alone.[17] Bupropion should also be avoided, as it can worsen anxiety in people with an anxiety disorder. E-cigarettes (Answer D) are neither recommended nor FDA-approved for smoking cessation.[17]

Key Learning Points

- Race is a social, NOT a biological, construct.

- Discrimination, racism, and implicit bias can lead to misdiagnosis, mismanagement, and worse health outcomes for patients with diabetes. Acknowledging biases can help providers deliver equitable care.

- Systemic racist policies, such as redlining or segregation, have been implicated in poorer health outcomes for marginalized communities.

- Assessing the social determinants of health allows health care providers to bridge the disparity gaps for marginalized communities.

References

1. Hoffman KM, Trawalter S, Axt JR, Oliver MN. Racial bias in pain assessment and treatment recommendations, and false beliefs about biological differences between blacks and whites. *Proc Natl Acad Sci U S A.* 2016;113(16):4296-4301. PMID: 27044069

2. Tuchman AM. *Diabetes: A History of Race and Disease.* Yale University Press; 2020.

3. Golden SH, Joseph JJ, Hill-Briggs F. Casting a health equity lens on endocrinology and diabetes. *J Clin Endocrinol Metab.* 2021;106(4):e1909-e1916. PMID: 33496788

4. Hsu WC, Araneta MRG, Kanaya AM, Chiang JL, Fujimoto W. BMI cut points to identify at-risk Asian Americans for type 2 diabetes screening. *Diabetes Care.* 2015;38(1):150-158. PMID: 25538311

5. Xu Z, Qi X, Dahl AK, Xu W. Waist-to-height ratio is the best indicator for undiagnosed type 2 diabetes. *Diabet Med.* 2013;30(6):e201-e207. PMID: 23444984

6. Young C, Myers AK. Racial and ethnic disparities in diabetes clinical care and management: a narrative review. *Endocr Pract.* 2023;29(4):295-300. PMID: 36464131

7. Qiao Q, Nakagami T, Tuomilehto J, et al; DECODA Study Group. Comparison of the fasting and the 2-h glucose criteria for diabetes in different Asian cohorts. *Diabetologia.* 2000;43(12):1470-1475. PMID: 11151755

8. Marcondes FO, Cheng D, Alegria M, Haas JS. Are racial/ethnic minorities recently diagnosed with diabetes less likely than white individuals to receive guideline-directed diabetes preventive care? *BMC Health Serv Res.* 2021;21(1):1150. PMID: 34689778

9. Fathy C, Patel S, Sternberg Jr. P, Kohanim S. Disparities in adherence to screening guidelines for diabetic retinopathy in the United States: a comprehensive review and guide for future directions. *Semin Ophthalmol.* 2016;31(4):364-377. PMID: 27116205

10. Agarwal S, Schechter C, Gonzalez J, Long JA. Racial-ethnic disparities in diabetes technology use among young adults with type 1 diabetes. *Diabetes Technol Ther.* 2021;23(4):306-313. PMID: 33155826

11. Lai CW, Lipman TH, Willi SM, Hawkes CP. Racial and ethnic disparities in rates of continuous glucose monitor initiation and continued use in children with type 1 diabetes. *Diabetes Care.* 2020;44(1):255-257. PMID: 33177169

12. Ye Y, Acevedo Mendez BA, Izard S, Myers AK. Demographic variables associated with diabetes technology awareness or use in adults with type 2 diabetes. *Diabetes Spectr.* 2023;37(1):60-64. PMID: 38385093

13. Odugbesan O, Addala A, Nelson G, et al. Implicit racial-ethnic and insurance-mediated bias to recommending diabetes technology: insights from T1D exchange multicenter pediatric and adult diabetes provider cohort. *Diabetes Technol Ther.* 2022;24(9):619-627. PMID: 35604789

14. Gallagher KA, Mills JL, Armstrong DG, et al; American Heart Association Council on Peripheral Vascular Disease; Council on Cardiovascular and Stroke Nursing; Council on Clinical Cardiology; and Council on Lifestyle and Cardiometabolic Health. Current status and principles for the treatment and prevention of diabetic foot ulcers in the cardiovascular patient population: a scientific statement from the American Heart Association. *Circulation.* 2024;149(4):e232-e253. PMID: 38095068

15. Armstrong DG, Swerdlow MA, Armstrong AA, Conte MS, Padula WV, Bus SA. Five year mortality and direct costs of care for people with diabetic foot complications are comparable to cancer. *J Foot Ankle Res.* 2020;13(1):16. PMID: 32209136

16. Babb S, Malarcher A, Asman K, et al. Disparities in cessation behaviors between Hispanic and non-Hispanic White adult cigarette smokers in the United States, 2000-2015. PMID: 31999539

17. American Diabetes Association Professional Practice Committee. 5. Facilitating positive health behaviors and well-being to improve health outcomes: standards of care in diabetes-2025. *Diabetes Care.* 2025;48(Suppl 1):S86-S127. PMID: 39651983

18. Castera L, Cusi K. Diabetes and cirrhosis: current concepts on diagnosis and management. *Hepatology.* 2023;77(6):2128-2146. PMID: 36631005

19. Hong YR, Jo A, Cardel M, Huo J, Mainous AG. Patient-provider communication with teach-back, patient-centered diabetes care, and diabetes care education. *Patient Educ Couns.* 2020;103(12):2443-2450. PMID: 32507589

20. CoreData.nyc. Accessed January 24, 2025. http://coredata.nyc

21. Williams M. *Elevating the Voices of Women of Color in the Workplace.* IGI Global; 2024.

22. Boyko EJ, Zelnick LR, Braffett BH, et al. Risk of foot ulcer and lower-extremity amputation among participants in the diabetes control and complications trial/epidemiology of diabetes interventions and complications study. *Diabetes Care.* 2022;45(2):357-364. PMID: 35007329

23. Lin C, Liu J, Sun H. Risk factors for lower extremity amputation in patients with diabetic foot ulcers: a meta-analysis. *PLOS ONE.* 2020;15(9):e0239236. PMID: 32936828

24. Baker TB, Breslau N, Covey L, Shiffman S. DSM criteria for tobacco use disorder and tobacco withdrawal: a critique and proposed revisions for DSM-5. *Addiction.* 2012;107(2):263-275. PMID: 21919989

Recommended Reading

- Blackstock U. *Legacy: A Black Physician Reckons With Racism in Medicine.* Viking; 2024.
- Tuchman AM. *Diabetes: A History of Race and Disease.* Yale University Press; 2020.
- Washington HA. *Medical Apartheid: The Dark History of Medical Experimentation on Black Americans From Colonial Times to the Present.* Doubleday Books; 2006.

Management of Cystic Fibrosis–Related Diabetes

Melissa Putman, MD. Harvard Medical School, Diabetes Research Center, Massachusetts General Hospital; Email: msputman@mgh.harvard.edu

Educational Objectives

After reviewing this chapter, learners should be able to:

- Describe the prevalence, pathogenesis, and clinical significance of cystic fibrosis–related diabetes (CFRD).

- Highlight current approaches to screening, diagnosis, and management of CFRD.

- Discuss the role of diabetes technologies and alternative therapies in the management of CFRD.

Significance of the Clinical Problem

Cystic fibrosis (CF) is an autosomal recessive disorder affecting roughly 40,000 people in the United States and more than 100,000 worldwide. Defective function of the CF transmembrane conductance regulator (CFTR) protein leads to exocrine pancreatic insufficiency and progressive pulmonary decline, which is the primary cause of mortality in this patient population. Due to improved care and treatments available to people with CF, the median predicted survival has increased substantially over the past 3 decades, from 30 years of age for people born between 1989 and 1993 to the current 61 years for those born between 2019 and 2023.[1] As people with CF live longer, nonpulmonary complications of CF are becoming more prevalent and add significant morbidity and treatment burden.

Up to 20% of adolescents and 30% to 50% of adults with CF develop CFRD,[1] making this one of the most common nonpulmonary complications of CF. The etiology of CFRD is likely multifactorial and is not fully understood, but the primary driver is a progressive insulin secretory defect caused by β-cell dysfunction.[2] There is also a component of insulin resistance that occurs in CFRD, likely related to significant illness and inflammation, which can fluctuate over time based on clinical status. Risk factors for CFRD include pancreatic exocrine insufficiency, older age, severe lung disease, CF-related liver disease, and lung transplantation.[3] The diagnosis of CFRD has been associated with clinical decline in those with CF, including worsening lung function and nutritional status, as well as earlier mortality.[4]

Practice Gaps

- Diabetes screening tools for people with CF are limited, and new approaches are needed for screening and diagnosing CFRD.

- Diabetes-related tasks can add substantial treatment burden to a patient population that already carries a large medical burden related to lung disease and other comorbidities.

- Nutritional needs are changing in the postmodulator era with the rising prevalence of obesity in people with CF.

- As life expectancy continues to improve in people with CF, new complications of aging will likely arise, including increasing rates of microvascular and macrovascular disease.

Discussion

Given the often insidious onset of CFRD with the gradual development of brief prandial hyperglycemia with normal fasting glucose levels and no apparent symptoms, screening is important. Oral glucose tolerance testing (OGTT) is recommended for annual CFRD screening in all people with CF older than 10 years.[4] OGTT is the screening test of choice because the diagnosis of CFRD by this test has been correlated with important CF-specific outcomes, including pulmonary function and nutritional status. However, rates of screening with OGTT have been suboptimal over the past 20 years, and just over 30% of adults with CF underwent annual screening OGTT in 2023.[1] New screening approaches are urgently needed.

Insulin is the only recommended treatment for CFRD because this is the only therapy that has been shown to improve CF-specific clinical outcomes.[4] Recommended glycemic targets are the same as they are for type 1 and 2 diabetes; however, these targets were established based on the development of microvascular complications, and there are no data guiding whether CF-specific targets are needed for optimizing lung function and nutritional status. Diabetes tasks can add significant burden to an already burdensome disease, affecting quality of life in addition to CF-specific clinical outcomes.[5,6] In addition, there are other unique aspects of CFRD that can make management challenging[7]: (a) variable degree of endogenous insulin production, such that some patients may need small doses of only rapid-acting insulin with meals, whereas others may require a more typical basal-bolus insulin regimen; (b) fluctuating insulin requirements based on clinical status, with much more insulin needed when sick or receiving glucocorticoid treatment and much less required while healthy; (c) high calorie nutritional requirements to attain optimal BMI and nutritional status for optimizing lung function, which can often involve high carbohydrate intake; and (d) risk of spontaneous reactive hypoglycemia related to delayed first-phase insulin secretion followed by an exaggerated second-phase insulin release. A key priority identified by the CFF-NIH Workshop is to develop approaches to improve diabetes management and reduce treatment burden for people with CFRD.[8]

Since the introduction of ETI (elexacaftor/tezacaftor/ivacaftor) in 2019, there has been a significant increase in the prevalence of overweight and obesity in adults with CF in the United States, with most recent estimates from the Cystic Fibrosis Foundation Patient Registry reporting 13% with a BMI in the obesity range above 30 kg/m^2 and 28.4% with a BMI in the overweight range of 25 to 29.9 kg/m^2.[1] Moreover, data suggest that normal-weight obesity, defined as a normal BMI with elevated fat mass, has been reported to occur with a prevalence of more than 30% in this patient population.[9] Although data are limited, complications of obesity are being increasingly reported in the aging CF population, including hypertension, hepatic steatosis (which can exacerbate underlying CF-related liver disease), and cardiovascular disease.[10-12] Insulin resistance related to obesity may exacerbate β-cell dysfunction and further complicate diabetes management. *CFRD-metabolic syndrome* is terminology currently being used to describe patients with CF who have diabetes and also have evidence of insulin resistance and underlying type 2 diabetes phenotype. Whether noninsulin therapies will be safe and effective in treating obesity and insulin resistance this patient population is currently being investigated.

Historically, microvascular complications of diabetes were relatively rare occurrences in people with CFRD, primarily because the limited life expectancy meant that people were more likely to die of lung disease before developing these complications. However, this is changing in the postmodulator era, and further studies are needed to understand the best approach to screening, prevention, and management of diabetes complications in people with CFRD.

Clinical Case Vignettes

Case 1

A 17-year-old young man has a history of CF, pancreatic insufficiency, and malnutrition requiring a gastrotomy tube with overnight formula feeds. His BMI is low at the 10th percentile, but his pulmonary function is excellent with forced expiratory volume in 1 second (FEV1) percent predicted at 99%. He has had no recent pulmonary exacerbations, hospitalizations, or glucocorticoid treatment. Results of annual CFRD screening with OGTT are shown in the *Table*.

Why is hemoglobin A_{1c} falsely low in patients with CF?

A. Accelerated red blood cell turnover

B. Chronic hypoxia

C. Laboratory error

D. It's not falsely low

Answer: D) It's not falsely low

Hemoglobin A_{1c} has been shown to correlate strongly with average glucose values in adults with CF, and this relationship is the same as in other diabetes populations.[13,14] However, hemoglobin A_{1c} does not perform well as a screening test for CFRD because average glucose is often normal in early CFRD, which is marked by brief prandial excursions with episodes of reactive hypoglycemia and normal glucose levels overnight. Recent studies suggest that hemoglobin A_{1c} can be used as an initial test to identify those at very low risk of CFRD who may not need OGTT in an effort to improve overall screening rates.[15-17] The Canadian CF guidelines have recently incorporated a tiered screening approach, such that those with hemoglobin A_{1c} values below 5.5% (<37 mmol/mol) do not require further CFRD screening with OGTT.[18]

Case 1, Continued

The patient declines a repeat OGTT to confirm the diagnosis.

Which of the following should be recommended next for this patient?

A. Check fingerstick glucose before meals and 2 hours after meals to collect more data

B. Initiate continuous glucose monitoring to collect more data

C. Start insulin glargine, 0.1 units/kg per day

D. Start insulin lispro with a carbohydrate ratio of 1:30 with meals

Answer: B) Initiate continuous glucose monitoring to collect more data

Although in the past we relied on fingerstick glucose checks to determine the next steps in treatment, intermittent glucose checks can easily miss glycemic variability in early CFRD, which is characterized by brief glycemic excursion after meals often lasting less than 2 to 3 hours with normal fasting and premeal glucose levels. Continuous glucose monitoring (CGM) has significantly changed our approach to CFRD

Year	Fasting glucose	2-Hour glucose	Hemoglobin A_{1c}*	Glycemic category
Year 1	108 mg/dL (SI: 6.0 mmol/L)	78 mg/dL (SI: 4.3 mmol/L)	5.0% (31 mmol/mol)	Impaired fasting glucose
Year 2	111 mg/dL (SI: 6.2 mmol/L)	110 mg/dL (SI: 6.1 mmol/L)	4.9% (30 mmol/mol)	Impaired fasting glucose
Year 3	114 mg/dL (SI: 6.3 mmol/L)	149 mg/dL (SI: 8.3 mmol/L)	5.0% (31 mmol/mol)	Impaired fasting glucose/ impaired glucose tolerance
Year 4	102 mg/dL (SI: 5.7 mmol/L)	203 mg/dL (SI: 11.3 mmol/L)	5.0% (31 mmol/mol)	CFRD

*Despite the diagnosis of CFRD based on OGTT, his hemoglobin A_{1c} values have remained overall stable and well within the normal range.

management by providing comprehensive glycemic data that can be used to inform treatment. For example, if glucose levels overnight are within the normal range and postprandial reactive hypoglycemia is occurring, then starting long-acting insulin may lead to significant hypoglycemia. Similarly, if the patient is having prandial hyperglycemia with glucose values in the range of 200 to 300 mg/dL (11.1-16.7 mmol/L) lasting 3 hours or more, this may indicate that rapid-acting insulin with meals can be started to improve dysglycemia. Although there are currently no accepted CGM thresholds to diagnose CFRD, one study found that CGM measures of hyperglycemia could reliably distinguish between those with and without diabetes,[13] laying the groundwork for future prospective longitudinal studies investigating CGM as a diagnostic tool. Future studies are needed to determine CGM measures that correlate with long-term CF-specific outcomes, such as pulmonary function and nutritional status. However, CGM may still be very helpful for deciding the best treatment approach for those with abnormal OGTT results.

Case 1, Continued

He had started treatment with ETI in between his OGTTs in years 3 and 4 and is concerned that CFTR modulator therapy may have affected his glycemic control.

How does CFTR modulator therapy affect glycemia in people with CF?

A. Makes it much better

B. Makes it a little better

C. Makes it much worse

D. Makes it a little worse

E. Does not have an effect

Answer: B) Makes it a little better

CFTR modulator therapy has transformed the landscape of CF. Studies have shown an estimated 14% sustained improvement in FEV1 and significant reduction in pulmonary exacerbations

with treatment in those with 1 copy of delF508 or other responsive variant.[19] There was an immediate and rapid uptake in treatment in the United States upon approval in 2019, and at present more than 75% of the CF population is currently on CFTR modulator therapy.[1] There are now emerging studies providing insight into how CFTR modulator therapy affects CFRD. Early studies using CGM reported improvement in measures of hyperglycemia and glycemic variability without an effect on hypoglycemia after initiation of modulator therapy.[20] The largest study to date was the PROMISE Endocrine substudy, a multicenter longitudinal observational study following children and adults with CF starting treatment with ETI at 12 to 18 months and again at 24 to 30 months. This study found a small but significant improvement in hemoglobin A_{1c} from 5.7% to 5.5% over 2 years. However, glycemic categories as defined by OGTT (normal glucose tolerance, early glucose intolerance, impaired glucose tolerance, and CFRD) did not significantly change.[21] Overall, these data suggest that this treatment may lead to small improvement in glycemia but may not prevent the development or progression of abnormal glucose tolerance or CFRD.

Case 2

A 32-year-old man has CF, pancreatic insufficiency, and moderate lung disease and was diagnosed with CFRD at age 20 years based on OGTT. His CFRD has been managed with a basal-bolus insulin regimen of glargine and lispro for many years. However, he acknowledges that diabetes management has always been one of his greatest challenges. Consistent with this, his hemoglobin A_{1c} level is 12.2% (110 mmol/mol). He has had frequent admissions to the hospital for treatment of CF exacerbations and has intermittently required high-dosage prednisone tapers over the past year. His BMI is 19 kg/m^2, and his pulmonary function tests show a predicted FEV1 of 50%.

Despite counseling, education, and adjustments to his insulin regimen in attempt to optimize glycemic control, his hemoglobin A_{1c} ranges from 11% to 12% (97-108 mmol/mol) over the next year, primarily because he rarely checks fingerstick glucose and frequently misses short- and long-acting insulin injections.

Which of the following is the best recommendation now to help this patient with diabetes management?

A. Metformin

B. Repaglinide

C. Semaglutide or tirzepatide

D. CGM

E. Automated insulin delivery device

Answer: D) CGM

In this patient with a BMI below the recommended goal of 23 kg/m² and significant lung disease, medications that may result in further weight loss should be avoided, such as metformin (Answer A) or GLP-1 receptor agonists (Answer C). In a clinical trial comparing insulin or repaglinide (Answer B) vs placebo, repaglinide led to transient weight increase, but only insulin was associated with sustained weight gain over the course of the year-long study.[22] CGM (Answer D) has been validated in patients with CF.[23] Although there are no randomized clinical trials investigating CGM in the management of CFRD, a recent meta-analysis and systematic review found that use of CGM over at least 6 weeks was associated with a 0.4% improvement in hemoglobin A_{1c} compared with fingerstick glucose monitoring.[24] Automated insulin delivery (AID) systems (Answer E) have also been studied in the management of CFRD. However, it would be prudent to first initiate CGM before moving forward with an AID device.

Case 2, Continued

Although the patient is initially reluctant to be "attached to something all the time," he starts using CGM, which he finds very helpful for glucose monitoring and reminding him to take his insulin.

There is a temporary improvement in his glycemic control. However, a series of medical stressors take his attention away from diabetes management, and his hemoglobin A_{1c} returns to 11.6% (103 mmol/mol) 6 months later. At a telehealth appointment, the option of starting an AID device in conjunction with CGM is discussed.

Which of the following is true about the use of AID devices in people with CFRD?

A. There are no randomized trials investigating the use of AID devices in the CF population

B. Observational studies suggest that AID devices do not increase the percentage of time in the target range for people with CFRD

C. People with CFRD spend a greater percentage of time in hypoglycemic ranges with AID devices than people with type 1 diabetes

D. There are no FDA-approved AID devices for CFRD

Answer: D) There are no FDA-approved AID devices for CFRD

There are limited data on the use of AID devices in CFRD. Two retrospective studies investigating the Tandem TslimX2 with Control IQ[25] and the Omnipod 5[26] reported improvement in the percentage of time in target range of 70 to 180 mg/dL (3.0-10.0 mmol/L) and percentage of time in the hyperglycemic range without a significant change in the percentage of time in the hypoglycemic range after initiation of each of these devices. Another nonrandomized longitudinal study compared people on multiple daily injection regimens with those who switched to either sensor-augmented pump or AID devices (Medtronic 670G or 780G, Omnipod, Tandem TslimX2, or Accu-Chek) and reported improvement in hemoglobin A_{1c} over 2 years.[27] In a random-order cross-over design clinical trial, the iLet Bionic Pancreas led to improvement in average glucose and percentage of time in the target range with no change in the percentage of time in the hypoglycemic range over 4 weeks in 20 adults with CFRD.[28] A multicenter randomized clinical trial investigating the iLet is ongoing in the United States (NCT06449677), and another randomized clinical trial is ongoing in the United Kingdom with the CamAPS system (NCT05562492). Overall, the decision to trial AID devices requires education and discussion of potential risks and benefits, tailored to each individual.

Case 3

A 42-year-old woman has CF and pancreatic insufficiency. As a child, she was underweight and had difficulty gaining weight gain and maintaining a goal BMI at the 50th percentile, but this improved by young adulthood. After starting ETI in 2019, her lung function improved to over 90% predicted, but she gained a substantial amount of weight, bringing her current BMI to 38 kg/m^2. Despite efforts at diet and exercise over the past year, she has not been able to lose weight; she finds her current appearance very frustrating and distressing. Annual screening labs show a hemoglobin A_{1c} value of 6.7% (50 mmol/mol), increased from 5.9% to 6.3% (41 to 45 mmol/mol) over the past 2 years. She has not had a recent OGTT.

Which of the following is the best next step for further evaluation?

A. OGTT

B. Pancreatic antibodies

C. Repeat hemoglobin A_{1c} measurement

D. CGM

E. No need for further testing

Answer: C) Repeat hemoglobin A_{1c} measurement

Similar to the diagnosis of type 2 diabetes, at least 2 tests are needed to confirm the diagnosis of CFRD.[4] Although hemoglobin A_{1c} is not a sensitive test for CFRD screening, a value of 6.5% or above (≥48 mmol/mol) is consistent with the diagnosis of diabetes. In this case, it would be challenging to have the patient come in for an OGTT, and an easier confirmatory test would be

to measure hemoglobin A_{1c} again (Answer C). CGM could also be used, but because there are no universally accepted thresholds for confirming the diagnosis of CFRD, this tends to be more helpful for deciding if and how insulin should be started.

Case 3, Continued

Which of the following should be recommended next to manage this patient's obesity and CFRD?

A. Diet and exercise

B. Insulin glargine, 0.1 units/kg per day

C. Insulin lispro with a carbohydrate ratio of 1:30 with meals

D. Repaglinide

E. Semaglutide or tirzepatide

Answer: E) Semaglutide or tirzepatide

As illustrated in this case, there has been a significant increase in the prevalence of overweight and obesity since the introduction and rapid uptake of ETI in 2019.[1] Although insulin is the recommended treatment for CFRD, starting insulin would likely exacerbate her weight gain. Moreover, her pulmonary function is excellent, suggesting that insulin is not required to improve her lung disease. Diet and exercise are key aspects of obesity management, but they have not worked for her, with worsening hemoglobin A_{1c} despite attempts at lifestyle changes. Repaglinide may also worsen weight gain. Recent studies suggest that GLP-1 receptor agonist therapy (Answer E) may be effective for weight loss and diabetes management in people with CF,[29] and this would a reasonable option to try for this patient. However, there are important considerations for the use of these medications in this specific patient population. Many people with CF have a history of gastroesophageal reflux disease, delayed gastric emptying, and gastroparesis, which can be exacerbated by this therapy. Moreover, some patients with CF require frequent procedures (bronchoscopy and colonoscopy) and should be counseled on holding treatment in advance of needing anesthesia. People with CF are at risk for distal intestinal obstruction syndrome. Although not reported with GLP-1 receptor agonist use, it is conceivable that slowed gastrointestinal motility and worsening constipation could predispose to this complication, and constipation should be aggressively managed. Pancreatitis occurs more commonly in people with certain *CFTR* pathogenic variants, particularly in individuals with pancreatic sufficiency. Excessive weight loss to a BMI below the recommended goal of 22 kg/m^2 in women and 23 kg/m^2 in men should be avoided. Ongoing clinical trials are investigating noninsulin therapies, including semaglutide (NCT05788965) and SGLT-2 inhibitors (NCT 06149793) in the management of CFRD. In the meantime, GLP-1 receptor agonists may be a reasonable option for treating CFRD and obesity in carefully selected patients, with comprehensive counseling on potential risks and adverse effects.

Key Learning Points

- CFRD is common and is associated with decline in pulmonary function, compromised nutritional status, and earlier mortality.

- The recommended screening test for CFRD is OGTT, although national screening rates are very low and new approaches are needed.

- Insulin is the only recommended treatment for CFRD, and it has been shown to improve clinical status.

- Diabetes technology may help to improve glycemic management and reduce treatment burden in people with CFRD.

- Rising rates of obesity and metabolic syndrome raise the possibility for other treatment options (GLP-1 receptor agonists, SGLT-2 inhibitors, etc) for CFRD.

References

1. Cystic Fibrosis Foundation Patient Registry, Annual Data Report, 2023. Accessed Feburary 10, 2025.

2. Norris AW, Ode KL, Merjaneh L, et al. Survival in a bad neighborhood: pancreatic islets in cystic fibrosis. *J Endocrinol.* 2019;241(1):R35-R50. PMID: 30759072

3. Granados A, Chan CL, Ode KL, Moheet A, Moran A, Holl R. Cystic fibrosis related diabetes: Pathophysiology, screening and diagnosis. *J Cyst Fibros.* 2019;18(Suppl 2):S3-S9. PMID: 31679726

4. Moran A, Brunzell C, Cohen RC, et al; CFRD Guidelines Committee. Clinical care guidelines for cystic fibrosis-related diabetes: a position statement of the American Diabetes Association and a clinical practice guideline of the Cystic Fibrosis Foundation, endorsed by the Pediatric Endocrine Society. *Diabetes Care.* 2010;33(12):2697-2708.

5. Millington K, Miller V, Rubenstein RC, Kelly A. Patient and parent perceptions of the diagnosis and management of cystic fibrosis-related diabetes. *J Clin Transl Endocrinol.* 2014;1(3):100-107. PMID: 29159090

6. Kwong E, Desai S, Chong L, Lee K, Zheng J, Wilcox PG, Quon BS. The impact of cystic fibrosis-related diabetes on health-related quality of life. *J Cyst Fibros.* 2019;18(5):734-736. PMID: 30935840

7. Scully KJ, Marks BE, Putman MS. Advances in diabetes technology to improve the lives of people with cystic fibrosis. *Diabetologia.* 2024;67(10):2143-2153. PMID: 38995399

8. Putman MS, Norris AW, Hull RL, et al. Cystic fibrosis-related diabetes workshop: research priorities spanning disease pathophysiology, diagnosis, and outcomes. *Diabetes Care.* 2023;46(6):1112-1123. PMID: 37125948

9. Scully KJ, Jay LT, Freedman S, et al. The relationship between body composition, dietary intake, physical activity, and pulmonary status in adolescents and adults with cystic fibrosis. *Nutrients.* 2022;14(2):310. [PMID: 35057491

10. Gramegna A, Aliberti S, Calderazzo MA, et al. The impact of elexacaftor/ tezacaftor/ivacaftor therapy on the pulmonary management of adults with cystic fibrosis: an expert-based Delphi consensus. *Respir Med.* 2023;220:107455. PMID: 37926181

11. Gramegna A, Majo F, Alicandro G, et al. Heterogeneity of weight gain after initiation of Elexacaftor/Tezacaftor/Ivacaftor in people with cystic fibrosis. *Respir Res.* 2023;24(1):164. PMID: 37330504

12. Sandouk Z, Nachawi N, Simon R, et al. Coronary artery disease in patients with cystic fibrosis - a case series and review of the literature. *J Clin Transl Endocrinol.* 2022;30:100308. PMID: 36267108

13. Scully KJ, Sherwood JS, Martin K, et al. Continuous glucose monitoring and HbA1c in cystic fibrosis: clinical correlations and implications for CFRD diagnosis. *J Clin Endocrinol Metab.* 2022;107(4):e1444-e1454. PMID: 34850006

14. Chan CL, Hope E, Thurston J, Vigers T, Pyle L, Zeitler PS, Nadeau KJ. Hemoglobin A1c accurately predicts continuous glucose monitoring-derived average glucose in youth and young adults with cystic fibrosis. *Diabetes Care.* 2018;41(7):1406-1413. PMID: 29674323

15. Racine F, Shohoudi A, Boudreau V, et al. Glycated hemoglobin as a first-line screening test for cystic fibrosis-related diabetes and impaired glucose tolerance in children with cystic fibrosis: a validation study. *Can J Diabetes.* 2021;45(8):768-774. PMID: 33926819

16. Burgess JC, Bridges N, Banya W, et al. HbA1c as a screening tool for cystic fibrosis related diabetes. *J Cyst Fibros.* 2016;15(2):251-257.

17. Gilmour JA, Sykes J, Etchells E, Tullis E. Cystic fibrosis-related diabetes screening in adults: a gap analysis and evaluation of accuracy of glycated hemoglobin levels. *Can J Diabetes.* 2019;43(1):13-18. PMID: 30173928

18. Coriati A, Potter K, Gilmour J, et al. Cystic fibrosis-related diabetes: a first Canadian clinical practice guideline. *Can J Diabetes.* 2024;49(1):19-28.e16. PMID: 39260688

19. Middleton PG, Mall MA, Drevinek P, et al. Elexacaftor-tezacaftor-ivacaftor for cystic fibrosis with a single Phe508del allele. *N Engl J Med.* 2019;381(19):1809-1819. PMID: 31697873

20. Scully KJ, Marchetti P, Sawicki GS, et al. The effect of elexacaftor/tezacaftor/ivacaftor (ETI) on glycemia in adults with cystic fibrosis. *J Cyst Fibros.* 2022;21(2):258-263. PMID: 34531155

21. Chan CL, Shirley Bezerra M, Stefanovski D, et al. Glycemia and insulin secretion in cystic fibrosis two years after elexacaftor/tezacaftor/ivacaftor: PROMISE-ENDO. *J Clin Endocrinol Metab.* 2024:dgae857. PMID: 39657947

22. Moran A, Pekow P, Grover P, et al; Cystic Fibrosis Related Diabetes Therapy Study G. Insulin therapy to improve BMI in cystic fibrosis-related diabetes without fasting hyperglycemia: results of the cystic fibrosis related diabetes therapy trial. *Diabetes Care.* 2009;32(10):1783-1788. PMID: 19592632

23. O'Riordan SM, Hindmarsh P, Hill NR, et al. Validation of continuous glucose monitoring in children and adolescents with cystic fibrosis: a prospective cohort study. *Diabetes Care.* 2009;32(6):1020-1022. PMID: 19279304

24. Kumar S, Soldatos G, Ranasinha S, Teede H, Pallin M. Continuous glucose monitoring versus self-monitoring of blood glucose in the management of cystic fibrosis related diabetes: a systematic review and meta-analysis. *J Cyst Fibros.* 2023;22(1):39-49. PMID: 35906171

25. Scully KJ, Palani G, Zheng H, Moheet A, Putman MS. The effect of Control IQ hybrid closed loop technology on glycemic control in adolescents and adults with cystic fibrosis-related diabetes. *Diabetes Technol Ther.* 2022;24(6):446-452. PMID: 35020476

26. Scully KJ, Palani G, Zheng H, Moheet A, Putman MS. Effect of hybrid closed loop insulin delivery on glycemic control in adolescents and adults with cystic fibrosis-related diabetes. *Diabetes Technol Ther.* 2022;24(6):446-452. PMID: 35020476

27. Grancini V, Alicandro G, Porcaro LL, et al. Effects of insulin therapy optimization with sensor augmented pumps on glycemic control and body composition in people with cystic fibrosis-related diabetes. *Front Endocrinol (Lausanne).* 2023;14:1228153. PMID: 37720540

28. Sherwood JS, Castellanos LE, O'Connor MY, et al. Randomized trial of the insulin-only iLet Bionic Pancreas for the treatment of cystic fibrosis-related diabetes. *Diabetes Care.* 2024;47(1):101-108. PMID: 37874987

29. Park S, Jain R, Mirfakhraee S. Glucagon-like-peptide-1 agonist therapy in adults with cystic fibrosis. *J Cyst Fibros.* 2025;24(1):40-46. PMID: 39214747

Optimizing Health After Gestational Diabetes: What's Next?

Ellen W. Seely, MD. Endocrinology, Diabetes and Hypertension Division, Brigham and Women's Hospital/Mass General Brigham, Boston, MA; Email: eseely@bwh.harvard.edu

Educational Objectives

After reviewing this chapter, learners should be able to:

- Determine the risk of type 2 diabetes (T2D) following gestational diabetes mellitus (GDM).

- Institute prevention of T2D after GDM.

- Identify and manage risk for cardiovascular disease (CVD) after GDM.

When caring for patients with previous GDM, health care providers should implement:

- T2D screening.

- T2D prevention with either an intensive lifestyle program or metformin (not FDA approved for this indication but recommended by the American Diabetes Association).

- CVD risk factor screening and prevention.

Significance of the Clinical Problem

GDM (diabetes first diagnosed in pregnancy after the first trimester) affects 7% to 8% of pregnancies in the United States and approximately 14% of pregnancies globally.[1,2] GDM is associated with risk during pregnancy both to the mother and to the fetus/neonate, and these risks are attenuated by diagnosis and treatment of GDM. Although GDM resolves with delivery of the pregnancy, women with GDM have increased risk of future GDM with subsequent pregnancies,[3,4] as well as future T2D[5-8] and CVD.[9-12] However, most women with previous GDM do not receive counseling or referral to programs to decrease future risks.

Practice Gaps

- Despite the well-recognized risk of T2D following GDM, most providers do not solicit a pregnancy history of GDM.

- Women with previous GDM should receive regular screening for T2D.

- Women with previous GDM should receive advice about lifestyle modification and referral to a National Diabetes Prevention Program (DPP), or similar program, to prevent T2D or be prescribed metformin.

- Women with previous GDM should receive counseling about CVD prevention.

Discussion

The American Diabetes Association defines GDM as diabetes first diagnosed during pregnancy after the first trimester.[13] GDM is diagnosed by oral glucose tolerance testing (OGTT), usually at weeks 24 to 28 of gestation by either the 2-step test (50-g glucose load followed by 100-g OGTT using Carpenter Coustan criteria) or 1-step test (75-g OGTT using the International Association of the Diabetes and Pregnancy Study Groups [IAPDSG] criteria).[13] There is debate as to which, if either, of these criteria are superior. Mothers with GDM have increased risk for hypertensive disorders of pregnancy and cesarean delivery, and the fetus/neonate is at increased risk for macrosomia, shoulder dystocia, birth trauma, and neonatal hypoglycemia. Two large randomized controlled trials have demonstrated that diagnosis and treatment of GDM decreases adverse pregnancy outcomes.[14,15]

T2D After GDM

Since the 1980s,[5] it has been known that women with prior GDM have an increased risk of future T2D. This risk has been supported by many subsequent studies. Data support that up to 50% of women with previous GDM develop T2D, with many developing the condition within 5 years of the GDM pregnancy.[6] A meta-analysis demonstrated that women with previous GDM were 7 to 8 times more likely to develop T2D than those without previous GDM.[7,8] Within the population of women with a history of GDM, Hispanic and non-Hispanic, non-White women are more likely to develop T2D than non-Hispanic White women.[16] Another meta-analysis confirmed the magnification of conversion rate, finding a relative risk of 8.3 (95% CI, 6.5-10.6) among more than 300,000 women with a history of GDM.[8] Because of the high risk of T2D associated with a history of GDM, the American Diabetes Association[13] recommends OGTT 4 to 12 weeks post partum to determine whether the woman has T2D at that time. If she does not have T2D but has impaired fasting glucose (IFG) or impaired glucose tolerance (IGT), the recommendation is to screen annually. If the OGTT result is normal, the recommendation is to screen every 3 years. Unfortunately, many women do not return for the 6-week postpartum OGTT (<50%),[17] and many women do not receive the recommended long-term screening.[18] Thus, there is lost opportunity for early detection, prevention, and early treatment of diabetes in this high-risk population.

T2D Prevention After GDM

The good news is that we have known since 2008 that diabetes can be prevented or delayed in women with previous GDM. A post hoc analysis of 350 parous women who participated in the DPP and who self-reported GDM revealed that intensive lifestyle modification reduced rates of diabetes by 53% and metformin reduced rates of diabetes by 50%.[19] The study also confirmed the magnification of risk for T2D in women with a history of GDM, as the rates of T2D were 71% higher in women with previous GDM than in parous women without this history.

The Diabetes Prevention Program Observational Study, which followed DPP participants for 10 years, demonstrated persistent protection against the development of T2D in the population who received intensive lifestyle modification or metformin.[20] Even 10 years later, women with a history of GDM had a 35% reduction in diabetes progression with intensive lifestyle modification, and those who had received metformin had a 40% reduction. Interestingly, in women with no history of GDM, intensive lifestyle modification demonstrated an overall reduction of diabetes by 30%, whereas no reduction was seen in the group who had received metformin. These studies were performed in women remote from their GDM pregnancy (age 43 ± 7.6 years).

Weight gain subsequent to a GDM pregnancy appears to modify future risk of T2D. A prospective population-based analysis from the Nurses' Health Study II showed that in women with previous GDM, each 1 kg/m² increase in BMI was associated with a 16% increase in risk of developing diabetes.[21] More proximate to pregnancy, a longitudinal study that followed participants with previous GDM for 4 years post partum showed that the group with a decrease in BMI of −1.8 kg/m² had an 8.6% incidence of diabetes, while the group with an increase in BMI of +1.6 kg/m² had a 16.9% incidence of diabetes.[22] Therefore, loss of pregnancy weight gain may be an opportunity to decrease future risk of diabetes.

There has been interest in targeting postpartum weight retention as an opportunity to decrease progression to diabetes, as weight retained at 6 months post delivery is predictive of long-term weight gain.[23] Several studies have been designed to decrease postpartum weight retention in women with recent GDM, and some have been successful in that regard.[24,25] Whether this will translate into diabetes prevention is not known.

Intensive Lifestyle Programs

Many lifestyle programs are available that are based on the DPP. The most prominent, and endorsed by the Centers for Disease Control, are the National Diabetes Prevention Programs.[26] These programs are available nationwide in the United States and are commonly covered by insurance. They are based on the DPP curriculum and are available both in-person and online. A history of GDM is a qualifying diagnosis for entry into a National Diabetes Prevention Program. Women with previous GDM appear to benefit from participation in a National Diabetes Prevention Program, with a study[27] showing that younger women (age <40 years) with previous GDM who attended at least 1 session had greater weight loss (3.04% ± 0.59 vs 1.49% ± 0.11, $P = .010$) in covariate-adjusted models than other participants. Despite this promise, younger women with previous GDM are about 50% less likely to enroll in a National Diabetes Prevention Program than women without GDM.[28] Other countries have DPP programs similar to the National Diabetes Prevention Program, such as the United Kingdom's National Health System Diabetes Prevention Programme and Australia's Diabetes Australia, which are free of charge.

Metformin

The DPP demonstrated that metformin, 850 mg orally twice daily, was as effective as intensive lifestyle modification in reducing rates of diabetes in women with previous GDM.[19] It is important to note that although metformin is widely used for diabetes prevention, it does not have an FDA-approved indication for this purpose.. In the original DPP study,[19] metformin therapy reduced diabetes incidence in women with previous GDM by 50%, a similar reduction rate as that associated with intensive lifestyle modification. In the DPP Outcomes Study,[20] metformin at a dosage of 850 mg twice daily reduced progression to diabetes by 40% compared with placebo in women with a history of GDM, similar to intensive lifestyle modification, which reduced diabetes progression by 35% over 10 years. Some argue that in the real world, metformin is more effective than intensive lifestyle modification for diabetes prevention because it may be easier for individuals to take a medication than to be adherent to lifestyle change.

History of GDM and Future CVD

Women with previous GDM who develop T2D are at increased risk for CVD, as diabetes is an important risk factor for CVD. Several studies have demonstrated that even after accounting for the future development of T2D, women with previous GDM have increased CVD risk. A meta-analysis and systematic review of women with previous GDM demonstrated an almost 2-fold increased risk for cardiovascular events (fatal/nonfatal ischemic heart disease and cerebrovascular events) compared with risk of women without previous GDM.[9] Women with previous GDM who had not developed T2D demonstrated a relative risk for CVD events of 1.56 (95% CI, 1.04-2.32) compared with the risk of women without previous GDM. In a study using a large United Kingdom biobank, the hazard ratio for developing a cardiovascular outcome (coronary artery disease, peripheral artery disease, heart failure, mitral regurgitation, and atrial fibrillation) was 1.36 (1.18-1.55) in women with previous GDM compared with women without previous GDM, even after adjusting for the development of T2D, further supporting a direct pathway from GDM to CVD.[10] Because of this and other data, in 2011, the American Heart Association designated GDM as a major risk factor for CVD.[11] As opposed to the studies that support prevention of diabetes following GDM, there are no data specific to the prevention of CVD in this population. However, it makes sense to recognize this group of women as being at increased risk for CVD and address CVD risk factor reduction with them,[12] have a lower threshold for prescribing medications that decrease CVD risk, such as statins and antihypertensive agents. Risk factor reduction should include weight management, physical activity, and smoking cessation. Hemoglobin A_{1c} and blood pressure should be monitored.[12] Whether women with previous GDM should receive more intensive lipid screening is not well established.

Previous GDM and GDM Recurrence in Subsequent Pregnancy

Women with GDM have a high risk of being diagnosed with GDM in a subsequent pregnancy. In a meta-analysis and systematic review, the pooled GDM recurrence rate was 48% (95% CI, 41%-54%).[3] These numbers may be inflated in that many women with previous GDM start doing fingerstick glucose measurement using their home glucose meters from a prior pregnancy and report elevated glucose values to their provider, thus bypassing formal screening for GDM. Whether weight loss between pregnancies reduces recurrent GDM is unclear. In observational studies, women who enter a subsequent pregnancy at a lower weight than they did for their previous GDM pregnancy have lower rates of subsequent GDM.[4] In cross-sectional data, women who were at lower body weights at the time of their subsequent pregnancy were at lower risk of recurrent GDM. A randomized controlled trial[29] that compared lifestyle intervention with decreased weight preconception in women with previous GDM was successful at reducing weight, but it did not reduce rates of recurrent GDM compared with rates in the control group, perhaps due to reduced power, as there were 50% fewer pregnancies than had been planned for. However, regardless of group assignment, greater weight loss between study entry and last weight before pregnancy

was associated with a 21% lower odds of GDM recurrence. In some other studies of weight loss before pregnancy, no benefit in the rate of GDM was observed, perhaps because those assigned to the weight-loss intervention counteracted this benefit by gaining more weight during pregnancy.

Clinical Case Vignettes

Case 1

A 32-year-old woman (G1, P1) with Hashimoto thyroid disease (treated with levothyroxine, 100 mcg daily) presents for a return visit. She is having regular menses.

On physical examination, her blood pressure is 130/80 mm Hg, pulse rate is 72 beats/min, and BMI is 32 kg/m². The rest of the examination findings are normal, including a normal thyroid gland and no hirsutism.

At the end of the visit, she says, "I hope that when I see you next year, I will have had another baby." You realize you had never obtained a pregnancy history. She had GDM in her first pregnancy 3 years ago and required insulin.

In addition to measuring TSH, which of the following assessments should be ordered?

A. Testosterone measurement

B. LH measurement

C. Ovarian ultrasonography

D. Antimullerian hormone measurement

E. Hemoglobin A_{1c} measurement

Answer: E) Hemoglobin A_{1c} measurement

She is having regular menses and has no hirsutism on exam, so there is no suggestion of polycystic ovary syndrome. With her regular menses and a recent pregnancy, there is no reason to expect premature ovarian insufficiency.

It is crucial to screen women with a history of GDM for T2D, as many such women develop T2D, with the highest relative risk in the first 5 years after pregnancy. Even if this patient had been screened 4 to 12 weeks after delivery, she should have screening now based on the American Diabetes Association recommendation to screen all women with previous GDM every 3 years if testing is normal. If test results indicate prediabetes, she should be screened yearly. The most sensitive test is OGTT, but patients generally dislike the test, it is time consuming, and it cannot usually be done on the day of the visit because it must be done in the fasting state. Thus, hemoglobin A_{1c} measurement (Answer E) is the most practical test at this point.

Family planning should be discussed with all women with previous GDM, so they are aware of the importance of screening for T2D (hemoglobin A_{1c}, fasting blood glucose, or OGTT) when planning a pregnancy. If test results confirm T2D, the patient will need counseling to achieve a hemoglobin A_{1c} level less than 6.5% (48 mmol/mol) before conception. Unless screening for T2D in patients with previous GDM is routine, the patient in this scenario could have presented while pregnant and with T2D and less-than-optimal glycemic control.

Case 1, Continued

You ask the patient to step back into your office, reminding yourself you should have discussed family planning and future risk of T2D during the visit. You discuss the high recurrence rate of GDM and ask if she had been counseled about future long-term risks following GDM. She replies, "I was told that my diabetes would go away when I delivered." You counsel her about future T2D risk and the need for regular diabetes screening every 3 years if testing is normal and yearly if she has impaired fasting glucose, impaired glucose tolerance, or prediabetes according to hemoglobin A_{1c} measurement. She is planning a pregnancy, which prompts you to order hemoglobin A_{1c} measurement that day.

What is her chance of developing T2D?

A. 10%

B. 20%

C. 50%

D. 100%

E. 0% (her 6-week postpartum OGTT results in the electronic medical record confirm she did not have T2D at that time)

Answer: C) 50%

Women with previous GDM have a 50% chance of developing T2D (Answer C) with the increase in relative risk being the highest in the first 5 years following the GDM pregnancy. Because her risk is so high and because the DPP appeared to be effective in women with previous GDM, you discuss referral to a National Diabetes Prevention Program and use of metformin.

Case 1, Continued

That evening when you are completing your notes, her hemoglobin A_{1c} has come back at 5.8% (40 mmol/mol). You remember that you only counseled her about future risk of T2D and forgot other important counseling.

You enter a reminder in the electronic medical record to talk to her about which of the following at her next visit?

A. She has a very high risk of premature ovarian insufficiency because she has thyroid disease and had GDM

B. She will not need adjustment of her levothyroxine dosage during her planned pregnancy because her recent TSH value was normal

C. She only needs to worry about future CVD if she develops future T2D

D. She has an increased risk for CVD independent of the development of future T2D

E. Her risk of recurrent GDM is low because it is most common in a first pregnancy

Answer: D) She has an increased risk for CVD independent of the development of future T2D

Women with a history of GDM have an increased risk for future CVD independent of the future development of T2D (Answer D). The American Heart Association has endorsed GDM as a major risk factor for CVD. Recommendations are to screen women with previous GDM for other CVD risk factors. She does not have high risk of premature ovarian insufficiency with only Hashimoto thyroiditis. The GDM recurrence rate is very high.

Key Learning Points

- A pregnancy history of GDM should be obtained from all parous women.

- Women with a history of GDM should be screened regularly for T2D to allow to early diagnosis and treatment of diabetes and its comorbidities.

- Women with previous gestational diabetes should be referred to a National Diabetes Prevention Program or similar program or be prescribed metformin to help prevent or delay diabetes. Of note, metformin is not FDA approved for this indication but is endorsed by many organizations, including the American Diabetes Association.

References

1. Gregory EC, Ely DM. Trends and characteristics in gestational diabetes: United States, 2016-2020. *Natl Vital Stat Rep.* 2022;71(3):1-15. PMID: 35877134

2. Wang H, Li N, Chivese T, et al; IDF Diabetes Atlas Committee Hyperglycaemia in Pregnancy Special Interest Group. IDF Diabetes Atlas: estimation of global and regional gestational diabetes mellitus prevalence for 2021 by International Association of Diabetes in Pregnancy Study Group's Criteria. *Diabetes Res Clin Pract.* 2022;183:109050. PMID: 34883186

3. Schwartz N, Nachum Z, Green MS. The prevalence of gestational diabetes mellitus recurrence--effect of ethnicity and parity: a metaanalysis. *Am J Obstet Gynecol.* 2015;213(3):310-317. PMID: 25757637

4. Sorbye LM, Cnattingius S, Skjaerven R, et al. Interpregnancy weight change and recurrence of gestational diabetes mellitus: a population-based cohort study. *BJOG.* 2020;127(13):1608-1616. PMID: 32534460

5. O'Sullivan JB. Diabetes mellitus after GDM. *Diabetes.* 1991;40(Suppl 2):131-135. PMID: 1748242

6. Kim C, Newton KM, Knopp RH. Gestational diabetes and the incidence of type 2 diabetes: a systematic review. *Diabetes Care.* 2002;25(10):1862-1868. PMID: 12351492

7. Bellamy L, Casas JP, Hingorani AD, Williams D. Type 2 diabetes mellitus after gestational diabetes: a systematic review and meta-analysis. *Lancet.* 2009;373(9677):1773-1779. PMID: 19465232

8. Dennison RA, Chen ES, Green ME, et al. The absolute and relative risk of type 2 diabetes after gestational diabetes: A systematic review and meta-analysis of 129 studies. *Diabetes Res Clin Pract.* 2021;171:108625. PMID: 33333204

9. Kramer CK, Campbell S, Retnakaran R. Gestational diabetes and the risk of cardiovascular disease in women: a systematic review and meta-analysis. *Diabetologia.* 2019;62(6):905-914. PMID: 30843102

10. Lee SM, Shivakumar M, Park JW, et al. Long-term cardiovascular outcomes of gestational diabetes mellitus: a prospective UK Biobank study. *Cardiovasc Diabetol.* 2022;21(1):221. PMID: 36309714

11. Mosca L, Benjamin EJ, Berra K, et al. Effectiveness-based guidelines for the prevention of cardiovascular disease in women--2011 update: a guideline from the American Heart Association. *Circulation.* 2011;123(11):1243-1262. PMID: 21325087

12. Parikh NI, Gonzalez JM, Anderson CAM, et al. Adverse pregnancy outcomes and cardiovascular disease risk: unique opportunities for cardiovascular disease prevention in women: a scientific statement from the American Heart Association. *Circulation.* 2021;143(18):e902-e916. PMID: 33779213

13. Management of diabetes in pregnancy: standards of care in diabetes-2025. *Diabetes Care.* 2025;48(Suppl 1):S306-S320. PMID: 39651985

14. Crowther CA, Hiller JE, Moss JR, McPhee AJ, Jeffries WS, Robinson JS. Effect of treatment of gestational diabetes mellitus on pregnancy outcomes. *N Engl J Med.* 2005;352(24):2477-2486. PMID: 15951574

15. Landon MB, Spong CY, Thom E, et al; Eunice Kennedy Shriver National Institute of Child Health and Human Development Maternal-Fetal Medicine Units Network. A multicenter, randomized trial of treatment for mild gestational diabetes. *N Engl J Med.* 2009;361(14):1339-1348. PMID: 19797280

16. Bower JK, Butler BN, Bose-Brill S, Kue J, Wassel CL. Racial/ethnic differences in diabetes screening and hyperglycemia among US women after gestational diabetes. *Prev Chronic Dis.* 2019;16:E145. PMID: 31651379

17. Brown SD, Hedderson MM, Zhu Y, et al. Uptake of guideline-recommended postpartum diabetes screening among diverse women with gestational diabetes: associations with patient factors in an integrated health system in USA. *BMJ Open Diabetes Res Care.* 2022;10(3):e002726. PMID: 35725017

18. Zera CA, Bates DW, Stuebe AM, Ecker JL, Seely EW. Diabetes screening reminder for women with prior gestational diabetes: a randomized controlled trial. *Obstet Gynecol.* 2015;126(1):109-114. PMID: 26241263

19. Ratner RE, Christophi CA, Metzger BE, et al. Prevention of diabetes in women with a history of gestational diabetes: effects of metformin and lifestyle interventions. *J Clin Endocrinol Metab.* 2008;93(12):4774-4779. PMID: 18826999

20. Aroda VR, Christophi CA, Edelstein SL, et al. The effect of lifestyle intervention and metformin on preventing or delaying diabetes among women with and without gestational diabetes: the Diabetes Prevention Program outcomes study 10-year follow-up. *J Clin Endocrinol Metab.* 2015;100(4):1646-1653. PMID: 25706240

21. Bao W, Yeung E, Tobias DK, et al. Long-term risk of type 2 diabetes mellitus in relation to BMI and weight change among women with a history of gestational diabetes mellitus: a prospective cohort study. *Diabetologia.* 2015;58(6):1212-1219. PMID: 25796371

22. Moon JH, Kwak SH, Jung HS, et al. Weight gain and progression to type 2 diabetes in women with a history of gestational diabetes mellitus. *J Clin Endocrinol Metab*. 2015;100(9):3548-3555. PMID: 26171796

23. Rooney BL, Schauberger CW. Excess pregnancy weight gain and long-term obesity: one decade later. *Obstet Gynecol*. 2002;100(2):245-252. PMID: 12151145

24. Nicklas JM, Zera CA, England LJ, et al. A web-based lifestyle intervention for women with recent gestational diabetes mellitus: a randomized controlled trial. *Obstet Gynecol*. 2014;124(3):563-570. PMID: 25162257

25. Ferrara A, Hedderson MM, Brown SD, et al. The comparative effectiveness of diabetes prevention strategies to reduce postpartum weight retention in women with gestational diabetes mellitus: the Gestational Diabetes' Effects on Moms (GEM) Cluster Randomized Controlled Trial. *Diabetes Care*. 2016;39(1):65-74. PMID: 26657945

26. Centers for Disease Control. National Diabetes Prevention Program. 2025. https://www.cdc.gov/diabetes-prevention/index.html

27. Ritchie ND, Seely EW, Nicklas JM, Levkoff SE. Effectiveness of the National Diabetes Prevention Program After Gestational Diabetes. *Am J Prev Med*. 2023;65(2):317-321. PMID: 36918133

28. Ritchie ND, Sauder KA, Fabbri S. Reach and effectiveness of the National Diabetes Prevention Program for Young Women. *Am J Prev Med*. 2017;53(5):714-718. PMID: 28928038

29. Phelan S, Jelalian E, Coustan D, et al. Randomized controlled trial of prepregnancy lifestyle intervention to reduce recurrence of gestational diabetes mellitus. *Am J Obstet Gynecol*. 2023;229(2):158.e1-158.e14. PMID: 36758710

Integrating Quality Improvement into Inpatient Diabetes Care

Sonali Thosani, MD. Department of Endocrine Neoplasia and Hormonal Disorders, MD Anderson Cancer Center, Houston, TX. Email: Sthosani@mdanderson.org

Educational Objectives

After reviewing this chapter, learners should be able to:

- Outline the steps to follow to implement a successful quality improvement (QI) initiative.

- Discuss the different types of QI tools that are available.

- Identify the types of metrics that can be used for tracking improvement in inpatient care for patients with diabetes.

Significance of the Clinical Problem

Caring for hospitalized patients with diabetes is a complex process with many opportunities for QI to ensure that care delivery meets the 6 Institute of Medicine aims: safe, effective, timely, patient-centered, equitable, and efficient. Patients with diabetes often need significant change to their outpatient regimen upon admission and dynamic monitoring to ensure that their treatment plan is tailored to their ongoing inpatient clinical situation. Without appropriate safeguards in place, certain vulnerable patients, such as those who are postoperative or on high-dosage steroids, can develop hyperglycemic emergency during their hospital stay, which is considered a preventable adverse event. Furthermore, patients can also be at risk of hypoglycemia and its related adverse events due to inappropriate insulin dosing or disruption of meal or tube feeds.

Practice Gaps

- Lack of awareness of standardized protocols/policies for inpatient diabetes management.

- Lack of knowledge on how to initiate and sustain QI initiatives.

Discussion

There are some key steps to developing a successful glycemic control initiative for inpatient diabetes care. The Glycemic Control Online Toolkit is an excellent resource that is based on this guide and provides step-by-step methodology on how to improve inpatient glycemic control as recommended in the Society of Hospital Medicine guide.[1]

Step 1: Gain support and priority for the initiative from institutional leadership

Stakeholder engagement is the first and most important step for any QI initiative. Stakeholder engagement requires a clear understanding of who your audience is and what matters to them. If your project is based in a single unit or affecting just a few areas, then focusing on length of stay and discharge-related metrics might be a good way to get stakeholder buy-in. If it is a larger project involving all inpatient diabetes care, then engaging

C-suite leaders will likely require more buy-in through review of preventable adverse events and discussion of how current practice compares with benchmark standards for glycemic care.

Step 2: Create a multidisciplinary team that focuses on reaching glycemic targets

For any QI project, it is very important to identify a leader or co-leaders for an initiative with diverse representation from various frontline members in the multidisciplinary team. Any effective inpatient diabetes QI project will likely involve representatives from nursing, pharmacy, diabetes educators, patient care technicians or medical assistants, clinical providers, informatics, and data analyst team. Input from various perspectives in developing the project and planning the intervention is key to ensuring that all facets of the problem have been considered and that intervention does not disrupt the workflow of any team members.

Step 3: Assess the current state of glycemic management in your facility through use of QI tools and methodology

Using QI Tools

The QI Essentials Toolkit from the Institute for Healthcare Improvement[2] provides a great summary of various tools that can be used for QI work (*Table 1*).

Step 4: Develop specific aims, or goals, that are time-defined, measurable, and achievable

Every QI initiative should have an aim statement that is Specific, Measurable, Attainable, Relevant, and Time bound (SMART). This statement is a clear summary of the magnitude of change that the intervention hopes to achieve in a specified amount of time and ensures ongoing stakeholder and team engagement. Aim statements can reflect 1 of the 2 types of measures that are used in health care analytics[3]:

- **Process measures:** These measures focus on the processes and systems that directly contribute to the desired outcomes. Example:

Table 1. QI Essentials Toolkit From the Institute for Healthcare Improvement

QI tool	Description	Utility in QI work
Process mapping	Flowchart outlining a complex process	Allows for shared understanding of workflow and can help identify bottleneck areas
Prioritization matrix	4 × 4 matrix that can help prioritize solutions/interventions based on effort and impact	Helps teams focus on "quick wins" (low-effort, high-impact) tasks, while setting aside time for high-effort/high-impact tasks
Pareto chart	According to Pareto principle, 80% of the effect comes from 20% of the causes; tool can identify which factors are contributing more often to problem	Helps teams concentrate their improvement areas on factors that will likely have the greatest impact
Ishikawa (fishbone) diagram	Cause-and-effect diagram that looks at the people, environment, materials, methods, and equipment related issues that are contributing to the problem	Helpful in identifying all the factors contributing to a problem
Staff and patient surveys	Questionnaires completed by staff and patients to gather more information of qualitative impact of initiative	Provides information on subjective effectiveness of the intervention and identifies challenges faced by frontline teams or impact of intervention on patient experience

measuring use of a new order set implemented to increase use of basal-bolus insulin therapy.

- **Outcome measures:** These measures reflect the impact on the patient and identify the result of improvement work. Example: measuring average glucose levels for patients on new order set compared with the benchmark target.

Step 5: Develop and track metrics that are relevant to your aim statement

There are many factors to consider when developing metrics related to inpatient diabetes care at any given institution, including ease of availability of data and access to a data analytics team and other resources to build a glycemic management dashboard. Metrics can focus on patient-days or on percentage of glucose values that meet a specified threshold. Metrics should be tracked over time with a control chart to allow study of variation in data over time, which can help identify causes of variation, such as special and common cause variation.

Some standardized metrics are available, such as the electronic quality measures (eCQM) for hyperglycemia and hypoglycemia as developed by Centers for Medicare and Medicaid Services.[4] Another practical resource is glucometrics developed by the Society of Hospital Medicine Task Force (Glycemic Control eQUIPS program).[5] Metrics can be in any of the following categories: measurements of safety, measurements of glycemic control, measurements of insulin use, or other process measures as summarized in *Table 2*.[6]

Step 6: Use Plan-Do-Study-Act model to pilot interventions

The most common type of QI model is the Plan-Do-Study-Act (PDSA) model (*Figure, following page*).[7] In the "plan" stage, teams must determine what data to collect, clarify the aim statement, and

Table 2. Practical Recommendations for Glucometrics in the Hospital

Measurement Issue	Non–Critical Care Units	Critical Care Units
Patient inclusion and exclusion criteria	• *All patients with POC glucose testing (sampling acceptable)* • *Exclude patients with DKA or HHS or who are pregnant*	• *All patients in every critical care unit (sampling acceptable)*
Glucose reading inclusion and exclusion criteria	• *All POC glucose values*	• *All POC and other glucose values used to guide care.*
Measures of safety	*Analysis by patient-day* • *Percentage of patient-days with ≥1 values < 40, < 70, or > 300 mg/dL*	*Analysis by patient-day* • *Percentage of patient-days with ≥1 values < 40, < 70, or > 300 mg/dL*
Measures of glucose control	*Analysis by patient-day* • *Percentage of patient-days with mean < 140, < 180 mg/dL and/or* • *Percentage of patient-days with all values < 180 mg/dL* *Analysis by patient stay* • *Percentage of patient stays with mean < 140, < 180 mg/dL*	*Analysis by glucose reading* • *Percentage of readings < 110, < 140 mg/dL* *Analysis by patient-day* • *Percentage of patient-days with mean < 110, < 140 mg/dL, and/or* • *Percentage of patient-days with all values < 110, < 140 mg/dL* *Analysis by patient stay* • *3-day blood glucose average (3BG) for selected perioperative patients[4]: Percentage of patients with 3BG < 110, < 140 mg/dL* • *Mean time (hours) to reach glycemic target (BG < 110 or < 140 mg/dL) on insulin infusion*
Measures of insulin use	• *Percentage of patients on any subcutaneous insulin that has a scheduled basal insulin component (glargine, NPH, or detemir)*	• *Percentage of patients with ≥2 POC or lab glucose readings > 140 mg/dL on insulin infusion protocol*
Other process measures	• *Glucose measured within 8 hours of hospital admission* • *A1c measurement obtained or available within 30 days of admission*	• *Glucose measured within 8 hours of hospital admission*

Adapted from Schnipper JL et al. J Hosp Med, 2008; 3(5 Suppl): 66-75. © Society of Hospital Medicine. Published by Wiley InterScience.

develop a clear plan to test the change. In the "do" stage, the test is carried out at a small scale, with documentation of any obstacles and/or unexpected observations. In the "study" stage, data are analyzed and compared with assumed predictions with reflection on what is learned. In the "act" stage, stakeholders review results and plan for the next step based on what was learned from this test. The cycle is repeated multiple times for a QI initiative until the aim is achieved.

Figure. Plan-Do-Study-Act Cycle

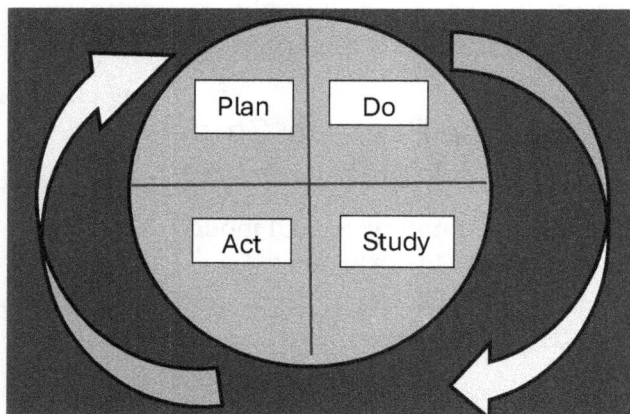

Reprinted from Barr E. & Brannan, GD. Quality Improvement Methods (LEAN, PDSA, SIX SIGMA), in *StatPearls*. 2025: Treasure Island (FL). © StatPearls Publishing LLC.

[Color—Print (Color Gallery page CG10) or web & ePub editions]

Step 7: Change and maintain a new culture of improvement

Although this is mentioned as the last step, it is the most challenging and requires continuous ongoing effort. At any institution, there are changing priorities as time progresses, and key partnerships with chief quality and patient safety officers can ensure ongoing project success. Maintaining ongoing, long-term stakeholder engagement can be very difficult. To plan for this, it is important to ensure that each area has a few champions who will continue to advocate for the needed changes. Project leaders should meet with the champions on a routine basis to ensure engagement. A safety reporting system and root causes analysis of high-harm events are also important in sustaining change, as it ensures identification of ongoing or new issues. If you can sustain the change in your area and want to work towards developing an institutional glycemic management program that meets best practice standards, you can consider working towards a disease state–specific certification through The Joint Commission for advanced inpatient diabetes management. This is a comprehensive program that is founded on the American Diabetes Association's Clinical Practice Recommendations and is linked to The Joint Commission standards. This certification represents a clinical program of excellence that can help improve care processes, care delivery, patient safety, and patient experience.[8]

Clinical Case Vignettes

Case 1

A 55-year-old woman with pancreatic cancer underwent the Whipple procedure 4 days ago. She has been initiated on tube feed therapy and is receiving a calorically dense formula, 1.5 Cal at 30 cc/h. She has been started on NPH insulin/regular insulin 70/30 every 6 hours along with correctional regular insulin via sliding scale every 6 hours. The patient's nurse administers 70/30 insulin at 6 PM and advances the feed to 40 cc/h. One hour later, the patient is vomiting and unable to tolerate feeds. Imaging shows that the tube has been dislodged and cannot be used until evaluation the next morning. The patient describes shakiness and dizziness around 10 PM, and a fingerstick glucose value is 40 mg/dL (2.2 mmol/L).

Based on review of the safety event system, the team identifies that there have been at least 15 other similar cases of hypoglycemia in patients receiving tube feeds.

Which QI tool would be best to analyze the most common contributing factors that led to hypoglycemia in these events?

A. Pareto chart

B. Ishikawa diagram

C. Process mapping

D. Staff survey

Answer: A) Pareto chart

A Pareto chart (Answer A) would be a good tool to determine which factors are leading to hypoglycemia in patients receiving tube feeds and to identify the most common cause. Ishikawa diagram (Answer B) is great at identifying all of the factors that may have a role in hypoglycemia development, but it cannot determine if one cause is more frequent than another. Process mapping (Answer C) can outline the workflow to prevent hypoglycemia in patients receiving tube feeds, but it is not able to determine the cause. Staff surveys (Answer D) may be helpful, but they are not objective measures to determine the most common cause.

Case 2

A 40-year-old man with known type 1 diabetes is admitted to the hospital with pyelonephritis. He has had significant nausea and vomiting in the last 24 hours and has not been able to eat much. At admission, electrolytes show no evidence of metabolic acidosis. Glucose values range from 90 to 120 mg/dL (5.0-6.7 mmol/L). He is treated with intravenous antibiotics. At home, the patient has been on insulin pump therapy and notes that his pump has been running in auto mode. The primary team orders CT for further evaluation, and the pump is removed before imaging. Due to unforeseen delay, the CT takes 2 to 3 hours longer than anticipated, and patient returns to his room at midnight and falls asleep without reconnecting his pump. The following morning, his glucose level is 425 mg/dL (23.6 mmol/L) with elevated anion gap, consistent with diabetic ketoacidosis.

Which of the following QI tools would be best to help us understand what steps should take place for a patient with an insulin pump who will be undergoing a diagnostic imaging study?

A. Fishbone diagram

B. Prioritization matrix

C. Process mapping

D. Staff and patient surveys

Answer: C) Process mapping

In this case, process mapping (Answer C) could be used to break down the complex process into simple steps to identify what did not happen correctly in this situation.

Case 2, Continued

Based on the event above, which of the following interventions would be most effective in preventing a similar event from happening again?

A. Development of periprocedural pump management protocol

B. Education of staff in diagnostic imaging

C. Education of staff in nursing unit

D. Safety alert within electronic health record to alert nursing staff to ensure that pumps are connected and functioning in patients who have had procedures requiring temporary pump removal

Answer: D) Safety alert within electronic health record to alert nursing staff to ensure that pumps are connected and functioning in patients who have had procedures requiring temporary pump removal

Creating a safety alert within electronic health record (Answer D) is likely the best way to prevent similar events from happening, as it is an alert that fires to remind any nurse who is in the patient's chart to ensure the insulin pump is connected and functioning after procedure. The other options could be helpful, but they unfortunately cannot guarantee that the teams will remember the education or protocol that applies to this patient's particular scenario.

Case 2, Continued

The team develops a project with an aim statement of "Increasing reconnection of insulin pump post diagnostic imaging by 50% from baseline by July 2025."

What type of measure is this aim statement?

A. Balance measure

B. Outcome measure

C. Process measure

Answer: C) Process measure

This is a process measure (Answer C), as reconnecting the insulin pump is a process that can help reduce the outcome of diabetic ketoacidosis that can result when insulin therapy is disrupted. A balance measure is typically looking for how one change impacts something downstream, which is not applicable here. Reconnecting the insulin pump is not an outcome measure.

Case 3

A 63-year-old man has a history of type 2 diabetes diagnosed at age 55 years and is admitted to the hospital for cholecystectomy. He does not have a strong family history of diabetes and was surprised that he required insulin therapy within 1 year of diabetes diagnosis. His BMI is 23 kg/m². His home regimen consists of insulin glargine and insulin lispro with recent hemoglobin A_{1c} measurement of 6.9% (52 mmol/mol). After surgery, he is placed on sliding-scale insulin therapy. On postoperative day 1, he has poor appetite, and his glucose levels range from 150 to 180 mg/dL (8.3-10.0 mmol/L). On postoperative day 2, his laboratory test results show development of mild metabolic acidosis with worsening hyperglycemia. Other results:

> C-peptide = 0.2 ng/mL (0.07 nmol/L)
> Glucose = 225 mg/dL (SI: 13.0 mmol/L)
> Glutamic acid decarboxylase 65 antibodies, positive

Which of the following is this patient's most likely underlying diagnosis?

A. Type 2 diabetes

B. Latent autoimmune diabetes

C. Ketosis prone diabetes

D. Steroid-induced diabetes

Answer: B) Latent autoimmune diabetes

This patient likely has underlying latent autoimmune diabetes (Answer B) given his positive antibody status and the history of needing insulin therapy within 1 year of diagnosis. He was assumed to have type 2 diabetes; however, the presence of diabetic ketoacidosis and low C-peptide concentration suggests that he likely has latent autoimmune diabetes. While ketosis-prone diabetes could be considered, the presentation is typically different and it does not happen in the postoperative setting. Steroid-induced diabetes is unlikely, as the patient has not received any steroids.

Case 3, Continued

Which of the following is the best QI tool to evaluate factors that contributed to this safety event?

A. Ishikawa diagram

B. Prioritization matrix

C. Process mapping

D. Develop a new policy

Answer: A) Ishikawa diagram

Many factors likely contributed to this safety event, and developing an Ishikawa diagram (Answer A) would be a helpful way to examine the various factors. A prioritization matrix is used to identify the best solutions. Process mapping is helpful for determining a current workflow and may not help with identifying the cause of this safety event. Policy creation is helpful after factors leading to the safety event are identified, and in the scenario of a gap being found between recommended standards and actual practice.

Case 3, Continued

A project is developed based on this safety event.

Which of the following would be an appropriate aim statement for this project?

A. Reduce inpatient diabetic ketoacidosis

B. Increase basal insulin use in patients with type 2 diabetes by 50%

C. Improve glycemic management in postoperative patients by May 2026

D. Decrease inpatient diabetic ketoacidosis in postoperative patients with type 2 diabetes by 10% from baseline by May 2026

Answer: D) Decrease inpatient diabetic ketoacidosis in postoperative patients with type 2 diabetes by 10% from baseline by May 2026

The aim statement in Answer D fulfills all the criteria of a SMART aim statement, which is specific, measurable, achievable, realistic, and timely. Answer A is partially correct but not time bound or specific. Answers B and C are also limited because they are missing all the elements of a SMART aim statement.

Key Learning Points

- QI projects require a methodical step-by-step approach to have impact and sustain change.

- Many useful QI tools are available to help identify the best methodology with which to approach a QI initiative.

- All QI projects need to have a SMART aim statement to ensure that there is a finite goal in mind that is agreed upon by all stakeholders.

References

1. Maynard G, Berg K, Kulasa K, O'Malley C, Rogers KM, eds. *The Glycemic Control Implementation Guide.* Society of Hospital Medicine; 2015.

2. Institute for Healthcare Improvement. *QI Essentials Toolkit.* Institute for Healthcare Improvement; 2017.

3. Preston K. Types of improvement measures in healthcare. LifeQI Blog. March 2020.https://blog.lifeqisystem.com/types-of-improvement-measures.

4. Khan SA, Zilbermint M. Centers for Medicare & Medicaid services' hospital harm measures for severe hypoglycemia and hyperglycemia: is your hospital ready? *Diabetes Spectr.* 2022;35(4):391-397. PMID: 36561656

5. Maynard G, Ramos P, Kulasa K, Rogers KM, Messler J, Schnipper JL. How sweet is it? The use of benchmarking to optimize inpatient glycemic control. *Diabetes Spectr.* 2014;27(3):212-217. PMID: 26246782

6. Schnipper JL, Magee M, Larsen K, Inzucchi SE, Maynard G, Society of Hospital Medicine Glycemic Control Task Force. Society of Hospital Medicine Glycemic Control Task Force summary: practical recommendations for assessing the impact of glycemic control efforts. *J Hosp Med.* 2008;3(Suppl 5):66-75. PMID: 18951387

7. Barr E, Brannan GD. Quality improvement methods (LEAN, PDSA, SIX SIGMA). 2024. Treasure Island (FL). StatPearls Publishing. PMID: 38261708

8. Arnold P, Scheurer D, Dake AW, et al. Hospital guidelines for diabetes management and the Joint Commission-American Diabetes Association Inpatient Diabetes Certification. *Am J Med Sci.* 2016;351(4):333-341. PMID: 27079338

Recommended Reading

- The Joint Commission. *Disease Specific Care Core and Advanced Certification Programs: Review Process Guide for Advanced Inpatient Diabetes.* The Joint Commission; 2024.

- Institute of Medicine (US) Committee on Quality of Health Care in America. *Crossing the Quality Chasm: A New Health System for 21st Century.* National Academies Press (US); 2001.

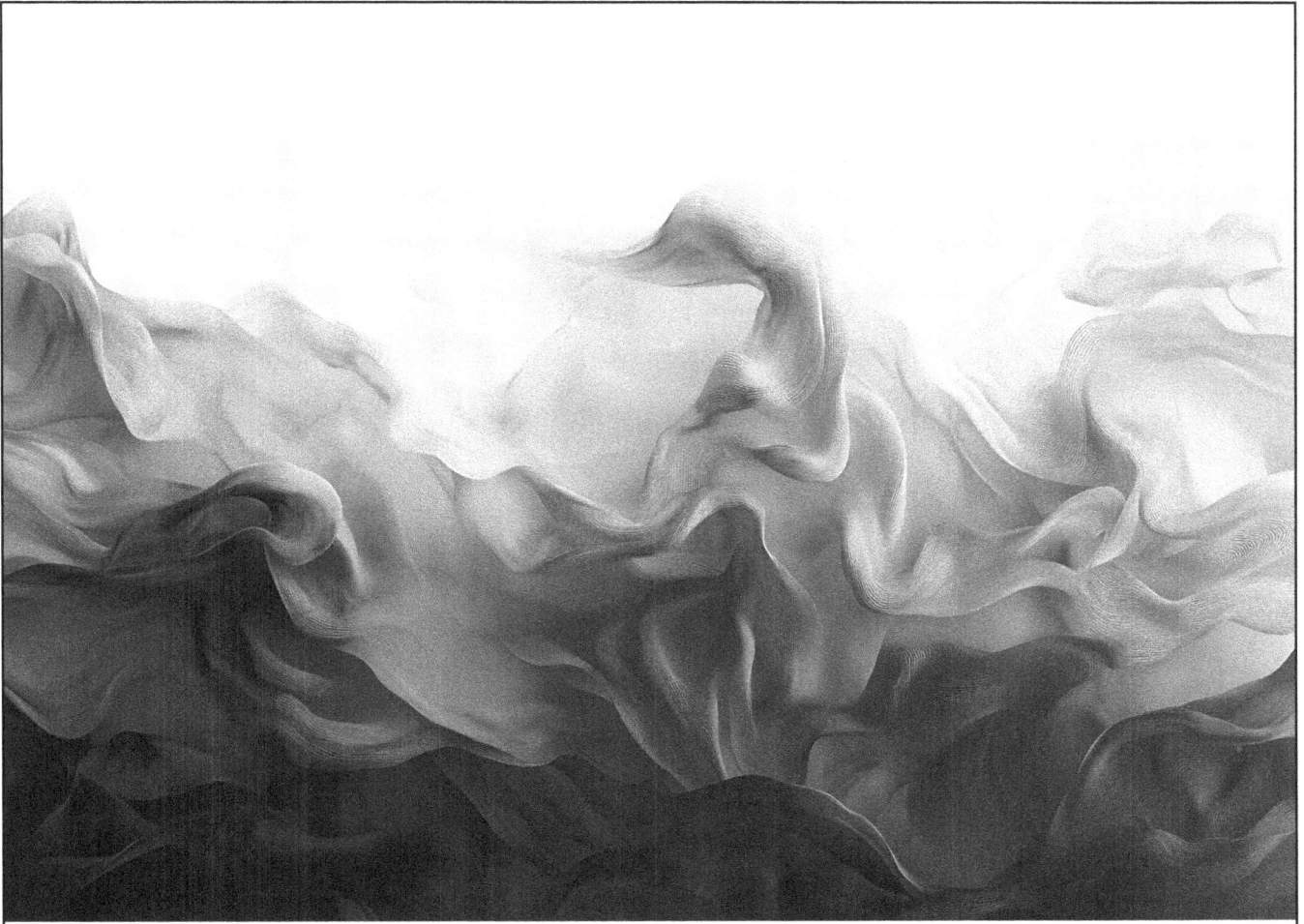

GENERAL
ENDOCRINOLOGY

Complications of Novel Nonimmunotherapy Cancer Treatments

Afreen Shariff, MD. Division of Endocrinology, Metabolism, and Nutrition, Duke University School of Medicine and Duke Cancer Institute, Durham, NC; Email: afreen.shariff@duke.edu

Randol Kennedy, MD. Division of Endocrinology, Metabolism, and Nutrition, Duke University School of Medicine, Durham, NC

Educational Objectives

After reviewing this chapter, learners should be able to:

- Identify mechanisms of endocrine complications associated with novel nonimmunotherapy-based cancer treatments.

- Recommend management and treatment options while considering the impact of treating endocrine complications of cancer therapies and vice versa.

- Describe and manage long-term sequalae of endocrine complications of nonimmunotherapy-based cancer treatments.

Significance of the Clinical Problem

Every 15 seconds, someone is diagnosed with cancer. Endocrine complications of cancer therapy are common and affect 10% of patients during treatment and up to 60% of survivors.[1,2] With cancer therapies rapidly evolving beyond traditional chemotherapy, radiation, and surgery, more than 80% of patients now face treatment-related adverse effects, some of them life-threatening. Early, effective management of these toxicities is critical to allow patients to continue life-saving therapies. As new treatments emerge, endocrinologists are stepping into a pivotal role by supporting both patients and oncologists to ensure safer, uninterrupted cancer care.

Practice Gaps

- There is lack of awareness of emerging cancer therapies and their impact on the endocrine system.

- There are training and education gaps on emerging toxicities and identification and management of endocrine toxicities.

- There are notable challenges with comanagement, evidence gaps, and coordinated care when working with complex, high-acuity oncology patients in the survivorship phase who continue to have persistent long-term endocrine complications.

Discussion

In 2024 alone, the US FDA granted approval for immunotherapy, combination immunotherapy, chemotherapy, and other agents for 62 new indications. While we continue to learn about endocrine immune-related adverse events, endocrinologists globally are being challenged with keeping abreast of the rapid adoption of novel cancer therapies, which is occurring at a much faster pace than evidence and expert guidelines can be generated to inform practice for these endocrine toxicities. In this chapter, we discuss novel cancer therapies targeting the insulin-signaling pathway, the cortisol synthesis pathway, and novel cancer delivery systems that are being adopted by oncologists globally.

Nonimmunotherapy Treatments

Inhibitors of the Phosphoinositide 3-Kinase/ Serine-Threonine Protein Kinase Akt/ Mammalian Target of Rapamycin (PI3K/ Akt/mTOR) Signaling Pathway

The interplay of metabolic disease, diabetes, and obesity strongly correlates with a greater risk for at least 13 different cancer types.[3] It is not surprising that patients can develop treatment-induced hyperglycemia when cancer treatment affects the insulin-signaling pathway.

The PI3K/Akt/mTOR signaling pathway is a highly conserved signal transduction network in eukaryotic cells that promotes cell survival, cell growth, and cell-cycle progression.[4] Regarding its role in gluconeogenesis, the mTOR pathway is also a modulator of insulin-mediated glucose metabolism and glycogen synthesis (*Figure 1*).[5,6] Deregulation of this pathway is a common and well-established mechanism for cancer growth. For example, pathogenic variants in the genes encoding PI3K/Akt/mTOR are the most frequent pathways of breast cancer tumorigenesis.[7] This, therefore, has led to evolution of cancer therapies, with more than 40 agents targeting this mechanism.[8,9] However, with the increased use of these therapies, there is an expectant increase in the number of hyperglycemia-related adverse

Figure 1. Simplified Schematic of the Intracellular Mechanism of the PI3K/Akt/mTOR Pathway

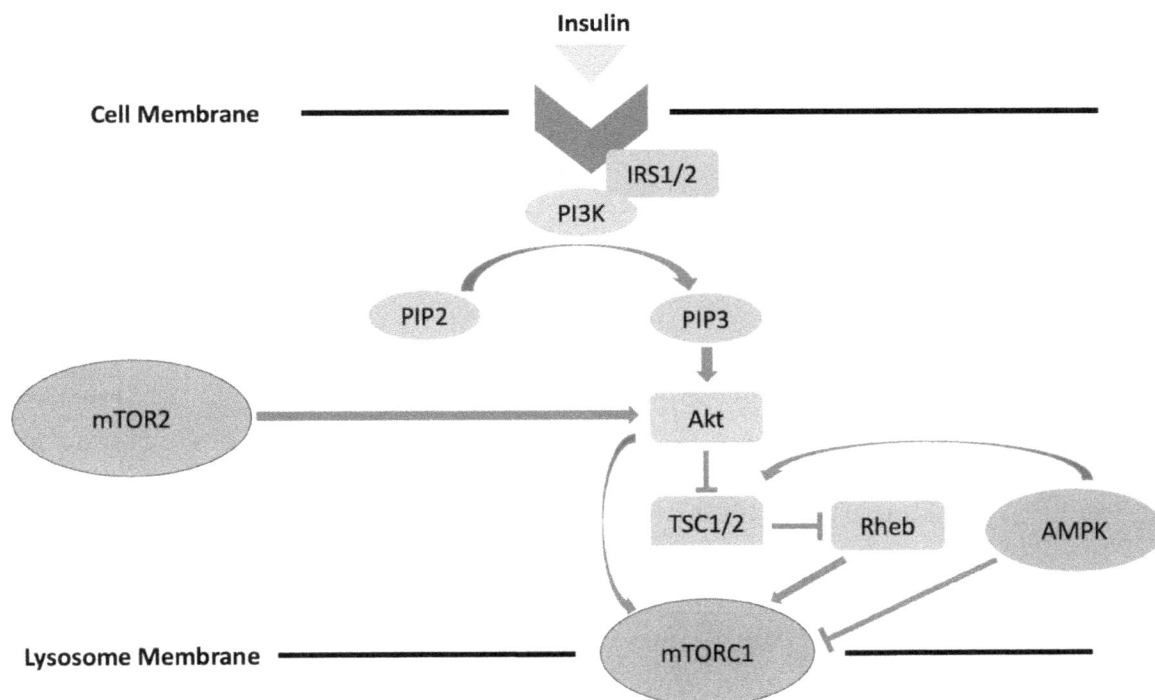

Insulin binding initiates autophosphorylation and activation of the tyrosine kinase component of the β domain. The activated tyrosine kinase phosphorylates IRS1, which, when triggered, activates PI3K that generates PIP3 from PIP2. PIP3 phosphorylates Akt/protein kinase B, which when activated, either indirectly affects mTORC1 through TSC2 or directly through PRAS40 (proline-rich Akt substrate of 40 kDa), leads to regulation of cellular metabolism and growth/proliferation. Activation is shown by arrowhead lines, whereas inhibition is indicated by 'T'-shaped lines. Abbreviations: AMPK, AMP-activated protein kinase; IRS1/2, insulin receptor substrate 1 and 2; mTORC1/2, mechanistic target of rapamycin complex 1 and 2; PI3K, phosphatidylinositide-3 kinase; PIP2, phosphatidylinositol 4,5-bisphosphate; PIP3, phosphatidylinositol 3,4,5-triphosphate; Rheb, Ras homolog enriched in brain; TSC1/2, tuberous sclerosis protein complex 1 and 2.

[Color—Print (Color Gallery page CG10) or web & ePub editions]

events. One drug class that will not be covered in this discussion because of its familiarity, but should be briefly mentioned in this context, is mTOR inhibitors (eg, sirolimus [rapamycin], temsirolimus, everolimus). Hyperglycemia is a relatively frequent adverse event associated with mTOR inhibitors, with reports that it affects as many as 50% of treated patients.[6] Less familiar but evolving targeted cancer therapies of the PI3K/Akt/mTOR signaling pathway include inhibitors of Akt and PI3K.

PI3K Inhibitors

Since the FDA approved idelalisib for chronic lymphocytic leukemia in 2014, there has been an upsurge in clinical trials and the use of PI3K inhibitors in cancer therapy. Currently, there are 5 FDA-approved drugs on the market (*Table 1*) with other clinical trials ongoing. PI3K inhibitors can be broadly characterized as pan-PI3K inhibitors (copanlisib), isoform selective (alpelisib, α isoform selective; idelalisib, δ isoform selective), and dual selective (duvelisib, δ and γ isoforms). Umbralisib is a unique dual inhibitor of the PI3K δ isoform and casein kinase-1ε. Interestingly, PI3K inhibitors with which the α isoform is spared (duvelisib, idelalisib, umbralisib) have not been associated with significant hyperglycemia.[6]

Hyperglycemia is the most frequent adverse event and the one of the most common reasons for PI3K inhibitor discontinuation.[10,11] While hyperglycemia with copanlisib infusion is usually transient (occurring within hours of infusion and resolving within 24 to 48 hours after infusion[12]), hyperglycemia with alpelisib is of slower onset, occurring days after drug initiation (*Table 1*).[11] Therefore, management of copanlisib-induced hyperglycemia may be brief, with fluid hydration during infusion and oral hypoglycemic agents or short-acting insulin as needed. Treatment with long-acting insulins is generally avoided due to risk of hypoglycemia. Hyperglycemia with alpelisib is generally approached with oral hypoglycemic agents as first-line treatment (metformin being the first agent of choice), with insulin regimens reserved for patients with severe hyperglycemia (*Figure 2, following page*).[6] Diabetic ketoacidosis has also been reported as a rare severe complication of alpelisib use.[13]

There is concern about the use insulin and sulfonylureas as part of hyperglycemia management in patients with PI3K-mediated cancer tumors, as this could potentially stimulate

Table 1. Incidence and Mechanism of Action of Hyperglycemia Associated With Cancer Therapies

Drug category	Drug name	Median onset/resolution of hyperglycemia	Mechanism of development of hyperglycemia	Reported incidence of hyperglycemia
Phosphatidylinositol IDE-1 kinase (PI3K) inhibitors	Idelalisib Duvelisib Copanlisib Alpelisib Umbralisib	Alpelisib Onset 15 days; resolution: 4-7 days[11] Copanlisib Onset, 5 hours after infusion; resolution: 24-48 hours after infusion	Blocking PI3K interferes with insulin signaling, resulting in insulin resistance	28% to 30%
Akt or protein kinase B inhibitors	Capivasertib	Onset, 15 days[15]	• Reduces hepatic glycogen synthesis • Induces hepatic glycogenolysis • Blocks insulin signaling, resulting in insulin resistance	2.3%
Antibody drug conjugates	Enfortumab vedotin	Onset, 19 days[22]	Unknown	14%

Figure 2. Algorithm for the Management of PI3K/Akt/mTOR–Induced Hyperglycemia

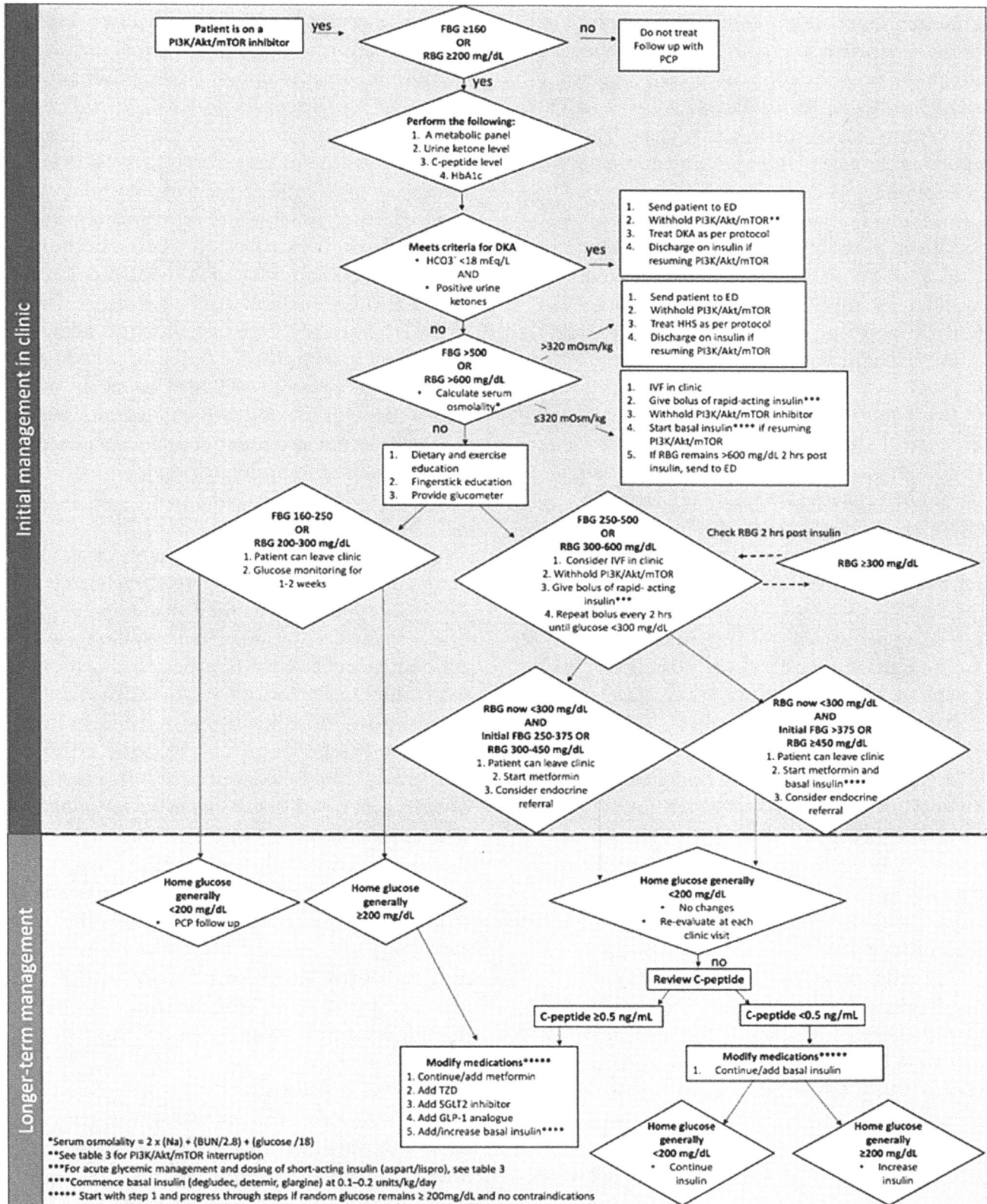

Abbreviations: DKA, diabetic ketoacidosis; ED, emergency department; eGFR, glomerular filtration rate; HCO3, bicarbonate; HHS, hyperglycemic hyperosmolar syndrome; IVF, intravenous fluids; MF, metformin; PCP, primary care provider; Na, serum sodium; TZD, thiazolidinediones; BUN, serum urea nitrogen.[6]

Reprinted from Cheung YM et al. *Curr Probl Cancer*, 2022; 46(1): 100776. © Elsevier Inc.

[Color—Print (Color Gallery page CG11) or web & ePub editions]

tumorigenesis through PI3K activation, based on the mechanism proposed above. However, this hypothesis remains speculative, with no evidence highlighting an association of cancer progression with high endogenous insulin use in these patients. However, there is a growing body of evidence supporting the role of hyperinsulinemic states in tumorigenesis.[6] As insulin is the most effective pharmacotherapy for severe hyperglycemia, especially in oncologic patients, exogenous insulin should also be used when clinically indicated. Sulfonylureas, however, should be discouraged in patients undergoing chemotherapy with PI3K/Akt/mTOR inhibitors.[6]

Akt Inhibitors

In November 2023, capivasertib became the first FDA-approved Akt inhibitor to be used in combination with fulvestrant (an estrogen receptor antagonist) in the treatment of breast cancer with biomarkers to Akt or the catalytic α-subunit on phosphoinositide 3-kinase (PI3KCA).[8] In the phase 3 trial leading to FDA approval, hyperglycemia of any grade occurred in 16.3% of patients (2.3% grade 3 or higher) in comparison with 3.7% of patients on placebo + fulvestrant (0.3% grade 3 or higher).[14] The median onset of hyperglycemia was 15 days, ranging from 1 to 51 days.[15] Although these incidences appear to be lower than that related to PI3K inhibitors, the authors did consider the intermittent use of capivasertib in the study as a contributing factor. Therefore, an increased incidence in clinical practice with more routine use of agents similar to PI3K inhibitors is a reasonable assumption.

Akt inhibition and its role in obesity and hyperglycemia has already been investigated in previous studies. For example, Cho et al demonstrated significant fasting hyperglycemia, as well as near 4-fold increase in islet mass consistent with β-cell compensation to insulin resistance.[16] Crouthamel et al also demonstrated a similar mechanism of hyperglycemia in vivo when GSK690693, a pan-AKT kinase inhibitor, was given to mice.[17] This Akt-induced hyperglycemia was demonstrated to be attenuated by fasting

before administration (to deplete liver glycogen stores), as well as by a low-carbohydrate diet. Interestingly, oral antidiabetes agents such as metformin, pioglitazone, and DPP-4 inhibitors did not completely attenuate prandial hyperglycemia, unlike the scenario with PI3K inhibitors. Despite these aberrancies in the response shown in vivo of oral hypoglycemic agents with Akt inhibitor–induced hyperglycemia, the approach to managing Akt inhibitor–induced hyperglycemia in clinical practice is similar to that of other forms of cancer therapy–induced insulin resistance. Oral hypoglycemic agents are first-line treatment, with or without insulin therapy (*Figure 2, preceding page*).[6] Hyperglycemia is usually reversible, with resolution after therapy discontinuation. Diabetic ketoacidosis has also been reported as a rare severe complication of Akt inhibitor use.[18]

Antibody Drug Conjugates

Targeted chemotherapies using monoclonal antibodies as a vector were introduced in the 1970s. By specifically binding an antigen on a cancerous cell, it was theorized that monoclonal antibodies could reduce nonspecific toxicities, target tumor cells, and either alter their signaling patterns towards a therapeutic outcome or direct an immune response toward the tumor cell.[19] Therefore, there is no surprise that this medium of cancer therapy has become more common, with approximately 13 antibody drug conjugates that are FDA approved for cancer therapy in the United Sates and more than 100 ongoing clinical trials.[20] However, in attempts to deliver the maximum dose for anticancer efficacy, antibody drug conjugates have been associated with unwarranted adverse events, leading to frequent therapy discontinuation.

Enfortumab Vedotin

Enfortumab vedotin is an antibody targeting the cell adhesion molecule nectin-4 linked to a microtubule inhibitor conjugate. This antibody drug conjugate was first granted accelerated FDA approval in 2019 for the treatment of urothelial carcinoma based on a phase 1 clinical trial.[21]

Pertinent to this discussion, severe hyperglycemia occurred in 5% of patients, and it was the only grade 3 or higher adverse event occurring in 5% or more of patients. In December 2023, enfortumab vedotin coupled with pembrolizumab (an inhibitor of programmed cell death protein-1/PD-1) was also FDA approved for the treatment of urothelial carcinoma.

In further clinical trials, hyperglycemia of any grade occurred in 14% of patients treated with enfortumab vedotin, with 7% of patients developing grade 3 to 4 hyperglycemia.[20,22] Median time of hyperglycemia onset was 19 days.[22] Hyperglycemia also occurred more frequently in patients with baseline hyperglycemia or BMI of 30 kg/m² or higher.[22] The mechanism of enfortumab-induced hyperglycemia is still unknown. Diabetic ketoacidosis has also been reported as a severe complication with high mortality.[23] Therefore, the FDA has issued guidelines related to monitoring for hyperglycemia while enfortumab is being used, with advice to hold enfortumab if the glucose concentration is greater than 250 mg/dL (>13.9 mmol/L).

Hepatic Intra-Arterial Chemotherapy

Lastly, hepatic intra-arterial chemotherapy was introduced in the early 1970s to deliver localized chemotherapy to the liver via the hepatic artery in an attempt to circumvent the toxic effects of systemic chemotherapy. The liver's dual blood supply preferentially delivers high doses of chemotherapeutic agents to the hepatic artery, and because the liver metabolizes the chemotherapy (first-pass effect), intra-arterial delivery diminishes the systemic toxic effects.[24] Cancers that could be treated using this medium includes hepatocellular carcinoma, metastatic colon cancer, and cholangiocarcinoma. Hepatic artery intra-arterial pump (HIAP) chemotherapy has become more frequently used as an option in treating unresectable disease.

HIAPs are implanted at specialized centers. Chemotherapy is instilled into the pump using infusion needles every 2 to 3 weeks, allowing for continuous rather than bolus infusions, thereby prolonging the exposure time of metastases to chemotherapy and decreasing systemic toxicity.[25] High-dosage intra-arterial dexamethasone commonly accompanies chemotherapy to reduce systemic toxicity.[24,25] Although clinical trials have not reported iatrogenic Cushing syndrome as a common adverse event of HIAP therapy, a few cases have been reported, suggesting a possible consequence of prolonged steroid exposure, as with other forms of high-dosage glucocorticoid steroid therapy.

Future Directions

Emerging cancer therapies continue to be more enhanced, personalized, and targeted, with several drugs in the pipeline for approval in the coming months to years. Importantly, these approvals are both as monotherapy and combination therapy that integrate radiation, chemotherapy, immunotherapy, and newer targeted therapies that can include vaccine therapies, bispecific agents, etc. Given the growth of oncology portfolio of therapies, treatments are being approved to manage early-stage cancers. This further expands the pool of individuals with cancer who are eligible to receive these treatments. The intertwined relationship of new endocrine toxicities and preexisting comorbidities, such as obesity, diabetes, and cancer, underscores the need to stay up to date with this intersecting field of oncology and endocrinology.

Clinical Case Vignettes
Case 1

A 73-year-old woman presents to the emergency department with a 3-week history of worsening fatigue, nausea, vomiting, increased thirst, and urination. She has no history of diabetes or no other notable endocrine issues. She does, however, have an oncologic history of ER/PR-positive, HER-2/neu-negative invasive ductal carcinoma of the left breast diagnosed 20 years ago. Treatment consisted of mastectomy, 4 cycles of dose-dense doxorubicin + cyclophosphamide with paclitaxel chemotherapy, radiation therapy, and 10 years of endocrine therapy (exemestane, then switched to letrozole therapy). After completion of endocrine therapy, she was found to have bone and lung metastases when she presented to the hospital for weight loss and dyspnea. Chemotherapy was reinitiated. Due to persistent disease, a liquid biopsy for tumor DNA analysis was performed, which identified pathogenic variants in the genes encoding PI3K and the estrogen receptor 1 (ESR1). She was therefore started on capivasertib and fulvestrant therapy 1 month before her current hospital presentation.

On physical examination, she appears ill. Her temperature is 98.9°F (37.2°C), blood pressure is 125/58 mm Hg, pulse rate is 94 beats/min, and oxygen saturation is 97% on room air. Her weight is 149.7 lb (67.9 kg) (BMI = 25.68 kg/m²). Mucous membranes are moist. Fine bibasilar crackles are audible and consistent with atelectasis. Examination findings are otherwise normal.

Laboratory test results:

> Sodium = 126 mEq/L (135-145 mEq/L)
> (SI: 126 mmol/L [135-145 mmol/L])
> Potassium = 4.5 mEq/L (3.5-5.0 mEq/L)
> (SI: 4.5 mmol/L [3.5-5.0 mmol/L])
> Chloride = 87 mEq/L (98-108 mEq/L)
> (SI: 87 mmol/L [98-108 mmol/L])
> Bicarbonate = 24 mEq/L (21-30 mEq/L)
> (SI: 24 mmol/L [21-30 mmol/L])
> Creatinine = 1.7 mg/dL (0.6-1.3 mg/dL)
> (SI: 150.3 μmol/L [53.0-114.9 μmol/L])
> Serum urea nitrogen = 37 mg/dL (7-20 mg/dL)
> (SI: 13.2 mmol/L [2.5-7.1 mmol/L])
> Glucose = 758 mg/dL (70-140 mg/dL)
> (SI: 42.1 mmol/L [3.9-7.8 mmol/L])
> Anion gap = 15 mEq/L (3-12 mEq/L) (SI: 15 mmol/L
> [3-12 mmol/L])
> β-Hydroxybutyrate = 0.4 mmol/L (<0.4 mmol/L)
> (SI: 400 μmol/L [<400 μmol/L])
> Hemoglobin A_{1c} = 5.5% (<5.7%) (37 mmol/mol
> [<39 mmol/mol])

Which of the following is the most likely mechanism explaining this patient's new-onset diabetes?

A. Autoantibody-mediated destruction of pancreatic β cells

B. Autoreactive T cell–mediated destruction of pancreatic β cells

C. Acquired adipolysis leading to hypoleptinemia and increased insulin resistance

D. Insulin resistance through direct inhibition of the insulin receptor–signaling pathway

E. Pathogenic variant in hepatocyte nuclear factor 1α leading to abnormal insulin secretion

Answer: D) Insulin resistance through direct inhibition of the insulin receptor–signaling pathway

This patient presented with symptoms concerning for diabetic ketoacidosis (polydipsia, polyurea, nausea, vomiting) with significant hyperglycemia. Although her biochemistry panel shows a mildly elevated anion gap, β-hydroxybutyrate and bicarbonate levels are normal, thereby ruling out diabetic ketoacidosis as a complication of severe hyperglycemia. She therefore likely has some preserved pancreatic β-cell function. Factors leading to pancreatic β-cell dysfunction are less likely to be the cause of this patient's new-onset diabetes. Type 1 diabetes is caused by autoantibody-mediated pancreatic β-cell destruction (Answer A), whereas the main proposed mechanism of immune checkpoint inhibitor–related diabetes is T cell–mediated destruction (Answer B). In both etiologies, diabetic ketoacidosis is a common presenting feature. Acquired generalized lipodystrophy is another rare cause of immune checkpoint inhibitors leading to hypertriglyceridemia and insulin resistance (Answer C). This patient is not on an immune checkpoint inhibitor, but rather a protein kinase B/Akt inhibitor (capivasertib), thereby leading to impaired insulin signaling through the PI3K/Akt/mTOR pathway (Answer D). This causes hyperglycemia with a median onset of 15 days. First-line treatments include oral hypoglycemic agents, such as metformin, unless there is a question of severe hyperglycemia. She was acutely managed with insulin and fluids with rapid improvement of glycemic control while capivasertib was briefly interrupted. Maturity-onset diabetes in the young (MODY), as its name implies, occurs in patients younger than 30 years who usually have a strong family history due to its autosomal dominant transmission (Answer E), which is not the case in this vignette.

Case 2

A 50-year-old man is referred for endocrinology consultation for 2 weeks of worsening fatigue. He has an oncologic history of colorectal adenocarcinoma with liver metastases diagnosed 2 years ago. Treatment consisted of folinic acid, fluorouracil, and oxaplatin (FOLFOX)-based chemotherapy and bevacizumab for 5 months, after which he underwent primary liver resection and placement of a HIAP with infusions of floxuridine (FUDR) and dexamethasone, 20 mg every 2 to 3 weeks, for 64 weeks. During treatment, the patient reported a 30-lb (14-kg) weight gain over 3 to 6 months. A random point-of-care glucose value of 500 mg/dL (27.8 mmol/L) during an outpatient follow-up visit prompted commencement of metformin and empagliflozin to address the new diagnosis of diabetes. HIAP therapy was discontinued 4 weeks before consultation whereby random point-of-care fingerstick glucose readings improved to 130 to 150 mg/dL (7.2-8.3 mmol/L).

On physical examination, his temperature is 98.9°F (37.2°C), blood pressure is 110/58 mm Hg, pulse rate is 80 beats/min, and oxygen saturation is 97% on room air. His weight is 219.8 lb (99.7 kg) (BMI = 34 kg/m²). Central obesity is noted with visible purple striae on the lower abdomen (*Figure 3*). Proximal muscle wasting is also noted in the extremities. Comparison staging CT of the abdomen and pelvis is shown (*Figure 4, following page*).

Which of the following is the most appropriate next step in this patient's management?

A. Order a basic metabolic panel and measure plasma renin and aldosterone

B. Order a cosyntropin-stimulation test

C. Initiate hydrocortisone, 20 mg in the morning and 10 mg in the afternoon

D. Measure 21-hydroxylase antibodies

E. Order a dexamethasone-suppression test

Answer: C) Start hydrocortisone, 20 mg in the morning and 10 mg in the afternoon

This patient has symptoms and signs of cortisol excess/Cushing syndrome related to HIAP dexamethasone infusion (weight gain, central obesity, proximal muscle wasting, purple striae, new-onset diabetes) and is now demonstrating central adrenal insufficiency because of abrupt discontinuation of intrahepatic dexamethasone infusion. Therefore, a diagnostic workup for

Figure 3.

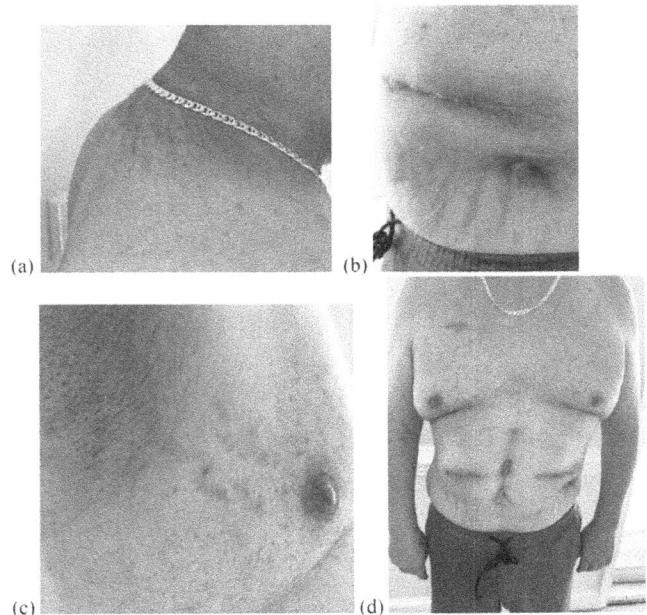

Physical exam findings include a dorsocervical fat pad ("buffalo hump") (*Panel A*), purple abdominal striae on the abdomen (*Panel B*) and under the armpit (*Panel C*), and truncal obesity 2 years after starting HIAP with dexamethasone, pictured here roughly 30 months after therapy initiation.[25]

Reprinted from Ferreira MS & Shariff AI. *Current Problems in Cancer: Case Reports*, 2022; 7(1): 100177. © The Authors. Published by Elsevier Inc.

[Color—Print (Color Gallery page CG12) or web & ePub editions]

Figure 4.

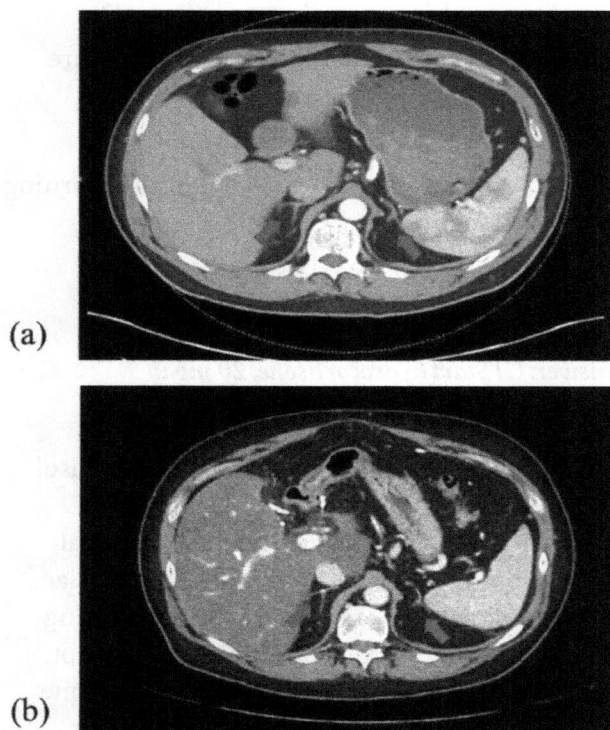

(a)

(b)

Contrast-enhanced abdominal CT of normal adrenal glands before initiation of floxuridine (FUDR) via HIAP (*Panel A*), and significant adrenal atrophy approximately 64 weeks after receiving 20 mg HIAP dexamethasone every 2 to 3 weeks (*Panel B*).

Reprinted from Ferreira MS & Shariff AI. *Current Problems in Cancer: Case Reports*, 2022; 7(1): 100177. © The Authors. Published by Elsevier Inc.

[Color—Print (Color Gallery page CG12) or web & ePub editions]

primary adrenal insufficiency (Answers A and D) should not be considered in this clinical scenario. Also, due to the patient's compelling signs and symptoms related to exogenous steroid use, a dexamethasone-suppression test (Answer E) is unnecessary. Although proof of adrenal insufficiency can be considered with laboratory testing, this patient's clinical scenario is convincing enough to forego further diagnostic laboratory workup. In cases of ambiguity, measurement of morning serum cortisol and ACTH would be the initial step, not a cosyntropin-stimulation test (Answer B), as this could be misleadingly normal in the setting of secondary adrenal insufficiency (if the adrenal cortex has not yet atrophied in the presence of prolonged steroid exposure). In this patient, the adrenal glands showed evidence of atrophy on interval imaging.

Key Learning Points

- Novel cancer therapies beyond immunotherapy—especially PI3K, Akt inhibitors, and antibody drug conjugates—are increasingly associated with serious endocrine toxicities, particularly hyperglycemia.

- Hyperglycemia is the most common and clinically significant endocrine adverse event associated with PI3K/Akt/mTOR inhibitors. Management requires tailored strategies based on the specific agents.

- Emerging treatments, such as HIAP chemotherapy, can lead to steroid-induced Cushing syndrome and secondary adrenal insufficiency, emphasizing the need for proactive monitoring and early intervention.

- Endocrinologists have a critical role in identifying, managing, and educating patients and clinicians about endocrine complications of cancer therapies to bridge gaps in survivorship care and help patients stay on life-saving treatments.

References

1. Hattersley R, Nana M, Lansdown AJ. Endocrine complications of immunotherapies: a review. *Clin Med (Lond)*. 2021;21(2):e212-e222. PMID: 33762389

2. Gebauer J, Higham C, Langer T, Denzer C, Brabant G. Long-term endocrine and metabolic consequences of cancer treatment: a systematic review. *Endocr Rev.* 2019;40(3):711-767. PMID: 30476004

3. Berrington de Gonzalez A, Hartge P, Cerhan JR, et al. Body-mass index and mortality among 1.46 million white adults. *N Engl J Med.* 2010;363(23):2211-2219. PMID: 21121834

4. Glaviano A, Foo ASC, Lam HY, et al. PI3K/AKT/mTOR signaling transduction pathway and targeted therapies in cancer. *Mol Cancer.* 2023;22(1):138. PMID: 37596643

5. Tremblay F, Gagnon A, Veilleux A, Sorisky A, Marette A. Activation of the mammalian target of rapamycin pathway acutely inhibits insulin signaling to

Akt and glucose transport in 3T3-L1 and human adipocytes. *Endocrinology.* 2005;146(3):1328-1337. PMID: 15576463

6. Cheung YM, McDonnell M, Hamnvik OR. A targeted approach to phosphoinositide-3-kinase/Akt/mammalian target of rapamycin-induced hyperglycemia. *Curr Probl Cancer.* 2022;46(1):100776. PMID: 34376311

7. Cancer Genome Atlas N. Comprehensive molecular portraits of human breast tumours. *Nature.* 2012;490(7418):61-70. PMID: 23000897

8. Mullard A. FDA approves first-in-class AKT inhibitor. *Nat Rev Drug Discov.* 2024;23(1):9. PMID: 38049466

9. Sirico M, D'Angelo A, Gianni C, Casadei C, Merloni F, De Giorgi U. Current state and future challenges for PI3K inhibitors in cancer therapy. *Cancers (Basel).* 2023;15(3):703. PMID: 36765661

10. Panayiotidis P, Follows GA, Mollica L, et al. Efficacy and safety of copanlisib in patients with relapsed or refractory marginal zone lymphoma. *Blood Adv.* 2021;5(3):823-828. PMID: 2021;5(3):823-828. PMID: 33560394

11. Rugo HS, Andre F, Yamashita T, et al. Time course and management of key adverse events during the randomized phase III SOLAR-1 study of PI3K inhibitor alpelisib plus fulvestrant in patients with HR-positive advanced breast cancer. *Ann Oncol.* 2020;31(8):1001-1010. PMID: 32416251

12. Patnaik A, Appleman LJ, Tolcher AW, et al. First-in-human phase I study of copanlisib (BAY 80-6946), an intravenous pan-class I phosphatidylinositol 3-kinase inhibitor, in patients with advanced solid tumors and non-Hodgkin's lymphomas. *Ann Oncol.* 2016;27(10):1928-1940. PMID: 27672108

13. Farah SJ, Masri N, Ghanem H, Azar M. Diabetic ketoacidosis associated with alpelisib treatment of metastatic breast cancer. *AACE Clin Case Rep.* 2020;6(6):e349-e351. PMID: 33244501

14. Turner NC, Oliveira M, Howell SJ, et al. Capivasertib in hormone receptor-positive advanced breast cancer. *N Engl J Med.* 2023;388(22):2058-2070. PMID: 37256976

15. Rugo HS, Oliveira M, Howell SJ, et al. Capivasertib and fulvestrant for patients with hormone receptor-positive advanced breast cancer: characterization, time course, and management of frequent adverse events from the phase III CAPItello-291 study. *ESMO Open.* 2024;9(9):103697. PMID: 39241495

16. Cho H, Mu J, Kim JK, et al. Insulin resistance and a diabetes mellitus-like syndrome in mice lacking the protein kinase Akt2 (PKB beta). *Science.* 2001;292(5522):1728-1731. PMID: 11387480

17. Crouthamel MC, Kahana JA, Korenchuk S, et al. Mechanism and management of AKT inhibitor-induced hyperglycemia. *Clin Cancer Res.* 2009;15(1):217-225. PMID: 19118049

18. Rodriguez YE, Batra R, Patel K, Martinez S. Capivasertib-induced diabetic ketoacidosis in a patient with estrogen receptor-positive/human epidermal growth factor receptor 2-negative (ER+/HER2-) metastatic breast cancer and no prior history of diabetes mellitus: a case report. *Cureus.* 2024;16(7):e63710. PMID: 39099917

19. Chau CH, Steeg PS, Figg WD. Antibody-drug conjugates for cancer. *Lancet.* 2019;394(10200):793-804. PMID: 31478503

20. Nguyen TD, Bordeau BM, Balthasar JP. Mechanisms of ADC toxicity and strategies to increase ADC tolerability. *Cancers (Basel).* 2023;15(3):713. PMID: 36765668

21. Rosenberg J, Sridhar SS, Zhang J, et al. EV-101: a phase I study of single-agent enfortumab vedotin in patients with nectin-4-positive solid tumors, including metastatic urothelial carcinoma. *J Clin Oncol.* 2020;38(10):1041-1049. PMID: 32031899

22. Powles T, Rosenberg JE, Sonpavde GP, et al. Enfortumab vedotin in previously treated advanced urothelial carcinoma. *N Engl J Med.* 2021;384(12):1125-1135. PMID: 38446675

23. Atemnkeng F, Aguilar F, Gupta S, Chugh S, Klein M. Diabetic ketoacidosis and acute kidney injury associated with enfortumab vedotin for urothelial carcinoma: a case report. *Kidney Med.* 2023;5(12):100737. PMID: 38028029

24. Franssen S, Soares KC, Jolissaint JS, et al. Comparison of hepatic arterial infusion pump chemotherapy vs resection for patients with multifocal intrahepatic cholangiocarcinoma. *JAMA Surg.* 2022;157(7):590-596. PMID: 35544131

25. Ferreira MS. Iatrogenic Cushing's syndrome presenting with adrenal insufficiency in 2 patients receiving dexamethasone for metastatic colorectal cancer through an intrahepatic arterial infusion pump. *Current Problems in Cancer: Case Reports.* 2022;7:100177.

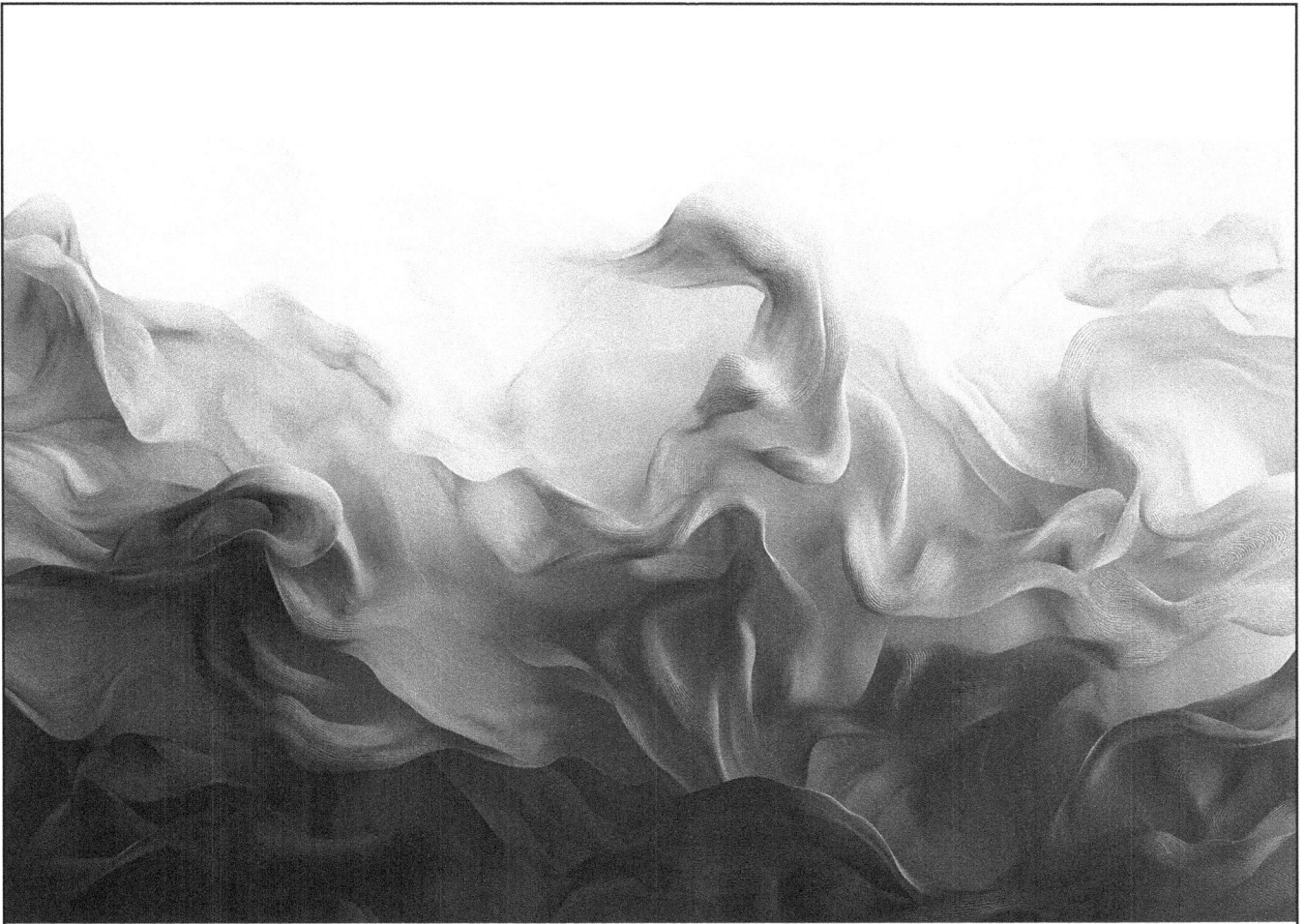

NEUROENDOCRINOLOGY AND PITUITARY

Challenging Cases of Hyponatremia

Mirjam Christ-Crain, MD, PhD. Department of Endocrinology, University hospital Basel, University of Basel, Switzerland; Email: mirjam.christ-crain@usb.ch

Educational Objectives

After reviewing this chapter, learners should be able to:

- Describe the clinical symptoms of acute and chronic hyponatremia.

- Construct the differential diagnosis of hyponatremia and distinguish various causes of chronic syndrome of inappropriate antidiuresis (SIAD).

- Recommend treatment options for acute severe hyponatremia and chronic hyponatremia.

Significance of the Clinical Problem

The prevalence of hyponatremia depends on the nature of the patient population studied (eg, hospitalized patients or outpatients) and the criteria used to define hyponatremia. Using a definition of hyponatremia of a sodium concentration less than 135 mEq/L (<135 mmol/L), it is the most common electrolyte disorder and affects more than 15% of hospitalized patients.[1] The prevalence rate is even higher (up to 30%) in acutely and chronically ill hospitalized patients.[1] The most common cause of hyponatremia is SIAD.

In acute hyponatremia (<48 hours), the brain's ability to compensate for the increased osmotic gradient across the blood-brain barrier is exceeded; water is osmotically shifted into the brain, and cerebral edema occurs. This can lead to increased intracranial pressure, which manifests as headaches, restlessness, and confusion. Brain herniation and death can occur if hyponatremia is not treated immediately. However, if hyponatremia develops over several days, sodium, followed by organic solutes, is extruded from the brain, decreasing intracerebral osmolality and preventing the development of cerebral edema. Due to this adaptive mechanism, chronic hyponatremia is often clinically asymptomatic.

A growing body of evidence has shown that chronic hyponatremia is associated with increased mortality and morbidity. A meta-analysis found that hyponatremia is significantly associated with overall mortality[2]; an increased risk of falling, osteoporosis, and fractures[3]; and attention deficit.[4] Multimorbid patients generally have a worse prognosis. However, it remains unclear whether these observations represent causality or are purely associations.

Practice Gaps

- Challenges in properly diagnosing the various etiologies of hyponatremia.

- Difficulty choosing the correct treatment for chronic hyponatremia.

- Challenges meeting the need to immediately treat patients with acute hyponatremia and severe symptoms.

Discussion

Diagnosis of Hyponatremia

Appropriate differential diagnosis is essential in hyponatremic patients because the treatment depends on the etiology. Once hypotonic hyponatremia is confirmed, urine osmolality should be measured, as it reflects arginine vasopressin (AVP) activity. Levels less than 100 mOsm/kg are indicative of suppressed AVP, such as in primary polydipsia, low solute intake, or beer potomania. Conversely, urine osmolality greater than 100 to 200 mOsm/kg reflects increased AVP activity, which can be nonosmotically triggered by cortisol deficiency or low effective arterial volume resulting from hypovolemia, heart insufficiency, or cirrhosis. However, AVP release can also be inappropriate with respect to plasma osmolality and hemodynamics as seen in SIAD.[5]

The clinical criteria necessary to diagnose SIAD go back to the definition by Schwartz and Bartter in 1967.[6] SIAD is considered a diagnosis of exclusion and is based on the evaluation of urine and serum osmolality and sodium in the setting of clinical euvolemia (*Box 1*).
SIAD has a variety of underlying causes (*Box 2*).

Treatment of Hyponatremia

Acute symptomatic hyponatremia is an emergency and must be treated immediately with hypertonic saline. American guidelines recommend intravenous infusion of 100 mL 3% hypertonic saline over 10 minutes up to 3 times.[7] European guidelines recommend intravenous infusion of 150 mL 3% hypertonic saline over 20 minutes followed by a second administration of 150 mL while checking plasma sodium, with the goal of reaching a 5 mmol increase and symptom improvement.[5]

In the management of chronic hyponatremia in patients with SIAD, fluid restriction is still the first-line therapy currently recommended by European Union and US hyponatremia guidelines.[5,7] Recommended fluid restrictions generally range from 500 to 1000 mL.[8] In patients with persistent SIAD not responding to fluid restriction, second-line therapy is required, such as urea (recommended as a second-line treatment after fluid restriction in both the European hyponatremia guidelines and the US expert panel recommendations).[5,7] Another second-line treatment option is vasopressin antagonists. Tolvaptan is an oral vasopressin V2-receptor antagonist that blocks AVP action in the kidneys, inducing water diuresis to raise serum sodium levels. The efficacy of tolvaptan vs placebo was established in the SALT-1 and SALT-2 trials in patients with chronic euvolemic and hypervolemic hyponatremia.[9] The results showed better improvement in serum sodium area under the curve with tolvaptan by day 4. The initial tolvaptan dosage was 15 mg daily. Based on this study, tolvaptan was approved by the US FDA in

Box 1. Diagnostic Criteria for SIAD

- Plasma osmolality <275 mOsmol/kg H_2O
- Urine osmolality >100 mOsmol/kg H_2O
- Clinical euvolemia
- Urinary sodium excretion >30 mmol/L with normal salt and water intake
- Exclusion of cortisol deficiency
- Normal kidney function
- Absence of diuretic use

Box 2. Etiologies of SIAD

- Malignancy: solid organ (particularly chest and nasopharyngeal), lymphoma
- Medications: antidepressants (eg, serotonin selective reuptake inhibitors), anticonvulsants, and antipsychotic agents
- Pulmonary disorders: infection, asthma, cystic fibrosis, respiratory failure
- Central nervous system disorders: infection, hemorrhage, thrombosis, trauma, tumor, hydrocephalus, autoimmune (multiple sclerosis/Guillain-Barre syndrome), multiple system atrophy, delirium tremens)
- Transient stimuli (secondary to nausea, pain, stress, prolonged endurance exercise, general anesthesia)
- Idiopathic
- Hereditary (eg, nephrogenic SIAD)

2009 to treat clinically significant hypervolemic or euvolemic hyponatremia.

Evidence supporting use of loop diuretics and salt tablets is limited. A recent randomized controlled trial comparing the effect of fluid restriction alone vs fluid restriction plus loop diuretics vs fluid restriction plus loop diuretics plus salt tablets did not show a significant additive effect of loop diuretics or salt tablets.[8]

SGLT-2 inhibitors are approved for use in diabetes and heart failure.[10,11] Because their mechanism of action leads to glycosuria and osmotic diuresis, they have also been investigated in euvolemic hyponatremia due to SIAD in hospitalized patients, but also in outpatients in whom 4 weeks of treatment with empagliflozin, 25 mg daily, increased sodium levels from a baseline of 131 mEq/L to 134 mEq/L (131 mmol/L to 134 mmol/L), corresponding to a serum sodium increase of 4.1 mEq/L (4.1 mmol/L), whereas no increase was seen with placebo.[12] Lastly, protein supplementation (90 g daily) increases plasma sodium by 3 mEq/L (3 mmol/L), while oral urea (30 g daily) increases plasma sodium by 2 mEq/L (2 mmol/L), thus pointing to a comparable effect of protein supplementation and urea.[13]

Clinical Case Vignettes

Case 1

A 47-year-old man is referred to the emergency department due to acute onset of headache, vomiting, and vertigo. He is otherwise healthy and takes no medications. In the first laboratory assessment, his sodium concentration is 112 mEq/L (SI: 112 mmol/L). His volume status is euvolemic.

Baseline laboratory test results:

Sodium = 112 mEq/L (136-145 mEq/L)
   (SI: 112 mmol/L [136-145 mmol/L])
Serum osmolality = 238 mOsm/kg (280-300 mOsm/kg)
   (SI: 238 mmol/kg [280-300 mmol/kg])
Hemoglobin = 14.2 g/dL (14.0-18.0 g/dL)
   (SI: 142 g/L [140-180 g/L])
Creatinine = 0.84 mg/dL (0.67-1.18 mg/dL)
   (SI: 74 µmol/L [59-104 µmol/L])
Urea = 1.7 mmol/L (3.2-7.3 mmol/L)

Glucose = 115.3 mg/dL (70.3-100.9 mg/dL)
   (SI: 6.4 mmol/L [3.9-5.6 mmol/L])
Urine osmolality = 298 mOsm/kg (200-1200 mOsm/kg)
   (SI: 298 mmol/kg [200-1200 mmol/kg])
Urinary sodium = 94 mmol/L (60-140 mmol/L)

Which of the following laboratory parameters is the most important to measure now?

A. TSH

B. Cortisol

C. Uric acid

D. Fractional excretion of urea

E. B-type natriuretic peptide

Answer: B) Cortisol

Case 1, Continued

Which of the following is the best treatment for this patient?

A. Urea, 15 g daily

B. Fluid restriction, <1 L per day

C. Vaptan, 7.5 mg daily

D. 3% saline, 100 mL bolus

E. Hydrocortisone, 100 mg intravenously

Answer: D) 3% saline, 100 mL bolus, and/or E) Hydrocortisone, 100 mg intravenously

This patient has acute onset of severe symptoms of hyponatremia. The laboratory parameters are consistent with SIAD. However, SIAD is a diagnosis of exclusion, and measurement of serum cortisol is important to exclude adrenal insufficiency. In one study, adrenal insufficiency was the underlying cause in 3.8% patients with euvolemic hyponatremia who were initially thought to have SIAD. A diagnostic cortisol cutoff value greater than 10.9 µg/dL (SI: >300 nmol/L) is recommended to exclude adrenal insufficiency.[14] There is only limited evidence that hypothyroidism contributes significantly to hyponatremia. Hyponatremia occurring in the setting of profound hypothyroidism may be a consequence of myxedema, cardiac failure, and systemic hypotension. An important study compared the serum sodium concentration of 999 patients with newly diagnosed hypothyroidism with that of 4875 euthyroid control participants. While there was a correlation, it amounted to a tiny 0.14 mEq/L (0.14 mmol/L) decrease in sodium levels for every 10 mIU/L rise in TSH, supporting the conclusion that there was no clinically relevant association between hypothyroidism and hyponatremia.[15]

This patient's serum cortisol value was 0.76 µg/dL (SI: 21 nmol/L) (reference range, 6.0-18.4 µg/dL [SI: 166-507 nmol/L]) and ACTH value was 7.8 pg/mL (SI: 1.7 pmol/L) (reference range, <60.5 pg/mL [SI: <13.3 pmol/L]), thus confirming the diagnosis of secondary adrenal insufficiency. Before cortisol levels were available from the lab, the patient was already transferred to the intensive care unit and treated with 3% saline infusion, which increased his sodium level from 112 mEq/L to 116 mEq/L (SI: 112 to 116 mmol/L) within the first 24 hours, thus significantly improving clinical symptoms. As soon as adrenal insufficiency was diagnosed, he received hydrocortisone (initially 150 mg daily). CT showed a pituitary macroadenoma (15 × 1 5 × 27 mm), and further laboratory assessment revealed secondary hypogonadism and secondary hypothyroidism in addition to secondary adrenal insufficiency. Treatment with levothyroxine and testosterone was started, and hydrocortisone was tapered as soon as his symptoms improved. Elective surgery was planned.

Case 2

A 32-year-old man is referred from a neurologist colleague. The patient has had epilepsy for several years and is treated with carbamazepine. While on this treatment, he developed chronic hyponatremia, with sodium values fluctuating between 123 and 127 mEq/L (SI: 123-127 mmol/L). Serum osmolality ranges between 250 to 260 mmol/kg, urine osmolality is 437 mmol/kg, and urinary sodium is 120 mEq/L (SI: 120 mmol/L). His cortisol concentration is 19.9 µg/dL (SI: 549 nmol/L), thus excluding adrenal insufficiency. Fluid restriction has been started, which increases his sodium

concentration to a maximum of 129 mEq/L (SI: 129 mmol/L). He poorly tolerates fluid restriction below 1.5 L per day.

Which of the following is the best next step in this patient's treatment?

A. No further treatment, as this hyponatremia is not relevant

B. Urea, 30 g daily

C. A vaptan, 7.5 mg daily

D. Salt tablets, 3 to 6 daily

E. Loop diuretics

Answer: B) Urea, 30 g daily or C) A vaptan, 7.5 mg daily

This patient has chronic hyponatremia due to SIAD. SIAD has multiple causes (*Box 2*), and one important cause is medication induced. Different medications can cause SIAD by stimulating AVP release (eg, antidepressant or antipsychotic agents), either by potentiating its action or by being a direct AVP analogue.[16] Thiazide diuretics are one of the most common causes of hyponatremia that can mimic SIAD. Anticonvulsant treatment in patients with epilepsy is another common cause of SIAD. Because of the association between hyponatremia and seizures, it is important to normalize sodium levels. Fluid restriction is the first-line treatment in SIAD. The efficacy of 1000-mL daily fluid restriction has been evaluated in a randomized trial in 46 patients, which showed a modest rise in serum sodium of 3 mEq/L (SI: 3 mmol/L) in fluid-restricted patients compared with 1 mEq/L (1 mmol/L) with no treatment. However, in this study, 39% of patients randomly assigned to fluid restriction did not respond to treatment.[17] Similarly, fluid restriction was unsuccessful in up to 50% of patients in larger observational trials and registries. Importantly, a high urine osmolality or high urine sodium level was shown to predict nonresponse to fluid restriction with high accuracy. In addition, fluid restriction is often poorly tolerated, as in this patient. Urea (Answer B) is a cheap alternative treatment option. It is a product of hepatic nitrogen metabolism that is renally excreted, exerting an osmotic effect and resulting in increased electrolyte-free water clearance. A recent systematic review, including 23 studies of 462 patients with SIAD treated with urea, showed that urea treatment increased sodium levels by a mean of 9.6 mEq/L (SI: 9.6 mmol/L) within a median treatment duration of 5 days. The mean increase in serum sodium after 24 hours was 4.9 mEq/L (4.9 mmol/L). Adverse events were few and mainly consisted of distaste or dysgeusia, and no instances of osmotic demyelination were reported.[18] The main limitations of urea are its limited availability and low palatability due to its bitter taste. Adherence can be improved by combining it with orange juice, citric acid, sucrose, and bicarbonate. Urea therapy increases the serum urea concentration and blood urea nitrogen, usually double baseline values, but this does not represent deterioration in kidney function or hypovolemia.[19] After failure of fluid restriction in this patient, urea was started at a dosage of 30 g daily, which increased sodium levels to 132 mEq/L (132 mmol/L). However, after a few days, the patient refused to continue treatment because the bitter taste of urea was causing nausea.

The patient's treatment was then transitioned to a vaptan, with a starting dosage of 7.5 mg daily, which was increased to 15 mg daily. The vaptan corrected the sodium level to 141 mEq/L (SI: 141 mmol/L). Vaptans are an efficient treatment option for chronic SIAD, but they are associated with risk for overcorrection and are expensive. While the SALT trials reported excessively rapid correction of hyponatremia in 1.7% of tolvaptan-treated patients, observational studies of tolvaptan have reported highly variable rates of overcorrection, ranging from 0% to 30%. Importantly, discontinuing fluid restriction when vaptans are started, initiating treatment in the hospital, and regularly monitoring sodium limits the risk for overcorrection. A lower initial dosage of tolvaptan, 7.5 mg daily, which has been associated with lower rates of overcorrection, should also be considered. Common adverse effects of tolvaptan include dry mouth, thirst, and

urinary frequency. Other concerns raised about tolvaptan include cost and risk of liver function derangement seen with sustained higher dosages for other indications (eg, autosomal dominant polycystic kidney disease). Alternative treatment options (*Figure*), which were not chosen for this patient, are SGLT-2 inhibitors (only off-label or in patients with concomitant diabetes type 2) and a high-protein diet. Evidence for loop diuretics (Answer E) and/or salt tablets (Answer D) is weak.

Figure. Treatment Options for SIAD

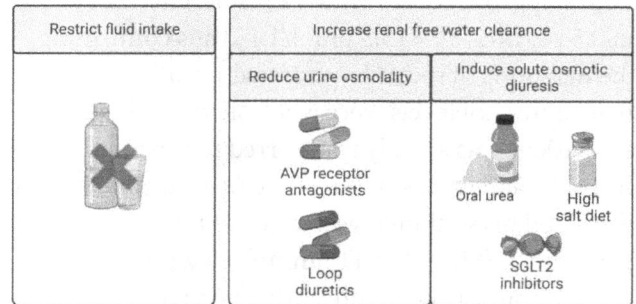

[Color—Print (Color Gallery page CG13) or web & ePub editions]

Case 3

A 47-year-old woman undergoes craniotomy to treat tuberculum sellae meningioma with visual field deficits. Her postoperative course is unremarkable, with sodium measured every day:

Date	Serum sodium
Day of surgery	140 mEq/L (SI: 140 mmol/L)
Day 1	141 mEq/L (SI: 141 mmol/L)
Day 3	138 mEq/L (SI: 138 mmol/L)
Day 4	139 mEq/L (SI: 139 mmol/L)
Day 4	**Discharge**
Day 8	123 mEq/L (SI: 123 mmol/L)
Day 9	128 mEq/L (SI: 128 mmol/L)
Day 11	140 mEq/L (SI: 140 mmol/L)

On postoperative day 8, she develops nausea, vomiting, and gait problems and is brought to the emergency department.

Laboratory test results:

Serum sodium = 123 mEq/L (SI: 123 mmol/L)
Serum osmolality = 258 mOsm/kg (SI: 258 mmol/kg)
Urine osmolality = 713 mOsm/kg (SI: 713 mmol/kg)
Urinary sodium = 224 mmol/L
Cortisol, normal

She is treated with 3% NaCl bolus therapy (total of 2 boluses), which increases her sodium concentration to 128 mEq/L (128 mmol/L) within 24 hours, followed by fluid restriction and normalization of her sodium concentration to 140 mEq/L (140 mmol/L). She is discharged after 3 days of hospitalization, on no treatment.

Which of the following is the best way to reduce the incidence of postoperative SIAD in patients who have undergone neurosurgery?

A. Hospitalization until the 10th postoperative day

B. Fluid restriction from hospital discharge until day 10

C. Vaptan, 7.5 mg daily, in all patients

D. No specific recommendation, as SIAD postoperatively is very rare

E. Informing patients about possible symptoms of hyponatremia and instructing to drink to thirst

Answer: B) Fluid restriction from hospital discharge until day 10 and E) Informing patients about possible symptoms of hyponatremia and instructing to drink to thirst

This patient has SIAD after pituitary surgery. In a recent meta-analysis,[20] delayed symptomatic hyponatremia was observed in 5.6% of patients who had undergone neurosurgery. Milder forms of postoperative SIAD can be found in up to 30% of patients. Hyponatremia typically develops between postsurgical days 4 and 14, peaking around day 7. While hyponatremia is generally mild and self-limiting, severe cases can arise, with symptomatic hyponatremia being one of the leading causes of hospital readmission after pituitary surgery. As most patients are discharged before SIAD develops, they must be educated to recognize symptoms of hyponatremia (eg, confusion, headaches, or nausea) and seek prompt medical attention if these symptoms develop. In recent years, preventive strategies have focused on implementing fluid-restriction protocols to mitigate the risk. Fluid restriction volumes and durations vary across studies, typically ranging from 1000 to 2500 mL/day for 1 to 2 weeks postoperatively. Matsuyama et al reported a reduction in SIAD incidence from 38% to 14% with fluid restriction of 1800 mL/day,[21] while another study observed a decrease in hospital readmissions from 8% to 2% using a 1500 mL/day restriction.[22] In addition, a study from 2021 demonstrated that a 7-day, 1000 mL/day fluid restriction reduced hyponatremia from 5% to 1%.[23] A meta-analysis including 1382 patients revealed a significant reduction in hyponatremia risk, with an odds ratio of 5.0 (95% CI, 2.2-11.7), favoring fluid restriction.[24] Despite these findings, no prospective randomized trials have established the optimal protocol.

Key Learning Points

- Adrenal insufficiency must be excluded before SIAD is diagnosed.

- Acute, severe symptoms of hyponatremia are a medical emergency due to cerebral edema, and immediate treatment is needed, usually with hypertonic saline and/or with hydrocortisone in case of adrenal insufficiency. One should be careful to avoid overcorrection!

- There are several treatment options of chronic SIAD. Fluid restriction is the first-line treatment, but it has a high rate of nonresponse. Main second-line treatment options are urea or vaptans.

- SIAD after pituitary surgery is often delayed. It is important to instruct patients about symptoms of hyponatremia and to drink to thirst. Preventive fluid restriction has been shown to reduce postoperative hyponatremia.

References

1. Upadhyay A, Jaber BL, Madias NE. Incidence and prevalence of hyponatremia. *Am J Med.* 2006;119(7 Suppl 1):S30-S35. PMID: 16843082

2. Corona G, Giulianai C, Parenti G, et al. Moderate hyponatremia is associated with increased risk of mortality: evidence from a meta-analysis. *PLoS One.* 2013;8(12):e80451. PMID: 24367479

3. Upala S, Sanguankeo A. Association between hyponatremia, osteoporosis, and fracture: a systematic review and meta-analysis. *J Clin Endocrinol Metab.* 2016;101(4):1880-1886. PMID: 26913635

4. Renneboog B, Musch W, Vandemergel X, Manto MU, Decaux G. Mild chronic hyponatremia is associated with falls, unsteadiness, and attention deficits. *Am J Med.* 2006;119(1):71.e71-e78. PMID: 16431193

5. Spasovski G, Vanholder R, Allolio B, et al. Clinical practice guideline on diagnosis and treatment of hyponatraemia. *Eur J Endocrinol.* 2014;170(3):G1-47. PMID: 24569125

6. Bartter FC, Schwartz WB. The syndrome of inappropriate secretion of antidiuretic hormone. *Am J Med.* 1967;42(5):790-806. PMID: 5337379

7. Verbalis JG, Goldsmith SR, Greenberg A, et al. Diagnosis, evaluation, and treatment of hyponatremia: expert panel recommendations. *Am J Med.* 2013;126(10 Suppl 1):S1-S42. PMID: 24074529

8. Krisanapan P, Vongsanim S, Pin-On P, Ruengorn C, Noppakun K. Efficacy of furosemide, oral sodium chloride, and fluid restriction for treatment of syndrome of inappropriate antidiuresis (SIAD): an open-label randomized controlled study (The EFFUSE-FLUID Trial). *Am J Kidney Dis.* 2020;76(2):203-212. PMID: 32199708

9. Schrier RW, Gross P, Gheorghiade M, et al. Tolvaptan, a selective oral vasopressin V2-receptor antagonist, for hyponatremia. *N Engl J Med.* 2006;355(20):2099-2112. PMID: 17105757

10. Zinman B, Wanner C. Lachin JM, et al. Empagliflozin, cardiovascular outcomes, and mortality in type 2 diabetes. *N Engl J Med.* 2015;373(22):2117-2128. PMID: 26378978

11. Wanner C, Inzucchi SE, Lachin JM, et al. Empagliflozin and progression of kidney disease in type 2 diabetes. *N Engl J Med.* 2016;375(4):323-334. PMID: 27299675

12. Refardt J, Imber C, Nobbenhuis R, et al. Treatment effect of the SGLT2 inhibitor empagliflozin on chronic dyndrome of inappropriate antidiuresis: results of a randomized, double-blind, placebo-controlled, crossover trial. *J Am Soc Nephrol.* 2023;34(2):322-332. PMID: 36396331

13. Monnerat S, Atila C, Baur F, et al. Effect of protein supplementation on plasma sodium levels in the syndrome of inappropriate antidiuresis: a monocentric, open-label, proof-of-concept study-the TREASURE study. *Eur J Endocrinol.* 2023;189(2):252-261. PMID: 37540987

14. Cuesta M, Garrahy A, Slattery D, et al. The contribution of undiagnosed adrenal insufficiency to euvolaemic hyponatraemia: results of a large prospective single-centre study. *Clin Endocrinol (Oxf).* 2016;85(6):836-844. PMID: 27271953

15. Warner MH, Holding S, Kilpatrick ES. The effect of newly diagnosed hypothyroidism on serum sodium concentrations: a retrospective study. *Clin Endocrinol (Oxf).* 2006;64(5):598-599. PMID: 16649984

16. Warren AM, Grossmann M, Christ-Crain M, Russell N. Syndrome of inappropriate antidiuresis: from pathophysiology to management. *Endocr Rev.* 2023;44(5):819-861. PMID: 36974717

17. Garrahy A, Galloway I, Hannon AM, et al. Fluid restriction therapy for chronic SIAD; results of a prospective randomized controlled trial. *J Clin Endocrinol Metab.* 2020;105(12):dgaa619. PMID: 32879954

18. Wendt R, Fenves AZ, Geisler BP. Use of urea for the syndrome of inappropriate secretion of antidiuretic hormone: a systematic review. *JAMA Netw Open.* 2023;6(10):e2340313. PMID: 37902751

19. Rondon-Berrios, H. et al. Urea for the Treatment of Hyponatremia. *Clin J Am Soc Nephrol.* 2018;13(11):1627-1632. PMID: 30181129

20. Yu S, Taghvaei M, Reyes M, et al. Delayed symptomatic hyponatremia in transsphenoidal surgery: systematic review and meta-analysis of its incidence and prevention with water restriction. *Clin Neurol Neurosurg.* 2022;214:107166. PMID: 35158166

21. Matsuyama J, Ikeda H, Sato S, Yamamoto K, Ohashi G, Watanabe K. Early water intake restriction to prevent inappropriate antidiuretic hormone secretion following transsphenoidal surgery: low BMI predicts postoperative SIADH. *Eur J Endocrinol.* 2014;171(6):711-716. PMID: 25227132

22. Deaver KE, Catel CP, Lillehei KO, Wierman ME, Kerr JM. Strategies to reduce readmissions for hyponatremia after transsphenoidal surgery for pituitary adenomas. *Endocrine.* 2018;62(2):333-339. PMID: 29961198

23. Snyder MH, Asuzu DT, Shaver DE, Vance ML, Jane JA. Routine postoperative fluid restriction to prevent syndrome of inappropriate antidiuretic hormone secretion after transsphenoidal resection of pituitary adenoma. *J Neurosurg.* 2021;136(2):405-412. PMID: 34330096

24. Castle-Kirszbaum M, Goldschlager T, Shi MDY, Kam J, Fuller PJ. Postoperative fluid restriction to prevent hyponatremia after transsphenoidal pituitary surgery: an updated meta-analysis and critique. *J Clin Neurosci.* 2022;106:180-184. PMID: 36369079

Stalk Lesions of the Pituitary Gland

Dana Erickson, MD. Division of Endocrinology, Metabolism, and Nutrition, Mayo College of Medicine, Rochester, MN; Email: erickson.dana@mayo.edu

Educational Objectives

After reviewing this chapter, learners should be able to:

- Identify the spectrum of etiologies contributing to imaging findings of pituitary stalk lesions (PSLs).

- Facilitate a logical and comprehensive diagnostic workup of etiologies and hormonal abnormalities in the setting of a PSL and recognize possible treatment pitfalls.

- Generate an effective management strategy, including conservative or necessary neurosurgical intervention.

Significance of the Clinical Problem

PSLs present a conundrum of challenges for clinicians from both diagnostic and therapeutic standpoints. They are sometimes discovered incidentally because advanced imaging techniques, such as MRI, are frequently used in clinical practice for the evaluation of chronic headaches or other issues. PSLs may also be identified during the evaluation of new-onset symptoms reflecting endocrinopathies or mass effect via optic chiasmal compression. The spectrum of clinical presentation varies by the extent of pituitary gland involvement, whether it is purely stalk or combination with extensive involvement of the hypothalamus and or other pituitary gland areas. Clinical context and the consideration of possible known or unknown systemic disorders are important.

Practice Gaps

- PSLs have many etiologies, and rare causes are often overlooked.

- The initial working diagnosis in patients with PSLs may be incorrect, and awareness of this phenomenon is important in clinical practice.

- Available data in the literature suggest that a significant proportion of patients with PSLs do not undergo comprehensive pituitary hormonal assessment in clinical practice (full assessment is reported in 48%-91%).[1]

- The rationale for tissue biopsy for PSL should be assessed on a case-by-case basis because it has the potential to cause new-onset pituitary hormonal deficiencies.

- There is no consensus on the recommended intervals for surveillance MRI.

Discussion

The prevalence of PSLs is difficult to estimate, but they are reported to be present in 0.1% to 0.2% of head MRI studies. In a retrospective study from Mayo Clinic (1987-2006) of 150,000 MRI studies, authors reviewed 2700 reports, and 152 patients harbored PSLs.[2] A study from Shanghai, China, identified 325 PSLs among 143,000 MRI studies (2012-2018).[1] The mean age of adults at presentation is 44 years, but large studies from Asia report an average of 30.5 years with a slight female predominance.[3] Interestingly, in males, there are 2 age peaks: age 6 to 18 years and 42 to 48 years.

The mode of incidental discovery varies, but up to 30% of PSLs are reported to be diagnosed incidentally.[1] Upon detailed further endocrine hormonal evaluation, 25% of patients with incidentally discovered PSLs have endocrine dysfunction. This underscores the necessity of a detailed workup and highlights the delicate location of the pituitary stalk and its importance from an anatomical and physiological standpoint. When symptoms are present, they can include headache (22%), visual field deficiencies (11%-25%), lethargy (14%), seizures or altered mental state (13%), poor appetite (8.3%), weight loss (14%), dizziness (11%), and others.[4]

Documentation of hypopituitarism varies from cohort to cohort of patients with PSLs. The prevalence of arginine vasopressin (AVP) deficiency ranges from 28% of a Mayo Clinic cohort to 69% in cohort from China[3] to 72% in a recent meta-analysis by Kim et al.[4] Anterior pituitary dysfunction is common when evaluated: 32% patients have a deficit in at least 1 hormonal axis and 21% of patients have a deficiency in 2 hormonal axes. Secondary hypogonadism can be present in up to 29% cases, secondary adrenal insufficiency in 15% to 25% of cases, and secondary hypothyroidism in 6.8% to 21% of cases. GH deficiency has not been evaluated in detail in many studies in adults with PSLs. Hyperprolactinemia occurs in 30% to 40% of patients. When AVP deficiency is documented, up to 94% of patients have additional anterior pituitary insufficiency, thus underscoring the necessity of testing.[1] Importantly, because patients with PSL are not always evaluated by an endocrinologist, hormonal evaluation might not be comprehensive (eg, in the Mayo cohort, 20% of patients lacked any hormonal evaluation).

In the setting of PSL, the frequency of hypopituitarism is associated with the extent of the lesion: 30% in pure stalk lesions, 73% in hypothalamic extension, 50% in sellar extension, and 100% when all sites are involved.[2] In a cohort from Shanghai, the degree of stalk thickening was associated with a higher incidence of hormone deficiencies (eg, for every 1 mm increase of pituitary stalk thickness in the group of patients with AVP deficiency, there was a 2.28-fold increase in the risk of anterior pituitary deficits), and stalk thickening greater than 4.5 mm was associated with the presence of AVP deficiency.[1]

The possible etiologies of PSL typically fall into 3 broad categories: (1) inflammatory/infiltrative processes; (2) neoplastic processes; and (3) congenital conditions (*Table 1*). In smaller cases

Table 1. Etiology of PSL Reported in Large Studies

Author	Year	Total, No.	Neoplastic, No.	Inflammatory*, No.	Congenital, No.	Unknown, No.
Hamilton et al	2007	44	16	19	9	Not included
Turcu et al	2013	152	49	30	13	60
Catford et al	2016	75	19	51	3	2
Sbardella et al	2016	26	3	8	4	11
Lee et al	2017	158	130**	28**		
Donec et al	2018	53	9	9	25	10
Zhou et al	2019	230	45	35	15	135
Ling et al	2019	325	56	14	Unknown	255
Devuyst et al	2020	38	11	27	0	0
Mean			30%	20%	6%	42%

Modified from Hana V et al. Neuroendocrinology, 2020; 110(9-10): 809-821. © S. Karger AG, Basel.

* Some authors include Langerhans cell histiocytosis in neoplastic group.

** Author provided diagnosis in some cases without tissue biopsy but based on follow-up.

series, neoplastic causes account for 29% of cases, while in larger series, 56% are reported to have a neoplastic etiology. The classification of Langerhans histiocytosis as a neoplastic process in some studies and as an inflammatory process in others obscures the data. A recent meta-analysis by Kim et al of 1368 patients confirmed the heterogeneity of this phenomenon with a pooled proportion of neoplasm of 45% (germ-cell tumors [14%], Langerhans histiocytosis [10%], metastasis [4.6%]).[4]

In most cohorts, only a proportion of patients undergo tissue biopsy of the stalk lesion (21%-46%). A working diagnosis is achieved when a systemic condition is established in a different locality, the patient is treated with empiric glucocorticoids for a presumed inflammatory etiology and lesion responds, or there is spontaneous regression of the lesion.[1-3]

Diagnostic clues have been explored by various investigators in several publications. While certain imaging features are more obvious and helpful to elucidate a particular disease process, others can be incredibly challenging. The average size of a normal pituitary stalk (transverse diameter) as seen on pituitary MRI is 2.4 to 3.25 mm at the level of the optic chiasm and 1.91 mm at the insertion on gland.[5] The most common cut off for abnormal size in a meta-analysis was greater than 3 mm.[4] The posterior pituitary is visible in 95% of the healthy population.

Turcu et al analyzed the various shapes of pituitary lesions on MRI (*Figure 1*), and the strongest association following gadolinium enhancement was seen in congenital lesions (round, presence of ectopic neurohypophysis), while neurosarcoidosis had a uniformly thickened stalk and xanthoma disseminatum had a pyramidal shape. Among neoplastic lesions, lymphomas had V-shaped pattern of PSL, while metastatic solid cancers had a V-shaped or round characteristic; however, there was overlap across the various etiologies. An interesting recent study used a model of recursive partitioning logistic regression analysis in 158 patients with PSL (and further validation in 63 patients) and described: (1) lack of extrasellar involvement; (2) stalk thickness less than 5.3 mm; and (3) presence of AVP deficiency as suggestive of nonneoplastic etiology (AUC 0.813).[6] Cystic changes, high T1 signal, presence of a diffusely thickened stalk, and gland involvement were of less discriminatory value. In contrast, in a smaller cohort,[7] the presence of

Figure 1. Illustration of Imaging Phenotypes of PSLs on MRI

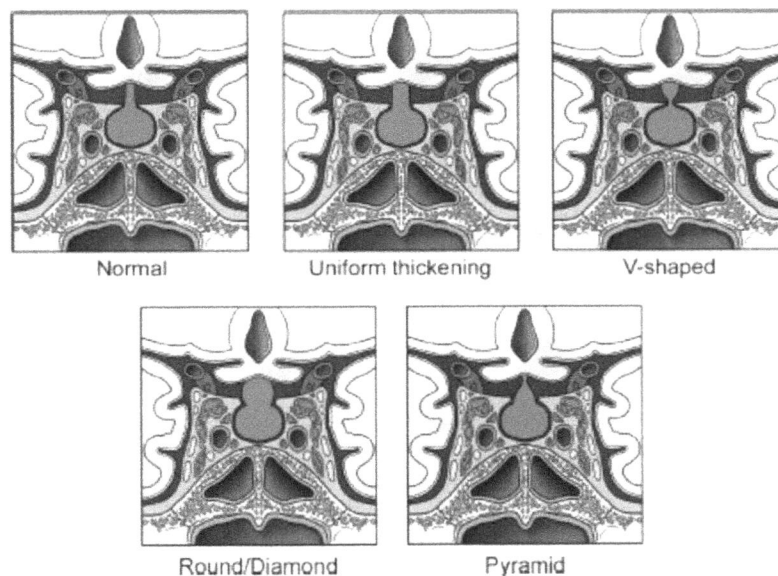

Normal Uniform thickening V-shaped

Round/Diamond Pyramid

Reprinted with permission from Turcu AF et al. *J Clin Endocrinol Metab*, 2013; 98(5): 1812–1818. © 2013 by The Endocrine Society.

AVP deficiency was more common in neoplastic etiologies along with texture heterogeneity on MRI. Ling et al developed a classifier model that considered important indicators differentiating neoplastic from inflammatory causes with variables, including sex, neutrophilic granulocytes percentage, serum sodium concentration, presence of AVP deficiency, and pituitary stalk, with patterns of thickening of stalk.[1] A study from Belgium and France suggested that higher degree of prolactin elevation might be associated with a neoplastic process (1.25 × upper normal limit; sensitivity, 95%; specificity, 67%).[8] Importantly, young patients tend to have intracranial germ-cell tumors and histiocytosis as leading causes of this clinical scenario.

Timing and necessity of tissue biopsy/surgical resection are challenging clinical dilemmas, and input from a multidisciplinary tumor board is the best approach for individual patients. In smaller lesions without severe endocrinopathies, tissue biopsy/surgical resection should be pursued only if it would change the course of treatment. For example, in a case series from Mayo Clinic, biopsy was necessary in 24% of patients, while it was performed in 40% to 65% of patients in other series.[6,9] The safety of this procedure has been recently analyzed in an elegant study by Kang et al[10] in 39 patients who underwent an endoscopic endonasal approach after multidisciplinary team recommendation (the most common pathological diagnosis was germinoma [46%]). In patients without preoperative hypopituitarism, 30% developed new AVP deficiency. Among those with at least 1 hormonal deficiency at baseline, 55% developed a new hormone deficiency. Finally, among 22 patients without preexisting AVP deficiency, new deficit of antidiuretic hormone developed in 9 (46%). While the diagnostic yield in this study was 100%, other series reported 10% nondiagnostic biopsies. Cerebrospinal fluid leak and infection can occur.[11]

As outlined in *Table 2*, the etiology of PSL is broad. Suggested workup and management are described in *Figure 2* (*following page*).[8] Constitutional symptoms (night sweats) should raise the possibility of hematologic malignancy or an infectious process. Concomitant autoimmune diseases or recent pregnancy point toward autoimmune hypophysitis. Hepatosplenomegaly and enlargement of lymph nodes can be seen in Langerhans histiocytosis or Erdheim-Chester disease. IgG4 disease serum titers should be measured in the setting of autoimmune pancreatitis and chronic sinusitis. A few tips include erythema nodosum skin lesions in sarcoidosis and concomitant pineal lesions in cases of germinoma. Serum α-fetoprotein and hCG are positive in a minority of patients harboring a germinoma, but hCG might be positive in two-thirds of such patients when analyzed in cerebrospinal fluid.[8] FDG-PET is important when evaluating infiltrative disorders and malignancies.

Treatment of PSLs can be surgical (craniopharyngioma, adenoma) or systemic (neoplasm, histiocytosis, neurosarcoidosis).

Table 2. Detailed Etiologies of PSL

Neoplastic	Inflammatory	Congenital
Germinoma	Hypophysitis (all types)	Ectopic neurohypophysis
Craniopharyngioma	Langerhans histiocytosis	Rathke cleft cyst
Metastases (breast, lung, kidney, melanoma, prostate, leukemia)	Neurosarcoidosis	Pituitary stalk interruption syndrome
Astrocytoma, glioblastoma	Erdheim- Chester disease	Vascular lesion
Primary CNS lymphoma	Tuberculosis	Duplication of stalk
Meningioma	Behcet disease	
Pituitary neuroendocrine tumor	Abscess	
Pituicytoma	Whipple disease, lupus	
	Granulomatosis with polyangiitis	

Autoimmune hypophysitis can be observed or treated with systemic glucocorticoids when mass effect or AVP deficiency effect is present. Other immunomodulating agents may be indicated if further progression occurs. Germinoma can be treated effectively with radiotherapy or chemoradiation.

The natural history of stalk lesions is underreported. Therefore, MRI at a short interval of 3 to 6 months is recommended, with further longitudinal follow-up depending on initial changes.

Of 106 patients with clinically indeterminate PSL pooled from 4 studies with a median follow-up of 3 to 7.6 years, 18.5% demonstrated progression (mean time to progression, 0.7-1.8 years), while 61% showed spontaneous regression of PSL.[4]

Hormonal function must be assessed longitudinally. Among patients with Langerhans cell histiocytosis, most develop at least 1 new hormonal dysfunction over 11 years of follow-up. However, normalization, especially of anterior pituitary function, has been reported in patients with lymphocytic hypophysitis.[12]

Clinical Case Vignettes

Case 1

Three months after delivering a healthy baby, a 30-year-old woman presents with symptoms of increased thirst, craving for water, fluid intake of 4 L per day, and frequent urination every 40 to 60 minutes (including at night). Menstrual cycles were initially normal until an intrauterine progesterone-containing device was inserted. She chose to nurse for 1 month.

There has been no unusual weight loss or weight gain. She has a normal appetite and blood pressure. There is no cold intolerance or skin dryness. She notes that she has frequent headaches. There is no history of recent head trauma. Mucous membranes and skin turgor are normal.

Initial laboratory evaluation reveals a normal serum sodium concentration. After a 6-hour fast, the following laboratory test results are documented:

Serum sodium = 146 mEq/L (SI: 146 mmol/L)
Serum osmolality = 315 mOsm/kg (SI: 315 mmol/kg)
Urine osmolality = 106 mOsm/kg (SI: 106 mmol/kg)
Arginine vasopressin = <0.5 pg/mL
Urine output = 150 cc/h

Figure 2. Suggested Stepwise Workup of PSLs or Pituitary Stalk Tumors

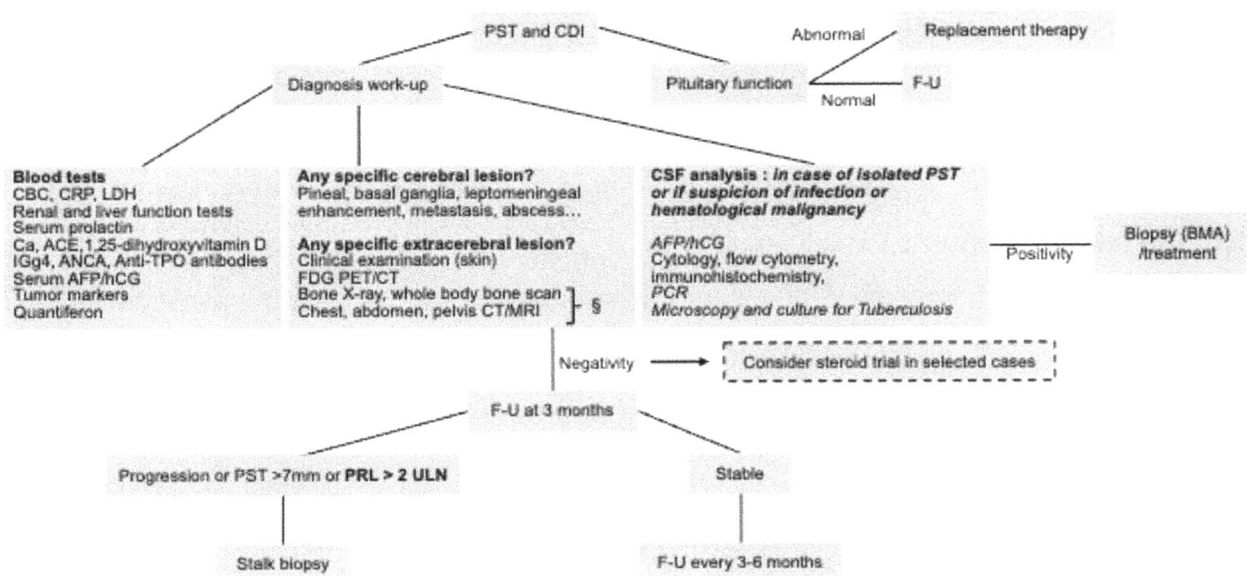

Modified from Devuyst F et al. *Eur J Endocrinol*, 2020; 181(3): 95-105. © European Society of Endocrinology.

Urine osmolality increases more than 100% following DDAVP administration.

Anterior pituitary function testing:

Thyroid function tests, normal
Cortisol (8 AM) = 13 µg/dL (SI: 358.6 nmol/L)
DHEA-S = 100 µg/dL (SI: 2.71 µmol/L)
ACTH = 26 pg/mL (SI: 5.72 pmol/L)
IGF-1 = 103 ng/mL (SI: 13.5 nmol/L)
Estradiol = 93 pg/mL (SI: 341.4 pmol/L)
Prolactin, normal

The initial diagnosis is isolated central AVP deficiency.

Findings on MRI of the pituitary gland (*Figure 3*) are consistent with stalk thickening of a globular shape, but the pituitary gland is not diffusely enlarged.

Figure 3.

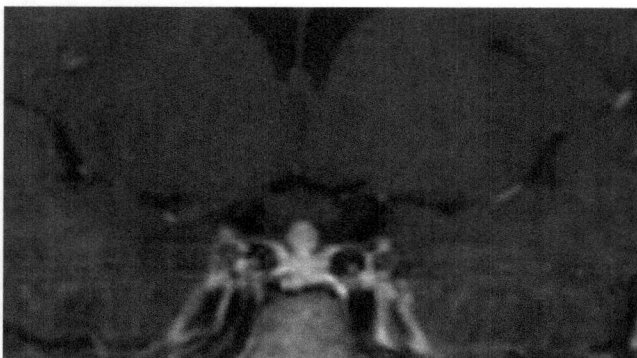

There is no evidence of other autoimmune disorders. Measurements of α-fetoprotein, hCG, and ACE are normal. Myeloperoxidase antibodies and proteinase 3 antibodies are negative. Findings on bone scan are negative.

Which of the following is the best next step?

A. Start replacement therapy with DDAVP only

B. Start replacement therapy with DDAVP and initiate a course of prednisone

C. Initiate rituximab

D. Perform biopsy

Answer: B) Start replacement therapy with DDAVP and initiate a course of prednisone

Central AVP deficiency was diagnosed, and DDAVP, 0.1 tablet at night, was initiated and uptitrated as needed to 3 tablets daily. A presumed diagnosis of autoimmune hypophysitis was established. A trial of prednisone, 40 mg over 3 weeks downtitrating, was also initiated, but she had no changes in her headache or degree of polyuria. She requested to discontinue prednisone given the adverse effects she was experiencing. Findings on follow-up MRI 4 months later were unchanged. One year later, there was a slight decrease in stalk thickening, and 2 years later, a further decrease was observed (*Figure 4*). AVP deficiency persisted. There were no new hormonal deficiencies.

Figure 4.

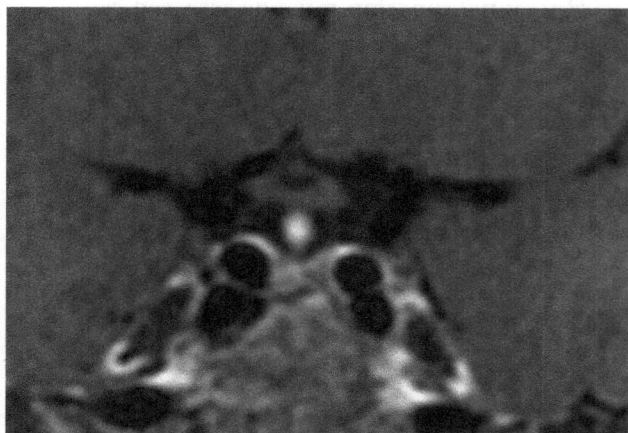

In this clinical situation, extensive workup for various causes of PSL was performed without a definitive secondary cause identified. Given the clinical scenario of postpartum presentation, her young age, and lack of other systemic involvement, the presumed diagnosis was lymphocytic hypophysitis. Unfortunately, we do not have clinically available pituitary antibodies, some studies reported limitations.[13] In the setting of significant headaches and a small prospective study suggestive of improvement in possible endocrinopathies and metanalysis of mostly retrospective data, a trial of glucocorticoids was initiated, but it was not well tolerated because of adverse effects.[12,14]

Critical follow-up imaging showed improvement of the degree of PSL, which indirectly confirmed the diagnosis of autoimmune or inflammatory origin.

Given the clinical stability of the patient, improvement in headaches, lack of PSL progression, and absence of other pituitary hormonal deficits, biopsy of this lesion was not justified as it could be associated with complications. Rituximab is second-line treatment in refractory cases. Although DDAVP would help with symptoms of polyuria, it would not help with symptoms of headaches from mass effect, although other medications for pain control could be considered.

Case 2

A 22-year-old man with a history of obstructive sleep apnea presents with concerns decreased libido, fatigue, poor appetite, nausea, vomiting, and weight loss (30 lb [13.6 kg] over the last 4 months). He has no headaches. Frequency of urination is increased (2 to 3 times per night). He notes increased thirst and fluid intake.

On physical examination, his BMI is 24 kg/m². Vital signs are normal, and visual fields are normal to confrontation. Physical findings are normal, including the skin and genitalia.

Laboratory test results:

LH = <0.3 mIU/mL (SI: <0.3 IU/L)
Testosterone = <7 ng/dL (SI: 0.24 nmol/L)
Prolactin = 89 ng/dL (SI: 3.9 nmol/L)
Cortisol (8 AM) = 9.2 µg/dL (SI: 253.8 nmol/L)
ACTH = 44 pg/mL (SI: 9.7 pmol/L)
Free T$_4$ = 0.8 ng/dL (SI: 10.30 pmol/L)
TSH = 2.9 mIU/L
IGF-1 = 75 ng/mL (SI: 9.8 nmol/L)
DHEA-S = 95 µg/dL (SI: 2.57 µmol/L)

Laboratory test results after 8 hours of fasting:

Urine osmolality = 414 mOsm/kg (SI: 414 mmol/kg)
Serum sodium = 151 mEq/L (SI: 151 mmol/L)
Serum osmolality = 302 mOsm/kg (SI: 302 mmol/kg)

Results of formal visual field testing are normal. Panhypopituitarism is diagnosed, including partial AVP deficiency. Treatment with hormone replacement therapy is initiated: hydrocortisone, 10 mg in the morning; levothyroxine, 100 mcg daily; testosterone gel; and DDAVP, 0.1 mg as needed at night. The patient reports feeling much better on this regimen.

MRI of the sella shows an enlarged gland with significant stalk thickening (*Figure 5*). Visual fields are normal.

Figure 5.

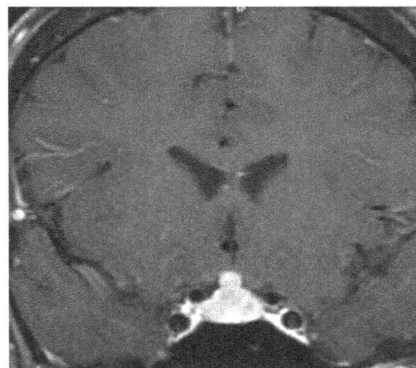

Additional laboratory test results:

Serum α-fetoprotein, normal
β-hCG, normal
C-reactive protein, normal
TPO antibodies, negative
ACE = 28 U/L (normal)
Calcium, normal
QuantiFERON for tuberculosis, negative
Syphilis, negative
Antineutrophil cytoplasmic antibodies, negative
Antinuclear antibodies, negative
Flow cytometry, negative for lymphoma
IgG4 = 78 mg/dL (normal)
Cytokine profile, negative

Cerebrospinal fluid analysis is negative for hCG and α-fetoprotein. There is a mild protein increase and nucleated cells.

No abnormal findings are identified on bone scan or whole-body PET. Biopsy via endoscopic endonasal approach is nondiagnostic. Three weeks later, a repeat biopsy documented the following pathology results: focal posterior pituitary tissue and anterior pituitary shows robust chronic inflammation, including multinucleated giant cells most consistent with granulomatous hypophysitis.

There is no evidence of lymphoma or other malignancies. GMS and AFB stains are negative.

Treatment is initiated with prednisone, 60 mg daily, with a slow taper. Three months later, there is slight improvement on imaging .The plan is to continue prednisone at the dosage of 15 to 20 mg daily for 12 months. Six months later, there is evidence of progression while on the lower dosage of prednisone, 15 mg daily (*Figure 6*).

Figure 6.

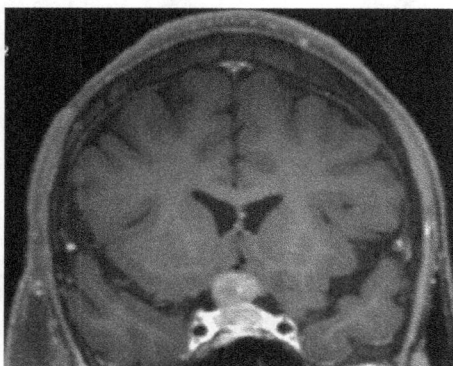

There are no clear-cut vision problems. The prednisone dosage is increased to 30 mg daily. Nine months after the initial biopsies, there is further progression of visual concerns (documented on visual field testing) (*Figure 7*).

Figure 7.

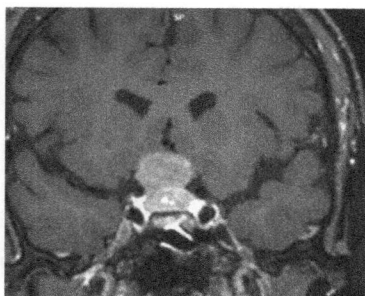

Which of the following should be done next?

A. Initiate very high-dosage methyprednisolone

B. Start other immunomodulators

C. Repeat biopsy

D. Administer radiation therapy

Answer: C) Repeat biopsy

The patient was started on high-dosage prednisone, 1000 mg for 5 days, and then 40 mg daily thereafter, and infliximab, 500 mg intravenously monthly. There was continued progression and new visual field defects. Twelve months since the previous biopsies, the patient underwent subtotal resection via an endoscopic endonasal approach (high-grade cerebrospinal fluid leak, repaired). Pathology documented a germ-cell tumor with T- and B-cell infiltrate in the background. Proton-beam radiation, 2340 cGY in 25 fractions, was administered to the area of lesion. Additional radiation was administered to the spine, 1620 GY in 9 fractions.

If a patient does not respond to standard therapies based on initial pathology, sampling error must be considered and eventually the biopsy should be repeated to confirm the correct tissue diagnosis.[15] Clinicians must recognize when the working diagnosis might be incorrect despite detailed investigation, including tissue biopsy. For this young man, germinoma should have been very high on the differential diagnosis list. Approximately 2.9% to 4.2% of intracranial germinomas could be masked by unspecific pathological findings of lymphocyte infiltration, fibrous tissue, and even granulomatous reaction, which are thought to reflect the host immune response to the neoplasm.[15] Thus, close follow-up is warranted when unspecified pathology is seen, and a second biopsy might be indicated, as highlighted in this case.

Key Learning Points

- PSLs can be discovered incidentally or after evaluation of new-onset symptoms reflective of endocrinopathies and/or local mass effect.

- Detailed hormonal workup of anterior and posterior pituitary function is necessary even for incidental lesions. AVP deficiency is reported to be present in 28% to 72% of patients with PSLs.

- Etiologies of PSLs include inflammatory/infiltrative processes, neoplastic processes, or congenital causes.

- Biopsy of PSLs should only be performed if extensive noninvasive testing does not reveal an etiology. Risks and benefits of this procedure must be weighed carefully.

- Treatment of PSLs includes hormonal replacement in the setting of hypopituitarism. Other systemic therapies are indicated depending on the etiology: immunomodulating agents for severe inflammatory processes, surgical decompression and/or radiation therapy, and chemotherapy for neoplastic processes. Observation might be an option for patients with certain nonneoplastic diagnoses (eg, congenital condition, autoimmune hypophysitis).

- PSLs are best managed by a multidisciplinary team.

References

1. Ling SY, Zhao ZY, Tao B, et al. Pituitary stalk thickening in a large cohort: toward more accurate predictors of pituitary dysfunction and etiology. *Endocr Pract.* 2019;25(6):534-544. PMID: 30865546

2. Turcu AF, Erickson BJ, Lin E, et al. Pituitary stalk lesions: the Mayo Clinic experience. *J Clin Endocrinol Metab.* 2013;98(5):1812-1818. PMID: 23533231

3. Zhou X, Zhu H, Yao Y, et al. Etiological spectrum and pattern of change in pituitary stalk thickening: experience in 321 patients. *J Clin Endocrinol Metab.* 2019;104(8):3419-3427. PMID: 30892632

4. Kim DY, Kim PH, Jung AY, et al. Neoplastic etiology and natural course of pituitary stalk thickening. J Clin Endocrinol Metab. 2021;107(2):563-574. PMID: 34614160

5. Hana V, Salenave S, Chanson P. Pituitary stalk enlargement in adults. *Neuroendocrinology.* 2020;110(9-10):809-821. PMID: 32074610

6. Lee JY, Park JE, Shim WH, et al. Joint approach based on clinical and imaging features to distinguish non-neoplastic from neoplastic pituitary stalk lesions. PLoS One. 2017;12(11):e0187989. PMID: 29140989

7. Sbardella E, Joseph RN, Jafar-Mohammadi B, Isidori Am, Cudlip S, Grossman AB. Pituitary stalk thickening: the role of an innovative MRI imaging analysis which may assist in determining clinical management. *Eur J Endocrinol.* 2016;175(4):255-263. PMID: 27418059

8. Devuyst F, Kazakou P, Baleriaux D, et al. Central diabetes insipidus and pituitary stalk thickening in adults: distinction of neoplastic from non-neoplastic lesions. *Eur J Endocrinol.* 2020;181(3):95-105. PMID: 32530258

9. Hamilton BE, Salzman KL, Osborn AG. Anatomic and pathologic spectrum of pituitary infundibulum lesions. *AJR Am J Roentgeno.*, 2007;188(3):W223-W232. PMID: 17312027

10. Kang H, Kim KM, Kim MS, Kim JH, Park CK, Kim YH. Safety of endoscopic endonasal biopsy for the pituitary stalk-hypothalamic lesions. *Pituitary.* 2022;25(1):143-151. PMID: 34471994

11. Catford S, Wang YY, Wong R. Pituitary stalk lesions: systematic review and clinical guidance. *Clin Endocrinol (Oxf).* 2016;85(4):507-521. PMID: 26950774

12. Donegan, D., et al., Outcomes of initial management strategies in patients with autoimmune lymphocytic hypophysitis: a systematic review and meta-analysis. *J Clin Endocrinol Metab.* 2022;107(4):1170-1190. PMID: 35137155

13. Chiloiro S, Capoluongo ED, Angelini F, et al. Autoantibody reactivity profile of primary autoimmune hypophysitis patients: preliminary results. *Endocrine.* 2022;76(1):224-227. PMID: 34797510

14. Chiloiro S, Tartaglione T, Capoluongo ED, et al., Hypophysitis outcome and factors predicting responsiveness to glucocorticoid therapy: a prospective and double-arm study. *J Clin Endocrinol Metab.* 2018;103(10):3877-3889.

15. Pal R, Rai A, Vaiphei K, et al. Intracranial germinoma masquerading as secondary granulomatous hypophysitis: a case report and review of literature. *Neuroendocrinology.* 2020;110(5):422-429. PMID: 31269501

Management of Pituitary Tumors During Pregnancy

Andrea Glezer, MD, PhD. Neuroendocrine Unit, Division of Endocrinology and Metabolism, University of São Paulo Medical School Hospital, São Paulo, Brazil; Email: andrea.glezer@hc.fm.usp.br

Educational Objectives

After reviewing this chapter, learners should be able to:

- Recognize that pituitary tumors can impair fertility and identify specific treatments for each type of tumor to be undertaken before pregnancy.

- Individualize the follow-up during pregnancy, depending on the type of pituitary tumor, tumor dimensions, and the patient's comorbidities.

- Reevaluate tumor status after delivery and individualize recommendations regarding breastfeeding, especially if clinical treatment is recommended.

Significance of the Clinical Problem

Pituitary tumors can cause hypogonadism and infertility. Hypogonadism can be caused by hyperprolactinemia (secondary to autonomous secretion or pituitary stalk effect), pituitary stalk disconnection, GH hypersecretion, hypercortisolism, pituitary damage due to direct tumor compression, neurosurgery, and/or radiotherapy. In women of childbearing age, prolactinomas are the most common pituitary tumor, followed by tumors causing acromegaly and rarely Cushing disease and nonfunctioning pituitary adenomas. Specific treatment for each pituitary tumor type is recommended, per guidelines, before pregnancy. In some cases, hypogonadism is irreversible, and assisted reproductive treatments are necessary.

The pituitary gland's function and size change during pregnancy. Pituitary volume increases due to normal lactotroph hyperplasia and hypertrophy with resultant hyperprolactinemia. Prolactinomas can grow during pregnancy because of estrogen stimulation, although symptoms related to mass effect usually occur in individuals with large prolactinomas. Therefore, tumor volume control is recommended before pregnancy in patients with macroprolactinomas.

Physiological hormonal changes during pregnancy make the diagnosis of GH and ACTH hypersecretion challenging. GH and ACTH hypersecretion increases adverse maternal-fetal outcomes such as arterial hypertension, diabetes mellitus, and spontaneous abortion rates. Hormonal hypersecretion should be controlled before and during pregnancy. Patients with tumor mass effect symptoms and/or severe repercussions of GH and ACTH secretion should be managed by an expert multidisciplinary team to individualize treatment, labor, and breastfeeding recommendations.

Practice Gaps

- Patients harboring pituitary tumors should be interviewed regarding fertility plans during routine follow-up appointments and, when indicated, should be treated before pregnancy, according to guidelines for the specific tumor type.

- Assisted reproductive techniques should be considered for patients with permanent hypogonadism.

- In patients with pituitary tumors, pregnancy can be safe and maternal-fetal outcomes are similar to those of the general population if hormonal hypersecretion and tumor volume are controlled before pregnancy.

- In patients with well-controlled disease, clinical treatment is typically withdrawn during pregnancy, and its maintenance should be discussed with a multidisciplinary care team.

Discussion

Pituitary tumors can cause hypogonadotropic hypogonadism and affect fertility. Fertility plans should be discussed routinely as part of follow-up for women of childbearing age with pituitary tumors. Treatment aimed at achieving hormonal and tumoral control should be offered before pregnancy. Hormonal deficiencies should be properly replaced and monitored during pregnancy. Pregnancy also influences normal pituitary size and function, which could lead to an increase in tumor dimension in some cases and add complexity to managing acromegaly and Cushing disease. This chapter reviews each type of pituitary tumor and their specific management during pregnancy.

Prolactinomas

Prolactinomas are the most common type of pituitary tumor, and they most often affect women in their third to fourth decades of life. Hyperprolactinemia can impair GnRH secretion and pulsatility, via kisspeptin reduction, causing hypogonadism, anovulation, and infertility. Dopamine agonists, mainly cabergoline, are the criterion standard treatment due to their efficacy in reducing tumor volume, promoting normal prolactin concentrations, and restoring gonadal axis.[1] Neurosurgery should be reserved for patients with dopamine agonist intolerance, dopamine agonist resistance, or expansive tumors with suprasellar expansion that do not shrink with clinical treatment.[2]

High estrogen levels during pregnancy increase serum prolactin and the size of the pituitary gland due to lactotroph hyperplasia and hypertrophy. Also, hyperestrogenism can increase prolactinoma volume. In microprolactinomas, symptomatic tumor growth occurs in less than 5% of cases, while in macroprolactinomas it is reported in 20% of cases.[3] Therefore, tumor size reduction before pregnancy is indicated for macroprolactinomas.

For microprolactinomas and intrasellar macroprolactinomas, treatment with dopamine agonists, at the lowest effective dosage, is recommended. However, treatment should be withdrawn after pregnancy confirmation to reduce fetal exposure to the drug.[4] Although there are more robust data with bromocriptine regarding pregnancy induction, there were no significant fetal and maternal adverse outcomes in the approximately 1000 pregnancies induced by cabergoline.[1,5,6] During pregnancy, patients with microprolactinomas should be followed up clinically in each trimester, whereas patients with expansive macroprolactinomas should be followed up monthly. Routine serum prolactin measurement is not indicated. In the presence of mass effect symptoms, sellar MRI without contrast and a neuro-ophthalmological evaluation should be performed. If, after evaluation, the symptoms are confirmed to be related to tumor size increase, dopamine agonist therapy must be reintroduced. Surgery should be performed in patients with significant vision deficiency despite dopamine agonist treatment, preferentially during the second trimester. If pregnancy is near term, possible delivery should be discussed with the multidisciplinary care team. After labor, breastfeeding is recommended, except in women for whom dopamine agonist therapy was necessary to control tumor volume during pregnancy. Prolactinoma status should be evaluated after delivery, as remission can occur. Dopamine agonist therapy should be reintroduced after labor (after breastfeeding cessation) in patients without remission.[7,8]

Acromegaly

Acromegaly is usually caused by somatotropinomas and mostly affects individuals in their fourth and fifth decades of life. Uncontrolled acromegaly can cause infertility due to hypogonadism, hyperprolactinemia, insulin resistance, and polycystic ovary syndrome.[9] Additionally, GH hypersecretion before pregnancy is associated with arterial hypertension and hyperglycemia, which could impact maternal and fetal outcomes.[10] Consequently, neurosurgery is recommended as first-line therapy for women with active acromegaly who desire pregnancy. When surgery is not an option, medical treatment with ligand somatostatin receptors or cabergoline can be used until pregnancy is confirmed.[4]

During pregnancy, the placenta secretes a GH variant that stimulates IGF-1 secretion. IGF-1 levels usually do not increase in pregnant women with untreated acromegaly, probably because of hyperestrogenism and the resistance that it can cause in hepatic IGF-1 production.[11] Mass effect symptoms are rare in pregnant women with acromegaly.

In patients with adequate hormonal and tumoral control, cessation of medical treatment should be considered before or right after pregnancy confirmation. Routine GH and IGF-1 measurement is not recommended during pregnancy.[4,12] Maternal outcomes such as diabetes and arterial hypertension can worsen or appear for the first time in pregnancy[13]; nevertheless, with recommended screening and treatment, there is no increase in maternal and fetal mortality.[10] In patients with expansive macroadenomas near the optic chiasm, periodic neuro-ophthalmological evaluation should be performed, and sellar MRI without contrast should be requested if mass effects symptoms are present. Clinical treatment should be initiated (or reinitiated) if the patient has neurological symptoms or severe clinical symptoms related to acromegaly. Neurosurgery, preferably during the second trimester, is indicated in patients with significant neurological symptoms and suboptimal response to medical treatment.[4] Acromegaly status should be reevaluated after delivery because rebound of disease activity can occur.[4] Breastfeeding should be discussed with the patient if medical treatment is indicated.

Cushing Disease

Pregnancy is rare in women with Cushing syndrome, and it is more likely to occur in women with adrenal tumors than in women with Cushing disease. In Cushing disease, infertility can be secondary to hypogonadism caused by hypercortisolism, hyperandrogenism, and hyperprolactinemia.[14] Pregnancy in patients with Cushing disease is associated with maternal and fetal morbidities such as preeclampsia, gestational diabetes, cardiac failure, poor wound healing after cesarean delivery, abortion, premature labor, intrauterine growth restriction, and perinatal death.[15] Therefore, patients with active Cushing disease desiring pregnancy should be treated, preferentially with neurosurgery, before attempting pregnancy.[4] For women with medically treated Cushing disease who would like to become pregnant, management by a multidisciplinary team, including those with expertise in high-risk pregnancy, is recommended.[16] Hypercortisolism diagnosis and evaluation during pregnancy is challenging because of placental corticotropin-releasing hormone production, physiological activation of the hypothalamic-pituitary-adrenal axis, and increased corticosteroid-binding globulin levels. Prophylactic anticoagulation should be considered, as hypercortisolism and pregnancy increase venous thrombosis risk. Transsphenoidal surgery, preferably during the second trimester, should be reserved for patients with severe disease that does not improve with medical treatment.[17] Tumor status should be reevaluated after delivery.[4]

Nonfunctioning Pituitary Adenomas

Nonfunctioning pituitary adenomas are rarely seen in the context of pregnancy. These tumors usually affect older individuals, and fertility is usually only impaired in patients with macroadenomas (which can cause hypogonadism, with or without hyperprolactinemia). Patients with macroadenomas should be treated surgically before attempting pregnancy.[4] Almost 30 cases were reported in the literature and approximately one-third were diagnosed before pregnancy.[18], During pregnancy, the normal pituitary gland can grow due to hyperestrogenism, potentially leading to mass effect symptoms. In the literature, 8 patients presented with mass effect symptoms, and most of them were successfully treated with dopamine agonist therapy.[18,19] However, if visual impairment does not improve, neurosurgery, preferably in the second trimester, or delivery if gestation is near term, should be discussed with a multidisciplinary care team.[4]

Clinical Case Vignettes

Case 1

A 29-year-old woman presents with 6 months of amenorrhea after stopping an oral contraceptive pill. She has no galactorrhea, comorbidities, or history of drug use.

Laboratory test results:

FSH = 8.0 mIU/mL (2.4-10.2 mIU/mL) (SI: 8.0 IU/L [2.4-10.2 IU/L])
LH = 3.5 mIU/mL (1.9-12.5 mIU/mL) (SI: 3.5 IU/L [1.9-12.5 IU/L])
Estradiol = 5.2 pg/mL (5.3-39.3 pg/mL) (SI: 19.0 pmol/L [19.5-144.2 pmol/L])
Prolactin = 217 ng/mL (4.2-24.2 ng/mL) (SI: 9.44 nmol/L [0.18-1.05 nmol/L])
TSH = 2.57 mIU/L (0.27-4.20 mIU/L)
Free T$_4$ = 1.08 ng/dL (0.93-1.70 ng/dL) (SI: 13.90 pmol/L [11.97-21.88 pmol/L])
IGF-1 = 243 ng/mL (83-259 ng/mL) (SI: 31.8 nmol/L [10.9-33.9 nmol/L])
Cortisol = 14.1 µg/dL (5.3-22.5 µg/dL) (SI: 389.0 nmol/L [146.2-620.7 nmol/L])

Sellar MRI identifies a macroadenoma (*Figure 1*), and macroprolactinoma is diagnosed.

Figure 1.

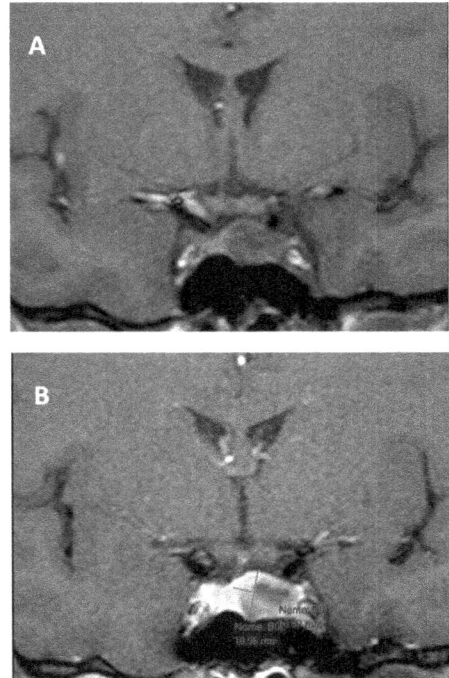

Sellar MRI, T1 coronal views, without contrast (*Panel A*) and with contrast (*Panel B*), showing a pituitary macroadenoma on the left with suprasellar expansion, not reaching the optical chiasma and in contact with the left cavernous sinus.

[Color—Print (Color Gallery page CG13) or web & ePub editions]

If the patient desires pregnancy, which of the following is correct?

A. Neurosurgery is the treatment of choice

B. Dopamine agonist therapy is the gold standard treatment and should be withdrawn after prolactin normalization, even before pregnancy, to avoid exposure during pregnancy

C. Radiotherapy is the treatment of choice

D. Pregnancy is not recommended for a patient with macroprolactinoma

E. Dopamine agonist therapy is the gold standard treatment, and barrier contraception is recommended until normoprolactinemia and tumor reduction are achieved

Answer: E) Dopamine agonist therapy is the gold standard treatment, and barrier contraception is recommended until normoprolactinemia and tumor reduction are achieved

Prolactinomas can cause a range of problems, from infertility to hypogonadism secondary to impairment of GnRH secretion. Fertility is usually restored after prolactin normalizes. Clinical treatment with dopamine agonists is the gold standard for both microprolactinomas and macroprolactinomas. In the setting of expansive macroprolactinomas, barrier contraception should be used until normoprolactinemia is achieved and tumor volume is reduced (Answer E). Although scarce, data show that dopamine agonist treatment for 12 to 24 months can reduce the risk of symptomatic tumor growth in patients with macroprolactinomas. Dopamine agonist therapy should be used at the lowest effective dosage and should be withdrawn after pregnancy confirmation. Surgery is reserved for patients who are intolerant of medical therapy or have treatment-resistant disease. Radiotherapy is contraindicated for patients desiring pregnancy in the next few months.

Case 1, Continued

After 4 months of cabergoline, 0.5 mg weekly, and subsequent normoprolactinemia and regular menses, pregnancy is confirmed. On sellar MRI performed just before pregnancy confirmation, the tumor volume had decreased to within sellar boundaries (*Figure 2*).

Which of the following is the best management after pregnancy confirmation?

A. Stop cabergoline

B. Switch cabergoline to bromocriptine

C. Follow-up during pregnancy with sellar MRI without contrast

D. Follow-up during pregnancy with serum prolactin evaluation each trimester

E. No follow-up is necessary during pregnancy; the risk of symptomatic tumor growth is less than 5%

Answer: A) Stop cabergoline

Figure 2.

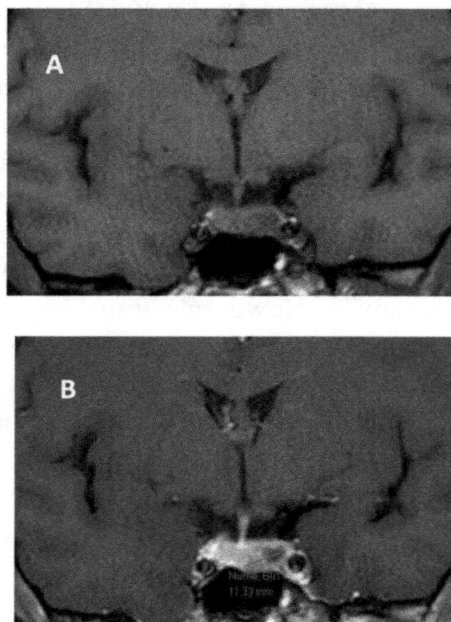

Sellar MRI, T1 coronal views without contrast (*Panel A*) and with contrast (*Panel B*), showing reduction of tumor dimensions and no suprasellar expansion.

[Color—Print (Color Gallery page CG13) or web & ePub editions]

Once normoprolactinemia is achieved and the macroprolactinoma volume is reduced to within sellar boundaries, dopamine agonist therapy should be withdrawn after pregnancy confirmation (Answer A). The patient should be followed up clinically each trimester, and if neurological symptoms develop, sellar MRI without contrast and neuro-ophthalmological evaluation must be done.

Case 1, Continued

During the 12th week of gestation, the patient starts experiencing severe headaches. Sellar MRI without contrast shows an increase in tumor volume (*Figure 3, following page*). Findings on neuro-ophthalmological evaluation are normal.

Which of the following is the best next step in management?

A. Refer for neurosurgery

B. Start bromocriptine

C. Reintroduce cabergoline

Figure 3.

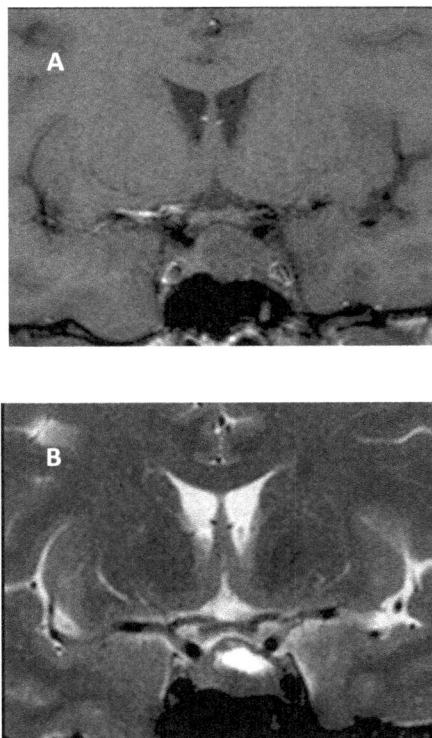

Sellar MRI, T1 coronal view without contrast (*Panel A*) and T2 coronal view (*Panel B*) showing an increase in tumor dimensions, with suprasellar expansion.

D. No specific management is necessary since there is no visual impairment

E. Evaluate for fetal maturity in anticipation of labor induction

Answer: C) Reintroduce cabergoline

In the presence of neurological symptoms due to an increase in tumor volume, the dopamine agonist should be reintroduced (Answer C) at the dosage that promoted tumor control before pregnancy—in this case, cabergoline, 0.5 mg weekly. Neurosurgery should be performed if there is visual impairment that does not improve with clinical treatment, preferentially during the second trimester. If the pregnancy is near term, and there has been no success with a dopamine agonist, delivery induction can be considered after assessment of fetal maturity and evaluation by a multidisciplinary team.

Case 2

Ten years ago, a 28-year-old woman presented with headache and diplopia. Cranial MRI showed a pituitary adenoma (4 cm in maximum diameter), with suprasellar expansion and right parasellar invasion (Knosp 4). She underwent transsphenoidal operations 10 years ago and 6 years ago, with partial debulking. Acromegaly was diagnosed 4 years ago. Lanreotide, 120 mg every 28 days, was initiated, but IGF-1 levels did not decrease. Cabergoline, 3.5 mg weekly, was added. There was no hormonal control or significant tumor volume reduction. Another neurosurgical operation was indicated. However, due to the COVID-19 pandemic, the procedure was postponed. Pegvisomant and pasireotide were not available.

The patient, now 38 years old, desires pregnancy. She takes levothyroxine to treat central hypothyroidism. There are no other hormone deficiencies. She does not have diabetes or arterial hypertension.

Current laboratory test results:

GH = 5.67 ng/mL (SI: 5.67 µg/L)
IGF-1 = 477 ng/mL (69-227 ng/mL) (SI: 62.5 nmol/L [9.0-29.7 nmol/L])
Prolactin = <1.5 ng/mL (SI: <0.07 nmol/L)

Current sellar MRI shows a pituitary tumor (3.4 cm in maximum diameter), with suprasellar extension and parasellar invasion.

In the context of the patient's desire for pregnancy, which of the following is correct?

A. Arterial blood pressure and glycemic parameters should be monitored to identify preeclampsia and gestational diabetes

B. Radiotherapy is indicated due to debulking difficulties of the parasellar tumor remnant

C. GH and IGF-1 should be periodically assessed during pregnancy

D. Neuro-ophthalmological evaluation is not necessary during pregnancy

E. Pregnancy is contraindicated for this patient

Answer: A) Arterial blood pressure and glycemic parameters should be monitored to identify preeclampsia and gestational diabetes

During pregnancy, evaluation of arterial blood pressure and assessment for hyperglycemia (Answer A) should be done periodically under the guidance of an obstetric team.

For patients with acromegaly desiring pregnancy, neurosurgery is the first treatment to be offered, and radiotherapy (Answer B) is contraindicated.

Once pregnancy is confirmed, routine GH and IGF-1 evaluations (Answer C) are not recommended and, in most cases, there is no increase in IGF-1 levels even after clinical treatment withdrawal.

For patients with large and invasive adenomas, especially those close to the optic chiasm, regular neuro-ophthalmologic evaluation is required and, if necessary, pituitary MRI without contrast should be performed (thus, Answer D is incorrect).

Pregnancy is not contraindicated (Answer E); however, fertility should be assessed to evaluate whether assisted reproduction technology may be needed to achieve pregnancy.

Another important issue is that clinical treatment does not control GH hypersecretion and does not decrease tumor dimensions. If the tumor increases during pregnancy and causes neurological symptoms, clinical treatment may or may not be effective, and neurosurgery during pregnancy may be indicated.

Case 2, Continued

The patient schedules a follow-up appointment after a positive home pregnancy test.

Which of the following statements is correct?

A. If there is tumor growth during pregnancy accompanied by neurological symptoms, pegvisomant should be prescribed
B. Breastfeeding is contraindicated
C. If she develops neurological symptoms, neurosurgery should be performed, regardless of trimester
D. Clinical treatment is contraindicated during pregnancy
E. Levothyroxine replacement should be maintained, and dosage adjustments may be necessary throughout pregnancy

Answer: E) Levothyroxine replacement should be maintained, and dosage adjustments may be necessary throughout pregnancy

During pregnancy, hypopituitarism should be treated with hormone replacement. The levothyroxine dosage should be adjusted according to free T_4 levels (Answer E).

If there are neurological symptoms due to tumor growth during pregnancy, clinical treatment can be tried, with first-generation somatostatin receptor ligands with or without cabergoline (thus, Answer D is incorrect).

Although use of pegvisomant has been reported in pregnancy, it does not act on tumor volume (thus, Answer A is incorrect).

If clinical treatment fails, neurosurgery should be performed, preferentially during the second trimester (thus, Answer C is incorrect).

Breastfeeding is not contraindicated in this setting, but recommendations should be individualized based on disease activity and drug treatment maintenance (thus, Answer B is incorrect).

Case 3

A 35-year-old woman presents with facial plethora, rounded face, violaceous striae, lower limb weakness, and amenorrhea.

Laboratory evaluation documents ACTH-dependent hypercortisolism.

Laboratory test results:

24-Hour urinary free cortisol = 85.6 µg/24 h (1750 mL), 83.4 µg/24 h (200 mL), and 697.9 µg/24 h (1700 mL) (reference range 3-43 µg/24 h)

Serum cortisol = 24.5 μg/dL (6.7-22.6 μg/dL)
(SI: 675.9 nmol/L [184.8-623.5 nmol/L])
Late-night salivary cortisol = 0.87 μg/dL (<0.2 μg/dL)
(SI: 24.0 nmol/L [<5.5 nmol/L])
ACTH = 87.0 pg/mL (7.2-63.3 pg/mL)
(SI: 19.1 pmol/L [1.6-13.9 pmol/L])

Sellar MRI reveals an 0.8-cm microadenoma, and she undergoes transsphenoidal neurosurgery. Postoperatively, she experiences clinical and hormonal remission, and sellar imaging 3 months later shows no tumor. Menses are regular, and she becomes pregnant 7 months after surgery, while on no medications. During the eighth week of gestation, she presents with signs and symptoms of hypercortisolism.

Laboratory test results:

Urinary free cortisol = 231 μg/24 h (28.5-213.7 μg/24 h) (1.08 times the upper normal limit) (SI: 637.6 nmol/d [78.7-589.8 nmol/d])
Late-night salivary cortisol = 0.61 μg/dL (<0.2 μg/dL) (3 times the upper normal limit) (SI: 16.8 nmol/L [<5.5 nmol/L])

Which of the following is correct regarding the diagnosis of hypercortisolism during pregnancy?

A. Low-dosage dexamethasone-suppression test (1 mg) is the method of choice

B. Late-night salivary cortisol increases early in the timeline of hypercortisolism recurrence

C. Urinary free cortisol is very sensitive, and slight increases are diagnostic of Cushing syndrome

D. Serum cortisol is a good method for diagnosis during pregnancy

E. Corticotropin-releasing hormone testing is easy and widely available

Answer: B) Late-night salivary cortisol increases early in the timeline of hypercortisolism recurrence

During pregnancy, hyperestrogenism increases cortisol-binding globulin levels, leading to inaccuracy in dexamethasone-suppression testing and random serum cortisol measurement. Additionally, in pregnancy, there is a physiological activation of the pituitary-adrenal gland, mostly due to corticotropin-releasing hormone placental secretion. Urinary free cortisol and late-night salivary cortisol increase throughout normal pregnancy. Cushing syndrome is indicated by a urinary free cortisol value more than 2 to 3 times the upper normal limit and a late-night salivary cortisol value 1.4 times the upper normal limit in the second trimester and 2 times the upper normal limit in the third trimester. Corticotropin-releasing hormone testing is a high-cost test that is not available in many countries. In this case, the late-night salivary cortisol value 3 times higher than the upper normal limit in the first trimester suggests hypercortisolism recurrence.

Case 3, Continued

When hypercortisolism recurrence is diagnosed in pregnancy, which of the following is correct?

A. Neurosurgery is the first choice of treatment, especially during the second trimester

B. Clinical treatment can be used without reservations during pregnancy

C. Mifepristone is the gold standard treatment for women with gestational diabetes related to hypercortisolism

D. Mild hypercortisolism can be followed with obstetric care aiming to control comorbidities

E. Bilateral adrenalectomy should be performed in patients with severe hypercortisolism, especially in the first trimester

Answer: D) Mild hypercortisolism can be followed with obstetric care aiming to control comorbidities

Patients with mild hypercortisolism can be followed up with supportive medical and obstetric care (Answer D). In patients with moderate hypercortisolism, a multidisciplinary team should discuss recommendations for clinical treatment or neurosurgery. In patients with severe hypercortisolism and in those for whom clinical treatment fails or those who experience intolerance, neurosurgery should be performed, preferentially during the second trimester. Although clinical treatment is not approved for use in pregnancy, an expert team can individualize treatment. Mifepristone is abortive and absolutely contraindicated in pregnancy.

Key Learning Points

- Clinicians should be comfortable discussing routine fertility and pregnancy issues with women of childbearing age harboring pituitary tumors to plan specific treatment for each type of tumor.

- Clinicians should properly replace hormonal deficiencies before and during pregnancy, while considering the physiological modifications in this setting.

- In most patients with tumor control before gestation, clinical treatment can be withdrawn after pregnancy confirmation. Follow-up during pregnancy is important, and patients should be reevaluated after delivery.

References

1. Petersenn S, Fleseriu M, Casanueva FF, et al. Diagnosis and management of prolactin-secreting pituitary adenomas: a Pituitary Society international consensus statement. *Nat Rev Endocrinol*. 2023;19(12):722-740. PMID: 37670148

2. Glezer ABM. Prolactinomas and disorders of prolactin secretion. In: Robertson RP, ed. *DeGroot's Endocrinology: Basic Science and Clinical Practice*. 8th ed. Elsevier; 2022.

3. Huang W, Molitch ME. Pituitary tumors in pregnancy. *Endocrinol Metab Clin North Am*. 2019;48(3):569-581. PMID: 31345524

4. Luger A, Broersen LHA, Biermasz NR, et al. ESE clinical practice guideline on functioning and nonfunctioning pituitary adenomas in pregnancy. *Eur J Endocrinol*. 2021;185(3):G1-G33. PMID: 34425558

5. Sant' Anna BG, Musolino NRC, Gadelha MR, et al. A Brazilian multicentre study evaluating pregnancies induced by cabergoline in patients harboring prolactinomas. *Pituitary*. 2020;23(2):120-128. PMID: 31728906

6. Bandeira DB, Alves LS, Glezer A, Boguszewski CL, Dos Santos Nunes-Nogueira V. Disease activity and maternal-fetal outcomes in pregnant women with prolactinoma: a systematic review and meta-analysis. *J Clin Endocrinol Metab*. 2024;110(4):e1241-e1251

7. Glezer A, Bronstein MD. Prolactinomas in pregnancy: considerations before conception and during pregnancy. *Pituitary*. 2020;23(1):65-69. PMID: 31792668

8. Zhang CD, Ioachimescu AG. Prolactinomas: preconception and duringpPregnancy. Endocrinol Metab Clin North Am. 2024;53(3):409-419. PMID: 390848816

9. Pirchio R, Auriemma RS, Grasso LFS, et al. Fertility in acromegaly: a single-center experience of female patients during active disease and after disease remission. *J Clin Endocrinol Metab*. 2023;108(8):e583-e593. PMID: 36790068

10. Bandeira DB, Olivatti TOF, Bolfi F, Boguszewski CL, Dos Santos Nunes-Nogueira V. Acromegaly and pregnancy: a systematic review and meta-analysis. *Pituitary*. 2022;25(3):352-362. PMID: 35098440

11. Bronstein MD, Paraiba DB, Jallad RS. Management of pituitary tumors in pregnancy. Nat Rev Endocrinol. 2011;7(5):301-310. PMID: 21403665

12. Abucham J, Bronstein MD, Dias ML. Management of endocrine disease: Acromegaly and pregnancy: a contemporary review. *Eur J Endocrinol*. 2017;177(1):R1-R12. PMID: 28292926

13. Jallad RS, Shimon I, Fraenkel M, et al. Outcome of pregnancies in a large cohort of women with acromegaly. *Clin Endocrinol (Oxf)*. 2018;88(6):896-907. PMID: 29574986

14. Castinetti F, Brue T. Impact of Cushing's syndrome on fertility and pregnancy. *Ann Endocrinol (Paris)*. 2022;83(3):188-190. PMID: 35443159

15. Machado MC, Fragoso MCBV, Bronstein MD. Pregnancy in patients with Cushing's syndrome. Endocrinol Metab Clin North Am. 2018;47(2):441-449. PMID: 29754643

16. Gheorghiu ML, Fleseriu M. Conundrums of diagnosis and management of Cushing's syndrome in pregnancy. *Endocrinol Metab Clin North Am*. 2024;53(3):421-435. PMID: 39084817

17. Hamblin R, Coulden A, Fountas A, Karavitaki N. The diagnosis and management of Cushing's syndrome in pregnancy. *J Neuroendocrinol*. 2022;34(8):e13118. PMID: 35491087

18. Jallad RS GA, Machado MC, Bronstein MD. Pituitary disorders during pregnancy and lactation. In: *Maternal-Fetal and Neonatal Endocrinology Physiology, Pathophysiology, and Clinical Management*. Elsevier; 2020: 259-286.

19. Rosmino J, Tkatch J, Di Paolo MV, Berner S, Lescano S, Guitelman M. Non-functioning pituitary adenomas and pregnancy: one-center experience and review of the literature. *Arch Endocrinol Metab*. 2021;64(5):614-622. PMID: 34033303

Craniopharyngiomas in Adults: Modern Management and Changes in the Paradigm

Emmanuel Jouanneau, MD, PhD. Pituitary Center, Neurological Department, Groupement Hospital Est, Hospices Civils de Lyon, Lyon, France; Claude Bernard University, Lyon, France; Cancer Research Center of Lyon, Lyon, France; Email: emmanuel.jouanneau@chu-lyon.fr

Gerald Raverot, MD, PhD. Claude Bernard University, Lyon, France; Cancer Research Center of Lyon, Lyon, France; Endocrinology Department, Reference Center for Rare Pituitary Diseases HYPO, "Groupement Hospitalier Est" Hospices Civils de Lyon, Bron, France; Email: gerald.raverot@chu-lyon.fr

Educational Objectives

After reading this chapter, readers should be able to:

- Describe the overexpressed oncogenic pathways in craniopharyngiomas in adults and pathogenic variants based on histopathology.

- Explain the possibility of targeted therapy for craniopharyngiomas and data from recent reports and studies.

- Describe the concept of neoadjuvant therapy for craniopharyngiomas.

Significance of the Clinical Problem

Craniopharyngiomas are rare, accounting for 1.2% to 4.6% of intracranial tumors in adults and up to 11% in children. There are 2 craniopharyngioma subtypes: adamantinomatous craniopharyngioma (ACP), which is the only subtype found in children, and the papillary form (PCP), which represents 20% of craniopharyngiomas in adults.[1]

When feasible, gross total removal gives the best recurrence-free survival and overall survival, with significantly lower recurrence rates than those associated with subtotal resection (0%-50% vs 50%-100% at 10 years).[2] When the craniopharyngioma has invaded the third ventricle or the visual pathway, surgery should be subtotal, sparing the hypothalamus and favoring a combined strategy with radiotherapy. Numerous studies have demonstrated that adjuvant radiotherapy significantly improves long-term tumor control and overall survival rates after subtotal removal at 10 years when compared with subtotal resection alone, with results similar to those of gross total removal.[3]

The main issue with such tumors remains the hypothalamic involvement found in type C (suprasellar-pseudoventricular craniopharyngioma) and type D (infundibulo-tuberal craniopharyngioma) (Prieto classification) tumors, with the high posttherapeutic morbidity.[4] In these cases, even subtotal removal may be damaging, resulting in a low quality of life. In such cases or in the case of recurrence after surgery or failure of radiotherapy, there is a need for medical treatment to avoid invasive surgery. Recently, Brastianos et al identified the *BRAF* V600E pathogenic variant in PCPs.[5] Additionally, overexpression of IL6 and

VEGF has been identified in ACPs. These findings have given rise to targeted therapies, such as anti-BRAF in PCP and anti-IL6/VEGF in ACP and have prompted neuro-oncological concepts for managing craniopharyngioma.[6-8]

Practice Gaps

- Clinicians typically consider only surgery and radiotherapy for craniopharyngiomas.
- Hypothalamic morbidity remains the main concern of the disease.
- All clinicians caring for patients should be aware of recent advances in targeted therapy and the possibility of a neoadjuvant approach with such therapies.

Discussion

Despite improvements in surgery in the endoscopic era and in radiotherapy, clinicians still face the problem of craniopharyngioma recurrence.[9,10] Surgery must spare the hypothalamus to maintain patients' quality of life. In types C and D craniopharyngioma Prieto subtypes, surgery is therefore mainly partial and risky.

Since the first description of results with anti-BRAF in PCPs carrying the *BRAF* pathogenic variant, strong evidence has accumulated showing the efficacy of such therapy in recurrent or newly diagnosed PCPs. The *BRAF* V600E pathogenic variant is present in approximately 95% of PCPs.[5,11]

Recently, in 15 of 16 patients treated with anti-MEK and anti-BRAF combined therapy in a French national cohort, a tumor volume reduction of nearly 90% was reported.[12] Morbidity was acceptable, but it led to treatment discontinuation in 3 patients, mainly for a combination of fever/pneumopathy or fever, fatigue, headache, rash, or diarrhea. Liver enzyme elevation led to transient discontinuation in 2 patients. Targeted therapy was used in 3 separate groups: neoadjuvant (biopsy-only followed by targeted therapy), adjuvant (recurrence after surgery followed by targeted therapy before radiotherapy), and palliative (recurrence after surgery and radiotherapy). All groups showed an identical response. In the neoadjuvant group, the tumor reduction was impressive and rapid (decompressive results in 3 months, maximum reached at around 6 months) and patients were referred thereafter for radiotherapy. In a phase 2 trial, in a similar cohort, the efficacy and adverse effects of the combined therapy were exactly the same.[13] Interestingly, 6 of 7 patients who discontinued targeted therapy had no evidence of recurrence after 23 months of follow-up. In these 2 cohorts, the cystic components responded more slowly to therapy, but showed an equivalent response in the solid tumor components by the end of treatment.

These results have given rise to a new paradigm: for invasive unresectable hypothalamic craniopharyngiomas, surgery should be replaced by simple biopsy with neoadjuvant anti-BRAF debulking in the case of PCPs, with the goal of avoiding ineffective surgery and decreasing hypothalamic morbidity.[14] Biopsy continues to remain mandatory, as imaging or liquid biopsy cannot currently ensure an accurate diagnosis.

However, in most published cases, combined anti-MEK and anti-BRAF have been used to maximize efficacy and reduce toxicity. However, numerous questions remain, and further trials are required to determine the optimal treatment duration in cases of recurrence and in newly diagnosed craniopharyngiomas, the benefits of upfront vs delayed radiotherapy using a neoadjuvant approach, and the final target of radiotherapy (initial tumoral volume or the final contrast enhancement). Studies are also needed to determine the recurrence rate when targeted therapy is stopped, and the efficacy of such therapy when it is resumed due to recurrence.

In ACPs, the pathogenic variants in the *CTNNB1* gene are typical (occurring in 96% of ACPs), which drives accumulation of β-catenin in cells and inactivates the proteasomal degradation pathway.[5,15] There is currently no targeted therapy available for disease associated with *CTNNB1* pathogenic variants. However, in ACPs, overexpression of growth factors, including EGFR, VEGF, and the proinflammatory cytokine IL6, have been found, with the latter growth factors being in the liquid or wall of cysts. Notably, in a recent case report of recurrent ACP, anti-VEGF therapy showed a 50% tumor reduction and visual improvement before radiotherapy.[16] In 2 other studies, combined systemic therapy with anti-VEGF and anti-IL6 was used with encouraging results and dramatic cyst reduction.[17,18]

Oncological medical treatments are emerging for both craniopharyngioma subtypes. The field is clearly moving towards a neuro-oncological paradigm to address aggressive pituitary neuroendocrine tumors and craniopharyngiomas. This is exemplified by the concept of pituitary tumor centers of excellence, which rely on strong collaboration with oncologists.[8,19] Three years ago, following these recent developments in France, a monthly national multidisciplinary team was established to discuss craniopharyngiomas for which targeted therapy could be used.

Clinical Case Vignettes
Case 1

A 56-year-old man is referred with a 2-month history of total pituitary insufficiency. In the last several months, he experienced weight gain of 22 lb (10 kg). He has no visual symptoms. MRI reveals a type D craniopharyngioma (infundibulo-tuberal Prieto classification).

Is the best next step surgery to remove the tumor or a simple biopsy to further characterize the diagnosis?

Since a PCP was suspected, a simple biopsy was performed and a neoadjuvant anti-BRAF agent (dabrafenib, 150 mg twice daily) and an anti-MEK agent (trametinib, 2 mg once daily) were started. The solid part of the tumor decreased quickly over 2 months, while the cystic part continued to grow during the next 4 months and was managed by transventricular marsupialization into the third ventricle. Radiotherapy was finally initiated to treat the remaining contrast enhancement, and the tumor was optimally controlled at the last follow-up (2 years after diagnosis). *Figure 1* summarizes the tumor's evolution during the treatment course.

Figure 1.

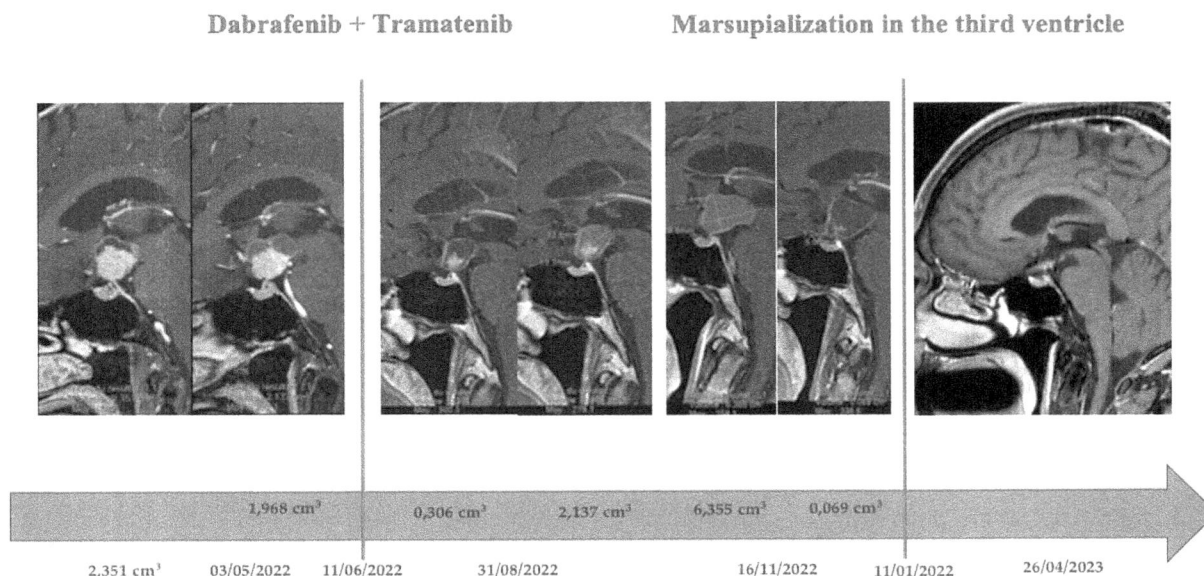

Dabrafenib + Tramatenib   Marsupialization in the third ventricle

2,351 cm³   03/05/2022   1,968 cm³   11/06/2022   0,306 cm³   31/08/2022   2,137 cm³   6,355 cm³   16/11/2022   0,069 cm³   11/01/2022   26/04/2023

Reprinted from De Rosa A et al. *Annales d'Endocrinologie*, 2023; 84(6):727–733. © Elsevier Masson SAS.

[Color—Print (Color Gallery page CG14) or web & ePub editions]

Case 2

A 68-year-old man is being monitored for multilocular sclerosis with an infundibulo-tuberal tumor (type D, Prieto and Pascal classification) discovered 3 years ago. The tumor has continued to grow over the last year. The occurrence of bitemporal hemianopsia prompts a treatment decision.

Considering the hypothalamus invasion, is the best next step surgery to remove the tumor or a simple biopsy with the aim of recommending targeted neoadjuvant therapy if a PCP is confirmed?
Considering the fast and effective tumor reduction achieved with anti-BRAF therapy, a simple biopsy should be chosen to avoid additional morbidity.

Once the diagnosis was confirmed, combined anti-BRAF and anti-MEK therapy (the same protocol used in the preceding case) was introduced, with visual improvement in 3 weeks, normalization in 3 months, and a 90% decrease in tumor volume in 3 months (*Figure 2*).

After a multidisciplinary meeting, the patient was referred to radiotherapy with optimal tumor control observed 1 year after treatment initiation. The patient had no hypothalamic symptoms.

Case 3

An 84-year-old man with poor clinical status presents with suspected recurrence of craniopharyngioma (the biopsy results from initial diagnosis are unavailable) and visual impairment. A transsphenoidal biopsy is performed, which confirms a final diagnosis of ACP.

Is the best therapeutic strategy to propose decompressive surgery or radiotherapy alone?
The patient's clinical status was poor, and he was not a candidate for decompressive surgery, so radiotherapy was proposed. The patient was almost blind within 4 weeks. After a multidisciplinary team meeting, anti-VEGF treatment was initiated, which had excellent clinical tolerance. After 4 weeks of treatment, the

Figure 2.

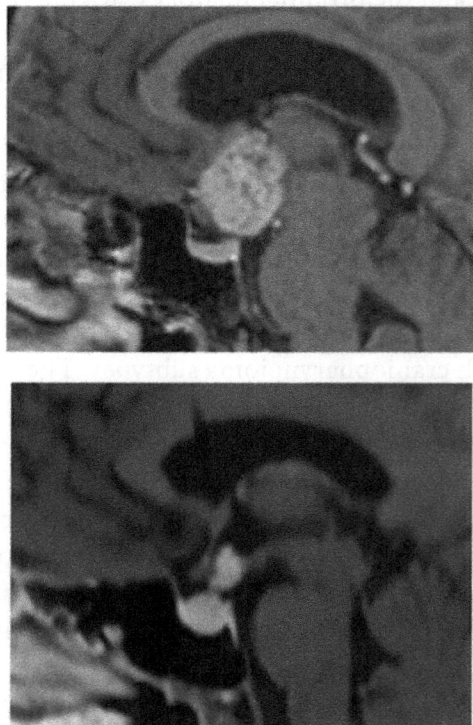

Reprinted from De Rosa A et al. *Annales d'Endocrinologie*, 2023; 84(6):727–733. © Elsevier Masson SAS.

patient was able to resume reading. He eventually had excellent visual recovery in 3 months in the right eye. Both the cystic and solid parts of the tumor shrank by 50% (*Figure 3, following page*). Radiotherapy was administered with subsequent good tumor control at 1 year follow-up.

Key Learning Points

- Craniopharyngiomas are benign tumors that can cause hypothalamic symptoms when invasive.

- All craniopharyngiomas in children are the adamantinomatous subtype; the papillary subtype represents 20% of craniopharyngiomas in adults.

- Ninety-five percent of PCPs have the V600E *BRAF* pathogenic variant and respond rapidly to combined anti-bRAF and anti-MEK therapy

Figure 3.

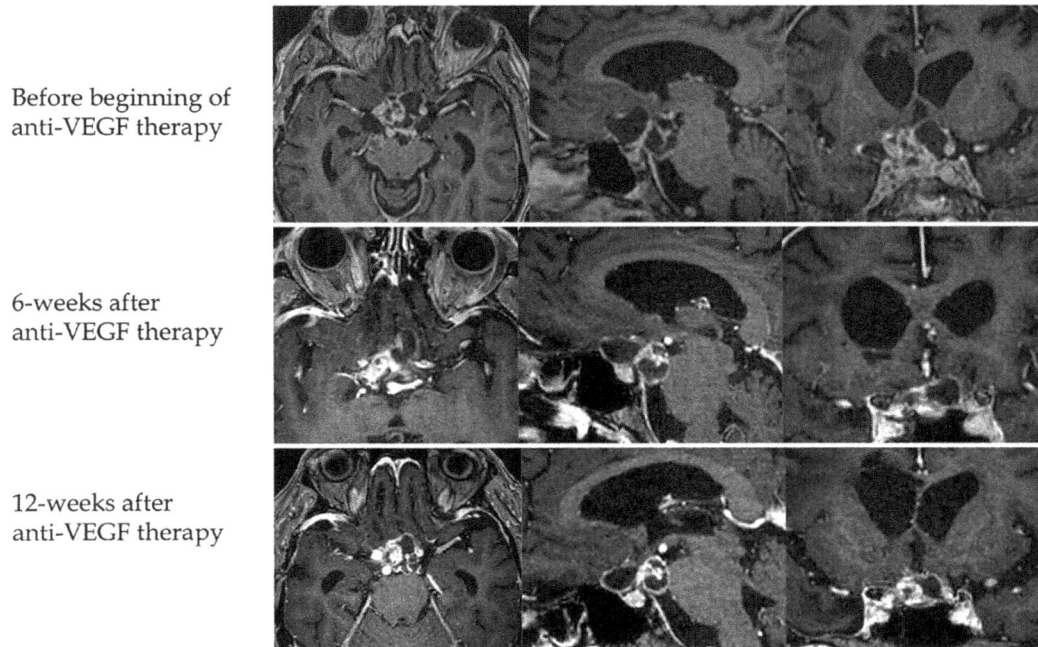

Before beginning of
anti-VEGF therapy

6-weeks after
anti-VEGF therapy

12-weeks after
anti-VEGF therapy

Reprinted from De Rosa A et al. *Annales d'Endocrinologie*, 2023; 84(6):727–733. © Elsevier Masson SAS.

in phase 2 and historical cohort studies (90% tumor volume reduction in a median time of 6 months).

- Overexpression of IL6 and/or VEGF in ACPs can be targeted by systemic therapy, as supported by encouraging findings published in case reports.

- Neoadjuvant targeted therapy for hypothalamic PCPs may replace surgery for tumoral debulking in the hope of decreasing final morbidity and improving oncological control.

- Multicentric trials are needed to answer questions about long-term outcomes and the exact role of targeted therapy.

- More pituitary centers of excellence are needed to treat these patients and incorporate neuro-oncological concepts into management.

References

1. Vasiljevic A, Villa. Histopathology and molecular pathology of craniopharyngioma in adults. In: Jouanneau E, Raverot G, eds. *Adult Craniopharyngiomas: Differences and Lessons From Paediatrics.* Springer; 2020:1-17.

2. Mortini P, Gagliardi F, Boari N, Losa M. Surgical strategies and modern therapeutic options in the treatment of craniopharyngiomas. *Crit Rev Oncol Hematol.* 2013;88:514-529. PMID: 23932582

3. Dandurand C, Sepehry AA, Asadi Lari MH, Akagami R, Gooderham P. Adult craniopharyngioma: case series, systematic review, and meta-analysis. *Neurosurgery.* 2018;83:631-641. PMID: 29267973

4. Prieto R, Pascual JM, Barrios L. Topographic diagnosis of craniopharyngiomas: the accuracy of MRI findings observed on conventional T1 and T2 images. *AJNR Am J Neuroradiol.* 2017;38(11):2073-2080. PMID: 28935625

5. Brastianos PK, Taylor-Weiner A, Manley PE, et al. Exome sequencing identifies BRAF mutations in papillary craniopharyngiomas. *Nat Genet.* 2014;46(2):161-165. PMID: 24413733

6. Martinez-Gutierrez JC, D'Andrea MR, Cahill DP, Santagata S, Barker FG, Brastianos PK. Diagnosis and management of craniopharyngiomas in the era of genomics and targeted therapy. *Neurosurg Focus.* 2016;41:E2. PMID: 24413733

7. Stec NE, Barker FG, Brastianos PK. Targeted treatment for craniopharyngioma. *J Neurooncol.* 2025;172(3):503-513. PMID: PMID: 39951179

8. Jouanneau E, Calvanese F, Ducray F, Raverot G. Pituitary tumor centers of excellence (PTCOE) should now include neuro-oncologic input. *Pituitary.* 2023;26(5):642-643. PMID: 37676531

9. Ghosh S, Goda JS, Chatterjee A, et al. Patterns of care in craniopharyngioma: clinical outcomes after surgery and radiation therapy in a real-world setting. *World Neurosurg.* 2024;181:e809e819. PMID: 37923012

10. Cappabianca P, Cavallo LM, Esposito F, De Divitiis E. Craniopharyngiomas. *J Neurosurg.* 2008;109(1):1-3. PMID: 18590426

11. Brastianos PK, Shankar GM, Gill CM, et al. Dramatic response of BRAF V600E mutant papillary craniopharyngioma to targeted therapy. *J Natl Cancer Inst.* 2016;108:djv310. PMID: 26498373

12. De Alcubierre D, Gkasdaris G, Mordrel M, et al. BRAF and MEK inhibitor targeted therapy in papillary craniopharyngiomas: a cohort study. *Eur J Endocrinol.* 2024;191(2):251-261. PMID: 39158090

13. Brastianos PK, Twohy E, Geyer S, et al. BRAF-MEK Inhibition in newly diagnosed papillary craniopharyngiomas. *N Engl J Med.* 2023;389(2):118-126. PMID: 37437144

14. Calvanese F, Jacquesson T, Manet R, et al. Neoadjuvant B-RAF and MEK inhibitor targeted therapy for adult papillary craniopharyngiomas: a new treatment paradigm. *Front Endocrinol (Lausanne).* 2022;13:882381. PMID: 35757402

15. Malgulwar PB, Nambirajan A, Pathak P, et al. Study of β-catenin and BRAF alterations in adamantinomatous and papillary craniopharyngiomas: mutation analysis with immunohistochemical correlation in 54 cases. *J Neurooncol.* 2017;133(3):487-495. PMID: 28500561

16. De Rosa A, Calvanese F, Ducray F, et al. First evidence of anti-VEGF efficacy in an adult case of adamantinomatous craniopharyngioma: case report and illustrative review. *Ann Endocrinol (Paris).* 2023;84(6):727-733. PMID: 37865272

17. Grob S, Mirsky DM, Donson AM, et al. Targeting IL-6 Is a potential treatment for primary cystic Craniopharyngioma. *Front Oncol.* 2019;9:791. PMID: 31497533

18. Webb LM, Okuno SH, Ransom RC, et al. Recurrent adamantinomatous craniopharyngioma stabilized with tocilizumab and bevacizumab: illustrative case. *J Neurosurg Case Lessons.* 2025;9(2):CASE24410. PMID: 39805108

19. Giustina A, Uygur MM, Frara S, et al. Pilot study to define criteria for Pituitary Tumors Centers of Excellence (PTCOE): results of an audit of leading international centers. *Pituitary.* 2023;26(5):583-596. PMID: 37640885

Therapeutic Use Exemption in Elite Sport: The Endocrinologist as the Expert for Hormonal Drugs

Alan D. Rogol, MD, PhD. Department of Pediatrics, University of Virginia, Charlottesville, VA; Email: adrogol@comcast.net

Educational Objectives

After reviewing this chapter, learners should be able to:

- Determine whether a patient/athlete requires a therapeutic use exemption (TUE) to compete in elite organized sport.

- Provide the appropriate medical information to the TUE Committee to permit them to concur with the medical diagnosis and issues a TUE.

Significance of the Clinical Problem

This Meet the Professor chapter is not about a specific disease and how to diagnose and manage it. It is about a process to help elite athletes/patients who have endocrine conditions that require a World Anti-Doping Agency (WADA)-banned drug obtain a TUE to compete. This means that the physician/endocrinologist should provide enough information to ensure that the athlete can obtain an exemption, specifically by meeting the following criteria of section 4.2 of the WADA code:

4.2a The *Prohibited Substance* or *Prohibited Method* in question is needed to treat a diagnosed medical condition supported by relevant clinical evidence.

[Comment to Article 4.2(a): The Use of the *Prohibited Substance* or *Prohibited Method* may be part of a necessary diagnostic investigation rather than a treatment per se.]

4.2b The Therapeutic Use of the *Prohibited Substance* or *Prohibited Method* will not, on the balance of probabilities, produce any additional enhancement of performance beyond what might be anticipated by a return to the Athlete's normal state of health following the treatment of the medical condition.

[Comment to Article 4.2(b): An Athlete's normal state of health will need to be determined on an individual basis. A normal state of health for a specific Athlete is their state of health but for the medical condition for which the Athlete is seeking a TUE.]

4.2c The *Prohibited Substance* or *Prohibited Method* is an indicated treatment for the medical condition, and there is no reasonable permitted Therapeutic alternative.

[Comment to Article 4.2(c): The physician must explain why the treatment chosen was the most appropriate, eg, based on experience, side-effect profiles, or other medical justifications, including, where applicable, geographically specific medical practice, and the ability to access the medication. Further, it is not always necessary to try and fail alternatives before using the *Prohibited Substance* or *Prohibited Method.*]

4.2d The necessity for the Use of the *Prohibited Substance* or *Prohibited Method* is not a consequence, wholly or in part, of the prior Use (without a TUE) of a substance or method which was prohibited at the time of such Use.

[Comment to Article 4.2: The WADA documents titled "TUE Physician Guidelines," posted on WADA's website, should be used to assist in the application of these criteria in relation to particular medical conditions. The granting of a TUE is based solely on consideration of the conditions set out in Article 4.2. It does not consider whether the *Prohibited Substance* or *Prohibited Method* is the most clinically appropriate or safe, or whether its use is legal in all jurisdictions.]

Practice Gaps

- Unfamiliarity with the TUE process.
- Unfamiliarity with the list of banned drugs or techniques.

Discussion

The World Anti-Doping Agency (WADA; in French, Agence mondiale antidopage [AMA]) is an international organization founded by more than 140 governments along with the International Olympic Committee (IOC) with headquarters in Montreal, Canada. Its purpose is to promote, coordinate, and monitor the use of drugs and illegal methods in sports. The agency's remit includes scientific research, education, development of anti-doping capacities, and monitoring of the World Anti-Doping Code (Code).

The Code is a document published by WADA to which hundreds of sports organizations are signatories.[1] This Code "harmonizes anti-doping policies, rules, and regulations within sport organizations and among public authorities" to "protect the athletes' multiple international standards

published by WADA covering multiple topics of prohibited substances, including Therapeutic Use Exemptions," the topic of this chapter.

TUE Guidelines

Introduction

The International Standard for Therapeutic Use Exemptions (ISTUE) was created to provide a detailed, fair, and understandable process for athletes, anti-doping organizations, physicians, and athlete support personnel to follow when situations arise where, due to illness or medical condition, an athlete may require the use of substances or methods that are specifically included in the WADA prohibited list (List).[2,3] The TUE application process provides athletes with an opportunity to apply for an exemption when medical treatment is required involving the use of a prohibited substance or prohibited method. This process promotes competition on a level playing field. If a TUE is granted, an athlete may continue, or start to use, the otherwise prohibited substance or method while competing without resulting in an Anti-Doping Rule Violation (ADRV) and sanction, if applicable. An athlete applying for a TUE must have a diagnosed medical condition, confirmed by relevant medical data that meet the ISTUE criteria for the granting of a TUE.[2] This mandatory documentation, provided by the athlete's physician, here likely an internal medicine or pediatric endocrinologist, must accompany the TUE application. This information should be guided by the relevant TUE Physician Guideline and Checklist.[4] For our purposes today, these guidelines and checklists cover diabetes mellitus, male hypogonadism (testosterone deficiency), and the use of GH for GH-deficient athletes, whether adolescent or adult, and for some adolescents with non–GH-deficient short stature.

> "An Athlete may be granted a TUE if (and only if) they can show, on the balance of probabilities, that each of the following conditions is met: a) The Prohibited Substance or Prohibited Method in question is needed to treat a diagnosed medical condition

supported by relevant clinical evidence. [Comment to Article 4.2(a): The Use of the Prohibited Substance or Prohibited Method may be part of a necessary diagnostic investigation rather than a treatment per se.] b) The Therapeutic Use of the Prohibited Substance or Prohibited Method will not, on the balance of probabilities, produce any additional enhancement of performance beyond what might be anticipated by a return to the Athlete's normal state of health following the treatment of the medical condition. [Comment to Article 4.2(b): An Athlete's normal state of health will need to be determined on an individual basis. A normal state of health for a specific Athlete is their state of health, but for the medical condition for which the Athlete is seeking a TUE.] c) The Prohibited Substance or Prohibited Method is an indicated treatment for the medical condition, and there is no reasonable permitted Therapeutic alternative. [Comment to Article 4.2(c): The physician must explain why the treatment chosen was the most appropriate, eg, based on experience, side-effect profiles or other medical justifications, including, where applicable, geographically specific medical practice, and the ability to access the medication. Further, it is not always necessary to try and fail alternatives before using the Prohibited Substance or Prohibited Method.] d) The necessity for the Use of the Prohibited Substance or Prohibited Method is not a consequence, wholly or in part, of the prior Use (without a TUE) of a substance or method which was prohibited at the time of such Use. [Comment to Article 4.2: The WADA documents titled "TUE Physician Guidelines", posted on WADA's website, should be used to assist in the application of these criteria in relation to particular medical conditions. The granting of a TUE is based solely on consideration of the conditions set out in Article 4.2. It does not consider whether the prohibited substance or prohibited method is the most clinically appropriate or safe, or

whether its use is legal in all jurisdictions. When an International Federation or Major Event Organization TUEC is deciding whether or not to recognize a TUE granted by another Anti-Doping Organization (see Article 7), and when WADA is reviewing a decision to grant (or not to grant) a TUE (see Article 8), the issue will be the same as it is for a TUEC that is considering an application for a TUE under Article 6, i.e., has the athlete demonstrated on the balance of probabilities that each of the conditions set out in Article 4.2 is met?]."[2,3]

Specific Endocrine Conditions

1. Diabetes mellitus[2-4]

a. Diabetes is diagnosed if the patient satisfies any 1 of the following criteria and, as in all cases of type 1 diabetes, treatment involves regular injections of insulin. TUE Physician Guidelines Diabetes Mellitus:

   a. Fasting plasma glucose ≥126 mg/dL (≥7.0 mmol/L); 2-hour plasma glucose ≥200 mg/dL (≥11.1 mmol/L) during oral glucose tolerance testing
   b. Hemoglobin A_{1c} ≥6.5% (≥48 mmol/mol)
   c. In a patient with classic symptoms of hyperglycemia or hyperglycemic crisis, a random plasma glucose value ≥200 mg/dL (≥11.1 mmol/L)

b. The drug of choice is insulin, which may be administered in multiple ways with multiple forms of longer- or shorter-acting insulin analogues.

c. Monitoring of blood glucose levels in real time and over months is beyond the scope of this discussion.

2. Male hypogonadism[2-4]

a. Organic hypogonadism with testosterone deficiency is the focus of this discussion. Low circulating testosterone without a clear pathological cause, in this context, is not considered to be hypogonadism. TUEs for androgen (testosterone) deficiency should not be approved in women.

b. Medical history: organic hypogonadism is usually long-lasting or permanent, while functional reductions in circulating testosterone are potentially reversible.

c. Primary hypogonadism may be due to:

   a. Genetic abnormalities
   b. Developmental abnormalities
   c. Bilateral testicular trauma
   d. Bilateral testicular torsion
   e. Orchitis

d. Secondary hypogonadism may be due to:

   a. Genetic abnormalities of pituitary and hypothalamus
   b. Pituitary or hypothalamic tumors
   c. Other anatomical (structural), destructive, and infiltrative disorders of the pituitary or hypothalamus.

3. Organic defects in androgen action or production (differences in sex development [46,XY DSD])

a. 46,XY DSD due to androgen receptor defects ranges from males with complete androgen insensitivity (CAIS, formerly known as testicular feminization) who have a near-normal female phenotype to males with mild androgen insensitivity (MAIS) who have a near-normal male phenotype. Individuals with partial androgen insensitivity syndrome (PAIS) have an intermediate level of androgen sensitivity and clinical phenotype.

b. 46,XY DSD due to 5α-reductase type 2 deficiency (5ARD2) or 17β-hydroxysteroid dehydrogenase type 3 (17HSD3) in genetic males who have atypical genitalia at birth.

4. Constitutional delay of puberty is viewed as a special category since TUE may be approved for treatment with testosterone even if the etiology may be temporary and reversible.

Clinical Case Vignettes
Case 1

A 23-year-old paralympic track and field athlete who sustained a blast injury to his lower body while deployed with the US Army in Iraq presents for the diagnosis and treatment of potential hypogonadism. He had 1 lower limb and both testicles removed immediately following the injury. After several years of physical therapy and training, he has become an elite paralympic shot putter.

Since he understands that a TUE is required, he asks for an evaluation and treatment recommendations, specifically with reference to testosterone therapy. He currently receives testosterone enanthate, 75 mg weekly subcutaneously.

On physical examination, he is a muscular male with 1 leg missing and normal external genitalia and pubic hair except for no palpable testicular tissue in a flat scrotum.

Previous laboratory data obtained before testosterone replacement confirm the diagnosis of primary hypogonadism:

Testosterone = 54 ng/dL (SI: 1.9 nmol/L)
LH = 50.0 mIU/mL (SI: 50.0 IU/L)
FSH = 91.0 mIUm/L (SI: 91.0 IU/L)

Twice-yearly laboratory data show the following average values:

Testosterone = 600 ng/dL (SI: 20.8 nmol/L)
LH = 8.0 mIU/mL (SI: 8.0 IU/L)
FSH = 23.0 mIU/mL (SI: 23.0 IU/L)

Should this athlete obtain a TUE for testosterone?
This is a "yes" or "no" answer, and the rationale involves the answers to the questions noted under 4.2a-d.

4.2a. The athlete has met the criterion of a proper medical diagnosis of primary hypogonadism based on the history of the injury, the surgical removal of the damaged testes, and low testosterone levels with elevated gonadotropin levels.

4.2b. The issue of enhancement vs return to normal state of health can be met by longitudinal history relevant to adverse events and serial measurements of testosterone as part of the athlete's biological passport.

4.2c. Testosterone is the appropriate therapy for this condition, and there is no other non-banned drug since other anabolic steroid hormones are not permitted for a TUE.

4.2d. There is no evidence that prior anabolic steroid therapy was responsible for this athlete's medical condition based on the history of injury and the operative notes.

Case 2

A 15-year-old elite tennis player presents to her pediatrician with a 1-month history of increasing fatigue and polyuria. She also has new-onset nocturia and polydipsia. She and her coaches have noted a drop-off in her usual energy level and ability to train or play during matches. Since she has a family history of type 1 diabetes (T1D), her pediatrician measures capillary glucose, which is documented to be 270 mg/dL (15.0 nmol/L). She is referred to a pediatric endocrinologist for precise diagnosis and therapy. The history obtained shows worsening symptoms over the last week. She has lost 5 lb (2.3 kg), but she continues to have regular menstrual cycles (menarche was at age 12 years).

On physical examination, she is a slightly lethargic adolescent girl. Her height is at the 50th percentile, and weight is at the 30th percentile. Basal heart rate is 80 beats/min, and blood pressure is 105/68 mm Hg. The rest of the findings are within normal limits except for a mild decrease in skin turgor.

Laboratory test results:

Glucose = 310 mg/dL (SI: 17.2 nmol/L)
β-Hydroxybutyrate = 2.1 nmol/L
Hemoglobin A$_{1c}$ = 7.1% (54 mmol/mol)

Two of 5 antibodies related to T1D are positive.

Should this athlete receive a TUE for insulin given the diagnosis of T1D?
This is a "yes" or "no" answer, and the rationale involves the answers to the questions noted under 4.2a-d.

4.2a. The athlete has met the criteria for the diagnosis of T1D as outlined by WADA. She has the appropriate history, severely elevated blood glucose level, elevated hemoglobin A$_{1c}$ level, likely mild ketoacidosis, and 2 of 5 positive antibodies (for T1D).

4.2b. The issue of enhancement vs return to state of normal health is easy for T1D because excessive insulin therapy, which may clearly be anabolic, causes hypoglycemia. Longitudinal monitoring, as is noted in multiple Endocrine Society guidelines, is key to the short-term and long-term health of these athletes/patients, especially for children and adolescents with decades of expected survival.

4.2c. There are no nonbanned primary drugs for T1D. Insulin in its many forms is the appropriate treatment, and the treatment regimen must account for rest, training, and competition days to ensure optimal health without hypoglycemia.

4.2d. This is usually not a problem with patients who have T1D.

Case 3

A 15-and-0/12-year-old national-level female tennis player (and thus subject to anti-doping rules) with GH deficiency presents to discuss obtaining a TUE for testosterone. Menarche was at age 13 and 0/12 years. She is otherwise well except for seasonal allergies for which she takes an antihistamine. Her parents and only sibling are at the 75th percentile for height, and no other members of the extended family have significant short stature. She is a good student and is considering international tennis competition.

She initially presented to a pediatric endocrinologist at age 9 and 6/12 years for short stature and faltering growth, at which time her height was −2.5 SD and weight was at the 10th percentile. She was prepubertal. Screening laboratory values were within normal limits. Her IGF-1 level was −1 SD for age. Bone age was interpreted to be 7 and 0/12 years. An arginine-glucagon test for GH documented peaks at 4.5 and 3.7 ng/mL (standard stimulation test for GH, since its normal levels are pulsatile [up and down], and one must stimulate the pituitary gland to secrete the already-made GH).

GH deficiency was diagnosed, and treatment was initiated with recombinant human GH, 30 mcg/kg daily. Catch-up growth was evident after GH therapy was started.

At today's appointment, her height is at the 60th percentile and weight is at the 50th percentile. Examination findings are normal, with no dysmorphic features. Sexual development is Tanner stage 5 at a chronologic age of 15 and 0/12 years, her bone age is mature, and her IGF-1 value is +0.9 SD for age and sex.

Should this athlete obtain a TUE for GH?
This is a yes or no answer, and the rationale involves the answers to the questions noted under 4.2a-d.

4.2a. The athlete was short and slowly growing at the time GH deficiency was diagnosed at 9 and 6/12 years. Her weight plotted slightly higher than her height at initial evaluation. The IGF-1 value was −1 SD, and the response to provocative stimuli was in the range of GH deficiency. In retrospect, she had marked catch-up growth when she began GH therapy. GH deficiency in children is characterized by growth failure and (usually) short stature. The diagnosis is based on the clinical history and auxology buttressed by biochemical data to rule out other diseases (eg, celiac disease or inflammatory bowel disease, kidney failure). The key data are those of the GH-IGF-1 axis, including GH responses to 2 provocative stimuli. Imaging analysis includes bone age and brain MRI. More recently, genetic panels have become available for some GH-related causes of short stature and, importantly, for the much more common causes of short stature that do not involve the GH-IGF-1 axis, such as genetic disorders of the growth plate. Catch-up growth during GH therapy to nearly the

midparental height is biological evidence of GH deficiency.

4.2b. The issue of enhancement vs return to state of normal health involves absence of adverse events, height velocity, IGF-1 levels within the upper normal range, and no rapid acceleration of bone age.

4.2c. Human GH is the appropriate therapy whether administered daily or with some of the newer longer-acting products. As noted above, its efficacy should be determined mainly by change in height velocity and IGF-1 concentration.

4.2d. As is usual for children, most of the diagnoses that fulfill the WADA requirements are not the result of abuse of drugs or methods.

Key Learning Points

- The TUE process is in place to permit athletes with diagnosed conditions that require banned drugs or methods to compete on a level playing field with other athletes.

- The medical practitioner working with the athlete is required to present enough information that a diagnosis can be made and that there is a rationale for the prescription of a banned substance.

- The TUE committee (TUEC) reviewing the data does not examine the patient and thus it is the sum of the history, physical examination, and laboratory/imaging data that must be consistent with the medical diagnosis and can convince a panel of experts in the field (TUEC) that the diagnosis is correct.

- The TUEC does not practice medicine for the patient/athlete. While it may appear that therapy is not optimal, the TUEC does not have all of the information that the physician has. The treatment needs to be reasonable (to the TUEC) and meets the a-d requirements of section 4.2.

- Embedded within the TUE process is therapy monitoring, which can differ by condition and age. For example, the long-term follow-up of a patient with GH deficiency differs greatly whether the patient is at adult height. In fact, there are 3 separate WADA TUE physician guidelines for human GH: children and adults with GH deficiency and a new one for children/adolescents with short stature, but who are not GH deficient.

- The transition from adolescent to adult care may require additional evaluation or change in therapy. For example, managing GH deficiency when near-adult height is attained or managing testosterone therapy for someone with transient hypogonadotropic hypogonadism (usually constitutional delay of growth and puberty).

References

1. World Anti-Doping Agency. The World Anti-Doping Code. https://www.wada-ama.org/en/what-we-do/world-anti-doping-code. Accessed November 2024.
2. World Anti-Doping Agency. International Standards. https://www.wada-ama.org/en/what-we-do/international-standards. Accessed November 2024.
3. World Anti-Doping Agency. Prohibited List. https://www.wada-ama.org/en/resources/world-anti-doping-code-and-international-standards/prohibited-list. Accessed November 2024.
4. World Anti-Doping Agency. WADA Publishes Updated Therapeutic Use Exemption Physician Guidelines and Checklists Reflecting Changes Concerning Injectable Glucocorticoids. https://www.wada-ama.org/en/news/wada-publishes-updated-therapeutic-use-exemption-physician-guidelines-and-checklists. Accessed November 2024.

Perioperative Management of Pituitary Tumors

Whitney W. Woodmansee, MD, MA. University of Florida Neuroendocrine/Pituitary Program, Department of Medicine, Division of Endocrinology, Diabetes, and Metabolism, University of Florida, Gainesville, FL; Email: whitney.woodmansee@medicine.ufl.edu

Educational Objectives

After reviewing this chapter, learners should be able to:

- Recommend the preoperative evaluation that should be performed before surgery for all patients with pituitary tumors.

- Manage immediate postoperative endocrine disorders.

- Provide postoperative management recommendations for ongoing care.

Significance of the Clinical Problem

Pituitary lesions are relatively common in the general population with prevalence estimates that 10% to 20% of the population have a visible lesion on imaging.[1] Although the differential diagnosis of a sellar mass is broad, most lesions are benign pituitary adenomas (>90%).[2] Patients can present with a wide range of signs and symptoms depending on the size of the tumor and whether it is disrupting normal pituitary hormonal systems. Symptoms may be related to mass effects, such as headaches, visual loss, or cranial nerve abnormalities. Some individuals with pituitary tumors are completely asymptomatic, while others may present with symptoms related to either hormonal excess or deficiency. The evaluation of patients with pituitary tumors can be quite complex, as many symptoms are nonspecific. A multidisciplinary team approach

is needed for treatment planning and long-term management. Evaluation involves assessing the extent of tumor burden and pituitary hyperfunction or hypofunction and includes clinical exams, hormonal testing, visual testing, and brain imaging. Many pituitary tumors are treated with surgical removal, and all require preoperative, perioperative, and postoperative management with long-term, ongoing follow-up for hormonal management and monitoring for tumor recurrence.

Practice Gaps

- Some clinicians see a low volume of patients with pituitary tumors in their clinical practice and thus have minimal experience performing the necessary perioperative management.

- Many outpatient endocrine clinicians are unfamiliar with optimal management of inpatients' acute postoperative endocrine issues.

- The importance of long-term follow-up for assessment of endocrine function and tumor recurrence can be under-appreciated by patients and clinicians.

Discussion

Pituitary lesions are the second most common intracranial tumor and represent approximately 18% of brain tumors reported in the recent US Central Brain Tumor Registry analysis.[3] Although most sellar masses are benign pituitary adenomas, the differential diagnosis includes cystic lesions (Rathke cleft cyst, craniopharyngioma), inflammatory lesions (hypophysitis, sarcoidosis, amyloidosis), nonadenomatous neoplasms, metastases, and vascular etiologies (apoplexy).[1,2] Pituitary lesions can present with mass effects (headaches, visual loss, cranial nerve dysfunction) and pituitary hormonal hypersecretion or deficiency (*Box 1*). Although medical therapy is often considered first-line management for prolactinomas, surgery is generally considered the treatment of choice for other endocrine-active pituitary adenomas (acromegaly, Cushing disease, and thyrotrope adenomas), as well as clinically nonfunctioning adenomas, pituitary apoplexy, Rathke cleft cysts, craniopharyngiomas, and other parasellar lesions causing mass effects. The decision to proceed with neurosurgical tumor resection can be quite complex and is best considered in a multidisciplinary clinical setting.[4] Once the decision has been made to proceed, all patients require preoperative evaluation, perioperative monitoring in an inpatient setting, and long-term follow-up (*Box 2 and Figure 1*).

Box 1. General Approach to Pituitary Disorders

Approach to Pituitary Disorders
Evaluate:
- Mass effects
- Pituitary hyperfunction
  - Baseline and "Suppression tests"
- Pituitary hypofunction
  - Baseline and "Stimulation tests"

Box 2. Perioperative Management of Pituitary Adenomas

Preoperative Evaluation:
Assess for mass effect and pituitary function:
- Brain imaging and visual assessment
- Replace deficiencies as needed. (thyroid & cortisol most important)
- Assess for pituitary hormonal hyperfunction
- Stress dosing glucocorticoids if necessary

Early Perioperative Management:
Assess for surgical complications:
- General: infection, DVT/PE
- Neurologic: hemorrhage, visual, CSF leak
- Endocrine
  - AVP deficiency
  - SIADH
  - Adrenal insufficiency

Postoperative Management:
- Patients typically evaluated 1, 6, 12 weeks post operatively.
- MRI typically repeated at 8-12 weeks postoperatively to serve as new baseline
- Annual follow-up recommended for all or as dictated by clinic status:
  - Hormonal assessments
  - Imaging - MRI
  - Vision
- Long-term assessment of hormonal status and tumor recurrence required

Figure 1. Perioperative Management Flowchart for Pituitary Adenomas

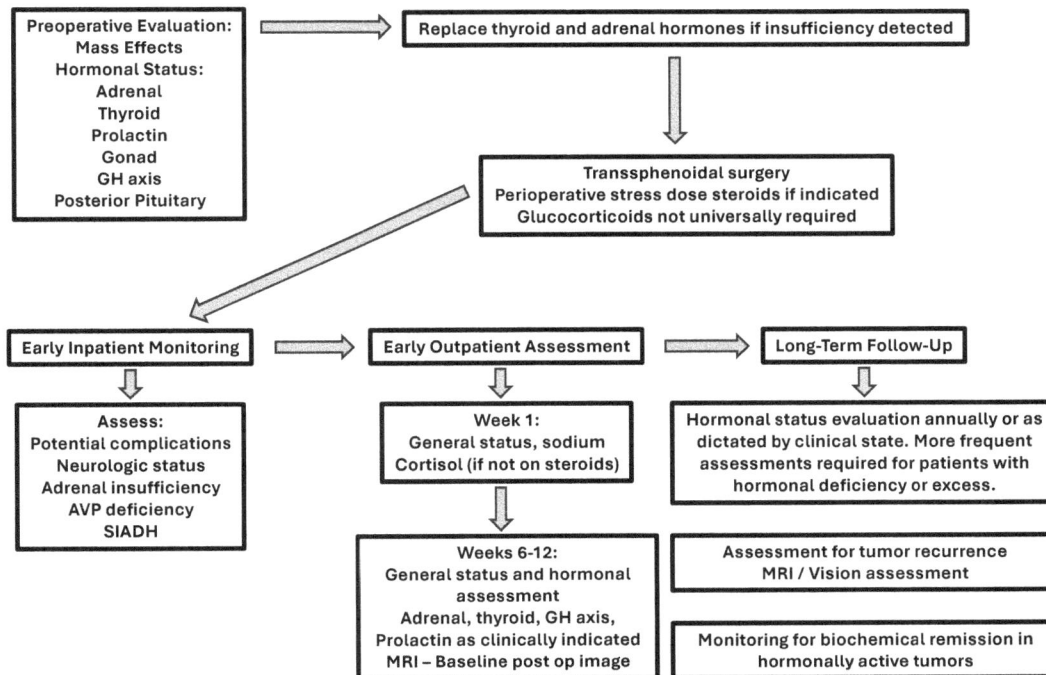

Preoperative Evaluation:
Mass Effects
Hormonal Status:
Adrenal
Thyroid
Prolactin
Gonad
GH axis
Posterior Pituitary

→ Replace thyroid and adrenal hormones if insufficiency detected

Transsphenoidal surgery
Perioperative stress dose steroids if indicated
Glucocorticoids not universally required

Early Inpatient Monitoring → Early Outpatient Assessment → Long-Term Follow-Up

Assess:
Potential complications
Neurologic status
Adrenal insufficiency
AVP deficiency
SIADH

Week 1:
General status, sodium
Cortisol (if not on steroids)

Weeks 6-12:
General status and hormonal assessment
Adrenal, thyroid, GH axis, Prolactin as clinically indicated
MRI – Baseline post op image

Hormonal status evaluation annually or as dictated by clinical state. More frequent assessments required for patients with hormonal deficiency or excess.

Assessment for tumor recurrence
MRI / Vision assessment

Monitoring for biochemical remission in hormonally active tumors

Adapted from Woodmansee WW et al. *Endocr Pract*, 2015; 21(7): 832-838. © Elsevier Inc.

Preoperative Evaluation

A full preoperative evaluation should include a thorough medical history, physical examination, laboratory testing, brain imaging, and neuro-ophthalmologic assessment with formal visual field testing if the lesion is close to the optic chiasm (*Box 2 and Figure 1*).[5,6] Assessment should include evaluation for signs and symptoms of pituitary hormonal deficiency or excess. It is critical to determine preoperatively if the lesion is a functional tumor (eg, prolactinoma, acromegaly, Cushing disease, or the rarely encountered thyrotropin-secreting tumor) or if any degree of hypopituitarism is present. Baseline laboratory testing of pituitary function should be performed in all patients. Typical preoperative baseline pituitary labs are listed in *Box 3* and include assessment of adrenal, thyroid, GH, prolactin, and reproductive axes. If Cushing disease or acromegaly is suspected, patients require more extensive confirmatory testing before consideration of surgical intervention. Prolactinomas are usually obvious based on prolactin levels, but sample dilution may be required in patients with large tumors and minimally elevated prolactin levels to rule out the "hook effect" that can occur in some laboratory assays, leading to artificially low prolactin levels.[7,8] In a recent Pituitary Society Delphi survey,[6] not all participants supported this preoperative laboratory assessment, citing the fact that the "hook effect" is less commonly observed with the newer automated prolactin immunoassays. However, not all clinicians have access to newer assays, so many

still recommend measurement of diluted prolactin in the setting of large tumors with mild prolactin elevation.[8] Confirmation of prolactinoma is an important diagnostic step, as this significantly affects treatment decisions.

Although neurologic assessment is critical for preoperative planning, it is also vital to assess and manage hypopituitarism preoperatively to achieve optimal outcomes. It is particularly important to identify deficiency of the adrenal and thyroid axes before surgery and to initiate replacement therapy preoperatively. Most patients with pituitary adenomas do not report signs or symptoms of arginine vasopressin (AVP) deficiency, but it is important to screen for the condition by taking an appropriate history (ask about thirst, polydipsia, polyuria). Measurement of serum electrolytes and urine specific gravity can also alert the clinician to this condition. Patients with adrenal insufficiency, hypothyroidism, and AVP deficiency should all receive replacement therapy before surgery. Preoperative replacement of gonadal hormones and GH is not required and can be considered later in the postoperative period.

All patients should also have their health optimized from a general medical standpoint and should be evaluated for other potential comorbidities. Individuals with acromegaly and Cushing disease are particularly prone to associated conditions, such as hypertension, cardiac dysfunction, hyperlipidemia, and diabetes, and thus benefit from preoperative medical management. It is recommended that thromboprophylaxis be considered for patients with Cushing disease.[9,10] There is no current consensus regarding preoperative disease-specific treatment of hyperfunctioning tumors to improve surgical cure rates or outcomes, but optimization of medical therapy for associated comorbidities may reduce perioperative complications and promote general postoperative recovery.[6,11,12]

Box 3. Standard Pituitary Laboratory Tests

Standard Pituitary Laboratory Tests

- Adrenal
  - ACTH, Cortisol

- Thyroid
  - TSH, Free T_4

- Reproductive
  - Prolactin (with dilution if macroadenoma)
  - FSH, LH, testosterone (men) or estradiol (women)

- GH
  - IGF-I, GH

| Critical to assess prolactin prior proceeding to surgery |
| Extra tests required if GH or ACTH excess or deficiency is suspected. |

Perioperative Management

All patients with preoperatively identified adrenal insufficiency and hypothyroidism require hormone replacement therapy before surgery. Adrenal-insufficient patients should receive stress-dosing glucocorticoids on the day of surgery and taper postoperatively to presurgical home doses as clinical status allows. For patients with normal preoperative adrenal function, there is no clear consensus on administration of glucocorticoids perioperatively. Perioperative steroids are a common component of pituitary surgical care with the goal to treat or prevent potential iatrogenic adrenal insufficiency and they may reduce edema. However, many centers follow a steroid-sparing protocol both perioperatively and postoperatively to avoid unnecessary glucocorticoid exposure. The literature suggests that withholding perioperative steroids in patients with known intact hypothalamic-pituitary-adrenal function can be an acceptable approach with appropriate clinical monitoring.[13,14]

Postoperative Management

Postoperative management occurs in 2 general phases: the immediate inpatient postoperative period and the longer-term outpatient follow-up that includes the early outpatient evaluation and chronic disease management and monitoring for recurrence.

Immediate Postoperative Management

Patients are generally monitored for immediate postoperative complications in an intensive care unit setting with close observation for potential surgical or endocrine complications. Fortunately, serious complications following pituitary adenoma surgery are relatively uncommon, particularly with an experienced surgical team.[15,16] The most serious early surgical complications include sellar hematoma, meningitis, CSF leakage, sinusitis, and epistaxis. Patients should be monitored closely for potential neurologic or ophthalmologic changes and urgent imaging should be performed if deterioration is detected.

The most important potential endocrine complications in the immediate postoperative period are fluid and electrolyte abnormalities and acute adrenal insufficiency. AVP/antidiuretic hormone insufficiency or excess (syndrome of syndrome of inappropriate antidiuretic hormone secretion [SIADH]) is not uncommon, and patients require close monitoring of fluid intake, urine output, and volume status, along with serial sodium and urine specific gravity or osmolality.[17] AVP deficiency most often develops within the first 48 hours after pituitary surgery and occurs in up to 25% of patients.[17] Fortunately, AVP deficiency is usually transient with only 2% to 5% of cases becoming permanent.[18,19] It is thought to occur from manipulation, traction, or disruption of the pituitary stalk during tumor removal leading to interruption of AVP release. It is more common in patients undergoing surgery for Rathke cleft cysts or craniopharyngiomas.[19] AVP deficiency can be managed with desmopressin (DDAVP), and since this condition is usually temporary, standing scheduled DDAVP doses are not recommended. Patients may also develop isolated SIADH leading to symptomatic and delayed hyponatremia.[20] It is recommended that sodium levels be checked every few days for 7 to 10 days to avoid missing delayed hyponatremia in the outpatient setting. Mild hyponatremia (ie, 130-135 mEq/L [130-135 mmol/L]) may be managed by fluid restriction as an outpatient, but severe or symptomatic hyponatremia (sodium typically <125 mEq/L [<125 mmol/L]) requires hospitalization for more aggressive management.

Finally, the clinician should be aware of the critical need to monitor adrenal function and replace glucocorticoids if deficiency is detected. As previously noted, there is a lack of consensus regarding glucocorticoid management in the perioperative and postoperative timeframes, ranging from glucocorticoid treatment at surgery with gradual tapering to steroid-sparing protocols with careful observation. Some clinicians choose to empirically treat all patients perioperatively with glucocorticoids at stress doses and others withhold glucocorticoids in patients with normal preoperative adrenal function. In the latter scenario, it is recommended that serial morning cortisol levels be monitored and glucocorticoids be initiated if the value is consistent with insufficiency. While measurement of basal morning cortisol is only suggestive of and not diagnostic of adrenal insufficiency, various cut points have been proposed, below which glucocorticoid replacement should be considered. Proposed cut points for guidance in management are based on studies that suggest a high likelihood of adrenal insufficiency with a morning cortisol level less than 5 μg/dL (<137.9 nmol/L) and low likelihood if the level is above 10 to 15 μg/dL (275.9-413.8 nmol/L).[21,22] There is no best approach, and many factors must be considered for an individual patient, but minimizing unnecessary glucocorticoid exposure is generally desired. If glucocorticoids are initiated in the perioperative period based on morning cortisol levels dropping below a specified cut point, then physiological replacement therapy should be maintained until further provocative testing (approximately 6 weeks postoperatively) can be performed to assess long-term replacement needs.

Finally, in patients with functional tumors, it is important to assess early biochemical remission following surgery.[6] For patients with acromegaly, Cushing disease, and prolactinomas, morning measurement of GH,[23] cortisol,[9,11] and prolactin,[24] respectively, on postoperative days 1 and 2 has been shown to be moderately predictive of early and long-term remission. In patients with acromegaly, IGF-1 levels should be measured 6 weeks postoperatively, and, if elevated, should be remeasured at 12 weeks before determining further interventions. After hospital discharge, patients are followed in the clinic and screened for potential surgical complications. As follow-up progresses in the ensuing months, the most active issues are usually related to pituitary function assessment and management (*Box 2 and Figure 1*) with either hormonal replacement of deficiencies (*Box 4*)[25] or ongoing assessment for biochemical remission in cases of hormonal excess.

Box 4. Management of Hypopituitarism

Hypopituitarism
Management

- Treatment based on correcting hormonal deficiencies.
  - *Thyroid* - levothyroxine (remember TSH cannot guide Rx, monitor free T_4 levels)
  - *Adrenal* – Hydrocortisone (preferred), prednisone. Use lowest dosage possible to control symptoms, avoid over or under replacement.
    - Central AI patients rarely need mineralocorticoid replacement.
    - Patients require education about stress dosing for illness
  - *Gonad* - Men often require testosterone, women may require HRT (OCP)
  - *Growth hormone* - Can treat with rhGH
  - *Prolactin* - no replacement available.
  - *Posterior pituitary* – Desmopressin (DDAVP)
    - Patient educated to drink to thirst. DDAVP primarily controls polyuria if thirst mechanism is intact. If thirst mechanism not functional, will need DDAVP and water intake recommendations
- Medical Alert Jewelry, especially if adrenal insufficiency

Early Postoperative Management (1-12 weeks)

It is generally recommended that all patients undergo a repeat full evaluation of pituitary function 6 to 12 weeks after surgery (*Figure 1*). As in the preoperative evaluation, all anterior pituitary hormonal axes are generally reevaluated to assess pituitary function integrity. Specifically, thyroid, adrenal, gonadal, and GH axes should be reassessed. Occasionally preoperative hormonal deficiencies recover after tumor resection.[26] Patients should be evaluated for hypothyroidism 6 to 8 weeks after surgery (timing based on the half-life of thyroid hormone). Adrenal function should be evaluated in all patients. If a patient was treated with glucocorticoids perioperatively, the long-term need for replacement therapy should be reassessed. If the screening morning cortisol value is not sufficient to rule out adrenal insufficiency (ie, >15 μg/dL [>413.8 nmol/L]), then dynamic endocrine testing for adrenal insufficiency should be performed (usually cosyntropin-stimulation test). Ongoing assessments are performed in functional tumors to determine biochemical remission persistence. GH and reproductive function are evaluated, and consideration for replacement therapy is performed at variable times after surgery. A postoperative MRI to serve as a new baseline image is typically obtained 8 to 12 weeks postoperatively to allow resolution of acute postoperative changes.

Long-Term Postoperative Management (Ongoing and Lifelong)

Periodic clinical assessment in the first year after surgery is dictated by the clinical status of the patient and the need for titration of hormonal replacement therapy or treatment of any persistent pituitary hormonal hyperfunction (*Box 4*). Generally, all patients are followed at least on an annual basis for evaluation of pituitary function. Since most pituitary adenomas grow very slowly, frequency of postoperative imaging must be tailored to the individual patient.[27,28] Imaging timing is dictated by consideration of patient and tumor characteristics, with larger, more aggressive tumors typically imaged at closer intervals than smaller, more stable microadenomas. Pituitary imaging for patients with hormonally hyperfunctioning tumors depends on tumor type, biochemical parameters, and overall disease activity. The main point to impress upon patients and clinicians is that all pituitary tumors, although usually benign, require long-term monitoring for pituitary function and tumor progression or recurrence. Long-term follow-up is critical, and patients require an individualized multimodality treatment program.

Clinical Case Vignettes

Case 1

A 69-year-old man with a history of hypertension, aortic stenosis, hyperlipidemia, nephrolithiasis, and prediabetes is referred for evaluation of a large sellar mass. He initially presented with vision loss and diplopia. He underwent cataract surgery last year with suboptimal vision improvement. He was seen by a retinal specialist who ordered MRI, revealing a large pituitary mass. He was then referred for further evaluation.

He reports headaches in addition to vision loss and acknowledges cold intolerance, mild constipation, and fatigue. He developed erectile dysfunction 8 years ago, and a low testosterone level was documented 2 years ago. He received testosterone replacement, but this was discontinued due to a rising PSA level. He has no symptoms of hypercortisolism or acromegaly. His medications are amlodipine and metformin.

Physical examination is notable only for bilateral visual field deficits.

Pituitary MRI demonstrates a 1.6 × 2.4 × 3.1-cm mass that compresses the optic chiasm and invades the right cavernous sinus (*Figure 2*). Preoperative formal visual field testing confirms bitemporal hemianopsia.

Figure 2.

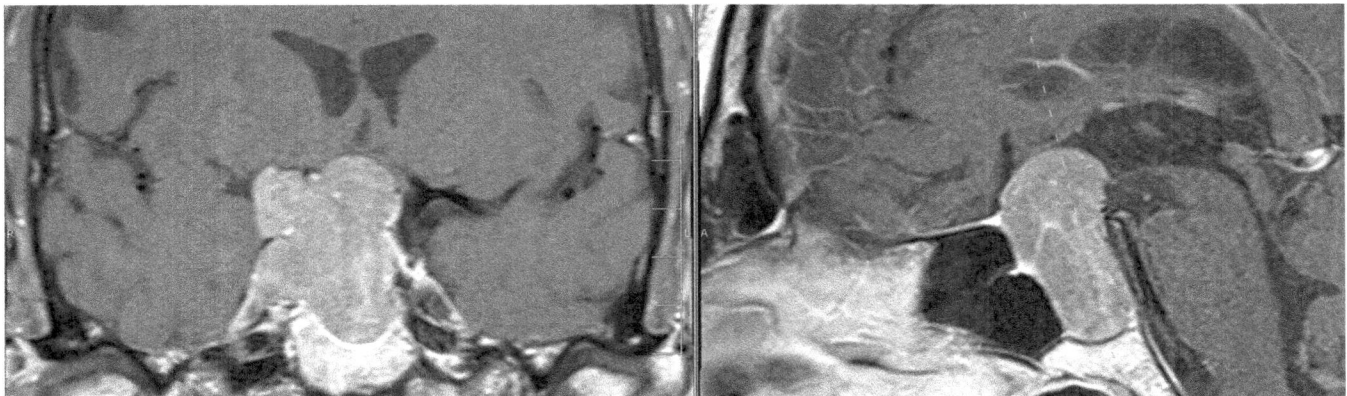

T1 postcontrast MRI demonstrating a large lobulated sellar mass invading the right cavernous sinus and compressing the optic chiasm.

[Color—Print (Color Gallery page CG14) or web & ePub editions]

Preoperative laboratory test results (sample drawn while fasting at 8:00 AM):

> Comprehensive chemistry panel (including sodium, kidney function, and liver function), normal
> Complete blood cell count, normal
> ACTH = 20.0 pg/mL (7.2-63.3 pg/mL) (SI: 4.4 pmol/L [1.6-13.9 pmol/L])
> Cortisol = 12.8 μg/dL (6.2-19.4 μg/dL) (SI: 353.1 nmol/L [171.0-535.2 nmol/L])
> TSH (third-generation assay) = 2.43 mIU/L (0.40-5.00 mIU/L)
> Free T$_4$ = 0.59 ng/dL (0.60-1.20 ng/dL) (SI: 7.59 pmol/L [7.72-15.44 pmol/L])
> Prolactin = 8.9 ng/mL (2.0-18.0 ng/mL) (SI: 0.39 nmol/L [0.09-0.78 nmol/L])
> FSH = 3.6 mIU/mL (1.0-19.0 mIU/mL) (SI: 3.8 IU/L [1.0-19.0 IU/L])
> LH = 1.6 mIU/mL (1.2-8.6 mIU/mL) (SI: 1.6 IU/L [1.2-8.6 IU/L])
> Testosterone = 82.0 ng/dL (230.0-800.0 ng/dL) (SI: 2.8 nmol/L [8.0-27.8 nmol/L])
> IGF-1 = 81 ng/mL (40-225 ng/mL) (SI: 10.61 nmol/L [5.24-29.48 nmol/L])
> Hemoglobin A$_{1c}$ = 6.1% (<5.7%) (43 mmol/mol [<39 mmol/mol])

Surgical resection is recommended given the large tumor size and impact on his vision.

Which of the following laboratory tests should be performed before considering surgery in this patient?

A. GH measurement

B. Oral glucose tolerance test

C. Diluted prolactin measurement

D. α-Subunit measurement

Answer: C) Diluted prolactin measurement

Many endocrinologists recommend measuring diluted prolactin (Answer C) in patients with macroadenomas to rule out the "hook effect" that can occur in some laboratory assays.[6-8,27] The "hook effect" results when the prolactin in the patient's serum is extremely high and in excess to the assay antibodies used to measure levels in vitro, and it can lead to artificially lower prolactin measurements. Accurate assessment of prolactin levels is imperative to help dictate treatment planning. This patient's prolactin measured

with serial dilution confirmed he did not have a prolactinoma.

GH can be measured preoperatively, but this is a pulsatile hormone and IGF-1 is the preferred hormone for assessing acromegaly preoperatively. Oral glucose tolerance testing is not required in this patient given that he already has a known diagnosis of prediabetes. This test would also not be needed to assess GH suppression following an oral glucose load given that his IGF-1 level was not elevated and clinically there was no concern for acromegaly. Finally, α-subunit can be measured, but its clinical utility does not add to this patient's management.

Case 1, Continued

Surgery is recommended for this patient due to large tumor size and his vision compromise. His laboratory tests confirm central hypogonadism and hypothyroidism. He is preoperatively started on levothyroxine replacement. His preoperative cortisol level suggests that his adrenal axis is functional, but he is started on preoperative empiric glucocorticoid replacement therapy to prevent the possibility that treating his central hypothyroidism will unmask adrenal insufficiency.

Immediate postoperative inpatient monitoring should include measurement of which of the following?

A. Daily fasting morning cortisol

B. Prolactin

C. Testosterone

D. Serial sodium and urine specific gravity

E. GH

Answer: D) Serial sodium and urine specific gravity

Perioperative monitoring for sodium disorders, including hypernatremia and hyponatremia, is critical in the postoperative period. Patients can develop AVP deficiency or SIADH in the early postoperative period. Monitoring sodium levels and urine specific gravity and/or urine osmolality and recording accurate oral fluid intake and urine output is recommended in the 24 to 72 hours immediately after surgery. Exact duration of intense monitoring depends on the patient, but it should usually be done at least for the first 24 to 48 hours and then periodically for the first 7 to 10 days after surgery. Most cases of AVP deficiency are transient and can be managed with on-demand desmopressin. Standing desmopressin doses are not recommended given the mostly transient nature (>95%)[19] of postoperative AVP deficiency.

Case 2

A 63-year-old man presents with concerns of progressive muscle weakness and fatigue. He was successfully treated for Cushing disease at age 35 years with transsphenoidal pituitary tumor resection. He has been on hormonal replacement therapy for panhypopituitarism since surgery, including levothyroxine, testosterone, and glucocorticoids (low-dosage prednisone). He notes having progressive weakness for the last several years. Earlier evaluations revealed deficiencies of vitamin B_{12} and vitamin D, but supplementation did not significantly improve symptoms. He had 2 episodes of unprovoked deep venous thrombosis with pulmonary embolism and developed a left biceps tear that required hospital admission. During admission, his muscle weakness was exacerbated by immobility, and he was subsequently referred to endocrinology for consideration of steroid-induced myopathy. At today's evaluation, he is able to ambulate with a walker but is unable to climb stairs or drive a car and requires assistance with activities of daily living. His only other symptoms are fatigue and insomnia.

Laboratory test results after holding prednisone:

ACTH = 128 pg/mL (6-50 pg/mL) (SI: 28.2 pmol/L [1.3-11.0 pmol/L])
Cortisol = 31.7 μg/dL (4.0-22.0 μg/dL) (SI: 875.5 nmol/L [110.3-606.9 nmol/L])
TSH (third-generation assay) = 0.01 mIU/L (0.40-5.00 mIU/L)
Free T_4 = 1.5 ng/dL (0.80-1.80 ng/dL) (SI: 19.3 pmol/L [10.30-23.17 pmol/L])
Prolactin = 4.9 ng/mL (2.0-18.0 ng/mL) (SI: 0.21 nmol/L [0.09-0.78 nmol/L])

FSH = <0.7 mIU/mL (1.0-19.0 mIU/mL) (SI: <0.7 IU/L [1.0-19.0 IU/L])
LH = <0.2 mIU/mL (1.2-8.6 mIU/mL) (SI: <0.2 IU/L [1.2-8.6 IU/L])
Testosterone = 85.0 ng/dL (230.0-800.0 ng/dL) (SI: 2.9 nmol/L [8.0-27.8 nmol/L])
IGF-1 = 55 ng/mL (41-279 ng/mL) (SI: 7.21 nmol/L [5.37-36.55 nmol/L])
Hemoglobin A_{1c} = 6.8% (<5.7%) (51 mmol/mol [<39 mmol/mol])

Given this patient's laboratory results and clinical presentation, what should be the initial approach to assess recurrent hypercortisolism after stopping prednisone?

A. Recheck cortisol and ACTH levels

B. Perform pituitary MRI

C. Perform 1 or more screening tests for hypercortisolism (eg, late-night salivary cortisol, 1-mg overnight dexamethasone-suppression test, and/or 24-hour urinary free cortisol with creatinine)

D. Perform inferior petrosal sinus sampling

E. Perform PET

Answer: C) Perform 1 or more screening tests for hypercortisolism (eg, late-night salivary cortisol, 1-mg overnight dexamethasone-suppression test, and/or 24-hour urinary free cortisol with creatinine)

One or more of the typical screening tests can be performed to confirm hypercortisolism (Answer C), and this should be the next step before other laboratory tests or additional imaging. It would be reasonable to simultaneously perform pituitary MRI since the patient has known history of confirmed Cushing disease, but the best answer in this case is to evaluate for recurrent hypercortisolism to determine the best treatment course.

Case 2, Continued

Prednisone is discontinued, and hypercortisolism is confirmed by a 1-mg overnight dexamethasone-suppression test that demonstrates lack of appropriate cortisol suppression and elevated 24-hour urinary free cortisol excretion. MRI confirms recurrent tumor (1.2 × 0.8 × 1.3 cm) extending into the right cavernous sinus (*Figure 3*). The patient undergoes repeat transsphenoidal tumor resection, and pathology confirms recurrent corticotrope adenoma. Postoperatively, he is in biochemical remission and there is no evidence of residual tumor on imaging.

What is the most sensitive test to monitor for recurrent hypercortisolism?

A. Fasting morning cortisol and ACTH measurement

B. 24-hour urinary free cortisol measurement

C. 1-mg overnight dexamethasone-suppression test

D. Late-night salivary cortisol level measurement (2-3 samples)

Answer: D) Late-night salivary cortisol measurement (2-3 samples)

All patients with pituitary tumors require long-term follow-up to monitor for recurrence or progression of residual disease. It is particularly important to follow patients with Cushing syndrome, as recurrence is associated with many comorbidities related to hypercortisolism. Although there is heterogeneity in presentation, it has been shown that late-night salivary cortisol levels (Answer D) tend to become abnormal earlier than other tests in cases of recurrent Cushing syndrome.[11,29,30] Unfortunately, this patient experienced a second recurrence 2 years later and was treated with radiation and medical therapy. This case highlights that patients with Cushing disease can have late recurrences and require long-term monitoring for return of hypercortisolism, even in cases of previous panhypopituitarism.

Key Learning Points

- Pituitary adenomas are relatively common, and diagnosis and treatment planning generally require a multidisciplinary team approach.

- All patients with pituitary tumors require full pituitary hormonal, visual, and brain imaging evaluations to help determine the best personalized treatment course. For many patients, surgical removal is the treatment of choice and, as such, they require care in the preoperative, perioperative, and postoperative periods.

- All patients with pituitary tumors require long-term follow-up for management and monitoring of hormonal status and tumor progression or recurrence.

Figure 3.

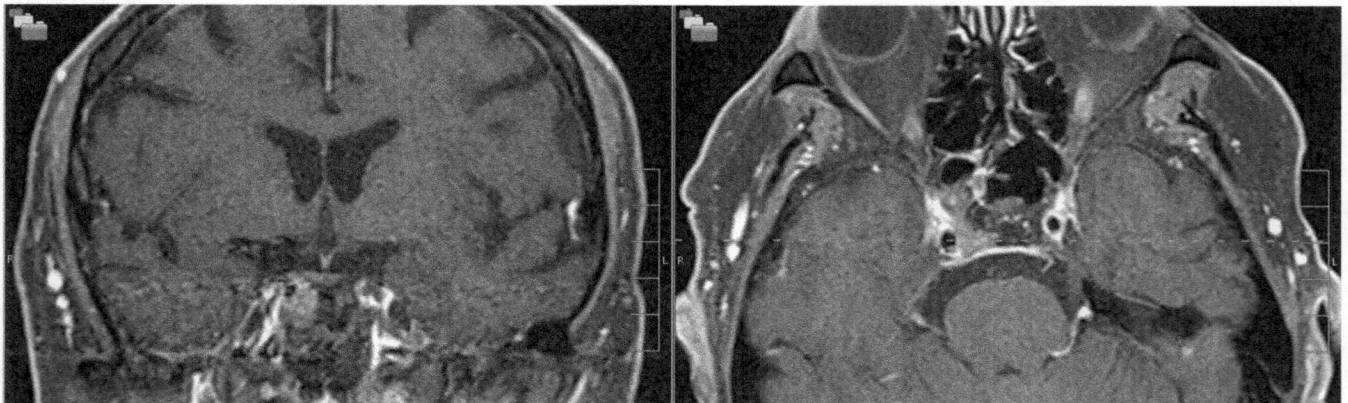

T1 postcontrast MRI demonstrating recurrent tumor invading the right cavernous sinus.

[Color—Print (Color Gallery page CG15) or web & ePub editions]

References

1. Giraldi E, Allen JW, Ioachimescu AG. Pituitary incidentalomas: best practices and looking ahead. *Endocr Pract*. 2023;29(1):60-68. PMID: 36270609

2. Freda PU, Post KD. Differential diagnosis of sellar masses. *Endocrinol Metab Clin North Am*. 1999;28(1):81-117. PMID: 10207686

3. Ostrom QT, Price M, Neff C, et al. CBTRUS statistical report: primary brain and other central nervous system tumors diagnosed in the United States in 2015-2019. *Neuro Oncol*. 2022;24(Suppl 5):v1-v95. PMID: 36196752

4. McLaughlin N, Laws ER, Oyesiku NM, Katznelson L, Kelly DF. Pituitary centers of excellence. *Neurosurgery*. 2012;71(5):916-924. PMID: 22902334

5. Woodmansee WW, Carmichael J, Kelly D, Katznelson L; AACE Neuroendocrine and Pituitary Scientific Committee. American Association of Clinical Endocrinologists and American College of Endocrinology disease state clinical review: postoperative management following pituitary surgery. *Endocrine Practice*, 2015;21(7):832-838. PMID: 26172128

6. Tritos NA, Fazeli PK, McCormack A, et al; Pituitary Society Delphi Collaborative Group. Pituitary Society Delphi Survey: an international perspective on endocrine management of patients undergoing transsphenoidal surgery for pituitary adenomas. *Pituitary*. 2022;25(1):64-73. PMID: 34283370

7. Melmed S, Casanueva FF, Hoffman AR, et al. Diagnosis and treatment of hyperprolactinemia: an Endocrine Society clinical practice guideline. *J Clin Endocrinol Metab*. 2011;96(2):273-288. PMID: 21296991

8. Mahmoud MM, Haj-Ahmad LM, Sweis NWG et al. Clinical features and hormonal profile of macroprolactinomas presenting with the hook effect: a systematic review. *Endocr Pract*. 2025;31(2) 215-225. PMID: 39542401

9. Varlamov EV, Vila G, Fleseriu M. Perioperative management of Cushing disease. *J Endocr Soc*. 2022;6(3):bvac010. PMID: 35178493

10. Isand K, Arima H, Bertherat J, et al. Delphi panel consensus on recommendations for thromboprophylaxis of venous thromboembolism in endogenous Cushing's syndrome: a position statement. *Eur J Endocrinol*. 2025;192(3):R17-R27. PMID: 39973025

11. Fleseriu M, Auchus R, Bancos I, et al. Consensus on diagnosis and management of Cushing's disease: a guideline update. *Lancet Diabetes Endocrinol*. 202;9(12):847-875. PMID: 34687601

12. Papaioannou C, Druce M. Preoperative medical treatments and surgical approaches for acromegaly: A systematic review. *Clin Endocrinol (Oxf)*. 2022;98(1):14-31. PMID: 35726150

13. Guo X, Zhang D, Pang H, et al; ZS-2608 Trial Team. Safety of withholding perioperative hydrocortisone for patients with pituitary adenomas with an intact hypothalamus-pituitary-adrenal axis: a randomized clinical trial. *JAMA Netw Open*. 2022;5(11):e2242221. PMID: 36383383

14. Batista S, Almeida JA, Koester S, et al. Safety of withholding perioperative steroids for patients with pituitary resection with an intact hypothalamus-pituitary-adrenal axis: ameta-analysis of randomized clinical trials. *Clin Neurol Neurosurg*. 2023;234:107974. PMID: 37797363

15. Barker FG 2nd, Klibanski A, Swearingen B. Transsphenoidal surgery for pituitary tumors in the United States, 1996-2000: mortality, morbidity, and the effects of hospital and surgeon volume. *J Clin Endocrinol Metab*. 2003;88(10):4709-4719. PMID: 14557445

16. Shahlaie K, McLaughlin N, Kassam AB, Kelly DF. The role of outcomes data for assessing the expertise of a pituitary surgeon. *Curr Opin Endocrinol Diabetes Obes*. 2010;17(4):369-376. PMID: 20453648

17. Loh JA, Verbalis JG. Diabetes insipidus as a complication after pituitary surgery. *Nat Clin Pract Endocrinol Metab*. 2007;3(6):489-494. PMID: 17515893

18. Nemergut EC, Zuo Z, Jane JA Jr, Laws ER Jr. Predictors of diabetes insipidus after transsphenoidal surgery: a review of 881 patients. *J Neurosurg*. 2005;103(3):448-454. PMID: 16235676

19. Burke WT, Cote DJ, Penn DL et al. Diabetes insipidus after endoscopic transsphenoidal surgery. *Neurosurgery*. 2020;87(5):949-955. PMID: 32503055

20. Hensen J, Henig A, Fahlbusch R, Meyer M, Boehnert M, Buchfelder M. Prevalence, predictors and patterns of postoperative polyuria and hyponatremia in the immediate course after transsphenoidal surgery for pituitary adenomas. *Clin Endocrinol (Oxf)*. 1999;50(4):431-439. PMID: 10468901

21. Marko NF, Hamrahian AH, Weil RJ. Immediate postoperative cortisol levels accurately predict postoperative hypothalamic-pituitary-adrenal axis function after transsphenoidal surgery for pituitary tumors. *Pituitary*. 2010;13(3):249-255. PMID: 20339931

22. McLaughlin N, Cohan P, Barnett P, Eisenberg A, Chaloner C, Kelly DF. Early morning cortisol levels as predictors of short-term and long-term adrenal function after endonasal transsphenoidal surgery for pituitary adenomas and Rathke's cleft cysts. *World Neurosurg*. 2013;80(5):569-575. PMID: 22902358

23. Krieger MD, Couldwell WT, Weiss MH. Assessment of long-term remission of acromegaly following surgery. *J Neurosurg*. 2003;98(4):719-724. PMID: 12691394

24. Amar AP, Couldwell WT, Chen JC, Weiss MH. Predictive value of serum prolactin levels measured immediately after transsphenoidal surgery. *J Neurosurg*. 2002;97(2):307-314. PMID: 12186458

25. Fleseriu M, Christ-Crain M, Langlois F, Gadelha M, Melmed S. Hypopituitarism. *Lancet*. 2024;403(10444):2632-2648. PMID: 38735295

26. Laws ER, Iuliano SL, Cote DJ, Woodmansee WW, Hsu L, Cho CH. A benchmark for preservation of normal pituitary function after endoscopic transsphenoidal surgery for pituitary macroadenomas. *World Neurosurgery*. 2016;91:371-375. PMID: 27113402

27. Tritos NA, Miller KK. Diagnosis and management of pituitary adenomas: a review. *JAMA*. 2023;329(16):1386-1398. PMID: 37097352

28. Constantinescua SM, Thierry Duprezb T, Bonnevillec JF, Maitera D. How often should we perform magnetic resonance imaging (MRI) for the follow-up of pituitary adenoma? *Ann Endocrinol (Paris)*. 2024;85(4):300-307. PMID: 38604408

29. Amlashi FG, Swearingen B, Faje AT, et al. Accuracy of late-night salivary cortisol in evaluating postoperative remission and recurrence in Cushing's disease. *J Clin Endocrinol Metab*. 2015;100(10):3770-3777. PMID: 26196950

30. Carroll TB, Javorsky BR, Findling JW. Postsurgical recurrent Cushing disease: clinical benefit of early intervention in patients with normal urinary free cortisol. *Endocr Pract*. 2016;22(10):1216-1223. PMID: 27409817

Additional Reading

- Ezzat S, Asa SL, Couldwell WT, et al. The prevalence of pituitary adenomas: a systematic review. *Cancer*. 2004;101(3):613-619. PMID: 15274075

- Scangas GA, Laws ER Jr. Pituitary incidentalomas *Pituitary*. 2014;17(5):486-491. PMID: 240522242

- Melmed S. Pituitary-tumor endocrinopathies. *N Engl J Med*. 2020;382(10):937-950. PMID: 32130815

- Fleseriu M, Lee M, Pineyro MM, et al. Giant invasive pituitary prolactinoma with falsely low serum prolactin: the significance of "hook effect." *J Neurooncol*. 2006;79(1):41-43. PMID: 16598425

- Vilar L, Vilar CF, Lyra R et al. Pitfalls in the diagnostic evaluation of hyperprolactinemia. *Neuroendocrinology*. 2019;109(1):7-19. PMID: 30889571

- Ben-Shlomo A, Melmed S. Clinical review 154: the role of pharmacotherapy in perioperative management of patients with acromegaly. *J Clin Endocrinol Metab*. 2003;88(3):963-968. PMID: 12629068

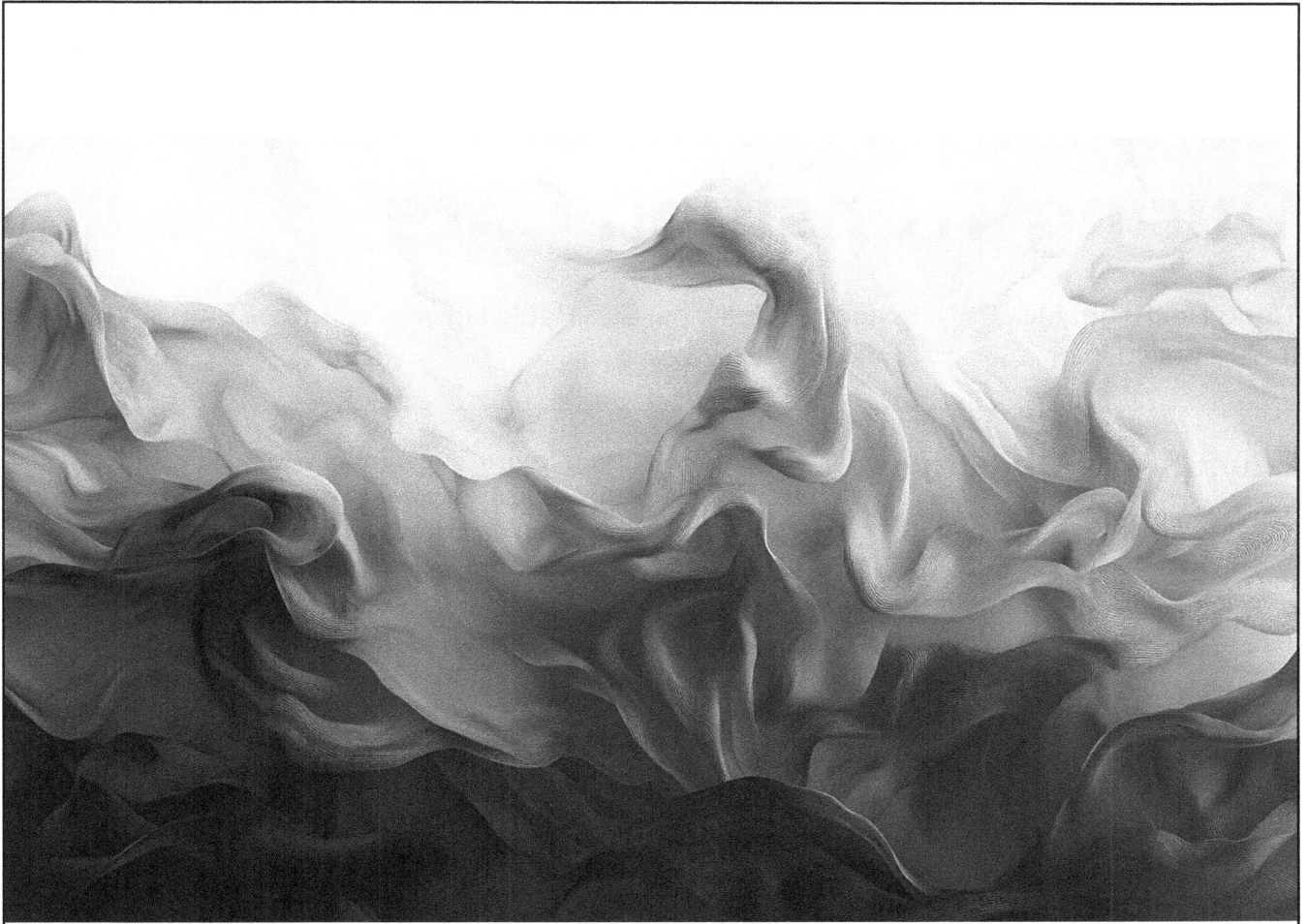

PEDIATRIC AND ADOLESCENT ENDOCRINOLOGY

Management of Patients With Congenital Adrenal Hyperplasia During Transition Care

Tânia Bachega, MD, PhD. School of Medicine, Sao Paulo University, Brazil; Email: tbachega@usp.br

Educational Objectives

After reviewing this chapter, learners should be able to:

- Highlight the importance of properly organizing the transition care of patients with congenital adrenal hyperplasia (CAH) in an individualized manner to ensure continuity of follow-up.

- Identify key points that should be evaluated in the transition care process, including glucocorticoid replacement therapy and comorbidities.

- Educate patients and their families about CAH, emphasizing measures to prevent adrenal crisis.

Significance of the Clinical Problem

CAH due to 21-hydroxylase deficiency is one of the most common autosomal recessive disorders and is characterized by impaired cortisol secretion. Depending on the degree of 21-hydroxylase impairment, aldosterone secretion may also be severely compromised, leading to adrenal insufficiency and salt-wasting crisis in the first weeks of life. In parallel, increased ACTH levels, secondary to loss of negative feedback of cortisol, result in excessive androgen secretion. This leads to prenatal external genital virilization in females and postnatal virilization in both sexes. In the simple virilizing form of CAH, some degree of residual enzyme activity may be sufficient to maintain aldosterone production; however, patients remain at risk of developing adrenal crises, particularly during stress conditions. The most severe cases of CAH are classified as the salt-wasting form, depending on the presence of hyponatremic dehydration and/or shock in the neonatal period. The classic forms are the most common cause of atypical genitalia in newborns with a 46,XX karyotype and of primary adrenal insufficiency in childhood.[1]

CAH is classified as a rare disease since it affects approximately 1:10,000 to 1:18,000 live births.[2] Therefore, in the absence of neonatal screening, most patients receive a delayed diagnosis and have many comorbidities, especially in developing countries,[3] highlighting the need for continuing education programs for health care professionals.

The primary goal of CAH therapy is to replace glucocorticoid and/or mineralocorticoid to prevent adrenal insufficiency and to avoid excessive secretion of adrenal androgens. Hydrocortisone is the preferred glucocorticoid therapy for pediatric patients, as the focus during childhood and adolescence is to optimize growth velocity and final height. In contrast, there is no consensus regarding the glucocorticoid regimen for adults, which varies significantly among centers.[4] Individuals with the salt-wasting form of CAH also require mineralocorticoid, typically fludrocortisone, alongside appropriate sodium intake. Dosage adjustments are based on adrenal androgens and steroid precursor levels. However, significant variability in individual glucocorticoid and mineralocorticoid metabolism and peripheral sensitivity makes achieving optimal therapeutic balance particularly challenging. A fundamental objective in managing CAH during transition care is to restore hormonal balance, which is frequently disrupted during puberty, by appropriately replacing glucocorticoids and mineralocorticoids, thereby preventing adrenal crises while minimizing androgen excess.[5]

Adolescence presents significant challenges, including psychological issues and maintaining treatment adherence. Additionally, this phase involves changes in steroid hormone metabolism, accompanied by the onset of gonadal sex steroid secretion. During transition care, support should be provided for monitoring and/or preventing metabolic complications; however, it is also essential to evaluate sexual function, provide guidance on contraceptive methods, assess the functionality of the genitalia (in patients who have undergone or not undergone feminizing genitoplasty), monitor menstrual patterns, and assess the risk of infertility (especially screening for the presence of testicular adrenal rest tumors [TARTs]). A flowchart for the multidisciplinary team can facilitate transition care by providing a clear, step-by-step visual guide to ensure a structured and efficient process. It helps health care providers navigate critical steps, reducing the risk of missed evaluations or delays. This process should be carefully planned, beginning at the onset of adolescence and extending into young adulthood if necessary. The primary goals are to empower young individuals through education, with open discussions of their medical history, to ensure proper follow-up while maintaining treatment adherence, and to facilitate access to multidisciplinary teams that address their individual needs.

Practice Gaps

- There is a lack of patient and family education and training regarding the continuous need for glucocorticoid replacement therapy and dosage adjustments during stress conditions.

- Deficiencies in communication and coordination between pediatric and adult teams may lead to loss of follow-up during the transition of care.

- Inadequate long-term health monitoring makes it difficult to systematically evaluate treatment adherence and the adverse effects of glucocorticoid therapy.

- Psychological support and quality of life assessment are often overlooked during the transition to adult care.

Discussion

Collaboration between pediatric and adult endocrinology services is crucial to ensure adequate transition care through the implementation of a structured transition program that incorporates joint consultations between pediatric and adult health care teams, enabling a gradual shift of responsibility to the patient and strengthening self-management skills. Young patients should acquire independence and autonomy. Therefore, the process should start gradually, be individualized, and include a multidisciplinary team.

The transition period is an important time to address the mental health of adolescents with chronic diseases and/or trauma related to the presence of genital atypia. In patients with CAH, anxiety, depression, and/or illicit drug use are not uncommon,[6] and therefore providing support to patients and caregivers is essential.

Clinical Case Vignettes

Case 1

A 19-year-old woman accompanied by her mother presents with concerns of menstrual irregularity and acne for the last year. Menarche occurred at age 12 years. She was diagnosed with salt-wasting CAH as a neonate. Her current treatment regimen is hydrocortisone, 25 mg daily (14 mg/m² per day), divided into 3 doses, and fludrocortisone, 75 mcg daily.

Her height is 63.8 in (162 cm) (target height = 65.4 in [166 cm]), and weight is 158.7 lb (72 kg) (BMI = 27.4 kg/m²).

Laboratory test results:

Serum 17-OHP = 10,502 ng/dL (follicular phase <110 ng/dL) (SI: 318.2 nmol/L [<3.3 nmol/L])
Androstenedione = 358 ng/dL (25-220 ng/dL) (SI: 12.5 nmol/L [0.87-7.68 nmol/L])
Total testosterone = 90 ng/dL (<63 ng/dL) (SI: 3.1 nmol/L [<2.2 nmol/L])
Plasma renin activity = 7.2 ng/mL per h (<5.8 ng/mL per h)

Which of the following is the best next step regarding her glucocorticoid regimen?

A. Continue hydrocortisone regimen and introduce low-dosage contraceptive pill

B. Continue hydrocortisone regimen and evaluate for polycystic ovary syndrome

C. Switch hydrocortisone to long-acting corticosteroid to improve adherence

D. Continue hydrocortisone regimen and increase fludrocortisone dosage

E. Discuss with the patient her therapeutic preferences regarding corticosteroid regimen and encourage lifestyle changes

Answer: E) Discuss with the patient her therapeutic preferences regarding corticosteroid regimen and encourage lifestyle changes

Glucocorticoid Therapy and Its Objectives

During transition care, once growth has ceased, a key step is to review glucocorticoid therapy with the patient, considering their expectations, adherence, and metabolic profile. For adults, there is still no consensus on the ideal glucocorticoid regimen. Some centers administer 2 glucocorticoid preparations, while others provide the higher dosage either at night or in the morning.[6] Hydrocortisone can be given in 2 doses or as a single dose of a longer-acting glucocorticoid to improve adherence. Prednisolone is often preferred for young adults due to its less frequent dosing requirements, while dexamethasone has been associated with greater steroid suppression and increased weight gain.[7] However, at our center, dexamethasone elixir is available, allowing for dose titration with good results.[8] New glucocorticoid formulations, such as modified-release hydrocortisone, appear to offer better hormonal control than conventional glucocorticoid therapy, although they are not yet widely available.[6]

Hormonal Control

Measurement of serum 17-OHP, androstenedione, and testosterone levels are the most widely used parameters to adjust glucocorticoid therapy. However, the optimal target levels of these steroids to prevent adverse metabolic outcomes remain unclear. According to the Endocrine Society guideline,[2] androstenedione levels should be referenced based on age- and sex-specific reference ranges, while upper-normal to mildly elevated 17-OHP levels are considered acceptable. Alternative target ranges, based on expert opinion, suggest 3 to 36 nmol/L or 12 to 36 nmol/L for 17-OHP, with the recommendation to normalize androstenedione within the sex- and age-specific range. In our center, after the achievement of final height, the primary goal is to normalize androstenedione and testosterone within the sex- and age-specific reference ranges to minimize glucocorticoid exposure.[8]

Recent advancements have broadened the understanding of androgen biosynthesis pathways, suggesting that 11-oxygenated androgens, originating from alternative androgen metabolites, may serve as more precise indicators of adequate hormonal regulation. However, they are not yet widely incorporated into routine clinical practice.[9]

The recommended hydrocortisone replacement dosage typically ranges from 10 to 15 mg/m² per day. However, higher dosages, between 12 and 18 mg/m² per day, have also been used. It is important to highlight that exceeding the dosage of 15 to 20 mg/m² per day increases the risk of adverse effects.[10]

Case 2

A 17-year-old girl presents to the emergency department with a history of persistent vomiting, lethargy, and poor feeding. She has the simple virilizing form of CAH and is regularly taking hydrocortisone, 20 mg daily, divided into 3 doses. She has been experiencing a cough and fever of 101.3°F (38.5°C) for the past 3 days, during which she doubled her daily hydrocortisone dose, but without improvement in her lethargy. Earlier this morning, her vomiting worsened, and she went to the emergency department where she was diagnosed with pneumonia. She showed her emergency letter to the health care team and received intravenous saline and was then discharged. She now returns for further evaluation due to severe weakness and worsening vomiting.

Her height is 65.0 in (165 cm), and weight is 130.1 lb (59 kg). Her blood pressure is 80/50 mm Hg, and pulse rate is 128 beats/min.

Which of the following is the best course of action?

A. Measure sodium and potassium levels to guide therapy

B. Triple the oral hydrocortisone dosage

C. Evaluate for sepsis

D. Administer intravenous saline and hydrocortisone (50-100 mg/m^2)

E. Exercise caution when administering corticosteroids due to the pulmonary infection

Answer: D) Administer intravenous saline and hydrocortisone (50-100 mg/m^2)

Adrenal Crisis

Transition care is important for educating patients on the prevention of adrenal crises and how to adjust glucocorticoid therapy during sick day episodes. During childhood, this knowledge is usually under the caregivers' domain, making it essential to enhance the patient's understanding and autonomy regarding their condition as they transition to adulthood.

Although glucocorticoid therapy has significantly improved survival rates in people with CAH, the risk of acute adrenal insufficiency remains a major concern, and life expectancy remains lower than that of the general population. A Swedish nationwide CAH study identified adrenal crises as the primary cause of death,[11] and gastrointestinal infections are a frequent trigger.[12] Data from the I-CAH multicenter registry disclosed that the frequency of hospital admissions was higher in individuals with the salt-wasting form, and sick-day episodes were more prevalent among toddlers and late adolescents receiving higher glucocorticoid dosages.[12] Nonadherence to treatment during adolescence may be a key factor contributing to the increased occurrence of adverse events. Although patient-initiated stress dosing is a crucial intervention to prevent adrenal crises, these events continue to occur at an elevated rate. Preventing adrenal crises remains a top priority in CAH management. Discussions about sick-day management strategies should be prioritized at every clinical visit with young patients and their families, emphasizing the need to use bracelets or identification cards for emergencies.[13] Efforts should also be made to promote continuing education for health care professionals involved in emergency care about the immediate use of glucocorticoids in patients with adrenal insufficiency during stressful situations, even in infectious conditions. Educational booklets and easy access to emergency cards on medical and patient society websites may be useful (www.sbteim.org.br).

Outcomes for Assessment

Body Mass Index

Increased BMI and unfavorable body composition have been frequently reported in patients with CAH undergoing different glucocorticoid regimens[4]; however, it is not possible to conclude whether synthetic glucocorticoids contribute to a higher frequency of obesity. In our cohort, which included 60 adults with CAH who were exclusively treated with a low dosage of dexamethasone after reaching their final height, the prevalence of obesity and overweight was 27% and 35%, respectively, which is higher than the prevalence in the general population. However, the mean BMI standard deviation did not differ significantly between the time of dexamethasone initiation and the last evaluation, over an average follow-up period of 10 years.[8] Although most studies report a high prevalence of obesity in patients with CAH, it is likely that weight gain begins in childhood as a compensatory mechanism to mitigate androgen excess and control the bone age advancement.[14]

Body fat distribution also appears to be altered in patients with CAH, with increased visceral and subcutaneous adipose tissue on CT reported in a cohort of 28 adolescents and young adults.[15] In addition to glucocorticoid type and dosage, genetic factors modulating glucocorticoid metabolism and peripheral sensitivity may contribute to the development of an adverse metabolic profile. Measures to combat obesity should be routinely assessed during follow-up, and healthy lifestyle habits should be encouraged.

Blood Pressure

A normal resting and 24-hour blood pressure profile is generally observed in patients with CAH; however, a slight increase in diurnal and/or nocturnal blood pressure has also been reported.[4] An increased prevalence of hypertension was observed in a cohort of 545 Swedish patients with CAH,[16] with a higher frequency in women. As expected, the high prevalence of obesity among people with CAH negatively affects blood pressure values. Variability in blood pressure outcomes across studies is likely influenced not only by cumulative glucocorticoid and mineralocorticoid dosages, but also by different hormonal control strategies. Some centers aim to maintain renin in the upper half of the reference range, while others prioritize normalizing blood pressure and serum sodium levels. Considering the great variability of renin levels according to posture, timing of the last mineralocorticoid dose, adherence, and concomitant medications, data from the I-CAH registry suggest that mineralocorticoid titration should not be primarily based on serum renin levels, but also on clinical parameters, such as blood pressure and serum electrolytes.[17]

Metabolic Profile and Cardiovascular Risk

In a systematic review of 437 patients with CAH, there were no significant differences in fasting blood glucose and insulin levels compared with values in control participants, but a higher homeostatic model assessment of insulin resistance was observed in patients with CAH.[18] Findings on the lipid profile remain controversial; in this systematic review, total cholesterol, LDL cholesterol, HDL cholesterol, and triglyceride levels were comparable between patients and control participants. However, higher carotid intima thickness was observed in patients with CAH. A study focusing on young adults with CAH[19] also identified similar lipid profiles in comparison with control participants.

The introduction of glucocorticoid replacement has improved the lifespan of people with CAH. As individuals with CAH are now reaching adulthood, a higher frequency of cardiovascular risk factors has been observed compared with the frequency in the reference population. It remains to be determined whether individuals with CAH have an increased frequency of cardiovascular disease. Currently, it is difficult to reach a conclusion, as the studies comprise heterogeneous young cohorts who are treated with different glucocorticoid regimens and have different goals of hormonal control. However, in many studies, there is an evident effect of obesity on the development of cardiovascular risk factors. Lifestyle modifications and attempts to adjust glucocorticoid and mineralocorticoid dosages seem to be of great importance.[4]

Fertility in Women

During transition care, aspects related to sexual function and fertility become central. Increased adrenal androgen secretion contributes to menstrual irregularities, often leading to a polycystic ovary-like phenotype. It is essential to assess menstrual patterns in adolescents and young adults with CAH during each clinical visit.

In adolescent patients who have previously undergone feminizing genitoplasty, transition care should include an assessment of whether the urogenital sinus opening and/or vagina are adequate for sexual activity. In cases of stenosis, acrylic mold dilations should only be recommended when the patient expresses a desire to initiate sexual activity, and surgical dilation is reserved for more severe cases.[20]

The routine practice of performing genital surgery within the first year of life for infants with CAH and atypical genitalia has become increasingly debated. Concerns regarding genital sensitivity, potential long-term complications, and the frequency of reoperation in adulthood have prompted some researchers to reassess the timing of surgical intervention. The guideline from the Endocrine Society, along with a European expert consensus, emphasizes that parents should be informed about surgical options, including the possibility of postponing surgery and allowing observation until the child reaches an age where they can participate in the decision-making process.[2,21] Extensive discussions regarding risks and benefits, shared decision-making, review of potential complications, and fully informed consent need to occur before surgery. If surgery is delayed, the risk of hematocolpos should be assessed.

In recent decades, surgical techniques have been refined to reduce clitoral size while preserving sensitivity and enhancing both the cosmetic and functional aspects of female genitalia.[22] However, it is essential to emphasize that these procedures should be performed only in centers with experienced pediatric surgeons/urologists, pediatric endocrinologists, pediatric anesthesiologists, behavioral/mental health professionals, and social work services.[2] Despite these advancements, research on long-term patient satisfaction and functional outcomes remains limited. In a cohort of 36 female participants with CAH who underwent feminizing genitoplasty under the care of an interdisciplinary team, the findings indicated that the procedure did not negatively affect overall genital sensitivity compared with sensitivity in control groups in

adulthood. Additionally, both patient and parental satisfaction with the surgical outcomes was high, with the majority preferring the procedure to be performed during childhood.[22] These results are consistent with previous studies.[23] It is also worth highlighting the lack of long-term studies on the psychological aspects in adulthood of 46,XX individuals who grew up with atypical genitalia. The outcomes of delayed surgical intervention are also unknown.

Case 3

A 25-year-old man is referred due to primary infertility. At 4 years of age, he was diagnosed with the simple virilizing form of CAH. Treatment with hydrocortisone was started. The patient developed normally until 19 years of age, when he abandoned his treatment and was lost to follow-up consultations. He and his wife have been unable to achieve pregnancy after 2 years of trying. His height is 66 in (168 cm), and weight is 172 lb (78 kg) (BMI = 27.8 kg/m²). He has small, soft testicles compatible with testicular atrophy. Semen analysis reveals azoospermia.

Laboratory test results are suggestive of testicular failure:

> Very increased levels of serum ACTH, 17-OHP, LH and FSH
> Total testosterone = 320 ng/dL (240-816 ng/dL) (SI: 11.1 nmol/L [8.3-28.3 nmol/L])

Which of the following describes the best initial approach for this patient?

A. Perform bilateral testicular biopsy to evaluate for obstructive azoospermia

B. Reintroduce glucocorticoid treatment and request scrotal ultrasonography to screen for TARTs

C. Start testosterone replacement therapy

D. Start mineralocorticoid therapy

E. Perform analysis of sperm DNA integrity

Answer: B) Reintroduce glucocorticoid treatment and request scrotal ultrasonography to screen for TARTs

Fertility in Men

Gonadal dysfunction is frequently identified in male patients with CAH, either due to poor hormonal control, leading to hypogonadotropic hypogonadism, or the presence of TARTs.[2,5] Excess ACTH is thought to be a key driver in the development of TARTs. Neonatal trophic stimulation of testicular cells may even increase the pool of ACTH-sensitive cells, which could grow into significantly sized TARTs during periods of poor hormonal control. A delayed CAH diagnosis (more than 1 year after birth) has been associated with a higher risk of TART development. The tumors' mass effects may lead to testicular damage, resulting in primary hypogonadism, impaired fecundity, and infertility.[24]

There is limited published guidance on the prevention of TARTs. Regular screening should begin in adolescence or as early as age 8 years, with annual testicular ultrasonography, as the risk of TARTs is higher in patients with poor disease control or a late diagnosis.[5] Close surveillance of gonadal function, along with optimization of hormonal control, is a key goal in managing classic forms of CAH in boys during adolescence. However, suppressing ACTH stimulation through glucocorticoid therapy often leads to significant weight gain and/or cushingoid features. Since infertility is a major risk for patients with TARTs, appropriate counseling should be provided at a young age to improve treatment adherence, which may reduce the risk of further tumor growth. When appropriate, semen analysis and storage should also be considered.[6]

New Therapies

Patients with CAH typically receive long-term treatment with supraphysiological doses of glucocorticoid to reduce adrenal androgen secretion, raising concerns about long-term risks. Recently, new therapies have entered the experimental phase, aiming to reduce stimulation of androgen production. Crinecerfont, an oral corticotropin-releasing factor type 1 receptor antagonist, lowered androstenedione levels in patients with CAH in phase 2 trials and, in phase 3, enabled a significant reduction in glucocorticoid dosages.[25] Atumelnant is a potent, once-daily, orally bioavailable, nonpeptide, first-in-class competitive and selective melanocortin type 2 receptor antagonist. Results from a phase 2, open-label, dose-finding study (40 mg, 80 mg, or 120 mg) demonstrated rapid, substantial, and sustained reductions in serum androstendione and 17-OHP levels. Androstenedione levels were reduced from baseline by 60%, 70%, and 80%, respectively.[25] No serious adverse events were reported with either crinecerfont or atumelnant.

Key Learning Points

Effective transition care should encompass thorough education on CAH with the aims of:

- Empowering and educating young people to take responsibility for their health condition.

- Emphasizing the importance of adhering to glucocorticoid and mineralocorticoid therapies to prevent adverse outcomes.

- Providing patients with detailed guidance on stress dosing during illness or surgical procedures to reduce the risk of complications.

- Psychological support should be offered, as adolescents with CAH often face issues with body image, concerns about genital appearance and/or functionality, and difficulties with social relationships.

- Regular assessment of metabolic indicators is essential to fine-tune treatment plans and swiftly detect emerging health issues.

- Support and counseling should be provided for both patients and caregivers to assist with the process.

- Evidence from studies of patients with other chronic medical conditions confirms that openness in the sharing of information is associated with enhanced psychosocial adaptation.[26] Engaging patients/families as effective partners in care management and shared decision-making is vital to ensuring high-quality, appropriate care.

Conflict of Interest

Principal investigator for the phase 2 study that evaluated the safety, efficacy, and pharmacokinetics of CRN04894 (Atumelnant) in individuals with CAH.

References

1. White PC, Bachega TA. Congenital adrenal hyperplasia due to 21 hydroxylase deficiency: from birth to adulthood. *Semin Reprod Med.* 2012;30(5):400-409. PMID: 23044877

2. Speiser PW, Arlt W, Auchus RJ, et al. Congenital adrenal hyperplasia due to steroid 21-hydroxylase deficiency: an Endocrine Society clinical practice guideline. *J Clin Endocrinol Metab.* 2018;103(11):4043-4088. PMID: 30272171

3. Miranda MC, Haddad LBP, Madureira G, Mendonca BB, Bachega TASS. Adverse outcomes and economic burden of congenital adrenal hyperplasia late diagnosis in the newborn screening absence. *J Endocr Soc.* 2019;4(2):bvz013. PMID: 32047870

4. Gomes LG, Bachega TASS, Mendonca BB. Classic congenital adrenal hyperplasia and its impact on reproduction. *Fertil Steril.* 2019;111(1):7-12. PMID: 30611420

5. Balagamage C, Arshad A, Elhassan YS, et al. Management aspects of congenital adrenal hyperplasia during adolescence and transition to adult care. *Clin Endocrinol (Oxf).* 2024;101(4):332-345. PMID: 37964596

6. Merke DP, Auchus RJ. Congenital adrenal hyperplasia due to 21-hydroxylase deficiency. *N Engl J Med.* 2020;383(13):1248-1261. PMID: 32966723

7. Whittle E, Falhammar H. Glucocorticoid regimens in the treatment of congenital adrenal hyperplasia: a systematic review and meta-analysis. *J Endocr Soc.* 2019;3(6):1227-1245.

8. Seraphim CE, Frassei JS, Pessoa BS, et al. Impact of long-term dexamethasone therapy on the metabolic profile of patients with 21-hydroxylase deficiency. *J Endocr Soc.* 2019;3(8):1574-1582. PMID: 31384718

9. Turcu AF, Mallappa A, Nella AA, et al. 24-Hour profiles of 11-oxygenated C19 steroids and Δ5-steroid sulfates during oral and continuous subcutaneous glucocorticoids in 21-hydroxylase deficiency. *Front Endocrinol (Lausanne).* 2021;12:751191. PMID: 34867794

10. Bacila I, Freeman N, Daniel E, et al. International practice of corticosteroid replacement therapy in congenital adrenal hyperplasia: data from the I-CAH registry. *Eur J Endocrinol.* 2021;184(4):553-563. PMID: 33460392

11. Falhammar H, Frisén L, Norrby C, et al. Increased mortality in patients with congenital adrenal hyperplasia due to 21-hydroxylase deficiency. *J Clin Endocrinol Metab.* 2014;99(12):E2715-E2721. PMID: 25279502

12. Ali SR, Bryce J, Haghpanahan H, et al. Real-world estimates of adrenal insufficiency-related adverse events in children with congenital adrenal hyperplasia. *J Clin Endocrinol Metab.* 2021;106(1):e192-e203. PMID: 32995889

13. Lousada LM, Mendonca BB, Bachega TASS. Adrenal crisis and mortality rate in adrenal insufficiency and congenital adrenal hyperplasia. *Arch Endocrinol Metab.* 2021;65(4):488-494. PMID: 34283908

14. Sarafoglou K, Forlenza GP, Yaw Addo O, et al. Obesity in children with congenital adrenal hyperplasia in the Minnesota cohort: importance of adjusting body mass index for height-age. *Clin Endocrinol (Oxf).* 2017;86(5):708-716. PMID: 28199739

15. Kim MS, Ryabets-Lienhard A, Dao-Tran A, et al. Increased abdominal adiposity in adolescents and young adults with classical congenital adrenal hyperplasia due to 21-hydroxylase deficiency. *J Clin Endocrinol Metab.* 2015;100(8):E1153-E1159. PMID: 26062016

16. Falhammar H, Frisén L, Hirschberg AL, et al. Increased cardiovascular and metabolic morbidity in patients with 21-hydroxylase deficiency: a Swedish population-based national cohort study. *J Clin Endocrinol Metab.* 2015;100(9):3520-3528. PMID: 26126207

17. Pofi R, Prete A, Thornton-Jones V, et al. Plasma renin measurements are unrelated to mineralocorticoid replacement dose in patients with primary adrenal insufficiency. *J Clin Endocrinol Metab.* 2020;105(1):dgz055. PMID: 26126207

18. Tamhane S, Rodriguez-Gutierrez R, Iqbal AM, et al. Cardiovascular and metabolic outcomes in congenital adrenal hyperplasia: a systematic review and meta-analysis. *J Clin Endocrinol Metab.* 2018;103(11):4097-4103. PMID: 30272185

19. Vijayan R, Bhavani N, Pavithran PV, et al. Metabolic profile, cardiovascular risk factors and health-related quality of life in children, adolescents and young adults with congenital adrenal hyperplasia. *J Pediatr Endocrinol Metab.* 2019;32(8):871-877. PMID: 31271560

20. Sircili MHP, de Mendonca BB, Denes FT, Madureira G, Bachega TASS, d Queiroz e Silva FA. Anatomical and functional outcomes of feminizing genitoplasty for ambiguous genitalia in patients with virilizing congenital adrenal hyperplasia. *Clinics (Sao Paulo).* 2006;61(3):209-214. PMID: 16832553

21. Cools M, Nordenström A, Robeva R, et al. Caring for individuals with a difference of sex development (DSD): a consensus statement. *Nat Rev Endocrinol.* 2018;14(7):415-429. PMID: 29769693

22. Bag MJ, Inacio M, Bachega TASS, et al. Long-term outcomes of feminizing genitoplasty in DSD: genital morphology, sensitivity, sexual function, and satisfaction. *J Endocr Soc.* 2025;9(3):bvaf014. PMID: 39975957

23. Shalaby M, Chandran H, Elford S, Kirk J, McCarthy L. Recommendations of patients and families of girls with 46XX congenital adrenal hyperplasia in the United Kingdom regarding the timing of surgery. *Pediatr Surg Int.* 2021;37(1):137-143. PMID: 33230638

24. Schröder MAM, Neacsu M, Adriaansen BPH, et al. Hormonal control during infancy and testicular adrenal rest tumor development in males with congenital adrenal hyperplasia: a retrospective multicenter cohort study. *Eur J Endocrinol.* 2023;189(4):460-468. PMID: 37837609

25. Auchus RJ, Hamidi O, Pivonello R, et al; CAHtalyst Adult Trial Investigators. Phase 3 trial of crinecerfont in adult congenital adrenal hyperplasia. *N Engl J Med.* 2024;391(6):504-514. PMID: 38828955

26. Richard A, Trainer P, Lucas KJ, et al; TouCAHn study investigators. Interim Analysis From a 12-Week, Phase 2, Open-Label, Sequential Dose Cohort Study to Evaluate the Safety, Efficacy, and Pharmacokinetics of CRN04894 Treatment in Participants with Classical Congenital Adrenal Hyperplasia (TouCAHn). Poster presentation at Endo 2024, June 1-4, Boston, MA.

How to Approach Children With Short Stature Not Responding to Growth Hormone Treatment

Stefano Cianfarani, MD. Department of Systems Medicine, University of Rome 'Tor Vergata,' Endocrinology and Diabetes Unit, 'Bambino Gesù' Children's Hospital, IRCCS, Rome, Italy; and Department of Women's and Children's Health, Karolinska Institute, Stockholm, Sweden; Email: stefano.cianfarani@uniroma2.it

Educational Objectives

After reviewing this chapter, learners should be able to:

- Define a good response to GH treatment and describe the predictive variables.

- Identify causes of poor response to GH treatment.

- Select appropriate further evaluation and therapeutic strategies when patients do not respond to GH treatment.

Significance of the Clinical Problem

GH therapy has been approved worldwide for treatment of children with different conditions associated with short stature. However, the individual response to GH treatment is variable, especially in non–GH-deficient short children. A high rate of poor or unsatisfactory response to GH therapy is commonly observed in the clinical setting and, despite that, many physicians continue GH treatment until adult height is achieved. Some children diagnosed as having GH deficiency may not respond to GH therapy, often due to incorrect diagnosis or poor adherence to therapy.

Poor treatment response should prompt the physician to discontinue GH treatment and determine the cause of the suboptimal response, which may require challenging the initial diagnosis. In many cases, further investigations (mainly genetic) are needed to clarify the underlying condition leading to growth failure and nonresponse to GH treatment. Another pitfall in the evaluation of the response to GH therapy and, consequently, in the decision whether to continue treatment, is the value given to the first-year growth response. During the first year of GH therapy, most short children, independent of the diagnosis, show a satisfactory response that is not sustained over time, resulting in an adult height far below their target (midparental) height. Finally, once a short child has been identified as a nonresponder to GH, the choice of other growth-promoting medications to be used alone or in combination with GH is difficult due to the lack of robust evidence and specific guidelines.

Practice Gaps

- GH therapy is often based on results of laboratory tests or clinical characterization without a clear understanding of the underlying molecular mechanism.

- The definition of a good response to GH treatment is still arbitrary.

- The prediction of a good long-term response to GH is challenging because the available prediction models are based on the short-term (first-year) response.

- There are no guidelines for genetic testing in short children who do not respond to GH therapy.

- There are no guidelines for alternative treatments in short children who do not respond to GH therapy.

Discussion

Indications for GH Therapy and Prediction of Response

GH therapy is licensed by the European Medicines Agency (EMA) and the US FDA for treatment of GH deficiency, Turner syndrome, short stature in children born small-for-gestational age and children who have Prader-Willi syndrome, SHOX deficiency, chronic kidney insufficiency, or Noonan syndrome. In the United States, the FDA has additionally approved GH therapy for idiopathic short stature. Children with severe GH deficiency are highly responsive to GH replacement therapy, whereas children with the other conditions for which GH therapy is licensed show a variable response.[1-3] Individual variability in response to GH treatment may be secondary to an incorrect diagnosis, underlying genetic cause of short stature making GH therapy ineffective, poor adherence, suboptimal treatment dosage, or late initiation of treatment. Furthermore, individual genetic variants may affect the response to GH therapy by influencing drug absorption, distribution, metabolism, and excretion.

The need to identify responders to therapy has led to the development of many prediction models based on the response during the first year of treatment in children with GH deficiency, Turner syndrome, small-for-gestational-age, and idiopathic short stature. The main predictive factors of response to GH in the first year of treatment and variably included in the equations of the different models are chronological age, birth weight, height, height SDS minus target height SDS, GH peak to provocative tests, and GH dosage. Prediction models derived from the large KIGS database (Kabi Pharmacia International Growth Study, Pharmacia & Upjohn, Inc., International Growth Database) explain approximately 60% of the variability of response to GH therapy in patients with GH deficiency and 40% in individuals with idiopathic short stature.[4]

The addition of genomic markers may increase the accuracy of prediction models. For example, an exon 3 deletion polymorphism in the GH receptor, as well as a specific (-202 A) polymorphism in the *IGFBP3* gene promoter, is associated with a better therapeutic response.[5,6] Recently, pretreatment blood transcriptomics by next-generation RNA sequencing has been proposed as a predictive tool for first-year growth and IGF-1 response to GH therapy.[7] The assumption of most predictive models is that first-year response is predictive of long-term response to GH therapy. However, it is a common clinical experience to observe a satisfactory response during the first year of treatment, which does not persist in the following years.

Definition of Good Response to GH Therapy

A univocal definition of responsiveness to GH is still lacking. A good response in the first year of GH treatment may be defined by a height gain of 0.5 or more SDS and/or an increase in height velocity of 3 cm or more per year and/or a height velocity of 1 or more SDS.[8,9]

Common Causes of Poor Response to GH Therapy

The diagnosis of childhood-onset short stature is often challenging and should be based on a comprehensive clinical, anthropometric, biochemical, endocrine, radiological, and, in selected cases, genetic approach. The lack of such a comprehensive approach may lead to misdiagnosis and, consequently, ineffective therapies. A diagnosis of GH deficiency based only on the response to provocative tests may be misleading due to the high false-positive rate of such tests. Therefore, a poor response to GH therapy should prompt the clinician to reconsider the initial diagnosis.[10] The false-positive rate of GH-provocative tests is even higher in children with delayed puberty. Sex steroids increase pituitary GH release during puberty. Estrogens are the effectors of such action on the pituitary gland in both sexes, as testosterone in males is converted into estrogens through androgen aromatization. Estrogens stimulate GH secretion by (a) reducing somatostatin receptor expression, (b) increasing the number of GHRH binding sites, and (c) amplifying ghrelin-induced GH secretion.[11] Due to the crucial role played in GH secretion during puberty, sex steroid priming before provocative tests should be considered in prepubertal boys older than 11 years and in prepubertal girls older than 10 years, especially to distinguish GH deficiency from constitutional delay of growth and puberty (CDGP).[12,13]

Idiopathic short stature and small-for-gestational-age are clinical definitions that imply many different underlying molecular defects accounting for broad individual variability in response to GH therapy.[14-16]

Rarely, an insufficient GH dosage is the cause of a poor response. Depending on the patient's condition, the GH dosage varies from 25 mcg/kg per day to 67 mcg/kg per day (*Table*).

Distinguishing between nonresponsiveness to GH therapy and suboptimal response because of poor adherence is often difficult, and a thorough investigation into the regularity of GH injections is needed to identify the cause of nonresponse. Nonadherence to GH therapy is as high as 36% to 66%,[17,18] and it can be secondary to discomfort (eg, associated with daily injections), long-term treatment, complexity of treatment regimens, age (eg, adolescence), and the patient's or family's lack of understanding of treatment benefits and consequences of nonadherence. Poor adherence is associated with impaired growth outcome because

Table. Current Indications for GH Therapy

Current indications for GH therapy	Year of approval	Dosage
GH deficiency	1985	*Daily* • 23-43 mcg/kg per day (US) • 25-35 mcg/kg per day (EU) • 0.16-0.24 mg/kg per week (EU and US) *Weekly* • Somatrogon: 0.66 mg/kg per week (EU and US) • Somapacitan: 0.16 mg/kg per week (EU and US) • Lonapegsomatropin: 0.24 mg/kg per week (EU and US) • Jintrolong: 0.2 mg/kg per week (China) • Eutropin-plus: 0.5 mg/kg per week (South Korea and EU*)
Chronic kidney insufficiency	1993	50 mcg/kg per day (US) 45-50 mcg/kg per day (EU)
Turner syndrome	1997	47-67 mcg/kg per day (US) 45-50 mcg/kg per day (EU)
Prader-Willi syndrome	2000	34 mcg/kg per day (US) 35 mcg/kg per day (EU)
Small-for-gestational-age without catch-up growth	2001	67-69 mcg/kg per day (US) 35 mcg/kg per day (EU)
Idiopathic short stature	2003**	43-67 mcg/kg per day (US)
SHOX gene haploinsufficiency	2006	50 mcg/kg per day (EU and US)
Noonan syndrome	2007	35-66 mcg/kg per day (EU and US)

Abbreviations: EU, European Union; US, United States.

* Approved but not commercialized.

** In US only.

missing more than 1 GH dose each week can affect long-term efficacy.[18] Measurement of IGF-1 may provide information about adherence, especially when an unexpected drop in IGF-1 concentration is observed. Strategies to reduce nonadherence include (a) educating the patient and family on manage management; (b) emphasizing the importance of adherence at each outpatient visit; (c) addressing the choice of the injection device; (d) facilitating inclusion in a patient support program; and (e) use of electronic monitoring.[19] The recent availability of long-acting GH preparations, which decrease the frequency of injections from daily to weekly, might improve adherence to GH therapy and ultimately lead to better growth outcomes.[20]

The algorithm to be followed in case of nonresponse or poor response starts with checking the appropriate dosage and assessing adherence to GH therapy. In cases with confirmed adherence, the therapy should be stopped, the diagnosis should be challenged, and further tests (mainly genetic) should be performed (*Figure*).

Alternative Growth-Promoting Therapies in Short Children With Poor Response to GH Treatment

A poor response to GH treatment raises the problem of choosing effective alternative therapeutic strategies. Increasing the GH dosage is usually ineffective and is associated with the challenge of maintaining IGF-1 levels in the normal range, as well as high cost. The use of long-acting GH may improve adherence,[20] but long-acting GH has been approved only for patients with GH deficiency.

Another theoretical alternative is to combine GH with IGF-1 to treat patients who with poor response to GH therapy alone. IGF-1 has been approved for treating patients with primary IGF-1 deficiency, but it has also been used in combination with GH to treat children with idiopathic short stature in a randomized clinical trial.[25] However, the response to combination therapy was modest and only seen in the first year. Moreover, as expected, children receiving combination treatment experienced dramatic elevations in serum IGF-1.[25] In addition, IGF-1 therapy requires a twice-daily regimen and is associated with a high rate of hypoglycemic reactions (42%).

Figure. Algorithm for Evaluating Children With Poor Response to GH Therapy

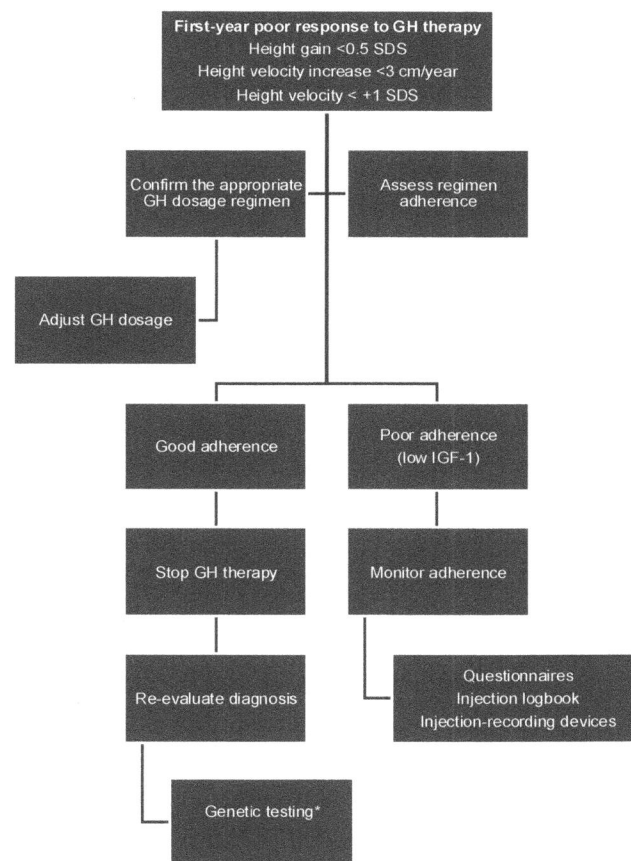

* Genetic testing includes karyotype analysis, comparative genomic hybridization array, single-nucleotide polymorphism array, whole-exome sequencing, whole-genome sequencing, and DNA methylation analysis.[21] More than one-third of children diagnosed as being small-for-gestational age or having idiopathic short stature have pathogenic variants, mainly in genes involved in growth cartilage physiology, such as *ACAN, COL2A1, FBN1, FGFR3, IHH, NPPC, NPR2,* and *SHOX*.[14,22,23] Some polymorphisms located in *GHR, IGFBP3,* and *SOCS2* reduce responsiveness to GH treatment.[24]

[Color—Print (Color Gallery page CG15) or web & ePub editions]

Genetic characterization of children with short stature can better personalize therapies. For example, children with gain-of-function pathogenic variants in the gene encoding fibroblast growth factor receptor 3 (*FGFR3*), causing hypochondroplasia and achondroplasia, respond to C-type natriuretic peptide analogues (eg, vosoritide) administered via daily subcutaneous injections.[26-28] A multicenter phase 2 clinical trial with vosoritide in children with idiopathic short stature is ongoing. Infigratinib is an oral tyrosine kinase inhibitor that counteracts FGFR3 hyperactivity by inhibiting its phosphorylation and therefore downstream signaling. Promising preliminary results have recently been reported in patients with achondroplasia.[29]

Another strategy to improve the growth outcome of short children who start GH therapy in puberty is to delay fusion of the growth plates either with GnRH analogues or aromatase inhibitors.[30] The use of GnRH analogues in combination with GH can promote growth in puberty in boys and girls with GH deficiency, small-for-gestational-age, and idiopathic short stature.[30] However, suppression of physiological puberty makes a pubertal child hypogonadal at a critical time of development. While treated with GnRH analogue therapy, the child will not only be short, but also sexually infantile compared with his/her peers, and this may impair psychological well-being. The high cost of such therapy is another limiting factor.

Aromatase inhibitors block estrogen and increase testosterone production, thus delaying growth plate fusion while GH promotes growth. Although safety and efficacy data of aromatase inhibitors used alone or in combination with GH in male children with GH deficiency and idiopathic short stature are promising, there is still little evidence because most reports are based on predicted rather than actual adult height. The potential detrimental effects of estrogen depletion and androgen increase on bone mineralization and virilization (increase in musculature and acne), respectively, should be closely monitored during aromatase inhibitor treatment.

Clinical Case Vignettes

Case 1

A 14-year-old boy diagnosed with GH deficiency is referred for short stature (height, −2.2 SDS) and poor response to GH therapy. He has been treated with GH for 1 year. The initial diagnosis of isolated idiopathic GH deficiency was based on subnormal peak GH responses to 2 different GH-stimulation tests. No sex steroid priming was performed before GH-provocative tests. During his first year of treatment, height gain was +0.3 SDS, height velocity was +0.2 SDS, and height velocity increase was +2.0 cm/year. His mother had menarche at age 14 years, and her height is −1.1 SDS. His father's height is −0.8 SDS. The patient's birth weight at 40 weeks' gestation was 6 lb 6 oz (2900 g), and birth length was 19.7 in (50 cm).

On physical examination, he has no dysmorphic features, testicular volume is 3 cc, and pubertal development is Tanner stage 2.

Bone age is 11.5 years. IGF-1 is +0.1 SDS. Results of endocrine and biochemical tests are in the normal range. Adherence to therapy is adequate according to his therapy logbook.

Which of the following is the best recommendation now?

A. Increase the GH dosage

B. Continue GH therapy for another year

C. Reassess the diagnosis of GH deficiency, stop GH therapy, and repeat GH-provocative testing after sex steroid priming

D. Continue GH therapy and add testosterone

E. Continue GH therapy and add a GnRH analogue

Answer: C) Reassess the diagnosis of GH deficiency, stop GH therapy, and repeat GH-provocative testing after sex steroid priming

This boy has had a poor response to GH therapy. Based on his family history, physical examination findings, delayed bone age, and normal IGF-1 concentration, the most likely diagnosis is constitutional delay of growth and development. Constitutional delay of growth and development is by far the most frequent cause of delayed puberty (absence of testis enlargement in boys at the age of 14 years or breast development in girls at the age 13 years) and transient growth retardation in both sexes. For unknown reasons, it is more common in boys than in girls. Boys with constitutional delay of growth and development are usually referred for short stature secondary to the delayed pubertal growth spurt, but their slow "tempo" of growth does not impair the achievement of a normal adult height corresponding to their genetic growth potential (midparental height). The patient's subnormal GH responses to provocative tests were misleading, suggesting impaired GH secretion. The false-positive rate of GH-provocative testing is high in children with delayed puberty. Sex steroids increase pituitary GH release during puberty, and sex steroid priming before provocative tests should be considered in prepubertal boys older than 11 years and in prepubertal girls older than 10 years to discriminate constitutional delay of growth and development from GH deficiency. Short courses of low-dosage testosterone may be indicated in boys with constitutional delay of growth and development who have a prolonged infantile phenotype to increase height velocity, accelerate sexual maturation, and improve psychosocial well-being without negative effects on bone maturation and adult height. The usual testosterone regimen is testosterone ester, 50 mg intramuscularly each month for 3 to 4 months, which can be repeated for another 3 to 4 months.

Case 2

An 8-year-old girl diagnosed with isolated idiopathic GH deficiency is referred for short stature (height, −3.2 SDS) and poor first-year response to GH therapy. During the first year of treatment, her height gain was +0.1 SDS, and height velocity was +0.3 SDS (+1.1 cm/year). The peak GH value in response to arginine-stimulation testing was 6.1 ng/mL (6.1 μg/L), and peak GH value in response to clonidine-stimulation testing was 6.7 ng/mL (6.7 μg/L). Her IGF-1 concentration was +2.0 SDS. MRI showed a normal hypothalamus and pituitary gland. Her GH dosage regimen is consistent with the diagnosis of GH deficiency: 0.2 mg/kg per week, and adherence to her treatment regimen is adequate according to her therapy logbook.

There is no relevant family history. Her mother's height is −2.9 SDS, and her father's height −1.6 SDS. At a gestational age of 39 weeks,

her birth weight was 4 lb 3 oz (1900 g), and length was 17.3 in (44 cm).

On physical examination, her BMI is +2.0 SDS. She is prepubertal and has no dysmorphic features.

Which of the following is the best next step in this patient's management?

A. Increase the GH dosage

B. Stop GH therapy and wait to see of spontaneous puberty occurs

C. Continue GH therapy and add an aromatase inhibitor

D. Continue GH therapy and add a GnRH analogue

E. Reassess the diagnosis of GH deficiency, stop GH therapy, and pursue further testing

Answer: E) Reassess the diagnosis of GH deficiency, stop GH therapy, and pursue further testing

The diagnosis of GH deficiency was based on the responses to provocative tests only, instead of a comprehensive clinical, anthropometric, biochemical, endocrine, radiological, and genetic approach. A GH dosage of 25 mcg/kg per day (0.18 mg/kg per week) is an adequate replacement regimen in GH-deficient children, leading to catch-up growth and achievement of adult height consistent with genetic potential (midparental height). A further increase in the GH dosage would not be advised in this case because the selected therapeutic regimen is appropriate and her IGF-1 concentration is in the upper normal range. Poor response to GH therapy, normal/high IGF-1 values, and normal pituitary and hypothalamus on MRI should strongly challenge the diagnosis of GH deficiency. Moreover, the patient's obesity may account for the blunted responses to GH-provocative tests. Her small size at birth and the degree of her mother's short stature suggest a genetic cause. The high IGF-1 levels are consistent with a pathogenic variant in the *IGF1R* gene. Most individuals carrying *IGF1R* variants are heterozygous with a single-nucleotide variant or deletions encompassing *IGF1R*. Only few patients with homozygous *IGF1R* variants or compound heterozygous *IGF1R* variants have been reported so far. In this case, the initial diagnosis of GH deficiency should be reassessed, and genetic tests (particularly focused on *IGF1R* variants) should be undertaken to elucidate the underlying cause of her short stature.

Case 3

An 8-year-old boy diagnosed with isolated idiopathic GH deficiency is referred for blunted response to GH therapy during the third year of therapy. His pretherapy GH responses to provocative tests were 1.4 ng/mL (1.4 μg/L) to arginine stimulation and 2.1 ng/mL (2.1 μg/L) to clonidine stimulation. His IGF-1 value was –2.1 SDS. Brain MRI showed ectopic posterior pituitary, pituitary stalk agenesis, and anterior pituitary hypoplasia. His pretherapy height was –3.5 SDS, and height velocity was –1.9 SDS. His first-year response to GH therapy was satisfactory with a height gain of +1.1 SDS, height velocity of +1.8 SDS, and height velocity increase of +4.5 cm/year. The good response was maintained during the second year of treatment. IGF-1 levels in the first and second year of GH therapy were +1.5 SDS and +1.2 SDS, respectively. Monitoring of thyroid function before and during GH therapy yielded normal results. Now, in his third year of treatment, he has had an unexpected drop in height velocity (–2.1 SDS), and IGF-1 concentration (–2.0 SDS). His GH dosage is appropriate for the diagnosis of GH deficiency (0.2 mg/kg per week). The rest of endocrine and biochemical test results are in the normal range.

Which of the following is the best next step in this patient's management?

A. Increase the GH dosage

B. Stop GH therapy and reassess the diagnosis of GH deficiency

C. Continue GH therapy and add an aromatase inhibitor

D. Explore the patient's adherence to therapy

E. Continue GH therapy and add a GnRH analogue

Answer: D) Explore the patient's adherence to therapy

The patient's anthropometry, responses to provocative testing, low IGF-1 concentrations, MRI findings, and the good response to GH therapy in the first and second year of treatment confirm the diagnosis of GH deficiency. The GH dosage is appropriate, as demonstrated by the initial satisfactory response to therapy and good response of IGF-1 levels. The sudden drop in height velocity and IGF-1 concentrations in the third year of treatment strongly suggest nonadherence to therapy.

Nonadherence in pediatric patients on GH therapy ranges from 36% to 66%. In general, adherence to therapy in patients with chronic diseases decreases with longer treatment duration. Multiple factors affecting patients and their parents impair long-term adherence, such as poverty, low literacy, unemployment, a weak social network, dysfunctional family relationships, unstable living conditions, cost of medicines and transportation, and principles and beliefs regarding the disorder and its treatment. Assessment of adherence is difficult and may be based on indirect or direct methods. Indirect methods include the verbal checks of the regularity of injections at each visit, as well as asking patients/families to fill in "ad hoc" questionnaires or therapy logbooks. Injection-recording devices represent direct methods to measure therapy adherence, but even these methods can be circumvented by fake injections. IGF-1 is probably the best biomarker of adherence to GH therapy, as was the case in this patient who had an initial increase of IGF-1 levels followed by a sudden drop. When interviewing his parents, it became apparent that there was a difficult parental separation in conjunction with the refusal to continue GH therapy.

Patient and parent education and communication between the pediatric endocrinologist and families are the pillars to improve the adherence to GH therapy. The recent introduction of long-acting GH with weekly, rather than daily, injections is another potentially effective tool to at least partially circumvent patient resistance to long-term GH therapy.

Key Learning Points

- GH is widely prescribed for children with short stature who have a range of growth disorders. A high rate of poor or unsatisfactory response to GH therapy (ie, not leading to significant catch-up growth) in terms of height gain and height velocity increase is observed in children with approved indications.

- A good response in the first year of GH treatment is defined by a height gain of 0.5 SDS or greater and/or height velocity increase of 3 cm/year or greater and/or a height velocity of 1 SDS or greater.

- The main predictive factors of the response to GH therapy are chronological age, birth weight, height, height SDS minus target height SDS, GH peak to provocative tests, and GH dosage.

- A poor response to GH therapy should lead clinicians to assess treatment adherence. Once good adherence is confirmed, the initial diagnosis should be reevaluated and further tests should be performed. Genetic variants affecting GH/IGF-1 axis function and growth plate physiology may account for poor response to treatment

- The use of long-acting GH preparations can be helpful in GH-deficient children with poor therapy adherence. Ongoing clinical trials are testing the efficacy and safety of long-acting GH preparations in children with Turner syndrome, small-for-gestational age, and idiopathic short stature.

- There are no valid alternatives to the use of daily or weekly GH for treating children with short stature (except for those with primary IGF-1 deficiency who can benefit from IGF-1 therapy). C-natriuretic peptide analogue therapy, previously shown to be effective in promoting growth in patients with achondroplasia and hypochondroplasia, is being tested in children with idiopathic short stature.

- When GH therapy is initiated in puberty, the use of GnRH analogues to suppress puberty or aromatase inhibitors to slow down growth plate maturation in association with GH may be an option to improve growth outcomes, but robust evidence for the long-term efficacy and safety of such combination treatments is still lacking.

References

1. Carel JC, Chatelain P, Rochiccioli P, Chaussain JL. Improvement in adult height after growth hormone treatment in adolescents with short stature born small for gestational age: results of a randomized controlled study. *J Clin Endocrinol Metab*. 2003;88(4):1587-1593. PMID: 12679443

2. Maiorana A, Cianfarani S. Impact of growth hormone therapy on adult height of children born small for gestational age. *Pediatrics*. 2009;124(3):e519-e531. PMID: 19706577

3. Deodati A, Cianfarani S. Impact of growth hormone therapy on adult height of children with idiopathic short stature: systematic review. *Bmj-British Medical Journal*. 2011;342:c7157. PMID: 21398350

4. Ranke MB, Lindberg A. Predicting growth in response to growth hormone treatment. *Growth Horm IGF Res*. 2009;19(1):1-11. PMID: 18824380

5. Dos Santos C, Essioux L, Teinturier C, Tauber M, Goffin V, Bougnères P. A common polymorphism of the growth hormone receptor is associated with increased responsiveness to growth hormone. *Nat Genet*. 2004;36(7):720-724. PMID: 15208626

6. 6.Costalonga EF, Antonini SR, Guerra-Junior G, Mendonca BB, Arnhold IJ, Jorge AA. The -202 A allele of insulin-like growth factor binding protein-3 (IGFBP3) promoter polymorphism is associated with higher IGFBP-3 serum levels and better growth response to growth hormone treatment in patients with severe growth hormone deficiency. *J Clin Endocrinol Metab*. 2009;94(2):588-595. PMID: 18984657

7. Garner T, Clayton P, Højby M, Murray P, Stevens A. Gene expression signatures predict first-year response to somapacitan treatment in children with growth hormone deficiency. *J Clin Endocrinol Metab*. 2024;109(5):1214-1221. PMID: 38066644

8. Bang P, Ahmed SF, Argente J, et al. Identification and management of poor response to growth-promoting therapy in children with short stature. *Clin Endocrinol (Oxf)*. 2012;77(2):169-181. PMID: 22540980

9. Cohen P, Rogol AD, Deal CL, et al; 2007 ISS Consensus Workshop Participants. Consensus statement on the diagnosis and treatment of children with idiopathic short stature: a summary of the Growth Hormone Research Society, the Lawson Wilkins Pediatric Endocrine Society, and the European Society for Paediatric Endocrinology Workshop. *J Clin Endocrinol Metab*. 2008;93(11):4210-4217. PMID: 18782877

10. Bright GM, Morris PA, Rosenfeld RG. When is a positive test for pediatric growth hormone deficiency a true-positive test? *Horm Res Paediatr*. 2021;94(11-12):399-405. PMID: 34856538

11. Partenope C, Galazzi E, Albanese A, Bellone S, Rabbone I, Persani L. Sex steroid priming in short stature children unresponsive to GH stimulation

tests: why, who, when and how. *Front Endocrinol (Lausanne)*. 2022;13:1072271. PMID: 36523598

12. Duncan G, Kiff S, Mitchell RT. Sex steroid priming for growth hormone stimulation testing in children and adolescents with short stature: A systematic review. *Clin Endocrinol (Oxf)*. 2023;98(4):527-535. PMID: 36515075

13. Grimberg A, DiVall SA, Polychronakos C, et al. Guidelines for growth hormone and insulin-like growth factor-I treatment in children and adolescents: growth hormone deficiency, idiopathic short stature, and primary insulin-like growth factor-I deficiency. *Horm Res Paediatr*. 2016;86(6):361-397. PMID: 27884013

14. Hauer NN, Popp B, Schoeller E, et al. Clinical relevance of systematic phenotyping and exome sequencing in patients with short stature. *Genet Med*. 2018;20(6):630-638. PMID: 29758562

15. Hokken-Koelega ACS, van der Steen M, Boguszewski MCS, et al. International consensus guideline on small for gestational age: etiology and management from infancy to early adulthood. *Endocr Rev*. 2023;44(3):539-565. PMID: 36635911

16. Cohen LE, Rogol AD. Children with idiopathic short stature: an expanding role for genetic investigation in their medical evaluation. *Endocr Pract*. 2024;30(7):679-686. PMID: 38679385

17. Haverkamp F, Johansson L, Dumas H, et al. Observations of nonadherence to recombinant human growth hormone therapy in clinical practice. *Clin Ther*. 2008;30(2):307-316. PMID: 18343269

18. Cutfield WS, Derraik JG, Gunn AJ, et al. Non-compliance with growth hormone treatment in children is common and impairs linear growth. *PLoS One*. 2011;6(1):e16223. PMID: 21305004

19. Wit JM, Deeb A, Bin-Abbas B, Al Mutair A, Koledova E, Savage MO. Achieving optimal short- and long-term responses to paediatric growth hormone therapy. *J Clin Res Pediatr Endocrinol*. 2019;11(4):329-340. PMID: 31284701

20. Pampanini V, Deodati A, Inzaghi E, Cianfarani S. Long-acting growth hormone preparations and their use in children with growth hormone deficiency. *Horm Res Paediatr*. 2023;96(6):553-559. PMID: 35220308

21. Collett-Solberg PF, Ambler G, Backeljauw PF, et al. Diagnosis, genetics, and therapy of short stature in children: a growth hormone research society international perspective. *Horm Res Paediatr*. 2019;92(1):1-14. PMID: 31514194

22. Inzaghi E, Reiter E, Cianfarani S. The challenge of defining and investigating the causes of idiopathic short stature and finding an effective therapy. *Horm Res Paediatr*. 2019;92(2):71-83. PMID: 31578025

23. Jee YH, Baron J, Nilsson O. New developments in the genetic diagnosis of short stature. *Curr Opin Pediatr*. 2018;30(4):541-547. PMID: 29787394

24. Braz AF, Costalonga EF, Trarbach EB, et al. Genetic predictors of long-term response to growth hormone (GH) therapy in children with GH deficiency and Turner syndrome: the influence of a SOCS2 polymorphism. *J Clin Endocrinol Metab*. 2014;99(9):E1808-E1813. PMID: 24905066

25. Backeljauw PF, Miller BS, Dutailly P, et al. Recombinant human growth hormone plus recombinant human insulin-like growth factor-1 coadministration therapy in short children with low insulin-like growth factor-1 and growth hormone sufficiency: results from a randomized, multicenter, open-label, parallel-group, active treatment-controlled trial. *Horm Res Paediatr*. 2015;83(4):268-279. PMID: 25765099

26. Galetaki D, Zhang A, Qi Y, et al. Phase 2 trial of vosoritide use in patients with hypochondroplasia: a pharmacokinetic/pharmacodynamic analysis. *Horm Res Paediatr*. 2024:1-7. PMID: 39427650

27. Savarirayan R, Irving M, Bacino CA, et al. C-type natriuretic peptide analogue therapy in children with achondroplasia. *N Engl J Med*. 2019;381(1):25-35. PMID: 31269546

28. Savarirayan R, Tofts L, Irving M, et al. Once-daily, subcutaneous vosoritide therapy in children with achondroplasia: a randomised, double-blind, phase 3, placebo-controlled, multicentre trial. *Lancet*. 2020;396(10252):684-692. PMID: 32891212

29. Savarirayan R, De Bergua JM, Arundel P, et al. Oral infigratinib therapy in children with achondroplasia. *N Engl J Med*. 2025;392(9):865-874. PMID: 39555818

30. Mauras N, Ross J, Mericq V. Management of growth disorders in puberty: GH, GnRHa, and aromatase inhibitors: a clinical review. *Endocr Rev*. 2023;44(1):1-13. PMID: 35639981

State-of-the-Art Management of Turner Syndrome

Claus H. Gravholt, MD, PhD. Department of Endocrinology and Department of Molecular Medicine, Aarhus University Hospital, Aarhus, Denmark; Email: claus.gravholt@clin.au.dk

Educational Objectives

After reviewing this chapter, learners should be able to:

- Identify and risk stratify patients with Turner syndrome (TS) at all ages.

- Continuously follow-up and regularly screen for relevant conditions occurring more frequently among patients with TS.

- Adequately treat comorbidities in patients with TS.

Significance of the Clinical Problem

Treatment with GH during childhood and adolescence allows a considerable gain in adult height. SHOX deficiency explains some of the phenotypic characteristics in TS, principally short stature. Puberty must be induced in most girls, and female sex hormone replacement therapy (HRT) should continue during the adult years. These issues are normally dealt with by pediatricians, but once a patient with TS enters adulthood, it is less clear who should be the primary care giver. Morbidity and mortality are increased, especially due to the risk of aortic dissection and other cardiovascular diseases, type 2 diabetes, hypertension, osteoporosis, thyroid disease, and other diseases.[1] The average loss of lifespan of women with TS is considerable and amounts to 13 to 15 years.[2] The comorbidities listed above and other conditions occur much more frequently in individuals with TS and also at a younger age

than normally seen in the general population.[3-5] This means that the clinician must be vigilant and expect the unexpected when dealing with patients who have TS. Furthermore, the clinical diagnosis of TS is often severely delayed,[6] despite the fact that textbook depictions of girls with TS describe a very distinct phenotypic presentation. However, many girls with TS present with fewer stigmata that may be easily overlooked, and the median age at diagnosis is 15 years.[6] An estimated 15% of all individuals with TS are never diagnosed.

Practice Gaps

- Diagnosis is delayed for many individuals with TS.

- Individuals with Turner syndrome almost always have comorbidities that often go undetected but should be diagnosed and treated. Known conditions, such as congenital heart malformations, also need correct treatment, including surgery, when necessary.

- Appropriate HRT should be given to all hypogonadal girls with TS starting around age 11 years to induce puberty and should be continued at least until the normal age of menopause (52-53 years), sometimes even longer. Some women with TS receive a suboptimal dosage or no HRT at all.

- Cardiovascular issues are common in women with TS, and they often interfere with other treatments, such as the possibility of becoming pregnant via oocyte donation.

Discussion

Consensus documents concerning the optimal treatment of Turner syndrome have been produced, but they are only fully implemented in a few clinics around the world.[3] Furthermore, a range of outstanding issues and questions remain unanswered, both when addressing problems relating to childhood and adolescence, as well as adulthood.

The 45,X karyotype is still the most common karyotype identified among individuals with TS; however, during recent decades, the number of individuals diagnosed with mosaic TS (45,X/46,XX) has increased.[6,7] Other karyotypes exist, including ring X chromosomes, iso chromosomes, deletions of part of the X chromosome, or karyotypes including part of a Y chromosome. Only 30% to 85% of all individuals with TS are ever diagnosed, with a wide range of age at diagnosis, from prenatally to after postmenopausal age.[6] There is no obvious explanation for this lack of diagnosis, but new avenues for better diagnostics, such as neonatal screening programs using genome sequencing, should probably be put in place.[1] The median age at TS diagnosis is 15 years, although it is younger in those with a 45,X karyotype or a mosaic karyotype, and older in those with other karyotypes.

TS is usually accompanied by hypergonadotropic hypogonadism, leading to low levels of estrogens and, compared with healthy girls, lower androgen levels.[8] Ovarian insufficiency leads to pubertal delay, primary or secondary amenorrhea, poor development of secondary sex characteristics, impaired sexual functioning, and in most cases infertility. The phenotype differentiates depending on karyotype, as individuals with 45,X have more pronounced symptoms. Gonadal functioning in TS is extremely variable and dependent on karyotype. Approximately 20% of girls with monosomy X enter puberty spontaneously, compared with 70% of girls with mosaicism. About one-third of girls with TS have spontaneous breast development, which is positively associated with the circulating antimullerian hormone concentration.[9] Regular menstrual cycles occur in 6% of girls with TS.[10]

Mosaic karyotypes are associated with a higher likelihood of preserved ovarian function, as determined by the frequency of spontaneous menarche. Women with TS are most often infertile, this being the greatest factor influencing their quality of life.[11] Very few can become pregnant with their own oocytes. Most women with TS are likely to experience premature ovarian insufficiency and are hence less likely to become pregnant. Spontaneous pregnancy occurs in 4.8% to 7.6% of women with TS,[12,13] and miscarriages are more frequent in such pregnancies.[14] According to the international TS guidelines,[1] it is recommended to initiate estrogen replacement when the patient is between 11 and 12 years of age, increasing to an adult dosage over 2 to 3 years. Low-dosage estradiol is recommended, and transdermal administration is preferred to oral use because of fewer adverse effects. Once bleeding occurs, progesterone should be added. With adequate hormone replacement, it is possible to stimulate uterine growth, which will then reach adult size and thus potentially be ready for oocyte donation from a foreign donor. It is also clear that pregnancy after oocyte donation carries a higher risk of pregnancy complications and spontaneous abortion than the rare spontaneous pregnancy among women with TS.[15]

The risk of both type 1 and type 2 diabetes is increased in women with TS.[5] Altered body composition associated with TS includes increased BMI, decreased muscle mass, and increased total fat mass and visceral fat mass.[16] Relatively sedentary lifestyle and decreased physical fitness have also been demonstrated.[17] In the face of widespread abnormalities of glucose homeostasis and increased risk of type 1 and type 2 diabetes, there is a need for persistent attention to these factors in clinical follow-up. Recommendations for diagnosis and treatment of diabetes adhere to general population guidelines and annual screening of fasting glucose and hemoglobin A_{1c} should be performed. Autoimmune thyroid disease is common in TS, with hypothyroidism occurring in up to 50% of women at age 50 years.[18] Hyperthyroidism also occurs more frequently than among control patients. Treatment of thyroid disease should follow clinical guidelines. In individuals with TS, the occurrence of all other autoimmune diseases is also increased in comparison with the background population risk, although the reason for this increase remains obscure.[19] Therefore, the clinician should be vigilant and examine women with TS if there is the slightest suspicion. Currently, there are recommendations for how a clinical care program should be tailored for adults with TS.[1] Some diseases, such as celiac disease, inflammatory bowel disease, and rheumatoid disease, occur frequently enough to warrant special attention. Peak bone mass depends on several factors, such as genetic background, nutrition, physical activity, local growth factors, and a spectrum of hormones. Estradiol secretion in TS is already deficient in childhood and adolescence, and children and younger and middle-aged adult patients with TS have low bone mineral density. Studies show that the risk of fracture and frank osteoporosis is increased in individuals with TS. Estrogen substitution therapy is crucial to attain maximal peak bone mass in adolescents and young adults.

Although cardiologists are the specialists treating aortic disease that is often present in TS, endocrinologists must also have knowledge of cardiac conditions. In early adult life, aortic dilatation and eventually aortic dissection is seen in significant numbers.[20] In clear contrast, aortic dissection is a disease mostly seen among elderly persons in the normal population. This is probably why aortic disease is misdiagnosed and mistreated in young women with TS, in whom the significance of aortic dilatation is underestimated and prophylactic surgery is often not offered in time. The presence of a bicuspid aortic valve is a major determinant for aortic dilatation, as well as for the presence of elevated diastolic blood pressure and aortic arch anomalies.[21] The current recommendation is to lower blood pressure with an angiotensin II receptor, ACE inhibitor, or β-adrenergic blocker. Hypertension is a common phenomenon in TS. The true prevalence is uncertain, but up to 50% of an adult population

with TS may have arterial hypertension.[22-24] The cause of hypertension in TS is likely multifactorial. The high prevalence of overweight and obesity in TS contributes significantly to the hypertension disease burden and to the association with type 1 and type 2 diabetes.[23]

Future Directions

Recently, new genes have been linked to TS. Tissue inhibitor of matrix metalloproteinases 1 (*TIMP1*) is an escape gene on Xp and is therefore normally expressed in duplicate. Females with TS have haploinsufficiency for this gene. *TIMP3* is a gene with partially overlapping function on chromosome 22 and haploinsufficiency of *TIMP1* and a certain risk single-nucleotide variant in *TIMP3* predisposes to developing typical hallmark signs of TS—aortic dilatation and bicuspid aortic valves. A decrease in TIMPs could lead to higher levels of MMP2 and MMP9, which are involved in the development of aortic dissection.[25] Recently, we showed increased levels of neutrophils and increased neutrophil activation, which may lead to neutrophil-driven inflammatory stress in TS (submitted manuscript). The increase in neutrophils was linked to increased expression of the X-Y homologous gene *TBL1X*, suggesting a genetic basis for the prevalence of neutrophil-driven chronic inflammatory diseases, such as autoimmune disorders and metabolic conditions in TS.[5,19] Similarly, the *SLC25A6* gene, also situated in the pseudoautosomal region of the X and Y chromosomes and normally expressed in 2 copies, is associated with increased QT interval in individuals with TS, who have just 1 copy.[26] Such new studies are fascinating because they may direct future therapies in TS, and knowledge of these genes could be used preventively.

Clinical Case Vignettes
Case 1

A 56-year-old woman has a complex medical history. She had menarche at age 11 years and regular menstruation until age 18 years. At age 23 years, her primary care provider initiated HRT. At age 29 years, she was reading a magazine story about a woman with TS. She recognized herself in this story and asked her primary care provider if she could be tested. The care provider told her that he had already tested her 5 years earlier with a confirmed karyotype of 45,X. She developed hypothyroidism at age 30 years, underwent hysterectomy at age 40 years because of profuse bleeding, and had a gall bladder operation at age 49 years, Hypertension was diagnosed at age 52 years. She retired early at age 54 years because of depression and burn-out; neurocognitive evaluation showed issues with executive functioning and multitasking. She recently had a knee replacement.

Current medications are lisinopril, citalopram, levothyroxine, and estradiol. Her weight is 176.4 lb (80 kg), and height is 58.7 in (149 cm) (BMI = 36.0 kg/m^2).

Continued treatment with estradiol is planned until at least 60 years of age.

Which of the following is the median age at diagnosis of TS?

A. Age 1 year

B. Age 5 years

C. Age 15 years

D. Age 27 years

Answer: C) Age 15 years

This vignette highlights problems with late diagnosis, which in this patient's case is likely related to the somewhat atypical normal menarche and ongoing menstruation until age 18 years. However, many girls with TS undergo menarche. The median age at diagnosis of TS is 15 years (Answer C). In addition, the vignette also illustrates the increasing comorbidity burden as women with TS age, and this necessitates ongoing vigilance on behalf of the caring physician.

Case 2

A woman was diagnosed with TS ((karyotype = 45,X) at age 10 years and subsequently received GH therapy. She did not have spontaneous menarche, so puberty was induced at age 14

years. Hypothyroidism was diagnosed at age 18 years. She had an uneventful early adulthood and successfully worked fulltime and led an active lifestyle. She received egg donation and had a healthy baby. She has always had delicate skin and psoriasis was diagnosed. She developed type 2 diabetes (no positive autoantibodies for type 1 diabetes) at age 51 years. At that time, her weight was 127.9 lb (58 kg) and height was 57.1 in (145 cm) (BMI = 27.6 kg/m^2). She developed angina when jogging. Coronary angiography showed constrictions of the left anterior descending artery (second branch); however, it was not possible to place a stent. She began treatment with metformin, statins, and acetylsalicylic acid. She did not tolerate acetylsalicylic acid, so this was replaced with clopidogrel. She developed severe exfoliative dermatitis and was twice hospitalized, needing high-dosage topical glucocorticoids. The psoriasis diagnosis was revised to pityriasis rubra pilaris and treated with methotrexate. She was determined to be probably likely allergic to statins, clopidogrel, acetylsalicylic acid, and possibly other medications. She developed hypertension at the age 52 years. She is currently being treated with metformin, a GLP-1 receptor agonist, methotrexate, bisoprolol, prasugrel (antithrombotic agent), topical steroids, HRT, and levothyroxine. She has lost weight and now weighs 119.1 lb (54 kg) (BMI = 25.7 kg/m^2).

Is metabolic syndrome more common in individuals with TS than in the general population?

A. Less common

B. Same frequency

C. More common

D. Type 1 diabetes, but not type 2 diabetes, is more common

Answer: C) More common

This vignette illustrates that metabolic syndrome sometimes develops with very slight weight increases in women with TS. This case also illustrates that despite an uneventful early adulthood, this patient developed a host of other comorbid conditions likely related to metabolic syndrome. We speculate that low-grade inflammation may be an integral part of TS.

Case 3

A 20-year-old woman with TS (karyotype = 45,X/46,XX) would like to know about her chances of fertility. She is on HRT to manage hypergonadotropic hypogonadism. She has bicuspid aortic valves and had an operation at age 4 months to address aortic valve stenosis. She is normotensive, but echocardiography shows moderate stenosis (30 mm Hg gradient), and subsequent MRI of the aorta shows a maximum dilatation of the ascending aorta of 4.5 cm (indexed aortic size is 2.58 cm/m^2). She also has ectatic truncus brachiocephalicus. The size is larger than normative data.[21] Her height is 60.6 in (154 cm), and weight is 167.6 lb (76 kg) (BMI = 32.1 kg/m^2).

Are congenital heart malformations problematic for individuals with TS?

A. No, these malformations are usually asymptomatic

B. Yes, they can be life-threatening, especially during pregnancy

C. Yes, they can be life-threatening and require lifelong monitoring

D. No, once they are identified and treated in infancy, no additional heart problems usually arise

Answers: B and C) Yes, they can be life-threatening, especially during pregnancy, and yes, they can be life-threatening and require lifelong monitoring

Cardiovascular issues are of great importance in the care of patients with TS, and they cause of 50% of excess mortality. Lifelong surveillance is necessary because during adulthood patients often develop issues with dilation of the aorta, bicuspid aortic valves, partial anomalous pulmonary return, etc. Therefore, endocrinologists must collaboration with knowledgeable cardiologists to keep patients healthy. Today, these cardiovascular issues should be viewed as preventable conditions that should not lead to premature death.

Key Learning Points

- TS is a chronic condition, often with numerous comorbidities that develop as patients age. It is important to be vigilant as the anchor physician and to diagnose such conditions during clinical follow-up. Morbidity and mortality are elevated in women with TS, and adulthood can be complicated by a host of conditions, such as osteoporosis, diabetes (both type 1 and 2), hypothyroidism, obesity, and other endocrine diseases. Prevention, intervention, and proper treatment are only just being recognized. Hypertension is common and can be a forerunner of cardiovascular disease. Aortic dilation and aortic dissection are frequently seen at a compellingly young age.

- The proper HRT dosage with female sex steroids has not been established, and, likewise, benefits and/or drawbacks of HRT have not been thoroughly evaluated. However, it is pivotal that patients with TS receive HRT for at least 42 years, which is equivalent to the normal length of time that women are exposed to endogenously produced estrogen.

- Fertility is an important issue for young adults, and many women with TS choose egg donation. Based on the latest literature, egg donation pregnancies may not be as risky as early reports suggested.

- The description of adult life with TS has been broadened, and medical, social, and psychological aspects are being added at a compelling pace. Proper care during adulthood should be studied, and a framework for care should be in place, since most morbidity is potentially amenable to intervention.

References

1. Gravholt CH, Andersen NH, Christin-Maitre S, et al. Clinical practice guidelines for the care of girls and women with Turner syndrome. *Eur J Endocrinol*. 2024;190(6):G53-G151. PMID: 38748847

2. Schoemaker MJ, Swedlow AJ, Higgins CD, Wright AF, Jacobs PA; United Kingdom Clinical Cytogenetics Group. Mortality in women with Turner syndrome in Great Britain: a national cohort study. *J Clin Endocrinol Metab*. 2008;93(12):4735-4742. PMID: 18812477

3. Viuff MH, Stochholm K, Gronbaek H, Berglund A, Juul S, Gravholt CH. Increased occurrence of liver and gastrointestinal diseases and anaemia in women with Turner syndrome - a nationwide cohort study. *Aliment Pharmacol Ther*. 2021;53(7):821-829. PMID: 33550624

4. Viuff MH, Stochholm K, Juul S, Graveholt CH. Disorders of the eye, ear, skin, and nervous system in women with Turner syndrome -a nationwide cohort study. *Eur J Hum Genet*. 2022;30(2):229-236. PMID: 34707298

5. Viuff MH, Berglund A, Juul S, Andersen NH, Stochholm K, Graveholt CH. Sex hormone replacement therapy in Turner Syndrome - impact on morbidity and mortality. *J Clin Endocrinol Metab*. 2020;105(2):dgz039. PMID: 31545360

6. Berglund A. Stochholm K, Gravholt CH. The epidemiology of sex chromosome abnormalities. *Am J Med Genet C Semin Med Genet*. 2020;184(2):202-215. PMID: 32506765

7. Tuke MA, Ruth KS, Wood AR, et al. Mosaic Turner syndrome shows reduced penetrance in an adult population study. *Genet Med*. 2019;21(4):877-886. PMID: 30181606

8. Viuff MH, Just J, Brun S, et al. Women with Turner syndrome are both estrogen and androgen deficient - the impact of hormone replacement therapy. *J Clin Endocrinol Metab*. 2022;107(7):1983-1993. PMID: 35302622

9. Hamza RT, Mira MF, Hamed A, Ezzat T, Sallam MT. Anti-müllerian hormone levels in patients with turner syndrome: relation to karyotype, spontaneous puberty, and replacement therapy. *Am J Med Genet A*. 2018;176(9):1929-1934.

10. Dabrowski E, Jensen R, Johnson E, Habiby RL, Brickman WJ, Finlayson C. Turner syndrome systematic review: spontaneous thelarche and menarche stratified by karyotype. *Horm Res Paediatr*. 2019;92;(3):143-149. PMID: 31918426

11. Sutton EJ, McInerney-Leo A, Bondy CA, Gollust SE, King D, Biesecker B. Turner syndrome: four challenges across the lifespan. *Am J Med Genet A*. 2005;139A(2):57-66. PMID: 16252273

12. Bryman I, Sylven L, Berntorp K, et al. Pregnancy rate and outcome in Swedish women with Turner syndrome. *Fertil Steril*. 2011;95(8)2507-2510. PMID: 21256486

13. Bernard V, Donadille B, Zenaty D, et al. Spontaneous fertility and pregnancy outcomes amongst 480 women with Turner syndrome. *Hum Reprod*. 2016;31(4)782-788. PMID: 26874361

14. Cauldwell M, Steer PJ, Adamson D, et al., Pregnancies in women with Turner syndrome: a retrospective multicentre UK study. *BJOG*. 2022;129(5):796-803. PMID: 34800331

15. Chevalier N, Letur H, Lelannou D, et al; French Study Group for Oocyte Donation. Materno-fetal cardiovascular complications in Turner syndrome after oocyte donation: insufficient prepregnancy screening and pregnancy follow-up are associated with poor outcome. *J Clin Endocrinol Metab*. 2011;96(2):E260-E267. PMID: 21147890

16. Gravholt CH, Eilersen Hjerrild B, Mosekilde L, et al., Body composition is distinctly altered in Turner syndrome: relations to glucose metabolism, circulating adipokines, and endothelial adhesion molecules. *Eur J Endocrinol*. 2006;155(4)583-592. PMID: 16990658

17. Santi M, Fluck CE, Hauschild M, Kuhlmann B, Kuehni CE, Sommer G. Health behaviour of women with Turner syndrome. *Acta Paediatr*. 2021;110(8):2424-2429. PMID: 33615554

18. Naessén S, Eliasson M, Berntorp K, et al. Autoimmune disease in Turner syndrome in Sweden: an up to 25 years ´controlled follow-up study. *J Clin Endocrinol Metab*. 2023;109(2):e602-e612. PMID: 37758506

19. Jorgensen KT, Rostgaard K, Bache I, et al. Autoimmune diseases in women with Turner's syndrome. *Arthritis Rheum*. 2010;62(3):658-666. PMID: 20187158

20. Alam S, Claxton JS, Mortillo M, et al. Thirty-year survival after cardiac surgery for patients with Turner syndrome. *J Pediatr*. 2021;239:187-192.e1. PMID: 34450123

21. Mortensen KH, Erlandsen M, Andersen NH, Gravholt CH. Prediction of aortic dilation in Turner syndrome--enhancing the use of serial cardiovascular magnetic resonance. *J Cardiovasc Magn Reson*. 2013;15(1):47. PMID: 23742092

22. De Groote K, Demulier L, De Backer J, et al. Arterial hypertension in Turner syndrome: a review of the literature and a practical approach for diagnosis and treatment. *J Hypertens*. 2015;33(7):1342-1351. PMID: 26039527

23. Fiot E, Zenaty D, Boizeau P, Haignere J, Dos Santos S, Leger J; French Turner Syndrome Study Group. X chromosome gene dosage as a determinant of congenital malformations and of age-related comorbidity risk in patients with Turner syndrome, from childhood to early adulthood. *Eur J Endocrinol*. 2019;180(6):397-406. PMID: 30991358

24. K. Sandahl, J. Wen, M. Erlandsen, N. H. Andersen, C. H. Gravholt, Natural History of Hypertension in Turner Syndrome During a 12-Year Pragmatic Interventional Study. *Hypertension*. 2020;76(5):1608-1615. PMID: 32895020

25. Corbitt H, Morris SH, Gravholt CH, et al; GenTAC Registry Investigators. TIMP3 and TIMP1 are risk genes for bicuspid aortic valve and aortopathy in Turner syndrome. *PLoS Genet*. 2018;14(10):e1007692. PMID: 30281655.

26. Skakkebæk A, Kjæ-Sorensen K, Matchkov VV, et al. Dosage of the pseudoautosomal gene SLC25A6 is implicated in QTc interval duration. *Sci Rep*. 2023;13(1):12089. PMID: 37495650

Pediatric Obesity: Challenges and Solutions

Ashley Shoemaker, MD, MSCI. Pediatric Endocrinology, Vanderbilt University Medical Center, Nashville, TN; Email: Ashley.H.Shoemaker@vumc.org

Educational Objectives

After reviewing this chapter, learners should be able to:

- Recognize patterns of abnormal weight gain in childhood.

- Identify appropriate pharmacologic options for treatment of pediatric obesity.

- Explain the role of genetic testing for the diagnosis of pediatric obesity.

Significance of the Clinical Problem

Pediatric obesity is an escalating problem, with a 2017-2020 prevalence of 19.7% among children and adolescents in the United States according to the Centers for Disease Control. The implications are far-reaching, with obesity-related comorbidities such as sleep apnea, type 2 diabetes, and metabolic dysfunction-associated steatotic liver disease, now prevalent among children. Traditional lifestyle interventions, including diet and exercise, have proven insufficient in combating pediatric obesity, often leading to frustration and a sense of hopelessness for both families and health care providers. This underscores the urgent need for enhanced efforts in obesity prevention and treatment.

Recent advancements in medical treatments offer promising solutions for pediatric obesity. Bariatric surgery and pharmacotherapy (particularly GLP-1 receptor agonists) have shown effectiveness in managing and reducing obesity in children, but physicians must be willing to integrate pharmacotherapy into their treatment plans. Additionally, incorporating genetic testing into diagnostic algorithms can further refine treatment selection as there are now drugs targeting leptin deficiency and MC4R pathway defects. Additional drugs are under development for treatment of Prader-Willi syndrome. By adopting a multifaceted approach, we can improve treatment efficacy and ultimately enhance the quality of life of children living with obesity and its associated complications.

Practice Gaps

- Many of the drugs used for treatment of pediatric obesity have been approved in the past 3 years; therefore, many physicians lack training in pharmacotherapy options for pediatric obesity.

- Inexpensive genetic obesity panels are now available, and physicians need additional education to understand how to incorporate these tools into their practice.

Discussion

Pediatric obesity is a growing public health concern, with significant implications for long-term health outcomes. It is critical that primary care physicians and subspecialists who manage obesity comorbidities become more comfortable with the diagnosis and treatment of pediatric obesity. Centers for Disease Control BMI growth charts are commonly used for diagnosis:

- Class 1 obesity: BMI ≥95th percentile
- Class 2 obesity: BMI ≥120% of the 95th percentile
- Class 3 obesity: ≥140% of the 95th percentile

There is a high correlation between pediatric and adult obesity, particularly in patients with early adiposity rebound.[1,2]

Intensive Lifestyle Programs

Intensive lifestyle programs are a cornerstone in the treatment of pediatric obesity. Intensive programs are defined as including 26 or more hours of face-to-face treatment over a period of 3 to 12 months. They focus on comprehensive behavioral interventions that include dietary changes, increased physical activity, and behavioral therapy. The American Academy of Pediatrics (AAP) and Endocrine Society guidelines recommend these programs for children and adolescents with obesity, emphasizing the importance of family involvement to support sustainable lifestyle changes.[3,4] Despite their intensive nature, the effectiveness of these programs can be modest. A review of 44 randomized controlled trials involving approximately 5000 adolescent participants found that lifestyle interventions resulted in a mean difference in BMI of only −1.18 kg/m².[5] This suggests that while lifestyle interventions are beneficial, they often need to be supplemented with other treatments for clinically meaningful results.

Pharmacotherapy

Pharmacotherapy is an important adjunct to lifestyle interventions for pediatric obesity. Numerous antiobesity medications are available for adults (*adult* defined by the US FDA as 17 years and older) and an increasing number are approved for use in children aged 12 years and older (*Table*). While medications such as orlistat

Table. FDA-Approved Antiobesity Medications

Drug	Approval date	Age range, y	Indication	Mechanism
Phentermine	1959	≥17	Obesity	Sympathomimetic amine that decreases appetite, approved for short-term (12 weeks) use only
Orlistat	1999	≥12	Obesity	Blocks intestinal lipase to reduce fat absorption
Phentermine/topiramate	2012 adults 2022 pediatrics	≥12	Obesity	Sympathomimetic amine plus topiramate (mechanism unknown)
Naltrexone/bupropion	2014	≥12	Obesity	Blocks autoinhibitory feedback and stimulates POMC neurons, possibly regulating reward pathways
Liraglutide	2014 adults 2020 pediatrics	≥12	Obesity	GLP-1 receptor agonist, increases satiety and decreases rate of gastric emptying
Metreleptin	2014	All	Congenital leptin deficiency	Leptin analogue, stimulates leptin receptor
Lisdexamfeta-mine	2015	≥17	Binge eating	Noncatecholamine sympathomimetic amine
Semaglutide	2021 adults 2023 pediatrics	≥12	Obesity	GLP-1 receptor agonist, increases satiety and decreases rate of gastric emptying
Tirzepatide	2023	≥17	Obesity	GLP-1 and GIP dual receptor agonist, increases satiety and decreases rate of gastric emptying
Setmelanotide	2020	≥2	Genetic obesity (biallelic PCSK1/LEPR/POMC deficiency, Bardet-Biedl syndrome)	α-Melanocortin stimulating hormone analogue, improves signaling through MC4R pathway

have been approved for decades, they were limited by lack of effectiveness and poor tolerability.[6] Incretin based therapies, such as GLP-1 receptor agonists, have revolutionized pharmacotherapy for obesity due to their dramatic improvement in efficacy. For example, 68 weeks of treatment with semaglutide resulted in a 15% mean decrease in BMI in adolescents.[7] Dual and triple incretins may have even better efficacy; trials are ongoing in children. The Endocrine Society guidelines recommend pharmacotherapy for children 12 years and older in children with obesity who have not responded to lifestyle interventions.[3] The 2023 American Academy of Pediatrics recommend use of pharmacotherapy for children 12 years and older with obesity and consideration of therapy for children 8 to 11 years old.[4]

Bariatric Surgery

For adolescents with severe obesity, bariatric surgery is a viable and effective treatment option. Procedures such as gastric bypass and sleeve gastrectomy have shown significant and sustained weight loss, along with improvements in obesity-related comorbidities such as type 2 diabetes and hypertension. Compared with adults, adolescents have similar 5-year outcomes, with an average weight loss of 26%, but adolescents are more likely to have resolution of comorbidities (type 2 diabetes, hypertension).[8] Referral for consideration of bariatric surgery is recommended by the AAP for adolescents (13 years and older) with a BMI greater than 120% of the 95th percentile/class 2 obesity. Challenges of bariatric surgery include access to pediatric bariatric surgery and insurance coverage.[9] Adolescents undergoing bariatric surgery need ongoing monitoring for nutritional deficiencies and long-term mental health support. Depression is often a comorbid condition with obesity. Mental health disorders are not a contraindication to bariatric surgery, unless there is active suicidality, active psychosis, or ongoing substance abuse.[10]

Genetic Obesity Syndromes

More than 80 genes have been identified as contributing to obesity risk, and screening patients for genetic obesity may improve treatment decisions. The Endocrine Society guidelines recommend considering genetic testing in patients with obesity onset before 5 years of age who have clinical features of genetic obesity syndromes, particularly extreme hyperphagia and/or a family history of extreme obesity.[3] It can be hard to determine obesity onset if early growth chart data are not available. At least 1 cohort found MC4R variants in greater than 5% of children with onset of severe obesity before 10 years old.[11] While children with genetic obesity may have associated short stature, their linear growth rate is usually normal.

Patients with syndromic obesity, such as Prader-Willi syndrome, Bardet-Biedl syndrome, and pseudohypoparathyroidism typically present with early-onset obesity, hyperphagia, developmental delays, and other congenital anomalies. Nonsyndromic obesity can present with childhood obesity alone. The most common cause of nonsyndromic obesity is due to deleterious variants in the MC4R gene, affecting approximately 1 in 100 persons with obesity.[12,13] When evaluating a patient with obesity, the severity of obesity alone is not a reliable indicator of a genetic cause; instead, a combination of early-onset and increased appetite should prompt genetic evaluation. The one exception is Prader-Willi syndrome, which has distinct nutritional phases, beginning with poor feeding and failure to thrive in infancy, not obesity. The classic extreme hyperphagia of Prader-Willi syndrome has an onset around 8 years old.[14]

Emerging treatments targeting genetic syndromes include the melanocortin 4 receptor (MC4R) agonist setmelanotide, which is approved for treatment of biallelic POMC, LEPR, or PCSK1 deficiency, as well as Bardet-Biedl syndrome. Recombinant human leptin is available for treatment of complete leptin deficiency.[15] Several drugs for Prader-Willi syndrome are in phase 3 clinical trials. Early genetic testing is crucial for identifying these syndromes and initiating appropriate interventions.

Conclusions

The treatment of pediatric obesity requires a multifaceted approach that includes intensive lifestyle programs, pharmacotherapy, and/or bariatric surgery. While lifestyle interventions form the foundation of treatment, their modest effectiveness highlights the need for additional therapeutic options. Pharmacotherapy and bariatric surgery offer significant benefits for selected patients, and advances in genetic research hold promise for personalized treatment strategies. Early identification and intervention are key to improving outcomes for children and adolescents with obesity.

Clinical Case Vignettes

Case 1

A 15-year-old boy presents for evaluation of type 2 diabetes. He has been overweight for several years, but reports gaining 30 lb (13.6 kg) over summer break that he attributes to more snacking while at home alone. At his well-child visit, his BMI is 40 kg/m² (class 3 obesity). The pediatrician sent screening labs which were significant for a hemoglobin A_{1c} value 7.5% (58 mmol/mol), mild mixed hyperlipidemia and elevated transaminases. There is a family history of obesity and type 2 diabetes in his father and maternal grandmother. Medical history is significant for an episode of supraventricular tachycardia and depression with a recent hospital admission for suicidality. He is asymptomatic without polyuria, polydipsia, or weight loss.

Which of the following antiobesity medications would you recommend as first-line treatment for this patient?

A. Semaglutide

B. Phentermine/topiramate

C. Setmelanotide

D. Metformin

E. Orlistat

Answer: A) Semaglutide

Semaglutide is approved for pediatric use and one of the more effective antiobesity medications and approved for treatment of both type 2 diabetes and obesity. Phentermine/topiramate is not recommended in a patient with a history of cardiac arrythmias. Setmelanotide is indicated for treatment of several genetic obesity syndromes but not common obesity. Metformin is an excellent first-line therapy for type 2 diabetes but has minimal antiobesity effects. Orlistat is typically less effective than semaglutide for treatment of adolescent obesity and does not lower hemoglobin A_{1c}.

Case 1, Continued

The patient has some weight loss with semaglutide (BMI now 37 kg/m²) but requires addition of basal insulin for persistent hyperglycemia. The family is interested in additional options for treatment of obesity.

Which of the following would represent a contraindication to bariatric surgery in this patient?

A. Age

B. Class 2 obesity

C. Depression with suicidality

D. Insulin-requiring type 2 diabetes

Answer: C) Depression with suicidality

The patient's age and degree of obesity meet criteria for referral for consideration of bariatric surgery. Type 2 diabetes, whether insulin dependent or not, and other obesity-related comorbidities are further indications for bariatric surgery. While a history of mental illness is not a contraindication for bariatric surgery, active psychosis, suicidality, and current substance abuse are reasons to delay referral.

Case 2

You are consulted for abnormal weight gain in an 8-year-old girl. Her weight is at the 99th percentile, and height is tracking along the 50th percentile. She has a history of developmental delays and a single kidney. She wears glasses and has some difficulty with night vision. Her parents report onset of obesity in the toddler years. She likes to snack and eats an adult portion at dinner. She participates in a Special Olympics softball program for exercise. There is no family history of consanguinity. She has 2 older siblings; both are healthy and do not have obesity.

Which of the following is the best laboratory test to order now for this patient?

A. Methylation testing of chromosome 15
B. Thyroid hormone levels
C. Targeted sequencing of *GNAS*
D. Genetic obesity panel
E. Midnight salivary cortisol level

Answer: D) Genetic obesity panel

This patient has clinical features of Bardet-Biedl syndrome, including early-onset obesity, developmental delays, kidney anomalies, and night blindness (early sign of rod-cone dystrophy). A genetic obesity panel is an appropriate next step, as there are more than 20 genes associated with Bardet-Biedl syndrome. Methylation testing of chromosome 15 is used in the diagnosis of Prader-Willi syndrome. Variants in *GNAS* can cause pseudohypoparathyroidism. A decrease in linear growth velocity would be expected from symptomatic hypothyroidism or hypercortisolism.

Case 2, Continued

The child is found to have 2 likely pathogenic variants in the *BBS2* gene. Ophthalmology consultation showed rod-cone dystrophy.

Which of the following medications is indicated for treatment of obesity in this child?

A. Semaglutide
B. Phentermine/topiramate
C. Setmelanotide
D. Tirzepatide
E. Orlistat

Answer: C) Setmelanotide

Setmelanotide is approved for treatment of obesity in patients 2 years and older with Bardet-Biedl syndrome. The other options are all antiobesity medications, but they are not approved for a child this young and not specifically indicated for her syndromic obesity.

Case 3

A child presents at 5 years old with class 3 obesity (BMI = 145% of the 95th percentile). She had rapid weight gain noted in early infancy, associated with severe hyperphagia. As an infant she would eat until she vomited. Now as a child she will sneak food at night and is never satiated. She is doing well in school without any developmental delays or other chronic medical problems. Her height is at the 95th percentile. She has acanthosis nigricans on exam but no other clinically significant physical or laboratory findings. The patient is adopted and family history is unknown.

Which of the following genetic obesity disorders is most likely in this patient?

A. Prader-Willi syndrome
B. Bardet-Biedl syndrome
C. MC4R deficiency
D. POMC deficiency
E. Leptin deficiency

Answer: C) MC4R deficiency

This patient has severe, early-onset obesity with hyperphagia, concerning for a genetic etiology. MC4R deficiency is the most common cause of nonsyndromic genetic obesity. Prader-Willi syndrome causes failure to thrive in infancy with hyperphagia onset later in childhood, as well as developmental delays. Bardet-Biedl syndrome is associated with numerous congenital anomalies, such as polydactyly, genitourinary anomalies, developmental delays, and rod-cone dystrophy. POMC deficiency is a rare autosomal recessive disorder associated with congenital adrenal insufficiency. Leptin deficiency is extremely rare, autosomal recessive, and often associated with frequent infections in childhood.

Key Learning Points

- Lifestyle modification is an important part of obesity management but is rarely sufficient as monotherapy.

- Several classes of antiobesity medications are approved for use in children.

- Bariatric surgery is an option for adolescents with class 2 obesity.

- Genetic testing can help determine the underlying cause of obesity.

- Some genetic obesity disorders have available targeted pharmacotherapies.

References

1. Whitaker RB, Pepe MS, Wright JA, Seidel KD, Dietz WH. Early adiposity rebound and the risk of adult obesity. *Pediatrics*. 1998;101(3):E5. PMID: 9481024

2. Serdula MK, Ivery D, Coates RJ, Freedman DS, Williamson DF, Byers T. Do obese children become obese adults? A review of the literature. *Prev Med*. 1993;22(2):167-77. PMID: 8483856

3. Styne DM, Arslanian SA, Connor EL, Farooqi IS, Murad MH, Silverstein JH, Yanovski JA. Pediatric obesity-assessment, treatment, and prevention: an Endocrine Society clinical practice guideline. *J Clin Endocrinol Metab*. 2017;102(3):709-757. PMID: 28359099

4. Hampl SE, Hassink SG, Skinner AC, et al. Clinical practice guideline for the evaluation and treatment of children and adolescents with obesity. *Pediatrics*. 2023;151(2):e202206040. PMID: 366221115

5. Al-Khudairy L, Loveman E, Colquitt JL, et al. Diet, physical activity and behavioural interventions for the treatment of overweight or obese adolescents aged 12 to 17 years. *Cochrane Database Syst Rev*. 2017;6(6):CD012691. PMID: 28639320

6. Sjostrom L, Rissanen A, Andersen T, et al. Randomised placebo-controlled trial of orlistat for weight loss and prevention of weight regain in obese patients. European Multicentre Orlistat Study Group. *Lancet*. 1998;352(9123):167-172. PMID: 9683204

7. Weghuber D, Barrett T, Barrientos-Perez M, et al; STEP TEENS Investigators. Once-weekly semaglutide in adolescents with obesity. *N Engl J Med*. 2022;387(24):2245-2257. PMID: 36322838

8. Inge TH, Courcoulas AP, Helmrath MAet al., Five-year outcomes of gastric bypass in adolescents as compared with adults. *N Engl J Med*. 2019;380(22):2136-2145. PMID: 31461610

9. Shoemaker AH, Chung ST, Fleischman A; Endocrine Society Obesity Special Interest Group. Trends in pediatric obesity management, a survey from the Pediatric Endocrine Society Obesity Committee. *J Pediatr Endocrinol Metab*. 2020;33(4):469-472. PMID: 32069245

10. Pratt JSA, Browne A, Browne NT, et al. ASMBS pediatric metabolic and bariatric surgery guidelines, 2018. *Surg Obes Relat Dis*. 2018;14(7):882-901. PMID: 30077361

11. Farooqi IS, Keogh JM, Yeo GSH et al. Clinical spectrum of obesity and mutations in the melanocortin 4 receptor gene. *N Engl J Med*. 2003;348(12):1085-1095. PMID: 12646665

12. Lubrano-Berthelier C, Dubern B, Lacorte J-M, et al. Melanocortin 4 receptor mutations in a large cohort of severely obese adults: prevalence, functional classification, genotype-phenotype relationship, and lack of association with binge eating. *J Clin Endocrinol Metab*. 2006;91(5):1811-1818. PMID: 16507637

13. Stutzmann F, Tan K, Vatin V, et al. Prevalence of melanocortin-4 receptor deficiency in Europeans and their age-dependent penetrance in multigenerational pedigrees. *Diabetes*. 2008;57(9):2511-2518. PMID: 185559663

14. Miller JL, Lynn CH, Driscoll DC, et al. Nutritional phases in Prader-Willi syndrome. *Am J Med Genet A*. 2011;155A(5):1040-1049. PMID: 21465655

15. Farooqi IS, Matarese G, Lord GM, et al. Beneficial effects of leptin on obesity, T cell hyporesponsiveness, and neuroendocrine/metabolic dysfunction of human congenital leptin deficiency. *J Clin Invest*. 200;110(8):1093-1103. PMID: 12393845

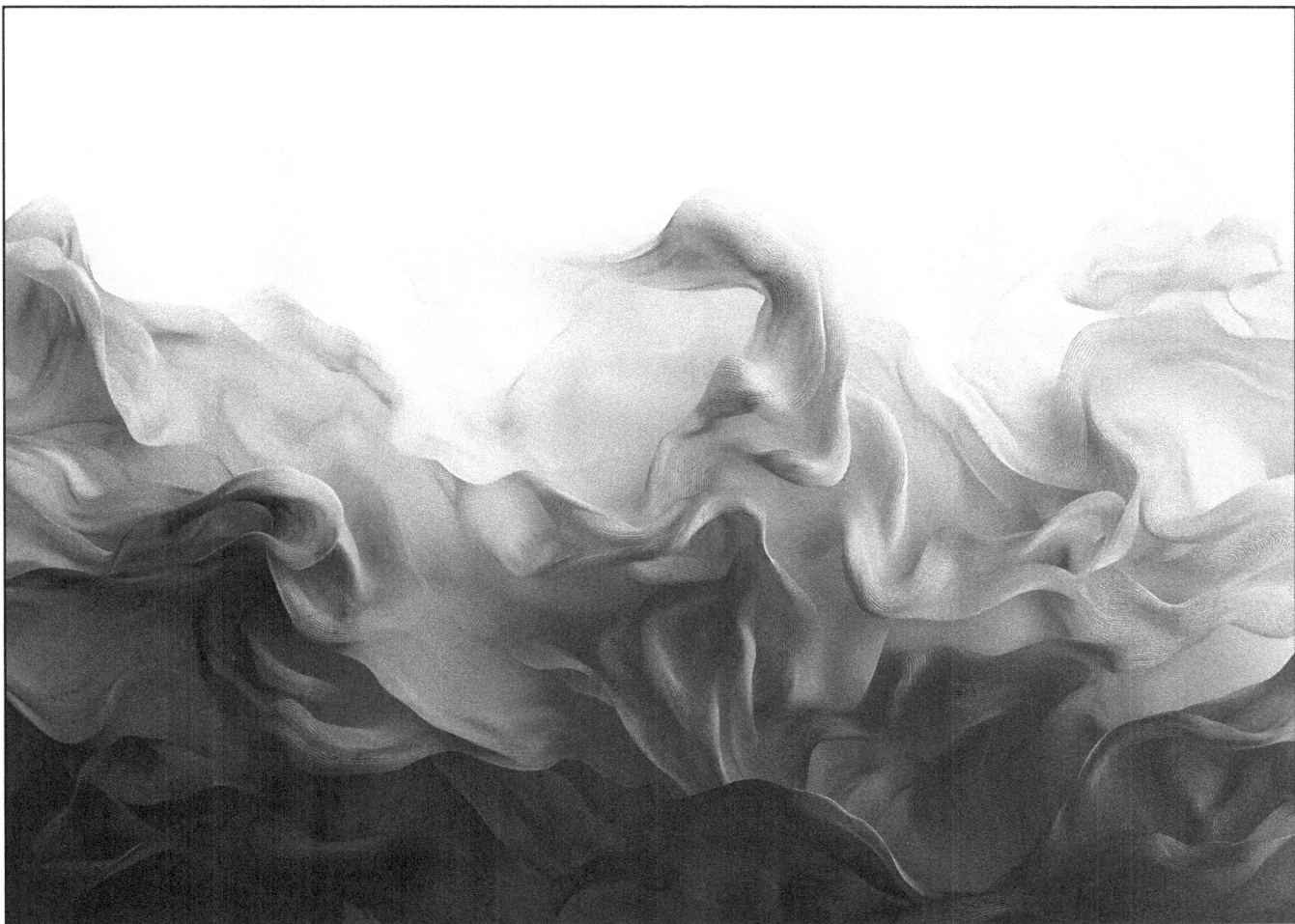

REPRODUCTIVE
ENDOCRINOLOGY

Hormone Management in Aging Transgender Patients

Danit Ariel, MD, MS. Division of Endocrinology, Gerontology and Metabolism. Stanford University School of Medicine, Stanford, CA; Email: dariel@stanford.edu

Micol S. Rothman, MD. Endocrinology, Diabetes, and Metabolism University of Colorado School of Medicine, Aurora; Email: Micol.Rothman@cuanschutz.edu

Educational Objectives

After reviewing this chapter, learners should be able to:

- Describe the effect that gender-affirming hormone therapy (GAHT) may have on cardiovascular disease risk factors in older transgender and gender-diverse (TGD) individuals.

- Implement osteoporosis screening appropriately in older TGD individuals.

- Explain the effect of GAHT on natural menopause in TGD patients designated female at birth.

Significance of the Clinical Problem

The proportion of people identifying as TGD ranges from 0.5% to 3% globally.[1-3] As the TGD population advances in age, health care systems must evolve to accommodate their distinct medical, psychosocial, and structural determinants of health. The confluence of aging and gender diversity necessitates a nuanced understanding of chronic disease burden, mental health trajectories, social determinants, and legal protections interwoven with GAHT.[4]

Despite the extensive number of studies focused on the health of TGD individuals in recent years, there remains a lack of studies focused on older adults. Moreover, despite guidelines for the initiation and monitoring of GAHT, there are no formal recommendations to guide management of GAHT for aging TGD individuals.

Practice Gaps

- No specific guidelines exist for the management of GAHT for older TGD individuals.

- No specific gender-affirming care guidelines exist for the management of the menopausal transition in older TGD individuals.

Discussion

Gender-affirming care remains a crucial component of health care for aging TGD individuals, necessitating a lifespan approach that incorporates both medical and psychosocial considerations. Long-term GAHT requires careful monitoring for potential effects on cardiovascular health, bone density, and metabolic function.[5] Feminizing GAHT has been associated with increased thrombotic risk and necessitates individualized cardiovascular screening protocols.[6] Similarly, masculinizing GAHT can influence lipid profiles, hematocrit levels, and bone mineral density, warranting continued endocrinological oversight.[8]

While there are not formal guidelines for cardiovascular screening or specific treatments for TGD people, studies have raised concerns about the risk of cardiovascular disease in transgender women, although results have varied in their findings based on the comparator groups chosen. The STRONG study, which is the largest US study, found 2.9 myocardial infarctions per 1000 patient-years in a cohort of 2842 transgender women.[6] This represented an increased risk compared with that of cisgender women (adjusted hazard ratio [aHR] = 1.8; 95% CI, 1.1-2.9) but not cisgender men (aHR = 0.9; 95% CI, 0.6-1.5).

A recent meta-analysis that included 10 studies with 15,781 transgender women from both Europe and the United States found a 1.2% incidence of myocardial infarction with a pooled relative risk of 1.0 (95% CI, 0.8-1.2) compared with cisgender men.[8] They found a higher incidence of stroke (1.8%; 1.3 times higher than that of cisgender men [95% CI, 1.0-1.8]) and venous thromboembolism (1.6%; 2.2 times higher than that of cisgender men [95% CI, 1.1-4.5]). Comparison was not made to cisgender women in this cohort. Given the heterogeneity of these and other results, this is certainly an area that needs more study. The role of minority stress and its impact on other risk factors must be considered as well.[9]

For transgender men, the data are generally reassuring. The STRONG study did not show an increased risk of venous thromboembolism, ischemic stroke, or myocardial infraction for comparator groups of both cisgender men and cisgender women.[6] The previously mentioned recent meta-analysis found the incidence of myocardial infarction was 0.6%, with a pooled relative risk of 1.7 (95% CI, 0.8-3.6) in the transgender male group compared with cisgender women.[8] Some studies have shown small rises in blood pressure, and testosterone is known to decrease HDL cholesterol. Longer-term studies with older adults are needed to know how best to counsel aging transgender men.

Cessation of ovarian function affects all persons with ovaries and may be relevant to older transgender people assigned female at birth who do not use GAHT. However, the term *menopause* is framed around cisgender women. Menopause in aging TGD individuals is a complex process at the intersection of gender identity and aging;

it is affected by one's physical, psychological, emotional, and cultural lens.

In a study examining transgender women's experience and belief about menopause, authors found that (1) menopause was generally not considered to be particularly relevant in light of biological differences between transgender and cisgender women; (2) most transgender women expected to use GAHT indefinitely; and (3) many expressed uncertainty regarding clinical management approaches at and beyond the "menopausal age," largely because of clinicians' inexperience with this clinical management.[10] There are no studies evaluating transgender men's personal experiences, beliefs, and expectations of menopause and GAHT.[11] However, transgender men are likely to have different experiences from those of transgender women depending on the level of their transitioning and history of gender-affirming surgery. For transgender women on estrogen-based GAHT who reach menopausal age, individualized shared decision-making is needed to determine next steps in their GAHT treatment. Depending on gonadectomy status, some women may decrease their estradiol dosage to be more in line with the steady decline of estradiol over a cisgender woman's lifespan. In this case, we would recommend a gradual decrease to minimize potential vasomotor symptoms. In addition, switching to a transdermal route of estradiol is recommended to reduce cardiovascular risk. Likewise, for transgender men on testosterone-based GAHT, it is important to consider the patient's personal goals and quality of life, comorbidities, and medical risks that increase with age when addressing continued GAHT. For those achieving target levels of total testosterone midcycle (400-700 ng/dL [13.9-24.3 nmol/L]), we would not expect menopausal symptoms, such as vasomotor symptoms. No vasomotor symptoms are expected because there is a stable exogenous source of sex hormones, so the decline in endogenous sex hormone production is irrelevant. Additionally, elevated levels of total testosterone have the potential to be aromatized to estradiol, which would provide estrogen to protect against vasomotor symptoms. Lastly, osteoporosis is also a disease impacted by age. Numerous studies have shown that transgender girls and women frequently have lower bone mineral density (BMD) than their peers of the same sex assigned at birth, even before initiating GAHT.[12] The etiology is not completely understood, but it may be related to decreased physical activity, low vitamin D, and other factors. Transgender youth who undergo treatment with GnRH agonists may have additional concerns for low peak bone mass. BMD typically improves with initiation of estrogen-based GAHT in adults, despite suppression of testosterone, but this generally levels off after a few years of treatment.[13] The only study with fracture data we have suggests that older transgender women may have increased fracture risk when compared with cisgender men of similar age, but there is no difference in fracture risk when compared with cisgender women of similar age.[14] Transgender boys and men are more likely to have baseline BMD similar to their cisgender peers, and addition of testosterone-based GAHT appears to maintain BMD despite relative suppression of estradiol. An exception to this may be in patients who undergo oophorectomy, but more data are needed in this population.[15]

Regarding interpretation of DXA in TGD people, the International Society of Clinical Densitometry released a position statement in 2019 on "Bone Densitometry in Transgender and Gender Non-Conforming (TGNC) Individuals.[16] When calculating the BMD Z-score in TGD individuals, they recommend "using the reference data (mean and standard deviation) of the gender conforming with the individual's gender identity."

Multiple guidelines suggest screening BMD at various ages for transgender women. Endocrine Society guidelines suggest considering screening transgender women with DXA as a baseline for patients at age 60 years, if GAHT is stopped after gonadectomy, or for those with other risk factors for low BMD.[17] International Society of Clinical Densitometry guidelines suggest baseline BMD testing for patients with (1) history of gonadectomy or therapy that lowers endogenous gonadal steroid levels before initiation of hormone therapy; (2) hypogonadism with no plan to take GAHT; and (3) other International Society of Clinical Densitometry indications for BMD testing, such as glucocorticoid use and hyperparathyroidism.[16] In our practice, we incorporate BMD data with a variety of risk factors to make decisions for individual patients regarding pharmacologic treatment options for low BMD.

Potential discontinuation of hormone therapy in later life introduces additional complexities. Some aging TGD individuals may face pressure to reduce or cease hormone therapy due to medical comorbidities, institutional policies in assisted living or long-term care settings, or provider biases. However, cessation of GAHT can lead to physical and psychological distress, including dysphoria, decreased muscle mass, osteoporosis risk, and mood instability. Expert opinion holds that GAHT should not be withheld solely based on age.[5] Multiple factors should affect decisions on continued or dose-adjusted GAHT, including comorbidities, risks, and patient preferences and goals. Thus, an individualized, patient-centered approach is essential to ensure continued access to GAHT while balancing overall health considerations.

Clinical Case Vignettes
Case 1

A 57-year-old transgender woman is seen in the clinic after hospital admission for myocardial infarction. At the time of admission, she was on a GAHT regimen consisting of oral estradiol, 6 mg daily, and micronized progesterone, 100 mg daily. She underwent orchiectomy and vaginoplasty several years before this admission. She underwent coronary artery stenting and has been prescribed appropriate lipid-lowering and blood pressure–lowering medications. Her estradiol and micronized progesterone were held at the time of admission, and she was told not to restart until seeing you. She is in no distress today and will be beginning cardiac rehabilitation, but she shares that she is experiencing hot flashes and fatigue.

Which of the following is true?

A. Standards of Care Version 8 guidelines suggest transgender women transition to injectable estrogen at age 55 years

B. Micronized progesterone is the optimal choice if she restarts GAHT

C. The antiandrogen spironolactone is the optimal choice if she restarts GAHT

D. Oral estrogen is the optimal choice if she restarts GAHT

E. Standards of Care Version 8 guidelines suggest transgender women transition to transdermal estrogen at age 45 years

Answer: E) Standards of Care Version 8 guidelines suggest transgender women transition to transdermal estrogen at age 45 years

As cardiovascular disease is a disease of aging, we are likely to encounter an increasing number of TGD patients who have had cardiac events. This is a challenging clinical scenario, and careful discussion should be had with the patient in conjunction with her cardiologist. If she is doing well with rehabilitation and is on adequate antiplatelet and lipid-lowering therapy, it may be reasonable to restart GAHT using low-dosage transdermal estrogen. The World Professional Association for Transgender Health (WPATH) Standards of Care Version 8 guidelines suggest transitioning all transgender women to transdermal estrogen at age 45 years (thus, Answer E is correct and Answers A and D are incorrect).[5]

Spironolactone (Answer C) is an antiandrogen that acts of the level of the testosterone receptor to block androgen action and also decrease testosterone levels to some degree. As this patient has already had an orchiectomy, it would not have a role in her gender-affirming care at this time.

Progesterone (Answer B) is not recommended as part of standard GAHT.[5] A recent systematic review did not find evidence for improved quality of life or breast development and raised concerns for increased risk of venous thromboembolism, as well as adverse effects on mood and decreased HDL cholesterol.[18] The studies reviewed typically used cyproterone or medroxyprogesterone, and some have questioned whether micronized progesterone could be a better choice with fewer adverse effects, but no data currently support this. Given this patient's recent cardiac event, it would seem prudent to continue withholding micronized progesterone at this time even if estrogen is reinitiated via the transdermal route.

Case 2

A 50-year-old healthy transgender man on masculinizing GAHT since age 30 years without interruption presents with vasomotor symptoms (hot flashes during the day and night sweats). He has not had removal of his uterus or ovaries. He reports no extraordinary social or economic stressors and states that these vasomotor symptoms are affecting his concentration at work and quality of sleep. His mother was 50 years old when she went through natural menopause, and he wonders whether this is what he is experiencing. He was taking testosterone cypionate, 100 mg intramuscularly once weekly, and another gender care clinic provider increased the dosage to 125 mg intramuscularly once weekly, with no symptom improvement, but worsening acne. The patient's midcycle total testosterone concentration was 769 ng/dL (26.7 nmol/L).

Which of the following is true?

A. His symptoms are likely related to natural menopausal

B. Low-dosage estradiol should be started to treat vasomotor symptoms

C. Evaluation should be done for other possible endocrine causes of hot flashes

D. Low-dosage progestogen should be started to treat vasomotor symptoms

E. Nonhormonal therapies, such as fezolinetant, selective serotonin reuptake inhibitor, serotonin and norepinephrine reuptake inhibitor, or gabapentin should be started to treat vasomotor symptoms

Answer: C) Evaluation should be done for other possible endocrine causes of hot flashes

Evaluation should be undertaken for other possible endocrine causes of hot flashes, including hyperthyroidism, hypoglycemia, pheochromocytoma, carcinoid syndrome, and anxiety (Answer C). The patient has been on longstanding and consistent masculinizing GAHT with testosterone, without a lapse in use. Therefore, we expect his endogenous estradiol to be suppressed through suppression of his hypothalamic-pituitary-ovarian axis. Moreover, laboratory studies demonstrate that he has adequate levels of circulating total testosterone. Thus, assuming his symptoms are due to natural menopause (Answer A) is incorrect, and his vasomotor symptoms should not be treated with estradiol, progestogen, or nonhormonal therapies (Answers B, D, and E) given that their etiology is likely another endocrine or nonendocrine cause.

In this patient's case, his masculinizing GAHT should be continued indefinitely with consideration of his goals, comorbid conditions, risks associated with GAHT, social or economic issues, and gender-affirming surgeries. If he wanted to eventually stop masculinizing GAHT at this age or beyond, no significant change would be expected in masculine secondary sex characteristics since endogenous estrogen production would remain low. In that case, GAHT should be gradually weaned to avoid signs and symptoms of sex hormone deficiency.

Case 3

A 66-year-old transgender woman presents for routine follow-up of GAHT. Her current medications include estradiol patch, 0.200 mg changed twice weekly; spironolactone, 100 mg daily; metformin, 1000 mg twice daily; lisinopril, 10 mg daily; and sertraline, 50 mg daily. She has a history of tobacco use (but does not currently smoke cigarettes). She exercises twice weekly and has never had a fracture.

She mentions that her 89-year-old mother recently died after complications of a hip fracture.

She wonders whether she should have DXA to assess her BMD.

Which of the following is true?

A. Since she was assigned male at birth, DXA screening is not recommended at any age
B. She should have DXA with Z-scores from the male reference database
C. She should have DXA with Z-scores from the female reference database
D. The FRAX calculator has an option to calculate fracture risk outside the gender binary
E. Transgender women typically have better BMD than their cisgender peers before starting GAHT

Answer: C) She should have DXA with Z-scores from the female reference database

There are concerns that transgender women have lower BMD than their cisgender peers (thus, Answer E is incorrect) and screening would be recommended (thus, Answer A is incorrect). Currently, the FRAX calculator does not have options outside the gender binary (thus, Answer D is incorrect). The International Society of Clinical Densitometry suggests that BMD, and specifically Z-scores, in people on GAHT be interpreted using gender identity (thus, Answer C is correct and Answer B is incorrect). The T-score reference is typically female in all comers, so this would not be affected by gender identity.

Key Learning Points

- Long-term GAHT requires careful monitoring for potential effects on cardiovascular health, bone density, and metabolic function.

- GAHT should not be withheld solely based on age.

- The World Professional Association for Transgender Health Standards of Care Version 8 guidelines suggest transitioning all transgender women to transdermal estrogen at age 45 years.

- Menopause in aging TGD individuals is a complex process at the intersection of gender identity and aging, impacted by one's physical, psychological, emotional, and cultural lens,

and shared-decision making must be used in creating an individualized treatment plan.

- Older transgender women may have increased fracture risk when compared with risk of similarly aged cisgender men, but there is no difference in fracture risk when compared with cisgender women of similar age.

References

1. Herman J, Flores A, O'Neill K. How many adults and youth identify as transgender in the United States? [Internet]. UCLA School of Law Williams Institute; 2022. Available from: https://williamsinstitute.law.ucla.edu/wp-content/uploads/Trans-Pop-Update-Jun-2022.pdf

2. Spizzirri G, Eufrásio R, Lima MCP, et al. Proportion of people identified as transgender and non-binary gender in Brazil. *Sci Rep.* 2021;11(1):2240. PMID: 33500432

3. Ipsos Global Advisor. LGBT+Pride 2023 Global Survey Report [Internet]. Ipsos; 2023. Available from: https://www.ipsos.com/sites/default/files/ct/news/documents/2023-05/Ipsos%20LGBT%2B%20Pride%202023%20Global%20Survey%20Report%20-%20rev.pdf

4. Witten TM, Eyler AE. *Gay, Lesbian, Bisexual, and Transgender Aging: Challenges in Research, Practice, and Policy.* Johns Hopkins University Press, 2012.

5. Coleman E, Radix AE, Bouman WP, et al. Standards of care for the health of transgender and gender diverse people, version 8. *Int J Transgend Health.* 2022;23(Suppl 1):S1-S259. PMID: 36238954

6. Getahun D, Nash R, Flanders WD, et al. Cross-sex hormones and acute cardiovascular events in transgender persons: a cohort study. *Ann Intern Med.* 2018;169(4):205-213. PMID: 29987313

7. Irwig MS. Testosterone therapy for transgender men. *Lancet Diabetes Endocrinol.* 2017;5(4):301-311. PMID: 27084565

8. van Zijverden LM, Wiepjes CM, van Diemen JJK, Thijs A, den Heijer M. Cardiovascular disease in transgender people: a systematic review and meta-analysis. *Eur J Endocrinol.* 2024;190(2):S13-S24. PMID: 38302717

9. Iwamoto SJ, Defreyne J, Kaoutzanis C, Davies RD, Moreau KL, Rothman MS. Gender-affirming hormone therapy, mental health, and surgical considerations for aging transgender and gender diverse adults. *Ther Adv Endocrinol Metab.* 2023;14:20420188231166494. PMID: 37113210

10. Mohamed S, Hunter MS. Transgender women's experiences and beliefs about hormone therapy through and beyond mid-age: an exploratory UK study. *Int J Transgend.* 2019;20(1):98-107. PMID: 32999597

11. Kelley C and Ariel D. A review of menopause in transgender and gender diverse individuals. *Curr Opin Obstet Gynecol.* 2025;37(2):83-96. PMID: 39970047

12. Rothman MS, Iwamoto SJ. Bone health in the transgender population. *Clin Rev Bone Miner Metab.* 2019;17(2):77-85. PMID: 31452648

13. Wiepjes CM, de Jongh RT, de Blok CJ, et al. Bone safety during the first ten years of gender-affirming hormonal treatment in transwomen and transmen. *J Bone Miner Res.* 2019;34(3):447-454. PMID: 30537188

14. Wiepjes CM, de Blok CJ, Staphorsius AS, et al. Fracture risk in trans women and trans men using long-term gender-affirming hormonal treatment: a nationwide cohort study. *J Bone Miner Res.* 2020;35(1):64-70. PMID: 31487065

15. Sanna E, Lami A, Giacomelli G, et al. Bone health in transgender assigned female at birth people: effects of gender-affirming hormone therapy and gonadectomy. *Front Endocrinol (Lausanne).* 2024;15:1416121. PMID: 39391880

16. Rosen HN, Hamnvik O-PR, Jaisamrarn U, et al. Bone densitometry in transgender and gender non-conforming (TGNC) individuals: 2019 ISCD Official Position. *J Clin Densitom.* 2019;22(4):544-553. PMID: 31327665

17. Hembree WC, Cohen-Kettenis PT, Gooren L, et al. Endocrine treatment of gender-dysphoric/gender-incongruent persons: an Endocrine Society clinical practice guideline. *J Clin Endocrinol Metab.* 2017;102(11):3869-3903. PMID: 28945902

18. Patel KT, Adeel S, Rodrigues Miragaya J, Tangpricha V. Progestogen use in gender-affirming hormone therapy: a systematic review. *Endocr Pract.* 2022;28(12):1244-1252. PMID: 36007714

Amenorrhea Management in Overweight and Underweight Women

Daniel A. Dumesic, MD. Department of Obstetrics and Gynecology, David Geffen School of Medicine at University of California Los Angeles, Los Angeles, CA; Email: ddumesic@mednet.ucla.edu

Educational Objectives

After reviewing this chapter, learners should be able to:

- Outline the diagnostic and laboratory assessment of women with hypothalamic amenorrhea.

- Describe the management of hypothalamic amenorrhea and its comorbidities.

- Distinguish amenorrhea due to obesity from that due to polycystic ovary syndrome (PCOS).

Significance of the Clinical Problem

Nutrition is important in human reproduction, with body fat mass being a crucial permissive signal governing the hypothalamo-pituitary-ovarian (HPO) axis.[1,2] Both insufficient and excessive body fat in women can disrupt metabolic-reproductive signaling and cause ovulatory dysfunction and amenorrhea, defined as absent menses for over a 6-month period or for at least 3 previous menstrual cycles (normal menstrual cycle duration: between 21 and 45 days from 1 to <3 years post menarche; between 21 and 35 days from ≥3 years post menarche to perimenopause).

Several mechanisms underlying nutrition, body fat, stress, and exercise contribute to amenorrhea. Hypothalamic amenorrhea accompanies suppression of circulating gonadotropin and estradiol levels without a central nervous system lesion and can occur in women who are underweight (<10% below ideal body weight). These women often report weight loss, emotional strain, and excessive exercise and can have an eating disorder, although no precipitating event may be identified.[2] Low bone mass from HPO suppression is a serious long-term complication. With undernutrition, anorexia nervosa (AN) can occur when weight loss of greater than 15% for height accompanies an altered body image and amenorrhea.

Conversely, obesity is now a global epidemic affecting 12% of the world's adult population. Amenorrhea due to obesity also disrupts HPO function through enhanced adipose aromatization of androgen to estrogen, altered adipokine production, and impaired ovarian function. Hyperinsulinemia from adipose-dependent insulin resistance increases androgen bioavailability through decreased hepatic SHBG, which can mimic or exaggerate PCOS expression.[3] Consequently, amenorrhea due to obesity can be easily confused with amenorrhea due to PCOS, with increased adiposity in both conditions increasing the risks of metabolic syndrome, cancers, and subfertility.[3,4]

Practice Gaps

- Lack of awareness exists regarding the diagnosis of hypothalamic amenorrhea in young women.

- Long-term adverse consequences of hypothalamic amenorrhea may be unrecognized.

- Distinguishing amenorrhea due to obesity from amenorrhea due to PCOS can be challenging.

- Personalized amenorrhea management should be established for overweight and underweight women.

Discussion

Functional hypothalamic amenorrhea (FHA) is a form of chronic anovulation associated with stress, weight loss, and/or excessive exercise without an identifiable organic cause.[2] Often accompanying an energy deficit below 30 kcals/kg (fat free mass), FHA is a diagnosis of exclusion that requires assessment of systemic and endocrine etiologies. Women with FHA have a higher prevalence of disordered eating patterns, stress, weight loss, or excess exercise, occasionally accompanied by an underlying genetic disorder.[5] Eating disorders are common in adolescent girls; in a cross-sectional study of girls (mean age 15.0 years), 23% had disordered eating and 4.1% had secondary amenorrhea.[6]

Adverse consequences of FHA involve metabolism, neuroendocrine function, and reproduction. Significant risks include delayed puberty, amenorrhea, infertility, and long-term consequences of hypoestrogenism, with a significant long-term risk being bone loss and/or inability to obtain peak bone mass despite exercise. Prolonged FHA also has adverse effects on metabolic, bone, cardiovascular, mental/cognitive, and reproductive health.[5,7] Women who conceive with a history of FHA are at risk for preterm labor, fetal loss, small-for-gestational-age infants, and cesarean delivery. Multidisciplinary care includes nutritional and psychological support, exercise modification, and hormone replacement.

Importantly, adipose serves as both energy storage and a dynamic endocrine organ. Subcutaneous adipose normally protects against insulin resistance through fat storage, while intra-abdominal adipose has the opposite effect. Normally, the anorexigenic hormone leptin and the orexigenic hormone ghrelin contribute to metabolism, energy homeostasis, and satiety, with contributions from enteroendocrine cells and gastrointestinal flora that affect the gut-brain relationship.[8] When energy intake exceeds the capacity to safely store fat, ectopic lipid accumulates in nonadipose tissue where it induces oxidative/endoplasmic reticulum stress linked with insulin resistance and inflammation (ie, lipotoxicity). Disruption of HPO function through increased adiposity can adversely affect puberty, fertility, menstrual cyclicity, endometrial development, and metabolism in women with or without PCOS. Although medications, hormonal managements, and bariatric surgery can improve some reproductive and metabolic consequences of obesity,[4,9,10] questions remain regarding adverse effects of obesity on oocyte quality and endometrial development in women wishing to conceive.

Clinical Case Vignettes
Case 1

A 17-year-old woman presents with secondary amenorrhea. She has no excess hair growth, galactorrhea, hot flashes, or headaches. Menarche occurred at age 11 years, and she had regular monthly menses until 6 months ago, when she lost more than 1 kg/week over 3 consecutive weeks while exercising 5 to 6 days weekly with heavy weights and running 10 miles weekly. She does not eat red meat, dairy, or eggs. She does not take any medications and uses condoms for contraception. Her medical history is notable for an altered body image and depression.

On physical examination, she is afebrile, blood pressure is 80/40 mm Hg, and pulse rate is 39 beats/min. Her BMI is 17 kg/m². She has normal breast and pelvic development.

Laboratory test results:

LH = 1.5 mIU/mL (2.0-8.0 mIU/mL [follicular])
  (SI: 1.5 IU/L [2.0-8.0 IU/L])
FSH = 4.0 mIU/mL (3.0-10.0 mIU/mL [follicular])
  (SI: 4.0 IU/L [3.0-10.0 IU/L])
Estradiol = 20 pg/mL (20-400 pg/mL)
  (SI: 73.4 pmol/L [73.4-1468.4 pmol/L])
Hemoglobin = 8.5 g/dL (12.0-18.0 g/dL) (SI: 85 g/L
  [120-180 g/L])
Sodium = 123 mEq/L (135-146 mEq/L)
  (SI: 123 mmol/L [135-146 mmol/L])
Serum urea nitrogen = 15 mg/dL (7-22 mg/dL)
  (SI: 5.4 mmol/L [2.5-7.9 mmol/L])
Potassium = 2.4 mEq/L (3.6-5.3 mEq/L)
  (SI: 2.4 mmol/L [3.6-5.3 mmol/L])

Findings on MRI of the head are normal.

Which of the following endocrine changes is most likely to exist in this patient?

A. Decreased antidiuretic hormone

B. Decreased cortisol

C. Decreased ghrelin

D. Increased GH

E. Increased total thyroxine

Answer: D) Increased GH

AN is a condition of severe undernutrition characterized by altered body image, persistent food restriction, low body weight, and endocrine dysregulation.[11] Accompanied by neuropsychiatric comorbidities, AN occurs in 1% of adolescent girls and young women.[12] Individuals with AN have HPO suppression with sex steroid deficiency, GH resistance (ie, increased GH secretion and decreased systemic IGF-1), hypercortisolism, low total T_4 (from its increased peripheral deiodination to reverse T_3), hyponatremia (from increased antidiuretic hormone), decreased leptin and insulin, and increased ghrelin.[11,12] These endocrine changes in hypothalamic hormones, adipokines, and appetite-regulating hormones can be in response to chronic nutritional deprivation.[11] Clinical effects include hypothalamic amenorrhea, bone loss, mood-affective symptoms, reduced fat/lean mass,

and disordered eating habits. Hospitalization for the treatment of severe AN may be necessary (*Table 1, following page*).[13] Approximately 50% of adults with AN recover following behavioral, psychiatric, and medical therapies; 30% experience only partial recovery; while the remaining have relapses or chronic disease.[11,12] Recovery can improve many, but not all, hormonal changes, with deficits in bone mass accrual due to multiple adaptive endocrine and neuropsychiatric comorbidities.[12,13]

Case 1, Continued

The patient is hospitalized, and cognitive behavioral therapy is started. Serum vitamin D, calcium, magnesium, and zinc concentrations are normal. DXA shows osteopenia of the spine and hip regions. You are consulted regarding hormone replacement.

Which of the following therapies should be started to prevent bone loss?

A. Transdermal estradiol with cyclic progesterone

B. Oral estrogen with cyclic progesterone

C. Oral contraceptives

D. Bisphosphate

E. Denosumab

Answer: A) Transdermal estradiol with cyclic progesterone

About 50% of girls with AN have a bone mineral density Z-score less than −2, with the spine being commonly affected. Transdermal estrogen can be used in teenagers who have completed growth and have a significant history of fracture or low bone density Z-scores. Transdermal estradiol and cyclic progesterone replacement increases spine and hip bone mineral density in adolescents with anorexia, although catch-up growth may not occur because of persistent hormone abnormalities (eg, cortisol) or frequent relapses. Oral estrogen administration is not effective in increasing bone density in these women, perhaps because it lowers hepatic IGF-1 levels as an important bone anabolic hormone.[11,12] The role of oral contraceptives in increasing bone density is controversial, likely for similar

Table 1. Risk Factors for Severity of AN at 17 Years of Age

Risk factor	Normal risk	Moderate risk	Severe risk
BMI percentile	≥fifth BMI percentile	First-fourth BMI percentile	<first BMI percentile
BMI	≥18.2 kg/m²	17.2-18.1 kg/m²	≤17.1 kg/m²
Weight loss	Stable	500 g to <1 kg/week for 3 weeks with <fifth BMI percentile	≥1 kg/week for 3 weeks with <fifth BMI percentile
Fluid intake	Little or no reduced fluid intake	Markedly reduced fluid intake or cessation of fluid intake for 12 to 24 h	Severe dehydration or cessation of fluid intake for >24 h
Food cessation	<12 h in a day	12-24 h	>24 h
Heart rate	Z-score > –1: >63 beats/min	Z-score –1 to –4: 40-62 beats/min	Z-score < –4: <39 beats/min
Systolic blood pressure	Z-score > –1 (106 mm Hg)	Z-score –1 to –4 (85-105 mm Hg)	Z-score < –4 (84 mm Hg)
Diastolic blood pressure	Z-score > –1 (63 mm Hg)	Z-score –1 to –4 (41-62 mm Hg)	Z-score < –4 (42 mm Hg)
Electrocardiography, QTc	<460 ms	<460 ms	>460 ms or electrocardiographic change not related to QTc
Syncope	No (pre)syncope	Dizziness, presyncope, or 1 syncope	Repeated syncopal episodes
Temperature	>36.0°C	<36.0°C to 35.5°C	<35.5°C
Laboratory findings	Normal phosphate, sodium, potassium, albumin, glucose, transaminases, leukocytes, and hemoglobin	Deviations from normal values still within the limits above severe values	Hypophosphatemia (phosphate <0.8 mmol/L) Hyponatremia (sodium <125 nmol/L) Hypokalemia (potassium <2.5 mmol/L) Hypoalbuminemia (albumin <30 g/L) Hypoglycemia (glucose <3 mmol/L) Transaminases > 3 times normal Leukocytes <2/nL Hemoglobin <10 g/dL

Modified from Hebebrand J et al. *Dtsch Arztebl Int*, 2024; 121(5): 164-174. Published by Deutsches Ärzteblatt International.

effects on lowering IGF-1 and free testosterone levels.[14] Adequate calcium (1200-1500 mg daily) and vitamin D (400-1000 international units [10-25 mcg]) intake is important,[5] and vitamin D levels should remain above 30 ng/mL (>74.9 nmol/L). Bisphosphates are not approved for women of childbearing age because they cross the placenta and can affect fetal development.[11] Denosumab, a human monoclonal antibody against receptor activator of nuclear factor-kB ligand, limits bone resorption by inhibiting osteoclast maturation. It has not been tested sufficiently in women with anorexia, and fetal exposure could potentially be teratogenic.[2]

Case 2

A 38-year-old nulliparous woman with obesity presents with a 4-month history of secondary amenorrhea that was preceded by irregular menstrual bleeding. Her medical history is notable for hypertension, hyperlipidemia, and migraine headaches with aura. She takes metformin, 1000 mg orally daily, and uses condoms for contraception.

On physical examination, she is afebrile, blood pressure is 135/85 mm Hg, and pulse rate is 90 beats/min. BMI is 31.5 kg/m². She has hirsutism and an abdominal circumference of 35.4 in (90 cm).

Laboratory test results:

LH = 15.0 mIU/mL (2.0-8.0 mIU/mL [follicular])
  (SI: 15.0 IU/L [2.0-8.0 IU/L])
FSH = 4.0 mIU/mL (3.0-10.0 mIU/mL [follicular])
  (SI: 4.0 IU/L [3.0-10.0 IU/L])
Testosterone = 72 ng/dL (9-55 ng/dL)
  (SI: 2.5 nmol/L [0.3-1.9 nmol/L])
Free testosterone = 0.85 ng/dL (0.08-0.74 ng/dL)
  (SI: 0.029 nmol/L [0.003-0.026 nmol/L])
DHEA-S = 4000 ng/mL (400-3600 ng/mL)
  (SI: 108.4 µmol/L [10.8-97.6 µmol/L])
Estradiol = 70 pg/mL (20-400 pg/mL)
  (SI: 257.0 pmol/L [73.4-1468.4 pmol/L])
Progesterone = 0.5 ng/mL (2.6-21.5 ng/mL [luteal])
  (SI: 1.6 nmol/L [8.3-68.4 nmol/L])
Fasting glucose = 104 mg/dL (<100 mg/dL)
  (SI: 5.8 mmol/L [<5.6 mmol/L])
Hemoglobin A_{1c} = 5.8% (<5.7%) (40 mmol/mol [<39 mmol/mol])
Total cholesterol = 207 mg/dL (<200 mg/dL)
  (SI: 5.36 mmol/L [<5.18 mmol/L])
HDL cholesterol = 40 mg/dL (>50 mg/dL)
  (SI: 1.04 mmol/L [>1.30 mmol/L])
LDL cholesterol = 124 mg/dL (<100 mg/dL)
  (SI: 3.21 mmol/L [<2.59 mmol/L])
Non–HDL-cholesterol = 154 mg/dL (<130 mg/dL)
  (SI: 3.99 mmol/L [<3.37 mmol/L])
Triglycerides = 162 mg/dL (<150 mg/dL)
  (SI: 1.83 mmol/L [<1.70 mmol/L])
Hemoglobin, normal
Electrolytes, normal
Complete metabolic panel, normal
Prolactin, normal
17-Hydroxprogesterone, normal
Thyroid function, normal
Overnight dexamethasone-suppression test, normal
Pregnancy test, negative

Transvaginal ultrasonography shows a 9-mm endometrium, a normal right ovary, and a 12 cc³ left ovary with 22 antral follicles. Results of a Papanicolaou test are normal.

Which of the following is the best next step?

A. Dilation and curettage

B. Endometrial biopsy

C. Hysteroscopy

D. Laparoscopy with hysteroscopy

E. Sonohysterography

Answer: B) Endometrial biopsy

Abnormal uterine bleeding (AUB) can occur due to polyps, adenomyosis, leiomyoma, endometrial hyperplasia/malignancy, coagulopathy, and anovulation associated with unopposed estrogen stimulation of the endometrium. History, examination, and testing in the context of age-related causes include pregnancy testing, complete blood cell count, TSH measurement, cervical cancer screening, and coagulation studies (ie, von Willebrand-ristocetin cofactor activity, von Willebrand factor antigen, and factor VIII) if a bleeding disorder is suspected. Although many endometrial sampling techniques can be used, endometrial biopsy is generally the first-line procedure in women with AUB who are older than 45 years or who are younger than 45 years with unopposed estrogen exposure from obesity and/or PCOS. This patient has PCOS by Rotterdam criteria with at least 2 of the following 3 features: (1) clinical/biochemical hyperandrogenism, (2) oligo-anovulation, and (3) polycystic ovaries, excluding other endocrinopathies.[15] Given her metabolic dysfunction, she is at increased risk for endometrial hyperplasia and carcinoma,[16] so an endometrial biopsy is indicated. With sufficient tissue, endometrial biopsy can detect endometrial disease throughout the uterine cavity but may not detect disease occupying less than 50% of the endometrial surface area.

Persistent bleeding despite a benign endometrial biopsy, or without sufficient tissue, requires further testing, including sonohysterography, dilation and curettage, and/or hysteroscopy to rule out isolated intrauterine pathology. MRI is not a primary imaging modality for AUB, although it may help guide treatment of multiple leiomyomata. Laparoscopy is not indicated since transvaginal ultrasonography shows a left polycystic ovary with no masses.[15]

Case 2, Continued

Histological examination of the biopsy tissue shows endometrial hyperplasia without atypia.

Which of the following is the best next step?

A. Endometrial ablation

B. Hysteroscopic-guided uterine sampling

C. Levonorgestrel-releasing intrauterine device

D. Micronized progesterone

E. Oral contraceptives

Answer: D) Micronized progesterone

Endometrial hyperplasia is classified as benign endometrial hyperplasia or atypical endometrial hyperplasia/endometrial intraepithelial neoplasia.[17] Benign endometrial hyperplasia rarely progresses to endometrial cancer, with a 20-year progression risk of less than 5%. It often is a noninvasive abnormal endometrial proliferation from chronic anovulatory unopposed estrogen exposure, although rare genetic factors exist. Women with PCOS are about 3 times more likely to develop endometrial cancer.

Benign endometrial hyperplasia in reproductive-aged women is usually managed with progestins (ie, medroxyprogesterone acetate, 10 to 20 mg daily; norethindrone acetate, 2.5 to 10 mg daily; micronized progesterone, 100 mg 2 to 3 times daily; megestrol acetate, 40 to 200 daily) or a levonorgestrel-releasing intrauterine device to antagonize estrogen action on endometrial proliferation and induce atrophy. The levonorgestrel-releasing intrauterine device has a 96% success rate of treating benign endometrial hyperplasia.[18] Progestins used in a continuous manner over 3 to 6 months, however, may be a better option than a levonorgestrel-releasing intrauterine device for women who wish to conceive, although their adverse effects include bloating, nausea, headaches, and mood swings.[17] Occasional bleeding may be more common with intrauterine devices, while nausea may be more associated with oral progestins. Oral contraceptives are avoided in women with migraines and aura.

The 20-year progression risk of endometrial intraepithelial neoplasia to endometrial cancer is about 28%. Although progestins can also be used to treat endometrial intraepithelial neoplasia when

hysterectomy is not an option, an endometrial biopsy should be supplemented with dilation and curettage and/or hysteroscopic-guided uterine sampling to exclude malignancy. Relapse of endometrial hyperplasia after initial regression can occur. Long-term follow-up is advised, with weight loss and glycemic control used to improve overall health and decrease the risk of endometrial carcinoma. Endometrial ablation is not used in women with unresolved endometrial hyperplasia who may wish to conceive.

Case 2, Continued

The patient returns 1 year after weight loss. She wishes to conceive and has had unprotected intercourse for 3 months. Metabolic parameters have improved, but she has menses every 2 months. She has discontinued metformin.

On physical examination, she is afebrile, blood pressure is 125/80 mm Hg, and pulse rate is 90 beats/min. Her BMI is 27.5 kg/m².

Laboratory test results:

Testosterone = 58 ng/dL (9-55 ng/dL)
(SI: 2.0 nmol/L [0.3-1.9 nmol/L])
Free testosterone = 0.75 ng/dL (0.08-0.74 ng/dL)
(SI: 0.026 nmol/L [0.003-0.026 nmol/L])
DHEA-S =3600 ng/mL (400-3600 ng/mL)
(SI: 97.56 µmol/L [10.84-97.56 µmol/L])
Estradiol = 80 pg/mL (20-400 pg/mL)
(SI: 293.7 pmol/L [73.4-1468.4 pmol/L])
Progesterone = 0.7 ng/mL (2.6-21.5 ng/mL [luteal])
(SI: 2.2 nmol/L [8.3-68.4 nmol/L])
Hemoglobin A$_{1c}$ = 5.7% (<5.7%) (39 mmol/mol
[<39 mmol/mol])
Total cholesterol = 200 mg/dL (<200 mg/dL)
(SI: 5.18 mmol/L [<5.18 mmol/L])
HDL cholesterol = 50 mg/dL (>50 mg/dL)
(SI: 1.30 mmol/L [>1.30 mmol/L])
LDL cholesterol = 110 mg/dL (<100 mg/dL)
(SI: 2.85 mmol/L [<2.59 mmol/L])
Non–HDL-cholesterol = 140 mg/dL (<130 mg/dL)
(SI: 3.63 mmol/L [<3.37 mmol/L])
Triglycerides = 149 mg/dL (<150 mg/dL)
(SI: 1.68 mmol/L [<1.70 mmol/L])
Pregnancy test, negative

Which of the following is the best next step?

A. Continue lifestyle intervention

B. Order an oral glucose tolerance test

C. Restart metformin

D. Start a GLP-1 receptor agonist

E. Engage in timed intercourse for 3 more months

Answer: B) Order an oral glucose tolerance test

Obesity has serious adverse effects on maternal and neonatal outcomes.[4] The 2023 International Evidence-Based Guideline for the Assessment and Management of Polycystic Ovary Syndrome recommends oral glucose tolerance testing in women with PCOS who do not have preexisting diabetes when planning pregnancy, given their increased risk of hyperglycemia and pregnancy comorbidities.[15] GLP-1–based therapies enhance glucose-dependent insulin secretion, slow gastric emptying, reduce postprandial glucagon, and decrease food intake. Use of a GLP-1 receptor agonist with or without metformin in women with PCOS who are overweight or have obesity can improve both metabolism (ie, improve insulin sensitivity, reduce weight central/visceral adipose and liver fat, decrease total/LDL cholesterol and triglycerides, lower blood pressure, and increase SHBG) and reproductive parameters (ie, reduce ovarian/adrenal androgens, decrease ovarian size, improve menstrual frequency and ovulation, and increase natural conception).[9,10] Although preliminary data suggest that these medications may not cause major congenital malformations, the small number of exposed human pregnancies thus far does not rule out an increased risk for malformations or fetal growth abnormalities.[19] Therefore, these drugs should not be used in pregnancy.

Metformin, a biguanide that increases peripheral insulin sensitivity and inhibits hepatic glucose production, is commonly used to treat gestational diabetes. It can pass the placenta and enter the fetus with potential long-term consequences for offspring.[4,20] In a double-blind randomized controlled trial comparing metformin (2000 mg daily) with placebo in 257 pregnant women with PCOS, children in the metformin group had a higher BMI Z-score at age 5 to 10 years than those in the placebo group, suggesting a potential risk of altered cardiometabolic health in later life.[21] Deciding whether to restart metformin in pregnancy should be considered in the context of oral glucose tolerance testing.

Lifestyle interventions may increase natural conception, improve ovulation induction, and reduce pregnancy morbidities in anovulatory women with obesity.[4,22] Lifestyle interventions' effects, however, do not necessarily improve the live birth rate in ovulatory women or in women requiring assisted reproductive technology.[4] In a randomized controlled trial of infertile women with obesity, 6-month lifestyle intervention preceding infertility treatment did not improve the term singleton birth rate at 24 months vs the birth rate of women receiving prompt infertility treatment. Rather, it delayed the time to pregnancy by about 2 months, despite the increased frequency of natural conception.[23] Given the adverse effects of maternal age vs obesity on fecundity of this 39-year-old patient,[24] (*Table 2*, *following page*), continued lifestyle intervention would not be a better choice than ovulation induction if results from oral glucose tolerance testing are normal.

Timed intercourse alone is not recommended since it is unclear whether this patient is ovulating. Even if a serum progesterone value greater than 3 ng/mL (>9.5 nmol/L) confirms infrequent ovulation,[25] she remains oligo-ovulatory and should undergo ovulation induction.

Case 2, Continued

Which of the following is the best next step for ovulation induction?

A. Aromatase inhibitor

B. Dopamine agonist

C. Human menopausal gonadotropins

D. Recombinant FSH

E. Selective estrogen-receptor modulator

Answer: A) Aromatase inhibitor

Table 2. Failure to Achieve an Intrauterine Pregnancy by Assisted Reproduction Based on Autologous Oocytes From Women by Age and BMI*

BMI kg/m²	AOR**	95% CI
	Age < 35 years	
18.5-24.9	1.00	Reference
25.0-29.9	1.07	1.00-1.16
30.0-34.9	1.21	1.10-1.34
35.0-39.9	1.38	1.20-1.60
40.0-46.0	1.80	1.46-2.23
	Age > 35 years	
18.5-24.9	1.00	Reference
25.0-29.9	1.00	0.93-1.08
30.0-34.9	1.07	0.97-1.18
35.0-39.9	1.25	1.08-1.45
40.0-46.0	1.31	1.05-1.64

* Overall clinical intrauterine pregnancy, 44% per embryo transfer.

** Adjusted for women's race, ethnicity, day/number of embryos transferred, and infertility diagnosis. Failure to achieve a clinical intrauterine pregnancy increased with high BMI, but to a lesser extent in older women due to impaired age-related oocyte quality. Woman's age effect (AOR [95% CI]): <30 y (1.00 [reference]), 30-34 y (1.03 [95% CI, 0.91-1.18]), 35-39 y (1.48 [95% CI, 1.31-1.69]), 40-44 y (2.84 [95% CI, 2.40-3.36]), ≥45 y (7.19 [95% CI, 3.10-16.66]).

Modified with permission from Luke B et al. *Hum Reprod*, 2011; 26(1): 245-52. © The Authors. Published by Oxford University Press on behalf of the European Society of Human Reproduction and Embryology.

Although used off-label in many countries, the aromatase inhibitor letrozole is now the first-line pharmacological treatment for ovulation induction in infertile women with anovulatory PCOS (with no other infertility factors), since it is more effective than clomiphene citrate (a selective estrogen-receptor modulator).[15,25] In a double-blind randomized controlled trial of letrozole vs clomiphene citrate for ovulation induction in women with PCOS, cumulative live births over 5 cycles (letrozole, 27.5%; clomiphene citrate, 19.1% [*P* = .007]), ovulation rate/cycle (letrozole, 61.7%; clomiphene citrate, 48.3% [*P* < .001]), and ovulation rate/patient (letrozole, 88.5%; clomiphene citrate, 76.6% [*P* < .001) were higher for letrozole than for clomiphene citrate.[25] Unless other factors exist (ie, male-factor infertility, other reproductive or genetic diseases), gonadotropins are generally second-line pharmacological therapy for women with PCOS for whom first-line ovulation induction has been unsuccessful. The decision to use gonadotropins should consider cost, expertise required, availability of ultrasonography for monitoring, and minimal dosing to minimize a multiple pregnancy. Clinical efficacy is similar for various gonadotropin preparations.

The dopamine receptor 2 agonist cabergoline is used in women undergoing assisted reproduction who are at risk of ovarian hyperstimulation syndrome with increased vascular permeability from ovarian hypersecretion of vascular endothelial growth factor. In a prospective, randomized, double-blind study of women at increased risk for ovarian hyperstimulation syndrome undergoing assisted reproduction, cabergoline prevented increased vascular permeability via inactivation of the vascular endothelial growth factor receptor 2.

Key Learning Points

- Amenorrhea related to altered body weight requires prompt diagnosis, examination, and laboratory assessment to establish a management plan for the health of the woman and her future offspring.

- Functional amenorrhea can accompany stress, weight loss, and/or excessive exercise without an identifiable organic cause, but can signal anorexia in a woman with altered nutrition and body image.

- Functional amenorrhea accompanying AN requires a prompt multidisciplinary plan with nutritional consultation, psychological support, exercise modification, and sex steroid replacement.

- Amenorrhea associated with obesity can mimic or exaggerate PCOS expression with adverse effects on endometrial development, metabolic-reproductive function, and fertility.

- In amenorrheic women with obesity, fertility strategies should balance postponing ovulation induction to improve metabolic health with delaying conception, as maternal-fetal complications increase with age.

References

1. Dobranowska K, Plińska S, Dobosz A. Dietary and lifestyle management of functional hypothalamic amenorrhea: a comprehensive review. *Nutrients.* 2024;16(17):2967. PMID: 39275282

2. Gordon CM, Ackerman KE, Berga SL, et al. Functional hypothalamic amenorrhea: an Endocrine Society clinical practice guideline. *J Clin Endocrinol Metab.* 2017;102(5):1413-1439. PMID: 28368518

3. Dumesic DA, Oberfield SE, Stener-Victorin E, Marshall JC, Laven JS, Legro RS. Scientific statement on the diagnostic criteria, epidemiology, pathophysiology, and molecular genetics of polycystic ovary syndrome. *Endocr Rev.* 2015;36(5):487-525. PMID: 26426951

4. Practice Committee of the American Society for Reproductive Medicine. Obesity and reproduction: a committee opinion. *Fertil Steril.* 2021;116(5):1266-1285. PMID: 34583840

5. Sophie Gibson ME, Fleming N, Zuijdwijk C, Dumont T. Where have the periods gone? The evaluation and management of functional hypothalamic amenorrhea. *J Clin Res Pediatr Endocrinol.* 2020;12(Suppl 1):18-27. PMID: 32041389

6. Selzer R, Caust J, Hibbert M, Bowes G, Patton G. The association between secondary amenorrhea and common eating disordered weight control practices in an adolescent population. *J Adolesc Health.* 1996;19(1):56-61. PMID: 8842861

7. Saadedine M, Kapoor E, Shufelt C. Functional hypothalamic amenorrhea: recognition and management of a challenging diagnosis. *Mayo Clin Proc.* 2023;98(9):1376-1385. PMID: 37661145

8. Barakat GM, Ramadan W, Assi G, Khoury NBE. Satiety: a gut-brain-relationship. *J Physiol Sci.* 2024;74(1):11. PMID: 38368346

9. Cena H, Chiovato L, Nappi RE. Obesity, polycystic ovary syndrome, and infertility: a new avenue for GLP-1 receptor agonists. *J Clin Endocrinol Metab.* 2020;105(8):e2695-e2709. PMID: 32442310

10. Bednarz K, Kowalczyk K, Cwynar M, et al. The role of Glp-1 receptor agonists in insulin resistance with concomitant obesity treatment in polycystic ovary syndrome. *Int J Mol Sci.* 2022;23(8):4334. PMID: 35457152

11. Schorr M, Miller KK. The endocrine manifestations of anorexia nervosa: mechanisms and management. *Nat Rev Endocrinol.* 2017;13(3):174-186. PMID: 27811940

12. Misra M, Klibanski A. Endocrine consequences of anorexia nervosa. *Lancet Diabetes Endocrinol.* 2014;2(7):581-592. PMID: 24731664

13. Hebebrand J, Gradl-Dietsch G, Peters T, Correll CU, Haas V. The diagnosis and treatment of anorexia nervosa in childhood and adolescence. *Dtsch Arztebl Int.* 2024;121(5):164-174. PMID: 38170843

14. Indirli R, Lanzi V, Mantovani G, Arosio M, Ferrante E. Bone health in functional hypothalamic amenorrhea: what the endocrinologist needs to know. *Front Endocrinol (Lausanne).* 2022;13:946695. PMID: 36303862

15. Teede HJ, Tay CT, Laven JJE, et al. Recommendations from the 2023 International Evidence-based Guideline for the Assessment and Management of Polycystic Ovary Syndrome. *J Clin Endocrinol Metab.* 2023;108(10):2447-2469. PMID: 37580314

16. Shetty C, Rizvi SMHA, Sharaf J, et al. Risk of gynecological cancers in women with polycystic ovary syndrome and the pathophysiology of association. *Cureus.* 2023;15(4):e37266. PMID: 37162768

17. Nees LK, Heublein S, Steinmacher S, et al. Endometrial hyperplasia as a risk factor of endometrial cancer. *Arch Gynecol Obstet.* 2022;306(2):407-421. PMID: 35001185

18. Gallos ID, Ganesan R, Gupta JK. Prediction of regression and relapse of endometrial hyperplasia with conservative therapy. *Obstet Gynecol.* 2013;121(6):1165-1171. PMID: 23812448

19. Harris E. First large study of GLP-1 receptor agonists during pregnancy. *JAMA.* 2024;331(4):280. PMID: 38170560

20. Newman C, Dunne FP. Treatment of diabetes in pregnancy with metformin. *Obstet Gynecol.* 2024;144(5):660-669. PMID: 39208454

21. Hanem LGE, Salvesen Ø, Juliusson PB, et al. Intrauterine metformin exposure and offspring cardiometabolic risk factors (PedMet study): a 5-10 year follow-up of the PregMet randomised controlled trial. *Lancet Child Adolesc Health.* 2019;3(3):166-174. PMID: 30704873

22. Legro RS, Dodson WC, Kris-Etherton PM, et al. Randomized controlled trial of preconception interventions in infertile women with polycystic ovary syndrome. *J Clin Endocrinol Metab.* 2015;100(11):4048-4058. PMID: 26401593

23. Mutsaerts MA, van Oers AM, Groen H, et al. Randomized trial of a lifestyle program in obese infertile women. *N Engl J Med.* 2016;374(20):1942-1953. PMID: 27192672

24. Luke B, Brown MB, Stern JE, Missmer SA, Fujimoto VY, Leach R; SART Writing Group. Female obesity adversely affects assisted reproductive technology (ART) pregnancy and live birth rates. *Hum Reprod.* 2011;26(1):245-252. PMID: 21071489

25. Legro RS, Brzyski RG, Diamond MP, et al; NICHD Reproductive Medicine Network. Letrozole versus clomiphene for infertility in the polycystic ovary syndrome. *N Engl J Med.* 2014;371(2):119-129. PMID: 25006718

Recommended Reading

- Nass R, Evans WS. Physiological and pathophysiological alterations of the neuroendocrine components of the reproductive axis. In: *Yen and Jaffe's Reproductive Endocrinology: Physiology, Pathophysiology and Clinical Management, Ninth Edition.* Strauss JF III, Barbieri RL, Dokras A, Williams CJ, Williams SZ (eds). Elsevier Saunders, Philadelphia, 2024, pgs. 475-515.

- Misra M, Katzman D, Miller KK, et al. Physiologic estrogen replacement increases bone density in adolescent girls with anorexia nervosa. *J Bone Miner Res.* 2011;26(10):2430-2438. PMID: 21698665

- GBD 2015 Obesity Collaborators; Afshin A, Forouzanfar MH, et al. Health effects of overweight and obesity in 195 countries over 25 years. *N Engl J Med.* 2017;377(1):13-27. PMID: 28604169

- Brennan KM, Kroener LL, Chazenbalk GD, Dumesic DA. Polycystic ovary syndrome: impact of lipotoxicity on metabolic and reproductive health. *Obstet Gynecol Surv.* 2019;74(4) 223-231. PMID: 31344250

- Li S, Ma S, Yao X, Liu P. Effects of metabolic syndrome on pregnancy outcomes in women without polycystic ovary syndrome. *J Endocr Soc.* 2024;8(10):bvae143. PMID: 39224458

- Pape J, Herbison AE, Leeners B. Recovery of menses after functional hypothalamic amenorrhoea: if, when and why. *Hum Reprod Update.* 2021;27(1):130-153. PMID: 33067637

- McLaughlin T, Lamendola C, Liu A, Abbasi F. Preferential fat deposition in subcutaneous versus visceral depots is associated with insulin sensitivity. *J Clin Endocrinol Metab.* 2011;96(11) E1756-E1760. PMID: 21865361

- Cui H, López M, Rahmouni K. The cellular and molecular bases of leptin and ghrelin resistance in obesity. *Nat Rev Endocrinol.* 2017;13(6):338-351. PMID: 28232667

- Papaetis GS, Kyriacou A. GLP-1 receptor agonists, polycystic ovary syndrome and reproductive dysfunction: current research and future horizons. *Adv Clin Exp Med.* 2022;31(11):1265-1274. PMID: 35951627

- Chittenden BG, Fullerton G, Maheshwari A, Bhattacharya S. Polycystic ovary syndrome and the risk of gynaecological cancer: a systematic review. *Reprod Biomed Online.* 2009;19(3):398-405. PMID: 19778486

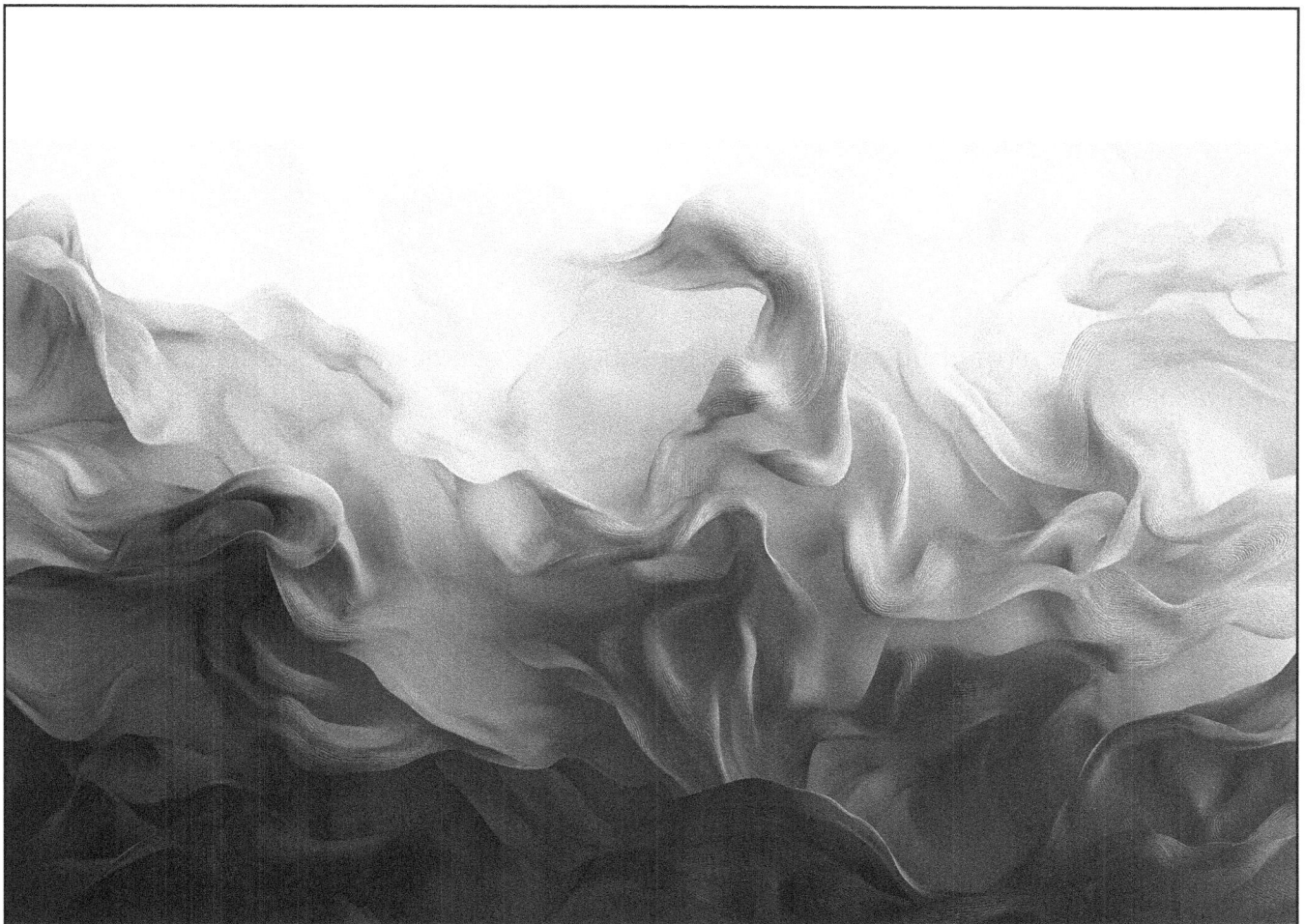

THYROID BIOLOGY AND CANCER

Management of Hyperthyroidism-Related Complications

Grigoris Effraimidis, MD, PhD. School of Health Sciences, University of Thessaly, Larissa, Greece; Department of Endocrinology and Metabolic Diseases, University General Hospital of Larissa, Larissa, Greece; E-mail: grigoris.effraimidis@gmail.com

Educational Objectives

After reviewing this chapter, learners should be able to:

- Identify the cardiac, electrolyte, and muscular complications associated with hyperthyroidism, including atrial fibrillation, thyrotoxic periodic paralysis, and thyroid storm.

- Diagnose hyperthyroidism-related complications using clinical features, laboratory findings, and diagnostic scoring systems.

- Manage hyperthyroidism-related atrial fibrillation, thyrotoxic periodic paralysis, and thyroid storm through targeted pharmacological and supportive therapies.

- Explain the role of anticoagulation in hyperthyroidism-related atrial fibrillation and the risks and benefits of direct oral anticoagulants vs warfarin.

Significance of the Clinical Problem

Hyperthyroidism is common, with an estimated global prevalence of 0.2% to 1.3% in its overt form and 0.7% to 1.8% in its subclinical form among iodine-sufficient populations.[1] It is a disorder affecting multiple organ systems.

Atrial fibrillation is the most common cardiac complication, occurring in 5% to 15% of hyperthyroid patients, compared with 1% to 3% in the general population, and it may be the initial presentation of hyperthyroidism.[2]

Thyrotoxic periodic paralysis is a rare but potentially life-threatening complication characterized by hypokalemia and muscle weakness that predominantly affects young Asian males. Without prompt recognition and treatment, thyrotoxic periodic paralysis can lead to cardiac arrhythmias and respiratory failure.

Similarly, thyroid storm represents a critical endocrine emergency with a high mortality rate, requiring immediate and aggressive intervention to prevent fatal outcomes.

These complications highlight the need for enhanced clinical awareness, prompt diagnosis, and effective management strategies to mitigate the risks.

Practice Gaps

- The optimal anticoagulation strategy for patients with hyperthyroid-related atrial fibrillation remains an area requiring further investigation.

- There is limited awareness and recognition of thyrotoxic periodic paralysis, resulting in delayed diagnosis and treatment, which increases the risk of cardiac arrhythmias or respiratory failure.

- Diagnosis can be challenging due to the inability of thyroid function tests to distinguish thyroid storm from uncomplicated thyrotoxicosis, as well as inadequate use of diagnostic scoring systems (eg, Burch-Wartofsky score) and standardized treatment protocols, which contributes to suboptimal management and higher mortality rates.

Discussion

Hyperthyroidism is associated with significant complications, including atrial fibrillation, thyrotoxic periodic paralysis, and thyroid storm, leading to increased morbidity and mortality if not promptly diagnosed and managed. Herein, we discuss the clinical manifestations, diagnostic approaches, and management strategies for these hyperthyroidism-related complications.

Atrial Fibrillation

Atrial fibrillation is the most common cardiac complication of hyperthyroidism and can be the first manifestation of hyperthyroidism, making routine thyroid function testing a significant diagnostic consideration in the evaluation of patients with new-onset atrial fibrillation. Individuals with Graves hyperthyroidism have a doubled risk of atrial fibrillation compared with risk of population controls.[3] Risk factors for atrial fibrillation in hyperthyroid patients do not differ from those in the general population (ie, age, male sex, ischemic heart disease, heart failure, and valvular heart disease). In addition, it has been found that subclinical hyperthyroidism, as well as free T_4 in the high-normal range, significantly increases atrial fibrillation risk.

Hyperthyroidism is a reversible cause of atrial fibrillation, with most patients spontaneously reverting to sinus rhythm within 4 to 6 months of achieving thyroid control, often even before full euthyroidism is reached. Therefore, control of thyroid hormone levels is the most important step in the management of hyperthyroidism-related atrial fibrillation, and euthyroidism should be achieved as soon as possible.

A holistic approach, similar to the management of atrial fibrillation in the general population, is recommended for hyperthyroidism-related atrial fibrillation. This approach is based on controlling rate and rhythm, avoiding stroke/thromboembolism, and managing cardiovascular risk factors and comorbidities, recognizing that hyperthyroidism is a modifiable risk factor for atrial fibrillation. Rate control with β-adrenergic blockers is central to the management of hyperthyroidism-related atrial fibrillation, by optimizing the ventricular response (optimal target <110 beats/min), relieving symptoms, and preventing cardiomyopathy. Rhythm control is generally reserved for hemodynamically unstable patients, or those in whom atrial fibrillation is persistent or recurrent after restoration of euthyroidism. The stroke and systemic embolism risk in hyperthyroidism-related atrial fibrillation remains a controversial topic. Decisions about anticoagulation should follow the general atrial fibrillation guidelines by using the CHA_2DS_2-VASc and HAS-BLED scores, although these scores may not fully account for hyperthyroidism-related atrial fibrillation–specific risks, as data are thus far inconclusive. Recent evidence suggests that both warfarin and direct oral anticoagulants are equally effective, but direct oral anticoagulants may potentially offer a lower bleeding risk. Finally, optimizing comorbidities (eg, hypertension, diabetes, obesity) and addressing modifiable risk factors, such as cigarette smoking and alcohol, is required (*Figure, following page*).

Thyrotoxic Periodic Paralysis

Thyrotoxic periodic paralysis is a rare endocrine emergency characterized by acute, reversible, painless muscle weakness and hypokalemia, predominantly affecting Asian individuals with thyrotoxicosis, with a reported incidence of 2% (compared with 0.1% to 0.2% in non-Asian individuals with thyrotoxicosis). More than 95% of thyrotoxic periodic paralysis cases occur in men, typically in those aged 20 to 40 years. Often, events

Figure. Management of Hyperthyroidism-Related Atrial Fibrillation

Figure.
Restoring euthyroidism is a critical first step in managing hyperthyroidism-related atrial fibrillation (AF), as controlling/normalizing thyroid function often leads to spontaneous conversion to sinus rhythm. Rate control, primarily using beta-blockers, is the initial strategy to manage symptoms and achieve a target heart rate (HR) of <110 bpm. Rhythm control, such as cardioversion or ablation, is considered secondary and reserved for cases where hyperthyroidism-related AF persists despite achieving euthyroidism. Given the clinical uncertainty regarding the benefits and harms of anticoagulation in patients with hyperthyroidism-related AF, stroke risk is evaluated using the CHA2DS2-VASc score, as in other patients with AF. Oral anticoagulation (OAC) is recommended based on stroke risk stratification. Finally, managing cardiovascular risk factors and concomitant diseases, such as hypertension, diabetes, and obesity, is essential to reduce overall cardiovascular risk in these patients. TOE: Transesophageal Echocardiography; LA: left atrial

Reprinted from Kostopoulos G & Effraimidis G. *Eur Thyroid J*, 2024; 13(2): e230254. © The Authors. Published by Bioscientifica Ltd. on behalf of The European Thyroid Association.

such as heavy exercise or high-carbohydrate meals precede the thyrotoxic periodic paralysis episodes.

Thyrotoxic periodic paralysis results from intracellular potassium movement, leading to hypokalemia, but the total body potassium is preserved. Episodes can range from mild muscle weakness to flaccid paralysis, primarily affecting proximal leg muscles, and occur only during thyrotoxicosis. Symptoms of thyrotoxicosis may precede, coincide with, or follow the onset of thyrotoxic periodic paralysis.[4] During attacks, serum potassium levels often drop below 3 mEq/L (<3 mmol/L), and sometimes less than 1.5 mEq/L (<1.5 mmol/L), risking cardiac arrhythmias or respiratory failure and making prompt diagnosis and treatment critical. Potassium chloride (10-200 mmol) should be administered cautiously to avoid rebound hyperkalemia. High-dosage nonselective β-adrenergic blockers, such as propranolol, are used in the treatment of thyrotoxic periodic paralysis due to their ability to suppress β2-adrenergic activity and inhibit insulin secretion, as hyperadrenergic activity and hyperinsulinemia are implicated in the pathogenesis of thyrotoxic periodic paralysis.

Further attacks can be prevented by managing the underlying cause of thyrotoxicosis (typically Graves hyperthyroidism), prescribing nonselective β-adrenergic blockers, and avoiding known precipitating factors.

Thyroid Storm

Thyroid storm is a rare, life-threatening condition characterized by severe thyrotoxicosis and high mortality rates. It is twelve times more likely to be fatal than uncomplicated thyrotoxicosis, and it typically results from untreated or poorly managed thyrotoxicosis, often triggered by factors such as infections, surgery, trauma, or iodine excess. All causes of thyrotoxicosis have been associated with thyroid storm, with Graves disease and multinodular goiter being the most common. Thyroid storm has also been reported as a complication of immune checkpoint inhibitor–mediated thyrotoxicosis.[5]

The diagnosis of thyroid storm is clinical, as thyroid function tests alone cannot distinguish thyroid storm from uncomplicated thyrotoxicosis, although free T_4 and free T_3 levels may be slightly higher in thyroid storm.[6] Scoring systems, such as the Burch-Wartofsky score and a Japanese system, assist in diagnosis, but clinical judgment is essential (*Table, following page*).[7,8] Symptoms include high fever, severe tachycardia, gastrointestinal manifestations (nausea, vomiting, diarrhea), and CNS disorders (irritability, confusion, coma).

Treatment of thyrotoxicosis in thyroid storm involves high-dosage antithyroid drugs to decrease production and secretion of thyroid hormones (propylthiouracil is preferred due to its inhibition of T_4 to T_3 conversion), β-adrenergic blockers to ameliorate manifestations of thyroid storm (particularly the cardiac ones), iodine to block thyroid hormone release, and glucocorticoids to inhibit extrathyroidal conversion of T_4 to T_3.[9] Supportive care should include cooling, fluids, intensive care unit monitoring, and appropriate treatment (eg, antibiotics) of the underlying precipitating factor. In refractory cases, plasmapheresis, hemoperfusion, or emergency thyroidectomy may be required. Early and aggressive treatment is crucial to reduce mortality.

Clinical Case Vignettes

Case 1

A 46-year-old man with no relevant medical history, aside from a history of smoking cessation, presents to his primary care physician with concerns of palpitations and fatigue following a 3-day viral illness characterized by fever, arthralgia, myalgia, and paroxysmal cough. On physical examination, an irregular heartbeat is noted, prompting referral to a cardiologist. The cardiologist diagnoses atrial fibrillation and admits the patient to the cardiology department. Treatment with a β-adrenergic blocker (bisoprolol, 10 mg daily) and anticoagulation (apixaban) is initiated.

Table. Scoring Systems to Diagnose Thyroid Storm

A. Burch-Wartofsky Point Scale

Temperature		CNS		GI/Liver		HR (bpm)		AFil		Heart Failure		Precipitant	
99-99.9 °F	5 pts	Absent	0 pts	Absent	0 pts	99-109	5 pts	Absent	0 pts	Absent	0 pts	Negative	0 pts
37.2–37.7 °C		Agitation	10 pts	Diarrhea,	10 pts	110-119	10 pts	Present	10 pts	Mild	5 pts	Positive	10 pts
100-100.9 °F	10 pts	Delerium,	20 pts	abdominal pain,		120-129	15 pts			Moderate	10 pts		
37.8-38.2 °C		psychosis		nausea/vomiting		130-139	20 pts			Severe	15 pts		
101-101.9 °F	15 pts	Seizure/Coma	30 pts	Jaundice	20 pts	≥140	25 pts						
38.3–38.8 °C													
102-102.9 °F	20 pts												
38.9–39.3 °C													
103-103.9 °F	25 pts												
39.4–39.9 °C													
>104.0 °F	30 pts												
≥ 40.0 °C													

<25 - unlikely to represent storm

25-44 - suggests impending storm

≥45 - highly suggestive of storm

B. Japan Thyroid Association Definition and Diagnostic Criteria for Thyroid Storm

Prerequisite for diagnosis

Presence of thyrotoxicosis with elevated levels of free triiodothyronine (FT3) or free thyroxine (FT4)

Symptoms

1. CNS manifestations: Restlessness, delirium, mental aberration/psychosis, somnolence/lethargy, coma (≥1 on the Japan or ≤14 on the Glasgow Coma Scale)
2. Fever : ≥ 100.4°F/ 38°C
3. Tachycardia : ≥ 130 beats per minute or heart rate ≥ 130 in atrial fibrillation
4. Congestive heart failure (CHF) : Pulmonary edema, moist rales over more than half of the lung field, cardiogenic shock, or Class IV by the New York Heart Association or ≥ Class III in the Killip classification
5. GI/hepatic manifestations : nausea , vomiting, diarrhea, or a total bilirubin level ≥ 3.0 mg/dL

Diagnosis

Grade of TS	Combinations of features	Requirements for diagnosis
TS1 (Definite TS)	First combination	Thyrotoxicosis and at least one CNS manifestation and fever, tachycardia, CHF, or GI/hepatic manifestations
TS1(Definite TS)	Alternate combination	Thyrotoxicosis and at least three combinations of fever, tachycardia, CHF, or GI/hepatic manifestations
TS2 (Suspected TS)	First combination	Thyrotoxicosis and a combination of two of the following: fever, tachycardia, CHF, or GI/hepatic manifestations
TS2 (Suspected TS)	Alternate combination	Patients who met the diagnosis of TS1 except that serum FT3 or FT4 level are not available

Exclusion and provisions

Cases are excluded if other underlying diseases clearly causing any of the following symptoms: fever (e.g., pneumonia and malignant hyperthermia), impaired consciousness (e.g., psychiatric disorders and cerebrovascular disease), heart failure (e.g., acute myocardial infarction), and liver disorders (e.g., viral hepatitis and acute liver failure). Therefore, it is difficult to determine whether the symptom is caused by TS or is simply a manifestation of an underlying disease; the symptom should be regarded as being due to a TS that is caused by these precipitating factors. Clinical judgment in this matter is required.

C. Comparison Burch-Wartofsky Point Scale vs Japan Thyroid Association (JTA) Criteria

Criterion	Burch and Wartofsky	JTA
Method	Quantitative	Not quantitative
Scoring system	Included	Not included
Exclusion criteria	Absence	Present
TFTs	Absence of TFTs in the criteria	Pre-requisite
Fever	≥ 99°F/ 37.2°C	≥ 100.4°F /38°C
Heart rate	≥ 90 bpm	≥ 130 bpm
Atrial fibrillation	Included	Not included
Heart failure	Pedal edema to pulmonary edema	NYHA classification class IV or Killip classification ≥III
Serum bilirubin concentrations	Not included	> 3 mg/dL
Jaundice	Included	Not included

CNS: central nervous system; GI: gastrointestinal; HR: heart rate; bpm: beats per minute; AFil: atrial fibrillation; CHF: Congestive heart failure;

TFTs: thyroid function test; NYHA: New York Heart Association

Thyroid function test results indicate autoimmune hyperthyroidism:

TSH = <0.01 mIU/L
Free T_3 = 15.6 pg/mL (1.6-3.9 pg/mL)
    (SI: 24.0 pmol/L[2.4-6.0 pmol/L])
Free T_4 = 2.9 ng/dL (0.7-1.5 ng/dL) (SI: 37.2 pmol/L
    [9.0–19.0 pmol/L])
TPO antibodies = 1050 IU/L
TRAb = 36.0 IU/L (<1.75 IU/L)

The cardiology team decides that cardioversion will be deferred until stabilization of thyroid function and consults an endocrinologist who starts methimazole, 10 mg twice daily, to manage hyperthyroidism.

Which of the following is the best recommendation?

A. Initiate anticoagulation as soon as possible due to high risk of embolism

B. Use warfarin only, as direct oral anticoagulants are contraindicated in hyperthyroidism

C. Follow standard atrial fibrillation guidelines using CHA_2DS_2-VASc and HAS-BLED scores to assess stroke and bleeding risk

D. Initiate aspirin instead of anticoagulation for stroke prevention

E. Use long-term anticoagulation even after thyroid function normalizes

Answer: C) Follow standard atrial fibrillation guidelines using CHA_2DS_2-VASc and HAS-BLED scores to assess stroke and bleeding risk

Hyperthyroidism is associated with a hypercoagulable state, as elevated levels of different clotting factors have been found in individuals with hyperthyroidism. However, epidemiological data on the association between hyperthyroidism, stroke, and thrombosis are inconclusive. Some studies suggest increased stroke risk in hyperthyroidism-related atrial fibrillation, while other studies show no increased risk, and sometimes even decreased risk, compared with risk in people with atrial fibrillation without hyperthyroidism.[10-12] These discrepancies may emerge from differences in study design and patient characteristics. Decisions regarding anticoagulation should follow general atrial fibrillation guidelines, using established stroke and bleeding risk assessment tools (CHA_2DS_2-VASc and HAS-BLED scores) (Answer C).

Since hyperthyroidism-related atrial fibrillation often resolves with control of hyperthyroidism, and patients experience a spontaneous return to sinus rhythm, recommendations for long-term anticoagulation follow those for the general population with atrial fibrillation.

Warfarin use in hyperthyroidism-related atrial fibrillation requires careful monitoring and regular dosage adjustments due to the increased breakdown of vitamin K-dependent clotting factors in hyperthyroidism. This results in lower warfarin dosage requirements to maintain a therapeutic INR.

The novel direct oral anticoagulants are not contraindicated in hyperthyroidism. Data on the comparison of direct oral anticoagulants with warfarin in hyperthyroidism-related atrial fibrillation suggests that direct oral anticoagulants are at least as beneficial as warfarin in this population but have a potential lower bleeding risk.

Aspirin is inferior to anticoagulants for stroke prevention in atrial fibrillation and is not recommended.

This patient became euthyroid 18 days after methimazole initiation (free T_4 = 1.4 ng/dL [17.8 pmol/L]) and experienced a spontaneous return to sinus rhythm at that time. His cardiologist had started apixaban at the time of atrial fibrillation diagnosis, which was not absolutely necessary given the CHA2DS2-VASc score of 0, indicating a stroke risk similar to that of persons without atrial fibrillation.

Case 2

A 42-year-old man of Chinese ancestry with a 1-year history of Graves disease presents to the emergency department with progressive weakness in his arms and legs. Thyroid tests 6 months earlier showed euthyroidism on methimazole, 5 mg daily. Symptoms began 2 weeks ago with episodic morning leg weakness that resolved spontaneously during the day. On the day of admission, the patient woke up with severe leg weakness, preventing him from getting out of bed. As the morning progressed, weakness extended to his arms, although less pronounced than in the legs.

On physical examination, muscle strength is 1-2/5 on knee flexion and extension, hip flexion, ankle dorsiflexion, and plantar flexion; 2/5 on abduction and on flexion of both shoulders; and 4/5 on extension of the elbows, wrists, and fingers. Muscle tone and deep tendon reflexes are normal. Sensation to light touch, pinprick, and temperature is intact.

Laboratory test results show severe hypokalemia (1.7 mEq/L [1.7 mmol/L]) and thyrotoxicosis. Electrocardiography reveals normal sinus rhythm.

Which of the following statements is correct?

A. The patient's Asian ethnicity and male sex are consistent with the typical epidemiology of thyrotoxic periodic paralysis

B. The patient's thyrotoxic state is unrelated to thyrotoxic periodic paralysis, as thyrotoxic periodic paralysis only occurs in euthyroid individuals

C. Genetic testing for variants in the gene encoding the Kir2.6 potassium channel is required to confirm the diagnosis of thyrotoxic periodic paralysis

D. Immediate first-line treatment is nonselective β-adrenergic blockers to correct hypokalemia and prevent paralysis

E. Prophylactic potassium supplementation is recommended to prevent future episodes of thyrotoxic periodic paralysis, even after achieving euthyroidism

Answer: A) The patient's Asian ethnicity and male sex are consistent with the typical epidemiology of thyrotoxic periodic paralysis

Thyrotoxic periodic paralysis predominantly affects Asian men, with a male-to-female ratio of 30:1, and 80% of first episodes present between 20 to 40 years of age. The patient's demographic profile aligns with the typical thyrotoxic periodic paralysis epidemiological pattern (Answer A). Nevertheless, it should be highlighted that thyrotoxic periodic paralysis can also occur in other ethnic groups. Raising awareness outside Asian populations is important to prevent delayed diagnosis.

Biochemical confirmation of thyrotoxicosis is essential for thyrotoxic periodic paralysis diagnosis, as paralysis only occurs in the thyrotoxic state.

Thyrotoxic periodic paralysis is an acquired disorder resulting in increased Na+/K+–ATPase sensitivity. Multiple susceptibility loci have been associated with thyrotoxic periodic paralysis, including a loss-of-function or dominant-negative variants in the gene encoding the skeletal muscle potassium channel Kir2.6 and variants in the *KCNJ2* gene that encodes the skeletal muscle potassium channel Kir2.1.[13] However, genetic testing is not required for diagnosis, which is primarily clinical. The hallmark is hypokalemia accompanied by thyrotoxicosis, triggered by conditions such as heavy exercise, high-carbohydrate meals, and, less often, trauma, respiratory infections, high salt intake, stress, alcohol, or medication. In this case, the patient reported no precipitating factors.[14]

Potassium correction is the primary treatment for acute thyrotoxic periodic paralysis episodes, while nonselective β-adrenergic blockers, such as propranolol, can be used at high dosages during acute episodes and at lower dosages to prevent recurrence.

Routine prophylactic potassium supplementation is not recommended, as there is no evidence supporting effectiveness in preventing thyrotoxic periodic paralysis episodes.

The patient was admitted for potassium correction, with a remarkable recovery following normalization of potassium levels (3.7 mEq/L [3.7 mmol/L]) 9 hours later. Strength fully returned to grade 5 in all extremities.

Case 3

A 47-year-old woman presents in a comatose state with tachycardia, hypertension, and pyrexia following a 5-day history of headache, cough, shortness of breath, nasal congestion, myalgias, and chills. Upon arrival at the hospital, tracheal intubation is required, and she is admitted to the intensive care unit with suspected meningoencephalitis. Initial hypertension progresses to hypotension, requiring noradrenaline infusion. Despite intervention, tachycardia and hyperpyrexia persist. The SARS-CoV-2 rapid nasal swab returns positive, and cerebrospinal fluid analysis is normal except for elevated lactate. Thyroid function tests reveal elevated free T_4 and free T_3 levels with undetectable TSH. A large goiter with bruit and positive TPO antibodies and TRAb support the autoimmune origin of hyperthyroidism. The Burch-Wartofsky score is 85, confirming the diagnosis of thyroid storm secondary to Graves hyperthyroidism. The patient is treated with propylthiouracil, 200 mg 4 times daily; propranolol, 40 mg 3 times daily; Lugol solution, 5 drops 4 times daily (60 minutes after administration of propylthiouracil); intravenous hydrocortisone, 200 mg bolus followed by 8 mg/h infusion; and cholestyramine, 3 g 3 times daily.

Which of the following statements is correct?

A. Thyroid storm's pathogenesis primarily involves increased serum catecholamine levels, making β-adrenergic blockers unnecessary in treatment

B. Diagnosis is based solely on elevated thyroid hormone levels (free T_4 and free T_3) and suppressed TSH, distinguishing thyroid storm from uncomplicated hyperthyroidism

C. Infections, including SARS-CoV-2 infection, do not act as a trigger, exacerbating thyroid hormone activity

D. Effective treatment requires high-dosage propylthiouracil, β-adrenergic blockers, iodine, glucocorticoids, supportive measures, and intensive care unit monitoring

E. Plasmapheresis is the standard first-line treatment for patients with thyroid storm resistant to medical therapy

Answer: D) Effective treatment requires high-dosage propylthiouracil, β-adrenergic blockers, iodine, glucocorticoids, supportive measures, and intensive care unit monitoring

Treatment guidelines recommend this comprehensive approach: high-dosage propylthiouracil, β-adrenergic blockers, iodine, glucocorticoids, supportive care, and treatment of the precipitating or underlying condition (Answer D). Thionamide antithyroid drugs are used to block new thyroid hormone synthesis, administered in high doses orally or via nasogastric tube, or, in selected patients, rectally as a suppository. Propylthiouracil is theoretically preferred to methimazole due to its additional inhibitory effect on peripheral T_4 to T_3 conversion. Iodide (Lugol solution or SSKI) is given to inhibit hormone release and must be administered an hour after the thionamide. Other treatment options include radiographic contrast agents (no longer available in the United States), lithium as an alternative to iodide in iodine-allergic patients or those with previous severe reactions to thionamides, cholestyramine (which works by decreasing reabsorption of thyroid hormone from the enterohepatic circulation), hemoperfusion and plasmapheresis in exceptional cases, and finally thyroidectomy, which is rarely performed during active thyroid storm as it is too risky before thyrotoxicosis is controlled.

The pathogenesis of thyroid storm is unclear, and very high thyroid hormone levels alone are insufficient to explain the condition. Decreased protein binding of thyroid hormones, resulting in higher free hormone levels, and increased peripheral tissue sensitivity to thyroid hormones can possibly be exacerbated by the precipitating or underlying conditions. Although symptoms resemble catecholamine excess, catecholamine levels are typically normal. However, drugs, such as propranolol, can dramatically improve symptoms, suggesting the involvement of the sympathetic nervous system.

Thyroid function tests in thyroid storm are often not different than those of uncomplicated hyperthyroidism. Diagnosis of thyroid storm relies primarily on recognizing the severity of thyrotoxic symptoms and signs, and it must be highlighted that the thyroid storm diagnosis should be based on clinical judgment, with the scoring systems being ancillary (Burch-Wartofsky score, Japanese Thyroid Association Criteria) (*Table*).

Thyroid storm can be triggered by an intercurrent illness or injury that worsens existing thyrotoxicosis. An acute event causing a sudden surge in thyroid hormone secretion, such as thyroidectomy or radioiodine therapy can (rarely) trigger thyroid storm. Infections are the most common trigger, but other illnesses, trauma (including surgery), and even certain toxins can also precipitate thyroid storm in individuals with underlying thyrotoxicosis. Distinguishing between symptoms of infection and impending thyroid storm can be challenging, but a disproportionately high fever and sweating may help to lead to the diagnosis.

As previously mentioned, hemoperfusion and plasmapheresis may be considered in exceptional cases.

This patient's tachycardia and pyrexia resolved within hours, and vasopressor support was discontinued. She was successfully extubated the following day and transferred to a general medical ward in stable condition.

Key Learning Points

- Hyperthyroidism can lead to severe complications, such as atrial fibrillation, thyrotoxic periodic paralysis, and thyroid storm, which require prompt recognition and management to prevent morbidity and mortality.

- Hyperthyroidism is a reversible cause of atrial fibrillation. Achieving euthyroidism is the most crucial step in the management of hyperthyroidism-related atrial fibrillation.

Rate control with β-adrenergic blockers is the mainstay of initial symptomatic treatment while rhythm-control is reserved in cases of hemodynamically unstable, persistent, or recurrent atrial fibrillation. Anticoagulation decisions should follow standard atrial fibrillation guidelines (CHA_2DS_2-VASc and HAS-BLED scores), with direct oral anticoagulants potentially offering a lower bleeding risk compared with that of warfarin. Further research is needed to optimize anticoagulation strategies in hyperthyroidism-related atrial fibrillation.

- Thyrotoxic periodic paralysis is a rare but life-threatening condition characterized by acute hypokalemia and muscle weakness, predominantly affecting young Asian males. Diagnosis is based on clinical presentation, hypokalemia, and thyrotoxicosis. Immediate potassium correction is critical, with cautious administration to avoid rebound hyperkalemia. Achieving euthyroidism is essential to prevent further episodes. Increased awareness of thyrotoxic periodic paralysis outside Asian populations is crucial to prevent delayed diagnosis.

- Thyroid storm is a critical endocrine emergency with high mortality, requiring aggressive treatment. Diagnosis relies on clinical judgment and scoring systems (eg, Burch-Wartofsky score), as thyroid function tests alone cannot distinguish thyroid storm from uncomplicated hyperthyroidism. Treatment involves high-dosage antithyroid drugs (propylthiouracil preferred), β-adrenergic blockers, iodine, glucocorticoids, and supportive care (eg, cooling, fluids, intensive care unit monitoring).

References

1. Wiersinga WM, Poppe KG, Effraimidis G. Hyperthyroidism: aetiology, pathogenesis, diagnosis, management, complications, and prognosis. *Lancet Diabetes Endocrinol.* 2023;11(4):282-298. PMID: 36848916

2. Kostopoulos G, Effraimidis G. Epidemiology, prognosis, and challenges in the management of hyperthyroidism-related atrial fibrillation. *Eur Thyroid J.* 2024;13(2):e230254. PMID: 38377675

3. Okosieme OE, Taylor PN, Evans C, et al. Primary therapy of Graves' disease and cardiovascular morbidity and mortality: a linked-record cohort study. *Lancet Diabetes Endocrinol.* 2019;7(4):278-287. PMID: 30827829

4. Chang CC, Cheng CJ, Sung CC, et al. A 10-year analysis of thyrotoxic periodic paralysis in 135 patients: focus on symptomatology and precipitants. *Eur J Endocrinol.* 2013;169(5):529-536. PMID: 23939916

5. Iwama S, Kobayashi T, Arima H. Management, biomarkers and prognosis in people developing endocrinopathies associated with immune checkpoint inhibitors. *Nat Rev Endocrinol.* PMID: 39779950

6. Brooks MH, Waldstein SS. Free thyroxine concentrations in thyroid storm. *Ann Intern Med.* 1980;93(5):694-697. PMID: 7212477

7. Burch HB, Wartofsky L. Life-threatening thyrotoxicosis. Thyroid storm. *Endocrinol Metab Clin North Am.* 1993;22(2):263-277. PMID: 17127140

8. Satoh T, Isozaki O, Suzuki A, et al. 2016 Guidelines for the management of thyroid storm from The Japan Thyroid Association and Japan Endocrine Society (First edition). *Endocr J.* 2016;63(12):1025-1064. PMID: 27746415

9. Ross DS, Burch HB, Cooper DS, et al. 2016 American Thyroid Association guidelines for diagnosis and management of hyperthyroidism and other causes of thyrotoxicosis. *Thyroid.* 2016;26(10):1343-1421. PMID: 27521067

10. Siu CW, Pong V, Zhang X, et al. Risk of ischemic stroke after new-onset atrial fibrillation in patients with hyperthyroidism. *Heart Rhythm.* 2009;6(2):169-173. PMID: 19187905

11. Friberg L, Rosenqvist M, Lip GYH. Evaluation of risk stratification schemes for ischaemic stroke and bleeding in 182 678 patients with atrial fibrillation: the Swedish Atrial Fibrillation cohort study. *Eur Heart J.* 2012;33(12):1500-1510. PMID: 22246443

12. Lin YS, Tsai HY, Lin CY, et al. Risk of Thromboembolism in Non-Valvular Atrial Fibrillation With or Without Clinical Hyperthyroidism. *Glob Heart.* 2021;16(1):45. PMID: 34211831

13. Allegretti AS, Czawlytko CL, Stathatos N, Sadow PM. Case 13-2024: a 27-year-old man with leg weakness. *N Engl J Med.* 2024;390(16):1514-1522. PMID: 38657248

14. Garvey LF, Bergmann NC, Worm D, Effraimidis G. Muscle weakness in the extremities in a man with Graves' disease. *Ugeskr Laeger.* 2022;184(18):V12210931. PMID: 35506625

Recommended Reading

- Wiersinga WM, Poppe KG, Effraimidis G. Hyperthyroidism: aetiology, pathogenesis, diagnosis, management, complications, and prognosis. *Lancet Diabetes Endocrinol.* 2023;11(4):282-298. PMID: 36848916

- Kostopoulos G, Effraimidis G. Epidemiology, prognosis, and challenges in the management of hyperthyroidism-related atrial fibrillation. *Eur Thyroid J.* 2024;13(2):e230254. PMID: 38377675

- Vanderpump M. Thyrotoxic periodic paralysis. In: Matfin G, ed. *Endocrine and Metabolic Medical Emergencies: A Clinician's Guide.* John Wiley & Sons Ltd; 2018:296-304.

- Angell TE, Lechner MG, Nguyen CT, Salvato VL, Nicoloff JT, LoPresti JS. Clinical features and hospital outcomes in thyroid storm: a retrospective cohort study. *J Clin Endocrinol Metab.* 2015;100(2):451-459. PMID: 25343237

Update on the Management of Nonhereditary Medullary Thyroid Carcinoma

Rossella Elisei, MD. Endocrine Unit, University Hospital of Pisa and University of Pisa, Pisa, Italy; Email: rossella.elisei@med.unipi.it

Educational Objectives

After reviewing this chapter, learners should be able to:

- Identify patients with sporadic medullary thyroid carcinoma (MTC) early, when the tumor is still intrathyroidal.

- Distinguish sporadic from hereditary forms of MTC by *RET* genetic screening.

- Recommend appropriate follow-up and choose the right drug at the right time in patients with metastatic disease that will be treated with systemic therapy.

Significance of the Clinical Problem

MTC is a well-differentiated thyroid tumor derived from parafollicular or calcitonin-producing C cells. Its neuroendocrine origin makes it a separate entity from other differentiated thyroid carcinomas. MTC is a unique model in that there is both a sporadic form (75%) and a hereditary form (25%). Regardless of whether it is sporadic or hereditary, the biological behavior of MTC is similar, and definitive cure essentially depends on early diagnosis when the tumor is still intrathyroidal.[1] Early diagnosis is achieved by measuring circulating calcitonin at the time of thyroid nodule diagnosis in the setting of sporadic disease[2] and by genetic screening for *RET* pathogenic variants in the case hereditary disease.[3]

The frequency of MTC in the general population is unknown, but it represents approximately 5% of all thyroid tumors and 0.4% to 1.4% of all thyroid nodules. Unlike differentiated thyroid carcinomas that are more common in women, MTC is not associated with a difference in distribution between the 2 sexes. The average age at diagnosis for the sporadic form is in the fourth and fifth decades, whereas the hereditary form has a wider range of age at diagnosis. Only the hereditary form affects children. Generally, the more aggressive the *RET* germline pathogenic variant responsible for the disease, the earlier MTC manifests.

To date, the risk factors that affect MTC development are unknown. However, its pathogenesis is very well understood, and it is due, in most cases, to activation of the *RET* oncogene by a pathogenic variant that constitutively activates the membrane tyrosine kinase receptor.[4] The *RET* pathogenic variant is present at the somatic level in 50% to 60% of sporadic cases and at the germline level in 98% of hereditary cases. The prevalence of *RET* somatic pathogenic variants increases in more aggressive cases. The biological behavior of MTC is less favorable than that of the other well-differentiated thyroid carcinomas, but it is more favorable than that of anaplastic carcinoma. Several series have reported a 10-year survival of approximately 50% in patients with MTC. Cure rate and survival of patients with MTC are positively affected by an early diagnosis.[1]

Practice Gaps

- The diagnosis of MTC is often late, and diagnosis may even occasionally occur after surgery performed for another indication, as serum calcitonin is not always measured in the workup of thyroid nodules.

- It is crucial that clinicians know how to interpret serum calcitonin values, especially when these values are between 20 and 50 pg/mL (5.8-14.6 pmol/L).

- There is a lack of awareness of the relevance of *RET* germline genetic analysis to distinguish sporadic from hereditary forms of MTC.

- Ideally, all patients with MTC at an advanced disease stage at diagnosis should rapidly have genetic testing to assess for the presence of somatic *RET* pathogenic variants.

Discussion

Clinical Presentation and Diagnosis

Sporadic MTC usually manifests as an isolated thyroid nodule or within a multinodular goiter. Except for the presence of diarrhea and/or flushing syndrome (*Figure 1*) (which is, however, rare and usually present only in advanced and metastatic cases), affected patients usually do not have specific symptoms. Neck ultrasonography is unable to identify or suggest the medullary origin of the nodule, and sonographic features of MTC are highly suspicious for malignancy in less than half of cases.[5] Thyroid scintigraphy, if performed, shows a "cold" nodule as is the case for most of thyroid malignancies. Cytologic examination of aspirate material from FNA of the nodule provides a diagnosis of MTC in only 50% of cases.[6] Since 1994, numerous studies have demonstrated that the routine measurement of serum calcitonin is the most accurate diagnostic tool for the correct diagnosis of MTC in patients with thyroid nodules.[7] Nevertheless, routine measurement

of serum calcitonin in all patients with thyroid nodules is still controversial[8] despite evidence that this approach allows for early diagnosis and treatment of MTC, which significantly improves the outcome of this potentially lethal disease.[2]

Figure 1.

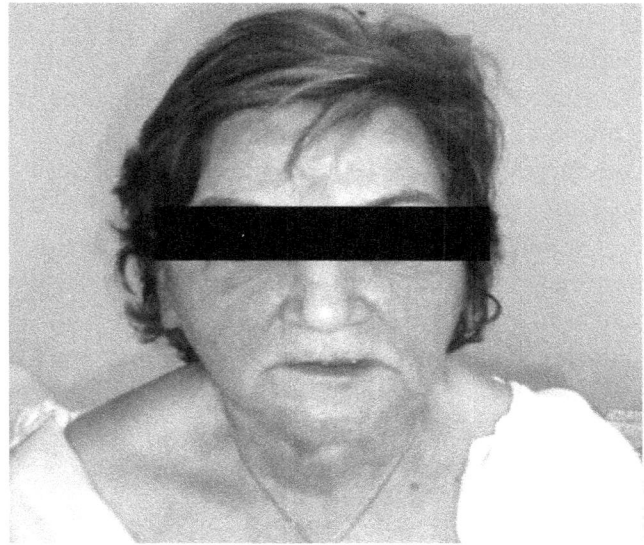

Patient with advanced MTC and flushing syndrome.

[Color—Print (Color Gallery page CG16) or web & ePub editions]

Surgical Treatment

According to current American Thyroid Association guidelines,[9] the elective intervention in the case of a presurgical MTC diagnosis is total thyroidectomy and central lymph node dissection. A bilateral or ipsilateral lateral cervical lymphadenectomy is indicated if neck ultrasonography shows the presence of metastatic lymph nodes. Thus, before the operation, it is necessary to perform accurate ultrasonography of the neck with evaluation of the lateral cervical lymph node compartments.

Recently, the scientific community has begun to consider the possibility of treating some selected patients with lobectomy and removal of the central lymph node hemicompartment.[10] This approach seems to be feasible in patients with sporadic MTC who have a single nodule, mildly elevated calcitonin values, and neck ultrasonography that is negative for extrathyroidal disease extension.

Postoperative Management and Follow-Up

Initial evaluation should be done approximately 3 months after surgery to assess circulating calcitonin and perform neck ultrasonography. The same response to therapy classification that has been applied to differentiated thyroid cancer can be also applied to MTC and used to guide clinical management during follow-up.[11] Patients with an excellent response must be followed for a few years with basal measurement of calcitonin and neck ultrasonography; action is only taken if calcitonin becomes detectable. Patients with biochemically persistent disease have a relatively high risk of developing structural disease over the years (30%-40%).[12] Thus, these patients must be followed with annual biochemical and imaging assessments. If calcitonin values remain stable, there is no need to perform imaging beyond neck ultrasonography. If calcitonin increases and neck ultrasonography does not show significant findings, it is best to perform second-level imaging. In this regard, it is important to remember that for circulating calcitonin values lower than 150 pg/mL (<43.8 pmol/L), it is very unlikely that even very sensitive imaging can identify the metastatic site.[9] Recently, ^{18}F-DOPA has been demonstrated to discover small metastatic lesions not detected by other imaging, indicating that its sensitivity and specificity are much higher (*Figure 2*).[13] Patients with incomplete removal of structural disease must be followed up given the risk that their disease will progress and require other therapies. In these cases, in addition to calcitonin measurement, it is advisable to measure carcinoembryonic antigen (CEA), which, although not specific for MTC, is strongly correlated with the tumor burden. The doubling time of both markers is important.[14]

Figure 2.

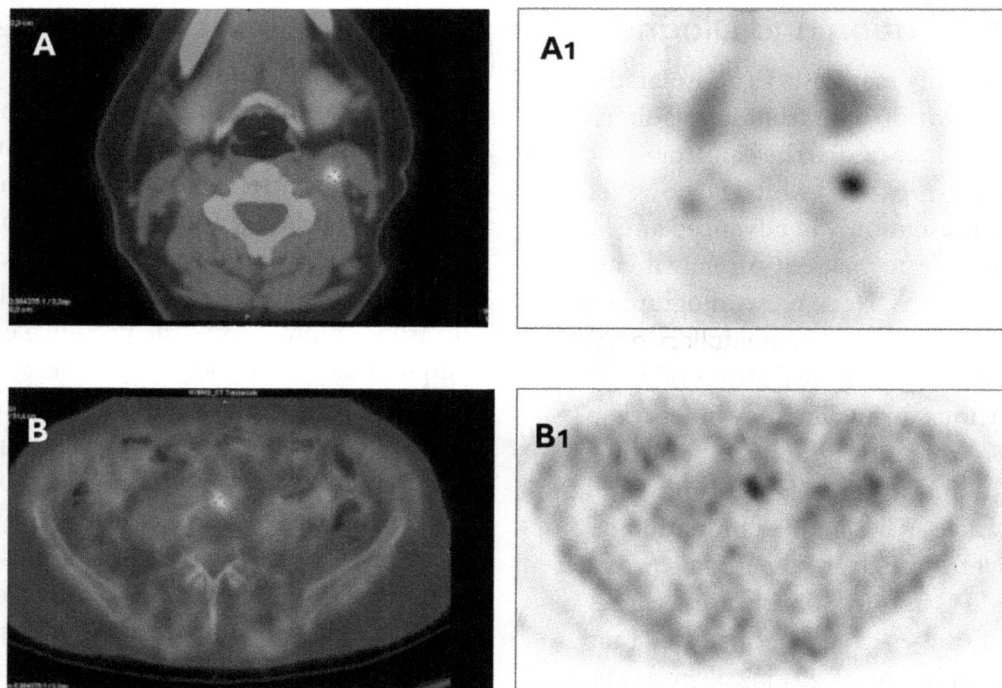

[18]DOPA PET showing a left latero-cervical lymph node (*Panel A*) and lesion in the anterior border of L4 (*Panel B*) and their CT coregistrations (*Panels A1 and B1*). Neither lesion had been previously identified on other imaging.

[Color—Print (Color Gallery page CG16) or web & ePub editions]

Therapies for Advanced and Progressive MTC

Advanced and progressive metastatic MTC can be treated with targeted therapies. The first-line drugs currently available are multikinase inhibitors, such as vandetanib[15] and cabozantinib,[16] and RET-specific inhibitors, such as selpercatinib[17] and pralsetinib.[18] Multikinase inhibitors inhibit various tyrosine kinase receptors involved in tumor cell growth and angiogenesis. They are essentially cytostatic drugs and are therefore able to inhibit tumor growth and stabilize disease, even for a long time. However, they are also strong antiangiogenic drugs, and their main target is the vascular growth factor receptor. Their efficacy has been well demonstrated in 2 international randomized phase 3 clinical trials,[15,16] which show significantly better progression-free survival in patients treated with the drugs than in those receiving placebo. However, because of their antiangiogenic action, the use of both multikinase inhibitors is burdened by numerous and varied adverse effects, which represent the main reason for the reduction or suspension of therapy over time.

The selective RET inhibitors selpercatinib and pralsetinib show great efficacy (*Figure 3*) and low toxicity as demonstrated in phase 1 and 2 clinical trials. Both selpercatinib and pralsetinib are very selective RET inhibitors that act on wild-type *RET*, *RET* fusions, and point variants and are also active against "gatekeeper" variants (eg, V804L, V804M) that induce resistance to vandetanib in in vitro studies.

Based on the results of the phase 1/2 trial, a randomized phase 3 study (LIBRETTO-531) was initiated comparing the efficacy and safety of selpercatinib vs standard therapy (vandetanib/cabozantinib) in the first-line treatment of patients with progressive *RET* variant–associated advanced MTC. Compared with standard therapy, selpercatinib demonstrated greater efficacy and better safety profile, and the drug has been approved in both first- and second-line treatment of advanced and progressive MTC. Manufacturers of pralsetinib subsequently decided to discontinue drug development, so selpercatinib is currently the only specific *RET* inhibitor that can be used in clinical practice.

Genetic Testing in the Era of Precision Therapy

The use of selective *RET* inhibitors in clinical practice raises the issue of genetic analysis; in particular, when and for whom it should be performed. Genetic screening on constitutive DNA is a standard test that must be performed in all patients of MTC, both in those who have hereditary disease and in those who have sporadic disease. Of those with sporadic disease, 7% to 8% of these cases may in fact be hereditary.[19] Still unresolved is the question of whether to perform the search for somatic variants in all sporadic cases or only in selected cases. Given the high frequency of *RET* somatic pathogenic variants in patients with sporadic disease and a worse prognosis,[20] genetic testing for somatic *RET* variants is

Figure 3.

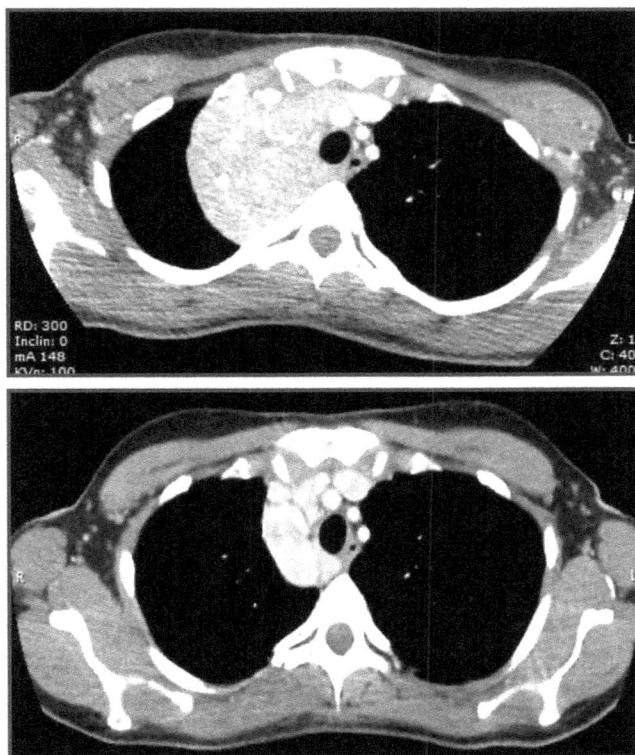

Large hilar lymph node metastasis before (*upper panel*) and 3 months after (*lower panel*) treatment with selpercatinib.

useful in patients with advanced and metastatic disease from the onset and in those patients not definitively cured by surgery who have risk factors for progression.[21]

Clinical Case Vignettes

Case 1

A 35-year-old woman presents for persistently elevated serum calcitonin values (35 pg/mL [10.2 pmol/L]) 3 months after total thyroidectomy. She had a 1-cm thyroid nodule diagnosed 5 years earlier and was followed up over time without further investigations. After 5 years, the nodule had grown to 2.5 cm. On neck ultrasonography, the nodule was isoechoic, had a well-defined border, had no microcalcifications, and, although fundamentally solid, had some anechoic areas. It was classified as EUTIRADS 3, which means low risk of malignancy. Although not fully recommended, FNA was performed because of the increasing volume, and findings on cytological examination were classified as Bethesda III. She chose to undergo total thyroidectomy. Histology showed that the nodule was malignant in nature (MTC), and several perithyroidal lymph nodes were already metastatic.

Which of the following diagnostic tools was missing in the workup of this nodule that could have led to a presurgical diagnosis of MTC and therefore to a more radical and likely curative intervention?

A. A second FNA

B. Elastosonography

C. Measurement of serum calcitonin

D. Thyroid scintigraphy

E. Doppler ultrasonography

Answer: C) Measurement of serum calcitonin

Calcitonin is the most specific and sensitive MTC marker, both before and after thyroidectomy. It is a small polypeptide hormone of 32 amino acids produced almost exclusively by C cells. Ten years after the recognition of MTC as a distinct histological type of thyroid carcinoma, high levels of calcitonin have been demonstrated to be present both in the tumoral tissue and serum of patients with MTC. Elevated basal levels of serum calcitonin, with few exceptions, are diagnostic of MTC. Mildly elevated calcitonin values in the presence of small thyroid nodules should represent an alert for the possibility of MTC, and additional evaluation should be performed, such as a calcium-stimulation test, measurement of calcitonin in the washout of the needle used for the cytology, and immunocytochemistry for calcitonin. If the serum calcitonin values are less than 50 pg/mL (<14.6 pmol/L) and the thyroid nodule is small, follow-up in 6 months could be recommended to ensure a definitive diagnosis.

Routine measurement of serum calcitonin in nodular thyroid diseases allows for preoperative diagnosis of unsuspected sporadic MTC. Calcitonin screening allows for early diagnosis of MTC, usually when the tumor is still at stage 1, thus favoring successful surgical treatment. In this patient's case, it is very likely that if the calcitonin had been measured when the nodule was first identified, even if centimetric, the MTC diagnosis could have been anticipated and the surgery could have been curative. Unfortunately, not all guidelines suggest screening patients with thyroid nodules with serum calcitonin measurement, but it remains undisputed that both ultrasonography and FNA with cytological examination have low sensitivity for finding MTC and may miss the correct diagnosis in many cases.

Case 2

A 47-year-old man with MTC who underwent surgical treatment 3 years ago is concerned because his postoperative calcitonin values have remained elevated in the absence of evidence of structural disease, as assessed by total-body CT. He asks what tests could be done to identify the source of calcitonin production. The calcitonin values, although elevated, have remained mostly stable (~60 pg/mL [17.5 pmol/L]). CEA has also had a similar trend with mean values of 7.5 ng/mL.

Which additional diagnostic tool could be used to look for the source of calcitonin production?

A. Nuclear magnetic resonance

B. ^{18}FDG

C. Bone scintigraphy

D. ^{18}F-DOPA

E. Octreotide scan

Answer: D) ^{18}F-DOPA

About 50% of patients with MTC who have persistently elevated serum levels of either basal or stimulated calcitonin after surgery have no evidence of metastatic disease when assessed with traditional imaging techniques. In the case of "biochemical disease" without evidence of metastatic lesions, the most widely accepted follow-up strategy is "wait and see." Detectable serum calcitonin is in fact compatible with long-term survival, as calcitonin may remain stable with time or slowly increase. The average time after which metastatic disease is detected is about 3 to 4 years. Typically, recurrence is in the neck, but it can also be distant. With very few exceptions, clinical manifestations of the disease correlate with the increase in serum markers (calcitonin and CEA) and, therefore, as long as they remain stable, it is very unlikely that the disease has manifested itself. In this regard, the doubling time of both calcitonin and CEA is very important: the shorter the doubling time, the faster the disease progression. Various studies suggest that if the serum calcitonin concentration is less than 150 pg/mL (<43.8 pmol/L), it is unlikely that second-level imaging techniques can identify the source of calcitonin production. However, ^{18}F-DOPA has shown a higher sensitivity and specificity than all other imaging techniques, especially in cases with detectable calcitonin and CEA values but in a medium-low range. Therefore, in this patient's case, PET ^{18}F-DOPA could be useful, but if findings are normal, no more second-level imaging should be performed unless calcitonin and CEA concentrations rapidly double.

Case 3

Five years after initial diagnosis of MTC, a 62-year-old man presents with progressive metastatic disease at the lung and bone level. The doubling time of calcitonin and CEA is 8 to 9 months, and the dimensional increase of the lung lesions is greater than 20%. These findings, therefore, represent a disease in progression according to the RECIST (Response Evaluation Criteria in Solid Tumors). Systemic therapy is recommended. No information is available regarding the *RET* status of the primary tumor, but the patient is trying to recover the paraffin-embedded tissues at the hospital where he underwent thyroidectomy.

Which of the following drugs would be best to treat this patient now?

A. Vandetanib

B. Cabozantinib

C. Selpercatinib

D. Either vandetanib or cabozantinib

E. Either vandetanib or selpercatinib

Answer: D) Either vandetanib or cabozantinib

Without knowing the molecular profile of the tumor or, in particular, the mutational status of *RET*, it is not possible to prescribe selpercatinib, which is a selective inhibitor of *RET*. To prescribe selpercatinib, one must demonstrate the presence of a *RET* pathogenic variant, either at the somatic or germline level. Therefore, in this patient's case, it would be necessary to start with a multikinase inhibitor, such as vandetanib or cabozantinb.

Recently, a randomized phase 3 study (LIBRETTO-531) comparing the efficacy and safety of selpercatinib vs standard therapy (vandetanib/cabozantinib) in the first-line treatment setting in patients with progressive *RET*-mutated advanced MTC clearly demonstrated higher efficacy and lower toxicity of selpercatinib. A total of 291 patients were included (selpercatinib to vandetanib/cabozantinib ratio of 2:1). At 12 months, the progression-free interval was 86.8% in the selpercatinib group and 65.7% in the control group. The objective response rate was 69.4% in the selpercatinib group and 38.8% in the control group. Adverse events led to dosage reduction in 38.9% of participants in the selpercatinib group and in 77.3% of participants in the control group and led to treatment discontinuation in 4.7% of participants in the selpercatinib group and in 26.8% of participants in the control group. Based on this study, selpercatinib has been approved as first-line treatment (it was already approved as second-line treatment) of advanced and progressive MTC. While selpercatinib represents an important opportunity for patients, its prescription, as already mentioned, requires the presence of a *RET* pathogenic variant. If the patient is able to locate the paraffin-embedded material and molecular analysis demonstrates the presence of a *RET* pathogenic variant, switching from the multikinase inhibitor to selpercatinib could be considered, especially if the patient were experiencing adverse effects during the treatment with the multikinase inhibitor. If, however, a *RET* pathogenic variant is not identified, the patient would continue therapy with the multikinase inhibitor already started. If there is disease progression, the patient could switch to the other multikinase inhibitor.

Therapeutic efficacy of the therapy should initially be monitored every 3 months with measurement of calcitonin and CEA and total-body CT with intravenous contrast medium. Both the medical staff and the patient must pay particular attention to the development of adverse events, so they can be treated immediately to ensure that it does not become so severe that treatment is interrupted. These patients should be followed in tertiary care centers that are experienced in the management of both the drug and the disease.

Key Learning Points

- MTC is a rare thyroid tumor that should be diagnosed as early as possible (when it is still intrathyroidal) for the best chance of complete cure. To diagnose MTC early, serum calcitonin should be measured in all patients with thyroid nodules. Although MTC's frequency is only 1 in 200 to 250 nodules, it has been very well demonstrated that screening is cost-effective.

- MTC can be either sporadic (in most cases) or hereditary. Since some cases appear to be sporadic but are actually hereditary (7%-8% of all sporadic forms), genetic testing for *RET* pathogenic variants should be performed in all newly diagnosed patients.

- Patients with MTC who are not cured completely by surgery but who have no obvious structural disease (ie, "biochemically persistent" disease) should have follow-up based on calcitonin and CEA values and their doubling time. As long as calcitonin levels remain less than 150 pg/mL (<43.8 pmol/L), identifying the source of production is very difficult. Performing ^{18}F-DOPA can be helpful.

- Patients with metastatic and progressive MTC can now be treated with molecularly targeted drugs, such as selpercatinib, which is very effective and has few adverse effects. If the pathogenic variant is not known or if no pathogenic variant is identified, the patient can be treated with 1 of the 2 multikinase inhibitors, vandetanib or cabozantinib.

References

1. Gharib H, McConahey WM, Tiegs RD, et al. Medullary thyroid carcinoma: clinicopathologic features and long-term follow-up of 65 patients treated during 1946 through 1970. *Mayo Clin Proc.* 1992;67(10):934-940, PMID: 1434853

2. Elisei R, Bottici V, Luchetti F, et al. Impact of routine measurement of serum calcitonin on the diagnosis and outcome of medullary thyroid cancer: experience in 10,864 patients with nodular thyroid disorders. *J Clin Endocrinol Metab.* 2004;89:163-168. PMID: 14715844

3. Wells SA Jr, Baylin SB, Leight GS, Dale JK, Dilley WG, Farndon JR. The importance of early diagnosis in patients with hereditary medullary thyroid carcinoma. *Ann Surg.* 1982;195(5):595-599. PMID: 7073356

4. Mulligan LM, Kwok JB, Healey CS, et al. Germ-line mutations of the RET proto-oncogene in multiple endocrine neoplasia type 2A. *Nature*. 1993;363(6428):458-460. PMID: 8099202

5. Matrone A, Gambale C, Biagini M, Prete A, Vitti P. Ultrasound features and risk stratification systems to identify medullary thyroid carcinoma. *Eur J Endocrinol*. 2021;185(2):193-200. PMID: 34010144

6. Essig GF Jr, Porter K, Schneider D, et al. Fine needle aspiration and medullary thyroid carcinoma: the risk of inadequate preoperative evaluation and initial surgery when relying upon FNAB cytology alone. *Endocr Pract*. 2013;19:920-927. PMID: 23757627

7. Pacini F, Fontanelli M, Fugazzola L, et al. Routine measurement of serum calcitonin in nodular thyroid diseases allows the preoperative diagnosis of unsuspected sporadic medullary thyroid carcinoma. *J Clin Endocrinol Metab*. 1994;78(4):826-829. PMID: 8157706

8. Deftos LJ. Should serum calcitonin be routinely measured in patients with thyroid nodules--will the law answer before endocrinologists do? *J Clin Endocrinol Metab*. 2004;89(9):4768-4769. PMID: 15356093

9. Wells SA Jr, Asa SL, Dralle H, et al; American Thyroid Association Guidelines Task Force on Medullary Thyroid Carcinoma. Revised American Thyroid Association guidelines for the management of medullary thyroid carcinoma. *Thyroid*. 2015;25(6):567-610. PMID: 25810047

10. Liang W, Shi J, Zhang H, et al: Total thyroidectomy vs thyroid lobectomy for localized medullary thyroid cancer in adults: a propensity-matched survival analysis. *Surgery*. 2022;172(5):1385-1391.PMID: 35995619

11. Tuttle RM, Ganly I. Risk stratification in medullary thyroid cancer: moving beyond static anatomic staging. *Oral Oncol*. 2013;49(7):695-701. PMID: 23601563

12. Prete A, Gambale C, Torregrossa L, et al. Clinical evolution of sporadic medullary thyroid carcinoma with biochemical incomplete response after initial treatment. *J Clin Endocrinol Metab*. 2013;108(8):e613-e622. PMID: 36722192

13. Beheshti M, Pocher S, Vali R, et al. The value of 18F-DOPA PET-CT in patients with medullary thyroid carcinoma: comparison with 18F-FDG PET-CT. *Eur Radiol*. 2009;19(6):1425-1434. PMID: 19156423

14. Laure Giraudet A, Al Ghulzan A, Auperin A, et al. Progression of medullary thyroid carcinoma: assessment with calcitonin and carcinoembryonic antigen doubling times. *Eur J Endocrinol*. 2008;158(2):239-246. PMID: 18230832

15. Wells SA, Jr., Robinson BG, Gagel RF, et al. Vandetanib in patients with locally advanced or metastatic medullary thyroid cancer: a randomized, double-blind phase III trial. *J Clin Oncol*. 2012;30(2):134-141. PMID: 22025146

16. Elisei R, Schlumberger MJ, Muller SP, et al. Cabozantinib in progressive medullary thyroid cancer. *J Clin Oncol*. 2013;31(29):3639-3646. PMID: 24002501

17. Hadoux J, Elisei R, Brose MS, et al; LIBRETTO-531 Trial Investigators. Phase 3 trial of selpercatinib in advanced RET-mutant medullary thyroid cancer. *N Engl J Med*. 2023;389(20):1851-1861. PMID: 37870969

18. Subbiah V, Hu MI, Wirth LJ, et al. Pralsetinib for patients with advanced or metastatic RET-altered thyroid cancer (ARROW): a multi-cohort, open-label, registrational, phase 1/2 study. *Lancet Diabetes Endocrinol*. 2021;9(8):491-501. PMID: 34118198

19. Romei C, Cosci B, Renzini G, et al. RET genetic screening of sporadic medullary thyroid cancer (MTC) allows the preclinical diagnosis of unsuspected gene carriers and the identification of a relevant percentage of hidden familial MTC (FMTC). *Clin Endocrinol (Oxf)*. 2011;74(2):241-247. PMID: 21054478

20. Elisei R, Cosci B, Romei C, et al. Prognostic significance of somatic RET oncogene mutations in sporadic medullary thyroid cancer: a 10-year follow-up study. *J Clin Endocrinol Metab*. 2008;93(3):682-687. PMID: 18073307

21. Matrone A, Prete A, Gambale C, et al. Timing and ideal patient for an appropriate search for somatic *RET* mutation in medullary thyroid cancer. *JCO Precis Oncol*. 2024;8:e2400017. PMID: 38709990

Oncocytic Thyroid Cancer

Ian Ganly, MD, MS, PhD. Department of Head and Neck Surgery, Memorial Sloan Kettering Cancer Center, New York, NY; Email: ganlyi@mskcc.org

Educational Objectives

After reviewing this chapter, learners should be able to:

- Describe the unique molecular, clinicopathologic, and genetic characteristics that differentiate oncocytic thyroid cancer (OTC) from other thyroid malignancies, including its classification as a distinct clinical entity by the World Health Organization.

- Identify the clinical features, preoperative investigations, and limitations in diagnosing OTC, including its typical presentation, imaging modalities, and cytological challenges.

- Analyze the current management options, including surgical approaches, systemic therapies, and the challenges posed by poor iodine avidity, while understanding the prognostic factors influencing disease-specific survival and recurrence.

Significance of the Clinical Problem

OTC, formerly known as Hürthle cell carcinoma, represents a rare but distinct type of thyroid malignancy. In recent years, the World Health Organization reclassified OTC as a separate clinical entity due to its unique molecular and clinicopathologic features.[1] Previously grouped with follicular thyroid carcinoma (FTC), OTC exhibits distinct genetic profiles, biological behavior, and clinical outcomes that necessitate tailored management strategies. This differentiation underscores the growing recognition of its specific pathologic and molecular hallmarks that set it apart from other differentiated thyroid cancers (DTCs).[2,3]

Despite accounting for only about 5% of all thyroid cancers, OTC poses significant clinical challenges due to its aggressive potential and relatively poor iodine avidity, which limits the efficacy of traditional radioactive iodine (RAI) therapy. The disease predominantly affects older individuals and can present with both locoregional and distant metastases, often at a more advanced stage compared with other DTCs.[4-8] These characteristics, coupled with the scarcity of specific epidemiologic and clinical data, highlight the need for a deeper understanding of OTC to optimize its diagnosis, treatment, and prognosis. This review synthesizes current literature on the molecular underpinnings, pathologic classifications, and clinical management of OTC.

Practice Gaps

- There is limited preoperative diagnostic accuracy for OTC. FNA cannot reliably distinguish between benign and malignant oncocytic thyroid neoplasms, as the diagnosis of OTC requires confirmation of capsular and/or vascular invasion. Additionally, current molecular testing methods, while improved, still face challenges in distinguishing benign from malignant oncocytic tumors. This diagnostic uncertainty complicates preoperative planning and management strategies.

- There is a lack of tailored treatment guidelines for OTC. Despite its distinct molecular profile, clinical behavior, and poor iodine avidity, OTC is often managed using the same guidelines as other DTCs. This approach fails to account for its unique characteristics, such as its limited response to RAI therapy and differences in surgical and systemic treatment efficacy.

- There are insufficient clinical trial data specific to OTC. Most clinical trials group OTC with other DTCs, leading to a lack of specific evidence regarding treatment efficacy for OTC. As a result, current systemic treatment options, including tyrosine kinase inhibitors, are extrapolated from broader DTC data and are limited by substantial adverse effects and suboptimal outcomes. Dedicated research is critically needed to inform evidence-based management of advanced and metastatic OTC.

Discussion

OTC is a distinct entity, previously classified under FTC, that is now recognized separately due to unique molecular, histopathologic, and clinical characteristics.[1-3]

Figure 1.

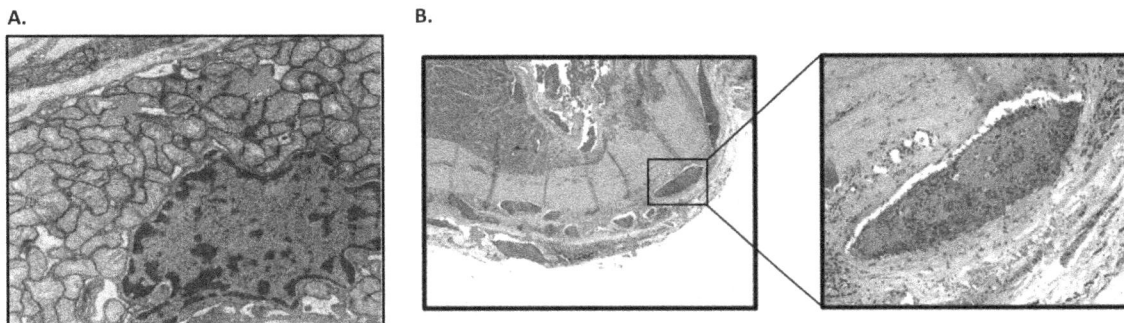

Panel A, Electron microscopy showing nucleus of cell surrounded by abundant mitochondria. Panel B, Hematoxylin and eosin slide showing vascular invasion in vessels surrounding a widely invasive OTC.

[Color—Print (Color Gallery page CG17) or web & ePub editions]

Figure 2.

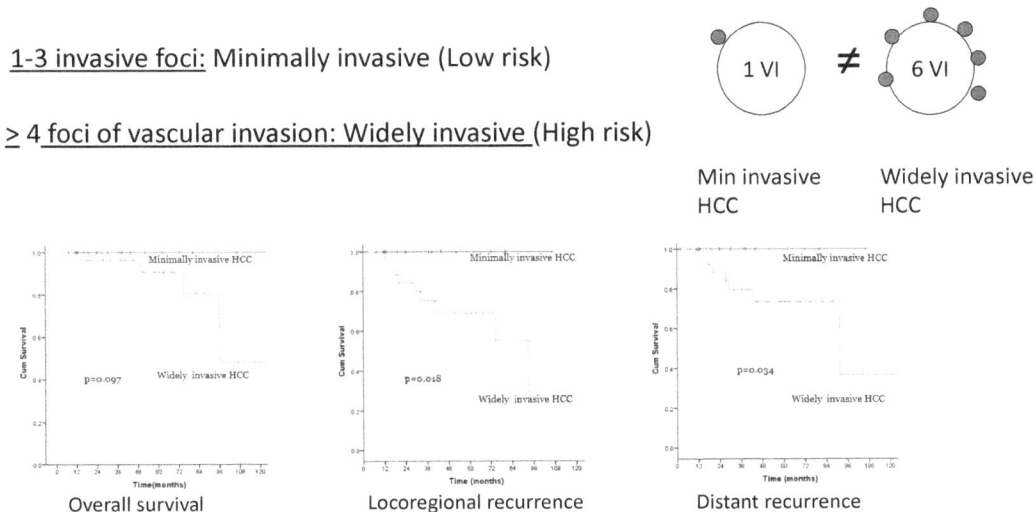

1-3 invasive foci: Minimally invasive (Low risk)

> 4 foci of vascular invasion: Widely invasive (High risk)

Overall survival   Locoregional recurrence   Distant recurrence

Panel A, Classification of OTC into minimally invasive and widely invasive by extent of vascular invasion. Panel B, Outcomes stratified by extent of vascular invasion showing poorer outcome with widely invasive carcinoma.

[Color—Print (Color Gallery page CG17) or web & ePub editions]

Gene	PTC	FTC	HCC
TERT promoter	9	18	22
ERCC5	0	0	13
EIF1AX	2	18	11
ERBB2	0	0	11
NRAS	8	21	9
NF1	1	4	9
HLA-A	0	0	9
TSC1/2	1	0	7
TP53	1	10	7
ALKBH7	0	0	7
FAT1	0	0	7
NBPF1	0	0	7
CREBBP	0	1	5
ATM	1	1	5
XPC	0	0	5
KRAS	1	4	4
HRAS	4	7	2
BRAF	62	2	0
RET fusions	7	0	0
PPARγ Fusions	1	27	0
PIK3CA	1	6	0

Table based on following manuscripts [2, 10-13]

Pathologic and Clinical Features

OTC consists of at least 75% oncocytic cells, characterized by eosinophilic granular cytoplasm due to mitochondrial proliferation (*Figure 1A, preceding page*). Malignancy is determined by capsular or vascular invasion (*Figure 1B, preceding page*). OTC was previously classified by extent of vascular invasion as widely invasive (>4 foci) and minimally invasive (<4 foci) (*Figure 2A, preceding page*). Biological behavior is determined by the extent of vascular invasion (*Figure 2B, preceding page*). The 2022 World Health Organization classification refines OTC into 3 prognostic subtypes.[9] Unlike FTC, OTC requires histological examination for diagnosis, as FNA alone is insufficient.

Clinically, OTC often presents at an advanced stage, spreading via hematogenous or lymphatic routes. Compared with FTC, OTC has a higher frequency of vascular invasion, increasing recurrence risk.[9]

Molecular Basis of OTC

OTC has a distinct genetic profile, differing from papillary thyroid carcinoma (PTC) and FTC (*Table*).[2,3,10-13] Whole-exome sequencing has identified pathogenic variants in *EIF1AX, MADCAM1, OR4L1, ATXN1, UBXN11, NRAS*, and other genes. Unlike FTC and PTC, OTC rarely harbors *BRAF, NRAS, HRAS, KRAS, PIK3CA*, or *RET* pathogenic variants or *PAX8-PPARG* fusions.

OTC is characterized by a high somatic mutational burden affecting the RAS/RAF/MAPK and PIK3CA/AKT/mTOR pathways (*Figure 3, following page*).

We identified *RTK* pathogenic variants (*ERBB2* in 11%), *RAS* pathogenic variants (15%), and tumor suppressor gene pathogenic variants in *NF1* (9%), *PTEN* (4%), and *TSC1/2* (6%). Chromosomal amplifications in *RICTOR* and *BRAF* contribute to oncogenesis. *EIF1AX* (11%) and *EIF3B* (overexpressed due to chromosome 7 duplication) influence translation dysregulation. OTC exhibits mitochondrial DNA pathogenic variants, including large deletions affecting the electron transport system (*Figure 4, following page*).[2,3] These variants disrupt oxidative phosphorylation, increasing reactive oxygen species and shifting metabolism to aerobic glycolysis (*Figure 5, following pages*).[14]

Metabolite quantification (*Figure 6, following pages*) confirms this metabolic shift.[15] This explains why OTCs are hypermetabolic on PET scans (*Figure 7, following pages*).

A unique OTC feature is genomic chromosomal loss of heterozygosity leading to chromosomal instability.[2,3] OTC has 3 phenotypes: diploid (minimally invasive), haploid, and polysomic (aggressive). Fluorescent in situ hybridization illustrates haploid and polysomic OTC (*Figure 8A and 8B, following pages*). Chromosome 7 preservation, housing

Figure 3.

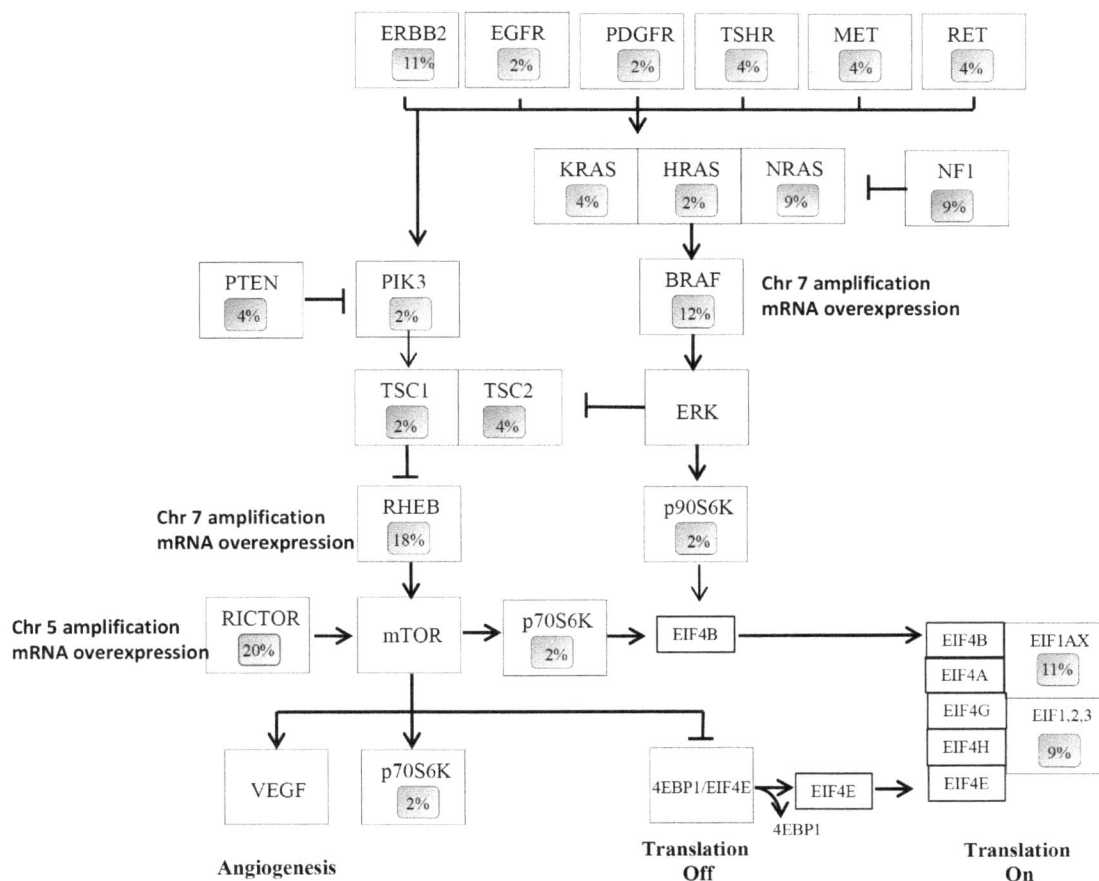

RTK/PIK3/RAS Pathway showing alterations in 60% of cancers

[Color—Print (Color Gallery page CG18) or web & ePub editions]

Figure 4.

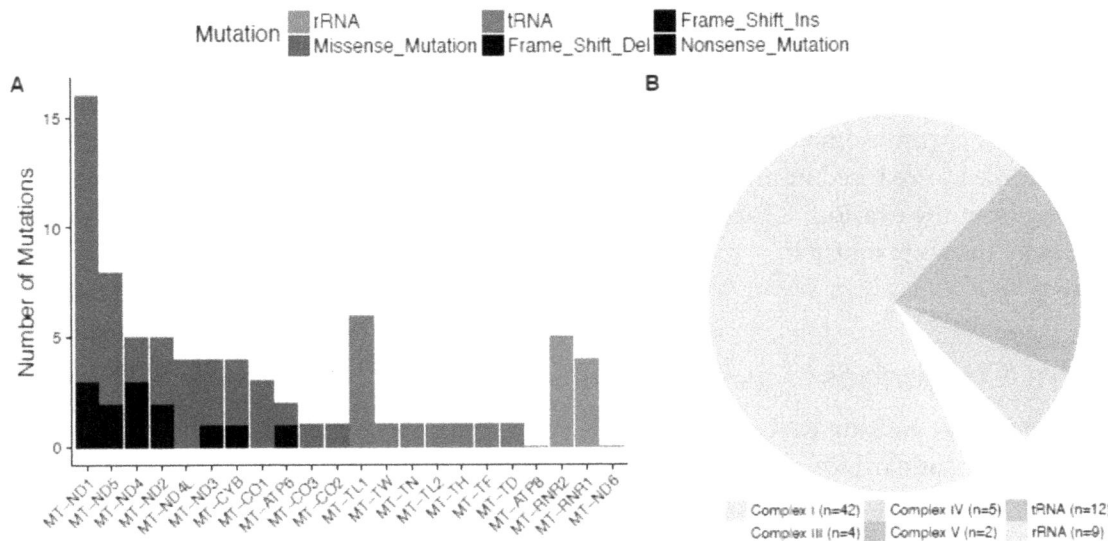

Panel A, Types of mitochondrial pathogenic variants observed in 56 OTCs.[2] Panel B, Mitochondrial variants categorized by electron transport complexes.

[Color—Print (Color Gallery page CG18) or web & ePub editions]

Figure 5.

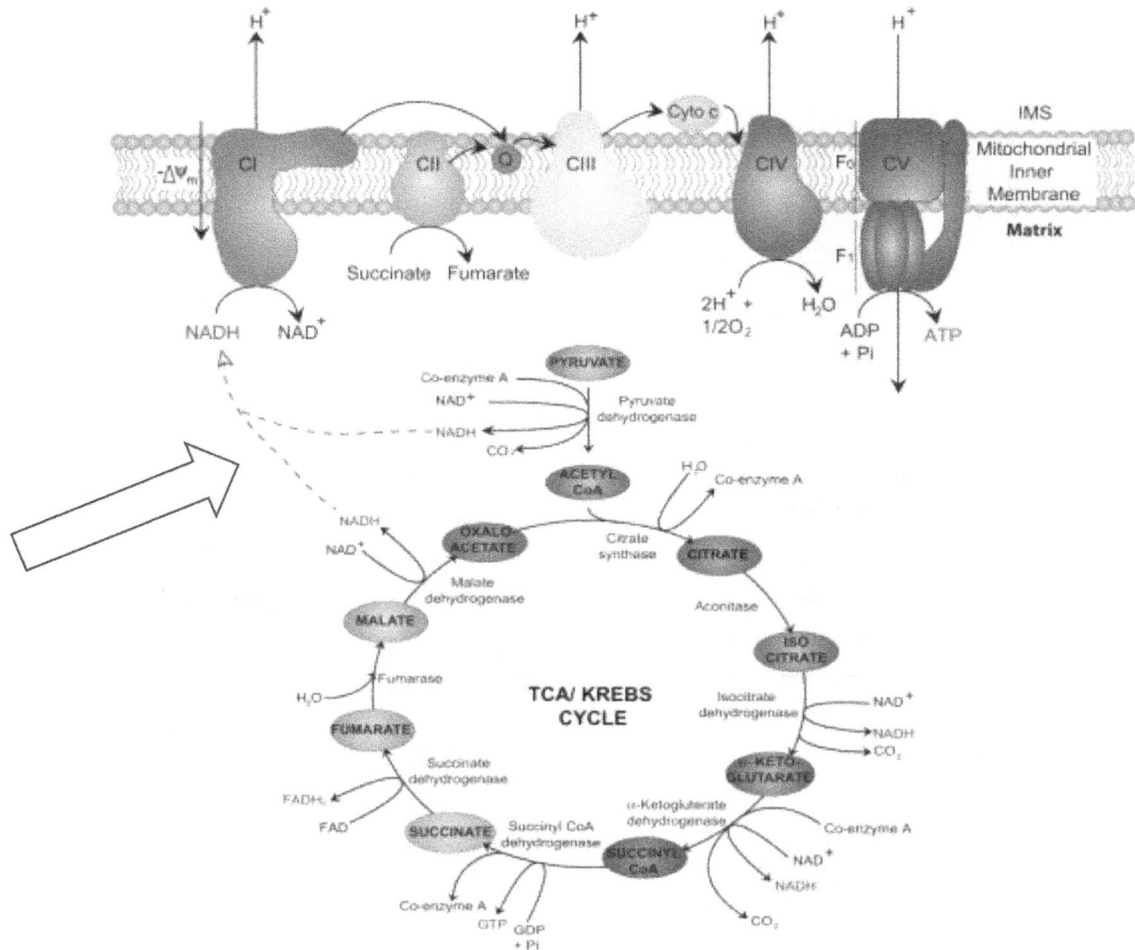

Electron transport chain showing interaction of complexes with Krebs cycle. The arrow indicates complex I is the first site of electron transport chain. Pathogenic variants in complex I disrupt electron transport chain, which in turn disrupts the TCA cycle.

[Color—Print (Color Gallery page CG19) or web & ePub editions]

key oncogenes *EGFR* and *BRAF*, may drive progression. Genomic chromosomal loss of heterozygosity is linked to reduced immune infiltration, aiding immune evasion.[16] Targeting the mTOR pathway shows promise in preclinical studies.[17]

Management Challenges

OTC is iodine-refractory, limiting RAI efficacy.[18] Total thyroidectomy is standard for advanced cases, while lobectomy suffices for minimally invasive tumors. Lymph node dissection is performed if metastases are present. Even when RAI uptake is detected, responses are rare. PET/

CT is preferred over whole-body iodine scans. Systemic therapy options are limited. Tyrosine kinase inhibitors (TKIs), such as sorafenib and lenvatinib, improve progression-free survival (DECISION, SELECT trials),[19,20] but overall survival benefits remain unclear. Ongoing trials targeting mTOR and immune checkpoints (nivolumab, ipilimumab) offer potential.[21,22] The ALLIANCE study showed improved survival with sorafenib and everolimus (*Figure 9, following pages*).[23]

Figure 6.

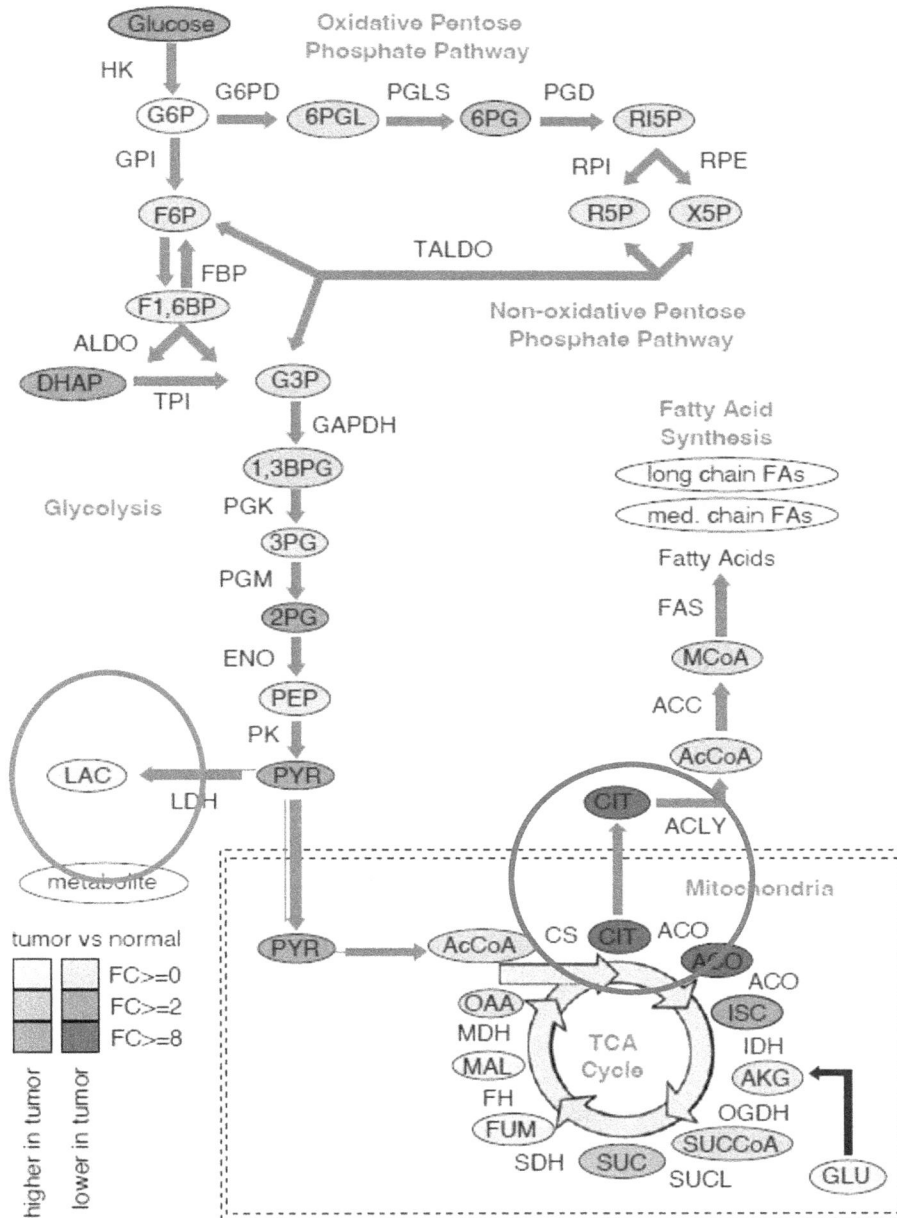

Metabolic alterations in 40 OTCs. Metabolites with less abundance to normal are shown in blue and those greater than normal are shown in red. The blue circle indicates the large decrease in citrate in the TCA cycle. The red circle indicates the increase in lactate due to increased aerobic glycolysis.

[Color—Print (Color Gallery page CG20) or web & ePub editions]

Prognosis and Future Directions

Prognosis varies based on invasiveness. Minimally invasive OTC has a 10-year disease-specific survival of ~100%, compared with ~70% for widely invasive cases. Iodine refractoriness in recurrent or metastatic OTC necessitates new therapies. OTC's distinct molecular and clinical features demand tailored management strategies. Advances in molecular characterization and targeted therapies offer hope for improved outcomes. Future research should focus on refining diagnostics and developing effective systemic treatments.

Figure 7.

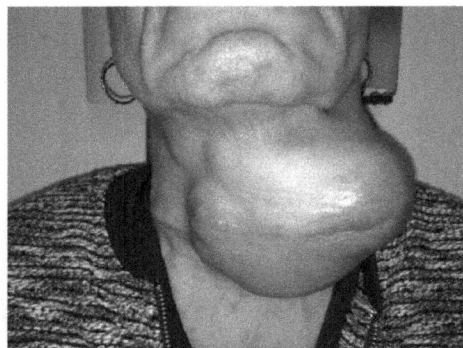

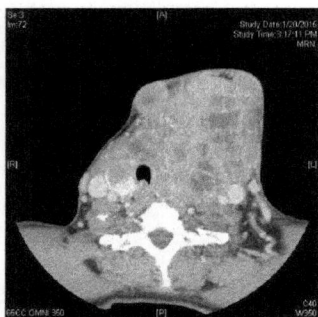
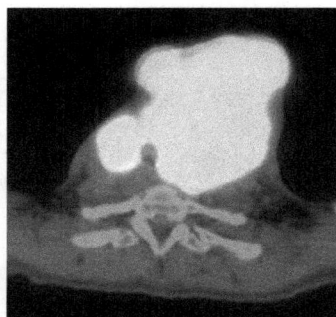
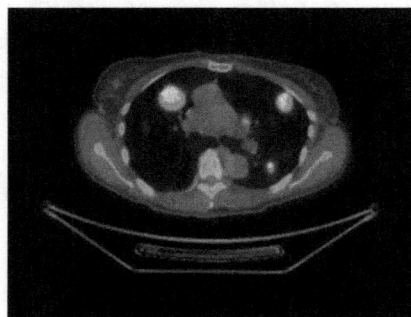

CT neck   PET/CT neck   PET/CT lung metastases

OTCs are hypermetabolic on FDG PET due to increased aerobic glycolysis. Imaging shows a large left thyroid lobe mass on CT and PET. The patient has multiple hypermetabolic lung metastases.

[Color—Print (Color Gallery page CG21) or web & ePub editions]

Figure 8.

A.

Haploid phenotype

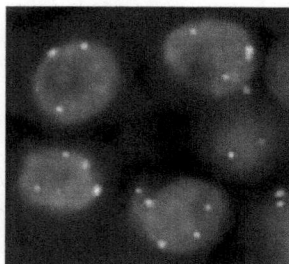

Chr 2 haploid (1 copy arrowed)
Chr 5 diploid
Chr 7 diploid

B.

Polysomic phenotype

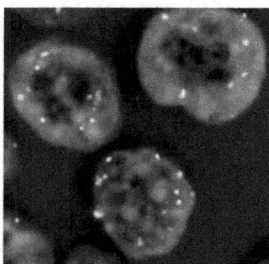

Chr 2 diploid
Chr 5 WCD (4 copies per cell)
Chr 7 WCD (>4 copies per cell)

∘chr2   chr5   ∘chr7

C.

➡ Global LOH

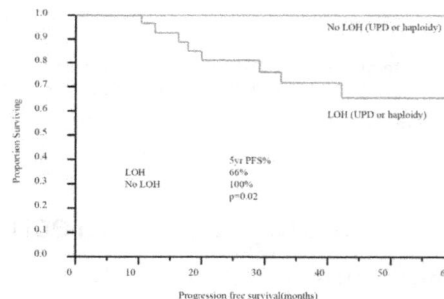

Panel A, Fluorescent in situ hybridization (FISH) staining of a haploid cancer showing 1 copy of chromosome 2 and 2 copies of chromosome 5 and 7. Panel B, FISH staining of a polysomic cancer showing 2 copies of chromosome 2 and 4 copies of chromosome 5 and 7. Panel C, Loss of chromosomes results in a global loss of heterozygosity (LOH). Cancers with global LOH have a poorer outcome as shown by the Kaplan Meier plot.

[Color—Print (Color Gallery page CG21) or web & ePub editions]

Figure 9.

A.

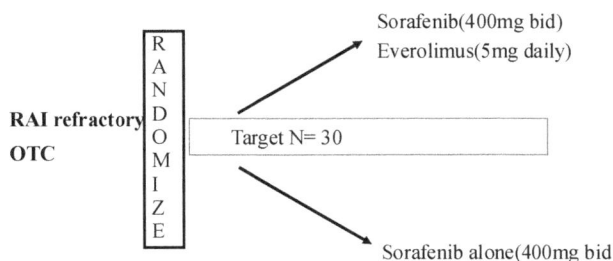

B.

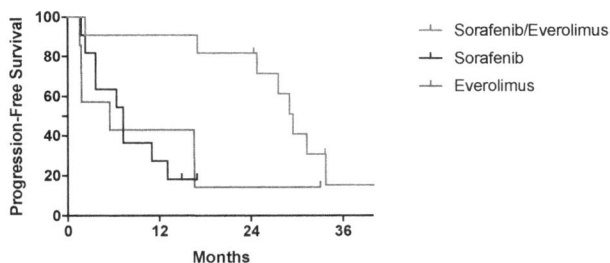

Panel A, Clinical phase 2 trial of patients with RAI-refractory OTC randomly assigning patients to sorafenib alone vs sorafenib/everolimus. Panel B, Patients treated with sorafenib/everolimus had increased progression-free survival.

[Color—Print (Color Gallery page CG22) or web & ePub editions]

Clinical Case Vignettes

Case 1

A 67-year-old woman with no notable medical history is referred for evaluation of a 2.8-cm thyroid nodule incidentally discovered during routine carotid ultrasonography. Physical examination reveals a palpable, nontender thyroid nodule without cervical lymphadenopathy. Thyroid ultrasonography shows an encapsulated 3-cm thyroid nodule with increased vascularity. There are no nodules in the contralateral lobe. There are no suspicious lymph nodes. FNA cytology is consistent with an oncocytic follicular neoplasm (Bethesda IV). A sample is sent for Thyroseq testing.

Which of the following best characterizes the differential diagnosis?

A. Oncocytic adenoma or oncocytic carcinoma

B. Follicular adenoma or follicular carcinoma

C. Papillary thyroid carcinoma

D. Follicular adenoma or oncocytic adenoma

E. Follicular adenoma, oncocytic adenoma, oncocytic carcinoma, or follicular carcinoma

Answer: E) Follicular adenoma, oncocytic adenoma, oncocytic carcinoma, or follicular carcinoma

Both benign and malignant oncocytic neoplasms could be reported as oncocytic follicular neoplasms. Oncocytic cells can also be present in follicular adenomas and carcinomas.

Case 1, Continued

If this were an oncocytic neoplasm, what would be the expected results with Thyroseq?

A. V600E *BRAF* positive

B. PPARG-PARP fusion positive

C. Amplification of chromosome 1q

D. Widespread copy-number alterations with amplification of chromosomes 5, 7, 12, 20

E. No pathogenic variants or copy-number alterations

Answer: D) Widespread copy-number alterations with amplification of chromosomes 5, 7, 12, 20

Oncocytic neoplasms can display distinct copy-number alterations characterized by amplification of chromosomes 5, 7, 12, and 20 and uniparental disomy of remaining chromosomes. These alterations are most pronounced in aggressive forms of oncocytic cancers, but they can also occur in more indolent forms. If copy-number alterations are absent, oncocytic neoplasms may have pathogenic variants in *NRAS*, *EIF1AX*, *PTEN*, *TSC1*, *TSC2*, and *mTOR*. *BRAF* pathogenic variants do not occur in OTC. Similarly, *PPARG-PARP* fusions occur in follicular neoplasms but not in oncocytic neoplasms.

Case 1, Continued

Diagnostic lobectomy is performed, and histopathology reveals a minimally invasive OTC with capsular invasion but no vascular invasion.

Which of the following treatments should be offered now?

A. None

B. Completion thyroidectomy

C. Completion thyroidectomy with ipsilateral central neck dissection

D. Completion thyroidectomy with ipsilateral central neck dissection and RAI

E. Completion thyroidectomy with bilateral central neck dissection and RAI

Answer: A) None

Given the absence of high-risk features, completion thyroidectomy is not indicated. Minimally invasive oncocytic carcinomas rarely metastasize to lymph nodes. This patient was monitored with periodic neck ultrasonography and serum thyroglobulin measurement, which remained undetectable over 3 years of follow-up.

Case 2

A 72-year-old man presents with a 3-month history of progressive dysphagia and hoarseness. Ultrasonography reveals a 5.5-cm hypoechoic left thyroid mass with extrathyroidal extension and suspicious cervical lymph nodes. Flexible laryngoscopy shows a paralyzed left vocal cord. FNA cytology suggests an oncocytic neoplasm, and subsequent core biopsy confirms widely invasive OTC with vascular invasion. Molecular testing reveals *TERT* and *mTOR* pathogenic variants, as well as widespread copy-number alterations of chromosomes 5, 7, 12, and 20.

Which of the following radiological tests should be done now?

A. PET and detailed ultrasound lymph node mapping of the neck

B. PET and contrast CT of the neck

C. Contrast CT of the neck

D. Contrast CT of the neck and chest

E. None

Answer: B) PET and contrast CT of the neck

Oncocytic neoplasms are very FDG-avid due to an extreme Warburg effect with a shift in metabolism from the Krebs cycle to aerobic glycolysis. Therefore, PET is a very effective method of detecting regional and distant metastatic spread. The presence of vocal cord paralysis and extrathyroidal extension on ultrasonography suggest invasion of the left recurrent laryngeal nerve, as well as possible involvement of the trachea and esophagus. A detailed contrast neck CT is required to evaluate the degree of extrathyroidal extension in this patient. PET is not sufficient to give this level of detail. Neck CT will also give more anatomical detail of regional lymph node spread and relationship to carotid artery and internal jugular vein. Thus, the best additional imaging for this patient is PET and contrast CT of the neck (Answer B).

Case 2, Continued

Imaging shows a large vascular left thyroid mass but no invasion of the trachea or esophagus. Multiple lymph nodes are present in the ipsilateral central neck, as well as in levels 2, 3, and 4 of the lateral neck. PET shows several small hypermetabolic subcentimeter pulmonary nodules suggestive of metastatic disease.

Which of the following treatments should be recommended now?

A. None; the patient should now be on palliative care

B. High-dose RAI

C. Surgery with left thyroid lobectomy and central and lateral neck dissection; observation of pulmonary metastases

D. Surgery with total thyroidectomy and central and lateral neck dissection; treatment of pulmonary metastases with lenvatinib

E. Lenvatinib alone

Answer: C) Surgery with left thyroid lobectomy and central and lateral neck dissection; observation of pulmonary metastases

As in all types of locally advanced thyroid cancer, the initial goal is to control the central neck to prevent airway compromise and asphyxiation. The presence of left vocal cord paralysis indicates extrathyroidal extension to the recurrent laryngeal nerve. Left thyroid lobectomy (Answer C) with central neck dissection would help control the central neck. Removal of lateral neck nodes can be done in the same operation. Total thyroidectomy is not required since widely invasive OTC are not RAI-avid. This also reduces the chance of any inadvertent injury to the contralateral right recurrent laryngeal nerve. The presence of multiple subcentimeter FDG-avid pulmonary nodules is not an indication for treatment at this stage. As in other forms of thyroid cancer, an initial period of observation with serial chest CT should be done to assess nodule growth. Distant metastatic disease can be treated with a tyrosine kinase inhibitor such as lenvatinib, which has strong VEGF inhibitor activity.

Case 2, Continued

Observation of the pulmonary nodules over 12 months shows rapid growth in both lungs. The patient also develops subcutaneous FDG-avid nodules in the operated neck 6 months after surgery.

Which of the following treatments should be offered now?

A. None; the patient should be on palliative care

B. Lenvatinib alone

C. Lenvatinib and everolimus

D. Everolimus alone

E. Lenvatinib and pembrolizumab

Answer: C) Lenvatinib and everolimus

The clinical and radiological findings show widespread distant metastases. OTCs, which are widely invasive, can recur as subcutaneous tumor deposits due to vascular and lymphatic permeation of the soft tissues. Metastases to lung and bone are common. Genomic analysis has shown upregulation of the mTOR pathway in 60% of widely invasive OTCs.[2] A randomized phase 2 trial has shown increased efficacy and prolonged progression-free survival with sorafenib in combination with the mTOR inhibitor everolimus.[23] There are no data to suggest that OTCs are sensitive to immune checkpoint inhibitor therapy. Recent research shows OTCs are immune-depleted tumors with increased immunosuppression in the more aggressive forms of OTC. Therefore, the use of immunotherapy alone is unlikely to have any activity. Thus, the best recommendation for this patient is lenvatinib and everolimus (Answer C).

Case 3

A 55-year-old woman undergoes total thyroidectomy for a presumed benign multinodular goiter. Pathology unexpectedly reveals a 5-cm, widely invasive OTC with vascular invasion.

Which of the following histological features are diagnostic of widely invasive OTC?

A. Abundant eosinophilic granular cytoplasm, encapsulated neoplasm, presence of vascular invasion (2 foci)

B. Abundant eosinophilic granular cytoplasm, encapsulated neoplasm, and presence of vascular invasion (5 foci)

C. Abundant eosinophilic granular cytoplasm, presence of vascular invasion (2 foci), extrathyroidal extension

D. Abundant eosinophilic granular cytoplasm, presence of vascular invasion (5 foci), extrathyroidal extension

E. Encapsulated neoplasm, presence of vascular invasion (5 foci)

Answer: D) Abundant eosinophilic granular cytoplasm, presence of vascular invasion (5 foci), extrathyroidal extension

Oncocytic neoplasms have granular eosinophilic cytoplasm due to the presence of 1000s of abnormal mitochondria. OTCs show invasion of the capsule +/- vascular invasion. The presence of fewer than 4 foci of vascular invasion occurs in encapsulated angioinvasive OTC. The presence of more than 4 foci with extrathyroidal extension occurs in the most aggressive OTC (widely invasive OTC) (Answer D).

Case 3, Continued

Postoperative ultrasonography shows no obvious metastatic lymph nodes.

Which of the following is the best way to manage the central neck and lateral neck?

A. Ipsilateral central neck dissection

B. Bilateral central neck dissection

C. Ipsilateral central neck dissection and ipsilateral lateral neck dissection

D. Bilateral central and lateral neck dissection

E. Observation

Answer: E) Observation

Metastatic spread of cancer to regional lymph nodes rarely occurs in minimally invasive OTC. However, it does occur in the more aggressive forms of OTC, particularly widely invasive cancers with extrathyroidal extension and vascular invasion. If present on lymph node mapping on ultrasonography or on contrast neck CT, regional lymph node dissection should be done of all involved lymph node levels.

Case 3, Continued

Should postoperative RAI treatment be given?

A. No because the postoperative thyroglobulin is undetectable

B. No because widely invasive OTCs are not RAI-avid

C. Yes; give low-dose 30 mCi since thyroglobulin is undetectable

D. Yes; give 100 mCi since thyroglobulin is detectable

E. Yes because it helps to reduce the incidence of distant metastases

Answer: B) No because widely invasive OTCs are not RAI-avid

As OTCs become more aggressive, they lose expression of the thyroid differentiation genes, including the sodium-iodide symporter gene (*NIS*). As a result, the widely invasive forms of OTC are not RAI-avid (Answer B). This is in contrast to minimally invasive OTC, which retains expression of the *NIS* gene and are RAI-avid. There is no evidence to suggest that RAI reduces the risk of distant metastases.

Key Learning Points

- OTC, formerly treated as a subtype of FTC, has been recognized by the World Health Organization as a distinct thyroid malignancy due to its unique molecular and clinicopathologic features. This change reflects advances in understanding OTC's genetic basis and distinct clinical behavior.

- OTC exhibits a unique genomic profile, including pathogenic variants in the genes involved in the RAS/RAF/MAPK and PIK/AKT/MTOR pathways and in genes controlling telomere elongation. Additionally, mitochondrial DNA pathogenic variants and genomic chromosomal loss of heterozygosity are hallmarks, with implications for tumor progression and therapeutic resistance.

- OTC typically presents at more advanced stages than other DTCs and is associated with worse survival outcomes. Diagnosis is challenging due to the inability of FNA to confirm capsular/vascular invasion. Furthermore, OTC is often iodine-refractory, limiting the efficacy of standard RAI therapy and necessitating alternative treatment strategies.

- Prognosis varies widely based on histopathologic features, with minimally invasive OTC showing excellent outcomes and widely invasive cases associated with significantly worse survival. Emerging therapies, such as mTOR inhibitors and combination systemic treatments, show promise in managing advanced or metastatic OTC but are constrained by limited data and substantial adverse effects.

References

1. Baloch ZW, Asa SL, Barletta JA, et al. Overview of the 2022 WHO classification of thyroid neoplasms. *Endocr Pathol.* 2022;33(1):27-63. PMID: 35288841

2. Ganly I, Makarov V, Deraje S, et al. Integrated genomic analysis of Hürthle cell cancer reveals oncogenic drivers, recurrent mitochondrial mutations, and unique chromosomal landscapes. *Cancer Cell.* 2018;34(2):256-70.e5. PMID: 30107176

3. Gopal RK, Kübler K, Calvo SE, et al. Widespread chromosomal losses and mitochondrial DNA alterations as genetic drivers in Hürthle cell carcinoma. *Cancer Cell.* 2018;34(2):242-55.e5. PMID: 30107175

4. Máximo V, Lima J, Prazeres H, Soares P, Sobrinho-Simões M. The biology and the genetics of Hürthle cell tumors of the thyroid. *Endocr Relat Cancer.* 2016;23(12):X2. PMID: 27807063

5. Ghossein RA, Hiltzik DH, Carlson DL, et al. Prognostic factors of recurrence in encapsulated Hurthle cell carcinoma of the thyroid gland: a clinicopathologic study of 50 cases. *Cancer.* 2006;106(8):1669-1676. PMID: 16534796

6. Shaha AR, Shah JP, Loree TR. Patterns of nodal and distant metastasis based on histologic varieties in differentiated carcinoma of the thyroid. *Am J Surg.* 1996;172(6):692-694. PMID: 8988680

7. Grossman RF, Clark OH. Hurthle cell carcinoma. *Cancer Control.* 1997;4(1):13-17. PMID: 10762998.

8. Lopez-Penabad L, Chiu AC, Hoff AO, et al. Prognostic factors in patients with Hurthle cell neoplasms of the thyroid. *Cancer.* 2003;97(5):1186-1194. PMID: 12599224.

9. Matsuura D, Yuan A, Wang LY, et al. Follicular and Hurthle cell carcinoma: comparison of clinicopathological features and clinical outcomes. *Thyroid.* 2022. PMID: 35078345

10. Cancer Genome Atlas Research Network. Integrated genomic characterization of papillary thyroid carcinoma. *Cell.* 2014;159(3):676-690. PMID: 25417114

11. Park H, Shin HC, Yang H, et al. Molecular classification of follicular thyroid carcinoma based on TERT promoter mutations. *Mod Pathol.* 2022;35(2):186-192. PMID: 34497362

12. Marques AR, Espadinha C, Catarino AL, et al. Expression of PAX8-PPAR gamma 1 rearrangements in both follicular thyroid carcinomas and adenomas. *J Clin Endocrinol Metab.* 2002;87(8):3947-3952. PMID: 12161538

13. Nikiforova MN, Lynch RA, Biddinger PW, et al. RAS point mutations and PAX8-PPAR gamma rearrangement in thyroid tumors: evidence for distinct molecular pathways in thyroid follicular carcinoma. *J Clin Endocrinol Metab.* 2003;88(5):2318-2326. PMID: 12727991

14. Frank AR, Li V, Shelton SD, et al. Mitochondrial-encoded complex I impairment induces a targetable dependency on aerobic fermentation in Hurthle cell carcinoma of the thyroid. *Cancer Discov.* 2023;13(8):1884-1903. PMID: 37262072

15. Ganly I, Liu EM, Kuo F, et al. Mitonuclear genotype remodels the metabolic and microenvironmental landscape of Hürthle cell carcinoma. *Sci Adv.* 2022;8(25):eabn9699. PMID: 35731870

16. Ganly I, Kuo F, Makarov V, et al. Characterizing the immune microenvironment and neoantigen landscape of Hürthle cell carcinoma to identify potential immunologic vulnerabilities. *Cancer Res Commun.* 2023;3(7):1409-1422. PMID: 37529400

17. Dong Y, Gong Y, Kuo F, et al. Targeting the mTOR pathway in Hurthle cell carcinoma results in potent antitumor activity. *Mol Cancer Ther.* 2022;21(2):382-394. PMID: 34789562

18. Bischoff LA, Ganly I, Fugazzola L, et al. Molecular alterations and comprehensive clinical management of oncocytic thyroid carcinoma: a review and multidisciplinary 2023 update. *JAMA Otolaryngol Head Neck Surg.* 2024;150(3):265-272. PMID: 38206595

19. Brose MS, Robinson B, Sherman SI, et al. Cabozantinib for radioiodine-refractory differentiated thyroid cancer (COSMIC-311): a randomised, double-blind, placebo-controlled, phase 3 trial. *Lancet Oncol.* 2021;22(8):1126-1138. PMID: 34237250

20. Brose MS, Nutting CM, Jarzab B, et al; DECISION investigators. Sorafenib in radioactive iodine-refractory, locally advanced or metastatic differentiated thyroid cancer: a randomised, double-blind, phase 3 trial. *Lancet.* 2014;384(9940):319-328. PMID: 24768112

21. Lorch JH, Barletta JB, Nehs M, et al. A phase II study of nivolumab (N) plus ipilimumab (I) in radioiodine refractory differentiated thyroid cancer (RAIR DTC) with exploratory cohorts in anaplastic (ATC) and medullary thyroid cancer (MTC). *J Clin Oncol.* 2020;38(15):6513-6513.

22. Sherman EJ, Dunn LA, Ho AL, et al. Phase 2 study evaluating the combination of sorafenib and temsirolimus in the treatment of radioactive iodine-refractory thyroid cancer. *Cancer.* 2017;123(21):4114-4121. PMID: 28662274

23. Sherman EJ, Foster NR, Su YB, et al. Randomized phase II study of sorafenib with or without everolimus in patients with radioactive iodine refractory Hurthle cell thyroid cancer. *J Clin Oncol.* 2021;39(15):6076-6076.

Special Diets for Thyroid Health: Fact or Fiction?

Angela M. Leung, MD, MSc. Division of Endocrinology, Diabetes, and Metabolism, Department of Medicine, University of California Los Angeles David Geffen School of Medicine, Veterans Affairs Greater Los Angeles Healthcare System, Los Angeles, California; Email: amleung@mednet.ucla.edu

Educational Objectives

After reviewing this chapter, learners should be able to:

- Describe the current understanding of trace mineral supplements use, thyroid autoimmunity, and thyroid dysfunction risk.

- Define the effects of various popular diets on thyroid autoimmunity and thyroid dysfunction.

- Summarize the associations between dietary patterns, risk of malignant thyroid nodules, and thyroid cancer behavior.

Significance of the Clinical Problem

Dietary supplements and restricted diets have become increasingly popular in recent years, with 52% of the US general adult population reporting use of a supplement in 2011-2012[1] and 17.1% of US adults 20 years or older reporting adherence to a specific diet in 2015-2018.[2] In particular, dietary supplements and dietary interventions aimed at improving thyroid health are becoming increasingly popular. Patients may be taking supplements or adhering to special diets, possibly in combination with prescribed thyroid or antithyroid medications, in an effort to maintain or decrease thyroid autoimmunity, preserve normal thyroid function, or mitigate the risks of thyroid nodules and thyroid cancer. A greater understanding of the benefits, potential harms, and uncertainties of various nonprescription supplements and diets is important when caring for patients with thyroid disease.

Practice Gaps

- There is a need for physicians to become more familiar with the literature addressing nonprescription supplements and diets that patients may be taking in an effort to improve or maintain normal thyroid health.

- Increased recognition of popular supplements and diets touted for thyroid health is an important component of shared decision-making between patients and clinicians.

- Discussion of the data gaps regarding the thyroidal benefits and potential harms of dietary supplements and interventions is an important component of managing thyroid issues.

Discussion

Dietary Supplements Commonly Used to Improve Thyroid Health

Autoimmune thyroid disease, also termed Hashimoto thyroiditis or chronic lymphocytic thyroiditis, and defined as the presence of serum thyroid autoantibodies, affects approximately 15% of individuals.[3] It is more common in persons with other autoimmune conditions, such as celiac disease, vitiligo, type 1 diabetes, and pernicious anemia. Women with thyroid autoimmunity have an approximately 2% per year risk of hypothyroidism compared with individuals without thyroid-antibody positivity.[4] It is not uncommon for patients with Hashimoto thyroiditis to inquire how they may mitigate the risk of developing hypothyroidism. Many supplements in this setting have been studied, including iodine, selenium, iron, magnesium, vitamin D, vitamin B_{12}, and others.

Iodine is a micronutrient required for thyroid hormone production that comes from dietary sources (eg, iodized salt and other foods) and iodine-containing supplements. Adequate iodine intake is particularly important in women during the preconception period, pregnancy, and the postpartum period because of the increased thyroid hormone requirements of the developing fetus during gestation. The World Health Organization recommends 150 mcg iodine daily in nonpregnant, nonlactating adults and 250 mcg iodine daily in pregnant women.[5] To help achieve this, pregnant women who may have risk of insufficient dietary iodine (ie, if they are following a restricted diet) should be advised to take a daily iodine supplement containing 150 mcg.[6,7] Patients should also be educated about the risk of thyroid dysfunction in the setting of iodine excess and advised to avoid supplements containing more than 500 mcg iodine.[8]

Special Diets Commonly Used to Improve Thyroid Health

There is increasing recognition that the composition of intestinal microbiota is related to health and disease, with some evidence suggesting that its alteration (ie, intestinal dysbiosis), bacterial overgrowth, and increased intestinal permeability may favor the development of thyroid autoimmunity.[9] Thus, the concept of addressing "leaky gut syndrome" has been proposed, in which diets that eliminate certain foods or food groups is thought to alter the risk of Hashimoto thyroiditis and potentially hypothyroidism. Elimination diets that omit or reduce gluten, lactose, dairy, grains,

and other items (including calories) have been studied for their effects on the thyroid. The data unfortunately remain sparse, and there are no consistent data supporting that such any specific type of elimination diets significantly reduces the risk of thyroid autoimmunity.[10]

Finally, there is some evidence suggesting that overweight and obesity may be independent risk factors for cancer development. Mechanisms underlying the higher risk of malignancy may be related to an inflamed white adipose tissue microenvironment, in which elevated insulin and IGF-1 can activate the PI3K/Akt/mTOR and Ras/Raf/MAPK pathways that stimulate tumor growth.[11] Although leptin is best understood as a signal of satiety, it can also stimulate TSH, and thus potentially represent a thyroidal growth factor.[12] In the United States, analysis of the NIH-AARP Diet and Health Study dataset suggests that higher BMI is a risk factor for both low- and high-risk thyroid cancers.[13] These findings are consistent with an animal study showing that mice fed a high-fat diet had higher mortality, larger thyroid tumors, and more histologic anaplastic changes compared with those fed a low-fat diet.[14] There is general understanding that a healthy, balanced diet rich in fruits and vegetables, whole grains, and lean proteins may diminish cancer risk. A survey study reported an inverse association between self-report of a Mediterranean-based diet and sonographically suspicious thyroid nodules,[15] while a large multicenter European study reported that consuming inflammatory foods was weakly positive for differentiated thyroid cancer risk.[16]

Clinical Case Vignettes
Case 1

A 32-year-old woman has a 10-year history of Hashimoto thyroiditis. Celiac disease was diagnosed 5 years ago, and she has since been strictly adherent to a gluten-free diet. She takes no medications. Her mother has hypothyroidism associated with Hashimoto thyroiditis and is taking levothyroxine, 100 mcg once daily. The patient is interested in learning about supplements she could take to reduce her risk of, or at least delay, developing hypothyroidism. She would like to avoid the need for future thyroid hormone replacement.

Which of the following is the best advice to provide this patient?

A. Start selenium, 200 mcg by mouth once daily

B. Start ferrous sulfate, 325 mg by mouth once daily

C. Start magnesium, 250 mg by mouth once daily

D. Start vitamin D, 25 mcg (1000 units) by mouth once daily

E. Measure TSH measurement if she develops any signs or symptoms of thyroid dysfunction

Answer: E) Measure TSH measurement if she develops any signs or symptoms of thyroid dysfunction

This patient has 2 autoimmune conditions: Hashimoto thyroiditis and celiac disease. She is thus at risk for developing additional autoimmune conditions. The diagnosis of Hashimoto thyroiditis confers an up to 2% per year added risk of developing hypothyroidism, compared with risk of individuals who do not have thyroid-antibody positivity.[4] Patients with Hashimoto thyroiditis often inquire how they may mitigate the risk of developing hypothyroidism.

Selenium (Answer A) is thought to have antiinflammatory properties that may protect against oxidative damage important for general health, and some selenoproteins (eg, glutathione peroxidase and iodothyronine deiodinases) have crucial roles in thyroid hormone metabolism. The US recommended daily allowance of selenium is 55 mcg daily in nonpregnant, nonlactating adults, with a tolerable upper limit set at 400 mcg daily.[6] Selenium-rich foods include seafood, organ meats, and mushrooms, with lower amounts found in breads, grains, meat, poultry, fish, and eggs. Although there are limited data showing that selenium supplementation (200 mcg daily) in small prospective cohorts of short duration (3-6 months) may decrease TPO-antibody and/or thyroglobulin-antibody levels, there is no known effect on thyroid function.[17,18] These negative findings thus do not support routine selenium supplementation for the purpose of improving thyroid health, outside of its selected use in some individuals with Graves ophthalmopathy.[19] This patient could be counseled that although sparse data suggest selenium supplementation may decrease some aspects of thyroid autoimmunity in the short term, its long-term benefits of altering the risk of thyroid dysfunction remain unknown, and it would not be recommended for this purpose (Answer A).

Iron is an important component of the thyroid synthesis pathway, as the heme-containing enzyme TPO is critical for thyroid hormone production, and deiodinase activity is altered in iron deficiency.[20] However, the evidence for an adverse thyroid impact resulting from iron deficiency is limited, and associations between iron deficiency, serum TPO-antibody and thyroglobulin-antibody positivity, higher TSH levels, and lower free T_4 levels are inconsistent.[21] As such, the thyroidal benefits of iron supplementation (Answer B) are not clear, and its routine use is not currently recommended for the purpose of supporting thyroid health.

Magnesium (Answer C) is thought have antiinflammatory properties, and low serum magnesium levels have been associated with markers of thyroid autoimmunity and an increased risk of hypothyroidism.[10] One Chinese study reported an up to 5-fold risk of hypothyroidism with severe magnesium deficiency, and limited data also show high magnesium levels may improve Graves disease.[10] However, supporting evidence is inconsistent, and thus routine magnesium supplementation is not recommended for its potential thyroid benefits.

Vitamin D (Answer D) has important roles in cell proliferation, differentiation, and immunomodulation, and limited data suggest that compared with healthy individuals, persons with Hashimoto thyroiditis have increased cytokines secreted by proinflammatory Th1 and Th17 cells (IFN-gamma and IL-17).[22] However, the specific benefit of vitamin D supplementation to alter thyroid autoimmunity remains unclear, and it is thus not recommended.

This patient may be advised that although she has a slightly higher risk of developing hypothyroidism[4] compared with individuals who do not have Hashimoto thyroiditis (and potentially an even higher risk given that she has coexisting celiac disease),[23] the benefit of supplements to mitigate this risk is unknown and they are not recommended. Serum TSH should be measured if she develops signs or symptoms of thyroid dysfunction (Answer E).

Case 2

A 49-year-old woman with no relevant medical history is seen for weight gain that she has noticed over the past 4 years. She reports that maintaining a normal weight is a constant struggle, despite adhering to healthy, low-fat, low-carbohydrate diet and a regular exercise regimen. She has heard about the connection between a "leaky gut" and autoimmune thyroid disease, which she is interested in preventing. Her serum TSH concentration is normal (1.4 mIU/L), and she has undetectable TPO antibodies. Her height is 62 in (157.5 cm), and weight is 130 lb (60.0 kg) (BMI = 23.8 kg/m^2).

Which of the following is the best advice to provide this patient?

A. Eliminate gluten from her diet

B. Reduce dietary intake by 500 calories per day

C. Avoid lactose-rich foods

D. Eat a paleo-style diet (ie, avoid grains and dairy products)

E. Reassure her that she has a normal BMI and recommend routine monitoring

Answer: E) Reassure her that she has a normal BMI and recommend routine monitoring

Obesity is a worsening epidemic, with approximately 42% of all US adults meeting criteria for obesity in 2016 (projected to increase to 50% by 2030).[24] The relationships between energy expenditure, metabolism, and the thyroid gland are complex. Only scarce evidence supports a predictable pattern of weight changes in the setting of thyroid dysfunction.[25] Compared with individuals who do not have thyroid-antibody positivity, women with thyroid autoimmunity have an up to 2% per year additional risk of developing hypothyroidism.[4] The risk of hypothyroidism may be independently associated with markers of obesity, such as waist circumference.[26]

Autoimmune thyroid disease commonly coexists with other autoimmune conditions. A systematic literature review and meta-analysis showed a greater than 3-fold risk of thyroid disease in persons with celiac disease. Mechanisms explaining the potential overlap between thyroid and celiac disease are not fully understood, but shared genetic factors are likely. HLA DQ2 and DQ8 are weakly associated with Hashimoto thyroiditis, and the haplotypes are overexpressed in celiac disease.[23] Furthermore, CTLA-4 is associated with both autoimmune thyroid and celiac disease.[23] A small, prospective, blinded interventional study showed that selenium supplementation given for 3 months significantly decreased serum TPO-antibody concentrations, but not thyroglobulin antibodies, compared with a placebo group.[17]

In summary, there are no consistent data demonstrating that adoption of a specific type of elimination diet is useful in this setting. The omission of gluten (Answer A), lactose (Answer C), and grains and dairy (Answer D) has not shown sustained benefits in individuals with autoimmune thyroid disease. Additionally, calorie reduction (Answer B) may be helpful in maintaining a net neutral energy balance depending on her level of daily physical activity, but it is not expected to, by itself, decrease her risk of developing autoimmune thyroid disease. This patient should be counseled that her weight is characterized as normal according to BMI definitions and routine screening with annual BMI assessment is recommended (Answer E).

Case 3

A 69-year-old man with no relevant medical history was diagnosed with papillary thyroid cancer 1 year ago. Surgical pathology was consistent with low-risk disease, and he was counseled that there is an estimated 5% risk of disease recurrence. He takes levothyroxine, 125 mcg once daily, and a multivitamin. His height is 70 in (177.8 cm), and weight is 168 lb (76.2 kg) (BMI = 24.1 kg/m^2). He is interested in learning about foods and dietary patterns that may be helpful in decreasing his risk of thyroid cancer recurrence.

Which of the following is the best advice to provide this patient?

A. Maintain a normal BMI through diet and exercise

B. Start a Mediterranean-based diet

C. Minimize intake of sugary foods

D. Avoid consuming cruciferous vegetables

E. Start a ketogenic high-fat, low-carbohydrate diet

Answer: A) Maintain a normal BMI through diet and exercise

The best advice is to encourage this patient to maintain a normal BMI through diet and exercise (Answer A), as there are some data showing a higher risk of malignancies among individuals with overweight or obesity due to the adverse metabolic and tumoral effects of an inflamed white adipose tissue microenvironment.[11] Evidence supporting that a specific diet, such as Mediterranean (Answer B), low-sugar (Answer C), or ketogenic (Answer E), confers a significantly decreased thyroid cancer risk is extremely limited or absent. Cruciferous vegetables (Answer D) (ie, those belonging to the *Brassica* genus) contain goitrogenic compounds that decrease the availability of iodine to the thyroid and thereby may pose a risk of hypothyroidism in individuals who ingest high amounts. However, consumption of cruciferous vegetables is not known to be associated with thyroid cancer, and in fact, may even decrease malignancy risk due to their antioxidant properties.

Key Learning Points

- Although thyroid autoimmunity is associated with an approximately 2% per year increased risk of developing hypothyroidism, the potential long-term benefits of various supplements, including iron, magnesium, and vitamin D, in altering thyroid autoimmunity and thyroid function remain unknown, and supplements are not recommended for this purpose.

- In small prospective cohorts of short duration, selenium supplementation has been shown to decrease TPO-antibody and/or thyroglobulin-antibody levels, but there are no effects on thyroid function. Current data do not support routine selenium supplementation for the prevention of thyroid dysfunction.

- The gut microbiome is important in health and disease. However, there are no consistent data that elimination diets (including the omission or reduction of gluten, lactose, dairy, grains, and caloric intake) significantly and durably reduce the risk of thyroid autoimmunity.

- Maintaining a normal BMI should be advised because overweight and obesity are independent risk factors for the development of some cancers, including thyroid cancer.

References

1. Kantor ED, Rehm CD, Du M, White E, Giovannucci EL. Trends in dietary supplement use among US adults trom 1999-2012. *JAMA.* 2016;316(14):1464-1474. PMID: 27727382

2. Stierman B, Ansai N, Mishra S, Hales C. Special diets among adults: United States, 2015-2018. NCHS Data Brief, no 389 Hyattsville, MD: National Center for Health Statistics. 2020.

3. Hollowell JG, Staehling NW, Hannon WH, et al. Iodine nutrition in the United States. Trends and public health implications: iodine excretion data from National Health and Nutrition Examination Surveys I and III (1971-1974 and 1988-1994). *J Clin Endocrinol Metab.* 1998;83(10):3401-3408. PMID: 9768638

4. Prummel MF, Wiersinga WM. Thyroid peroxidase autoantibodies in euthyroid subjects. *Best Pract Res Clin Endocrinol Metab.* 2005;19(1):1-15. PMID: 15826919

5. World Health Organization (WHO), United Nations International Children's Emergency Fund (UNICEF), and International Council for the Control of Iodine Deficiency Disorders (ICCIDD). Assessment of the iodine deficiency disorders and monitoring their elimination. Geneva: World Health Organization; 2007. Report No.: WHO/NHD/01.1.

6. Food and Nutrition Board, U.S. Institute of Medicine. Dietary reference intakes. National Academy Press; 2006: 320.

7. Alexander EK, Pearce EN, Brent GA, et al. 2017 Guidelines of the American Thyroid Association for the diagnosis and management of thyroid disease during pregnancy and the postpartum. *Thyroid.* 2017;27(3):315-389. PMID: 28056690

8. Sohn SY, Inoue K, Rhee CM, Leung AM. Risks of iodine excess. *Endocr Rev.* 2024;45(6):858-879. PMID: 38870258

9. Cayres LCF, de Salis LVV, Rodrigues GSP, et al. Detection of alterations in the gut microbiota and intestinal permeability in patients with Hashimoto thyroiditis. *Front Immunol.* 2021;12:579140. PMID: 33746942

10. Larsen D, Singh S, Brito M. Thyroid, diet, and alternative approaches. *J Clin Endocrinol Metab.* 2022;107(11):2973-2981. PMID: 35952387

11. Iyengar NM, Gucalp A, Dannenberg AJ, Hudis CA. Obesity and cancer mechanisms: tumor microenvironment and inflammation. *J Clin Oncol.* 2016;34(35):4270-4276. PMID: 27903155

12. Flier JS, Harris M, Hollenberg AN. Leptin, nutrition, and the thyroid: the why, the wherefore, and the wiring. *J Clin Invest.* 2000;105(7):859-861. PMID: 10749565

13. La Greca A, Grau L, Arbet J, et al. Anthropometric, dietary, and lifestyle factors and risk of advanced thyroid cancer: the NIH-AARP diet and health cohort study. *Clin Endocrinol (Oxf).* 2023;99(6):586-597. PMID: 37694684

14. Kim WG, Park JW, Willingham MC, Cheng SY. Diet-induced obesity increases tumor growth and promotes anaplastic change in thyroid cancer in a mouse model. *Endocrinology.* 2013;154(8):2936-2947. PMID: 23748362

15. Barrea L, Muscogiuri G, de Alteriis G, et al. Adherence to the Mediterranean diet as a modifiable risk factor for thyroid nodular disease and thyroid cancer: results from a pilot study. *Front Nutr.* 2022;9:944200. PMID: 35782938

16. Lecuyer L, Laouali N, Dossus L, et al. Inflammatory potential of the diet and association with risk of differentiated thyroid cancer in the European Prospective Investigation into Cancer and Nutrition (EPIC) cohort. *Eur J Nutr.* 2022;61(7):3625-3635. PMID: 35635567

17. Gartner R, Gasnier BC, Dietrich JW, Krebs B, Angstwurm MW. Selenium supplementation in patients with autoimmune thyroiditis decreases thyroid peroxidase antibodies concentrations. *J Clin Endocrinol Metab.* 2002;87(4):1687-1691. PMID: 11932302

18. Negro R, Formoso G, Mangieri T, Pezzarossa A, Dazzi D, Hassan H. Levothyroxine treatment in euthyroid pregnant women with autoimmune thyroid disease: effects on obstetrical complications. *J Clin Endocrinol Metab.* 2006;91(7):2587-2591. PMID: 16621910

19. Burch HB, Perros P, Bednarczuk T, et al. Management of thyroid eye disease: a consensus statement by the American Thyroid Association and the European Thyroid Association. *Thyroid.* 2022;32(12):1439-1470. PMID: 36480280

20. Beard JL, Brigham DE, Kelley SK, Green MH. Plasma thyroid hormone kinetics are altered in iron-deficient rats. *J Nutr.* 1998;128(8):1401-1408. PMID: 9687562

21. Garofalo V, Condorelli RA, Cannarella R, Aversa A, Calogero AE, La Vignera S. Relationship between iron deficiency and thyroid function: a systematic review and meta-analysis. *Nutrients.* 2023;15(22):4790. PMID: 38004184

22. Mikulska AA, Karazniewicz-Lada M, Filipowicz D, Ruchala M, Glowka FK. Metabolic characteristics of Hashimoto's thyroiditis patients and the role of microelements and diet in the disease management-an overview. *Int J Mol Sci.* 2022;23(12):6580. PMID: 35743024

23. Sun X, Lu L, Yang R, Li Y, Shan L, Wang Y. Increased incidence of thyroid disease in patients with celiac disease: a systematic review and meta-analysis. *PLoS One.* 2016;11(12):e0168708. PMID: 28030626

24. Ward ZJ, Bleich SN, Cradock AL, et al. Projected U.S. state-level prevalence of adult obesity and severe obesity. *N Engl J Med.* 2019;381(25):2440-2450. PMID: 31851800

25. Roa Duenas OH, Xu Y, Ikram MA, Peeters RP, Visser E, Chaker L. Thyroid function and anthropometric measures: a systematic review and meta-analysis. *Endocr Pract.* 2025;31(2):198-207. PMID: 39631665

26. Wen X, Mao Y, Li Z, Chen G, Zhou S. Association between weight-adjusted waist index and Hashimoto's thyroiditis: insights from NHANES 2007-2012. *Front Nutr.* 2024;11:1520440. PMID: 39834468

The Unhappy Patient With Hypothyroidism

Marco Medici, MD, PhD, MSc. Erasmus Medical Center, Rotterdam, Netherlands; Email: m.medici@erasmusmc.nl

Maria Papaleontiou, MD. Division of Metabolism, Endocrinology, and Diabetes, University of Michigan, Ann Arbor, MI; Email: mpapaleo@med.umich.edu

Educational Objectives

After reviewing this chapter, learners should be able to:

- Describe the prevalence and potential causes of persistent symptoms despite biochemical euthyroidism in levothyroxine (LT4)-treated patients with hypothyroidism.

- Describe the evidence regarding LT4/liothyronine (LT3) combination therapy and desiccated thyroid extract (DTE) use in patients with hypothyroidism who have persistent symptoms.

- Discuss the utility of addressing patient requests to assess unconventional clinical thyroid parameters (eg, reverse T_3) or genetic variants.

Significance of the Clinical Problem

Hypothyroidism has a prevalence of 3% to 8% in the general population, with thyroid autoimmunity being the cause for most patients. Hypothyroidism increases the risk of cardiovascular, metabolic, depressive, and anxiety disorders if it remains untreated.[1] Since the 1970s, synthetic LT4 has been the standard of care for thyroid hormone replacement in patients with hypothyroidism. This is because LT4 is cheap, has a long half-life allowing for once-daily dosing, and results in stable serum levels of thyroid hormones. It has generally been assumed that the peripheral conversion of LT4 into T_3 makes it unnecessary to add LT3 to the treatment regimen.

Despite normalized TSH levels that indicate biochemical euthyroidism, a substantial group of patients with hypothyroidism (~10%-15%) are "unhappy" because they do not feel well and report dissatisfaction with and reduced quality of life on LT4 monotherapy. These patients often exhibit persistent debilitating hypothyroid symptoms, including fatigue and weight gain, but also impaired neurocognitive function (brain fog), impaired psychological well-being, depression or anxiety, or other somatic hypothyroid symptoms.[2,3] As a uniform approach to these patients is still lacking, this clinical problem places a high burden on daily clinical practice, leads to patient dissatisfaction, and may challenge the relationship between patients and clinicians.

Practice Gaps

- There is lack of knowledge on the prevalence and potential causes of persistent symptoms despite biochemical euthyroidism in patients with hypothyroidism who are treated with LT4.

- There is lack of knowledge on the benefits and limitations of existing LT4/LT3 combination therapy and DTE for patients with hypothyroidism, leading to heterogeneity in their use among clinicians in clinical practice.

- It is crucial that clinicians can reassure patients and adequately address patient requests to test for nonconventional clinical thyroid parameters (eg, reverse T_3) or genetic variants.

Discussion

Excluding Concomitant Diseases

The most common cause of primary hypothyroidism is chronic autoimmune thyroiditis (Hashimoto disease). Up to 15% of patients with hypothyroidism have at least 1 concomitant autoimmune disease, including rheumatoid arthritis (up to 30%), type 1 diabetes (6%-24%), and celiac disease (3%), among others, and it can be a part of a polyglandular autoimmune syndrome. Concomitant autoimmune diseases in patients with hypothyroidism who are biochemically euthyroid may lead to persistent nonspecific symptoms and should be excluded. It is important to note that symptoms related to other nonautoimmune conditions, such as perimenopausal status, obstructive sleep apnea, and depression, may also overlap with hypothyroid symptoms, and these should be considered when evaluating these patients. In addition, a recent study has shown a high prevalence of somatic symptom disorder among patients with hypothyroidism.[4]

Levothyroxine Dosage Adjustments Within the Euthyroid Range

Anecdotal evidence has previously suggested that the well-being of patients with hypothyroidism may be improved by fine adjustments of the LT4 dosage, aiming for a serum TSH concentration in the lower end of the reference range. Walsh et al conducted a double-blind randomized controlled trial with a crossover design where 56 patients received 3 different LT4 dosages in 8-week courses (high, middle, and low in 25 mcg increments) in random order, aimed to achieve target TSH levels less than 0.30 mIU/L, 0.30 to 1.99 mIU/L, and 2.0 to 4.8 mIU/L, respectively.[5] Small changes in the LT4 dosage to achieve serum TSH concentrations in the lower reference range or slightly below did not lead to measurable changes in hypothyroidism

symptoms, well-being, or quality of life compared with targeting a TSH concentration in the upper reference range. Another study by Samuels et al randomly assigned 138 LT4-treated individuals with normal baseline serum TSH to receive an unchanged, higher, or lower LT4 dosage in double-blind fashion, targeting a TSH range of 0.34 to 2.50 mIU/L, 2.51 to 5.60 mIU/L, or 5.61 to 12.0 mIU/L.[6] Participants had their LT4 dosage adjusted every 6 weeks. After 6 months, there were no significant differences in health status, mood, memory, or executive function between the 3 treatment arms. However, even though patients could not ascertain how their LT4 dosages were adjusted, they preferred LT4 dosages that they perceived to be higher. These studies provide some preliminary data on the topic; however, they were limited by small sample sizes. In addition, these data do not address the possibility that differences in individual TSH setpoints may exist, such that the TSH concentration needed to achieve similar circulating thyroid hormone concentrations may differ between individuals and may lead to patients with similar TSH concentrations responding differently to treatment.

Synthetic LT4/LT3 Combination Therapy

Studies have shown that with LT4 monotherapy, normalization of serum T_3 and TSH levels can only be achieved at the expense of higher-than-normal free T_4 levels, leading to higher T_4 to T_3 ratios than those observed in healthy persons.[7,8] Therefore, the limitation of LT4 monotherapy is that it fails to mimic the physiological serum T_4 to T_3 ratio, which could be a plausible cause of the persisting hypothyroid symptoms. Animal studies have provided specific insights into the consequences of LT4 monotherapy on T_4 and T_3 concentrations in peripheral tissues. Escobar-Morreale et al showed that LT4 monotherapy in thyroidectomized rats did not, at any dose, result in normal T_4 and T_3 levels simultaneously in all tissues.[9] However, LT4/LT3 combination therapy was able to normalize T_4 and T_3 concentrations in plasma, as well as in all tissues, while also normalizing plasma TSH concentrations.

For these reasons, 19 clinical trials have investigated whether LT4/LT3 combination therapy has benefit over LT4 monotherapy in the treatment of patients with hypothyroidism. These studies show conflicting results with several meta-analyses showing no beneficial effects on various complaints.[1,10] However, several sources of heterogeneity in these trials must be considered. First, the largest limitation common to all studies was the lack of clear selection of patients with the highest potential benefit (ie, patients with persistent symptoms despite LT4 monotherapy). Second, many of the studies used LT4 to LT3 ratios ranging between 10:1 and 5:1. However, the average daily production of T_4 and T_3 by the thyroid is 56 and 3 μg/day/m², corresponding to a physiological T_4 to T_3 ratio of 16:1, which is therefore also the recommended ratio endorsed by various international guidelines.[11] Third, these studies used different nonthyroid-specific quality-of-life (QoL) questionnaires, while none used the well-validated and internationally accepted thyroid-specific ThyPRO QoL questionnaire. Finally, other sources of heterogeneity include the short duration of follow-up and large differences in sample sizes. However, when pooling the results of those studies that reported on treatment preference, 25% of the participants expressed no preference, 27% preferred LT4 monotherapy, and 48% preferred LT4/LT3 combination therapy.[11] Given these conflicting results, international guidelines recommend against the routine use of LT4/LT3 combination therapy, but state that a trial can be considered in select patients.

Desiccated Thyroid Extract

DTE was the standard of treatment for hypothyroidism until the mid 1970s, after which it was replaced by LT4. DTE is derived from the porcine or bovine thyroid gland and is commonly prescribed in grains, in which 1 grain typically contains approximately 38 mcg of T_4 and 9 mcg of T_3.[1] As for LT4/LT3 combination therapy, DTE is of potential interest in LT4-treated patients with persistent symptoms despite biochemical euthyroidism, as this patient population might be particularly sensitive to the relatively low T_3 levels inherent to LT4 monotherapy. While the dosing and stability are less of an issue nowadays, the largest concern with DTE remains its supraphysiological T_3 content, which might lead to transient thyrotoxicosis, with potential harmful effects on cardiovascular and skeletal tissues. The few small randomized controlled trials that have been performed do not support beneficial effects of DTE.[1] Its use is therefore not recommended by international guidelines, while it is frequently requested by patients due to social media attention.

Nonconventional Thyroid Parameters and Genetic Variants

Patient dissatisfaction with hypothyroidism management due to reduced QoL may lead to patient requests for nonconventional tests and treatments.[12] Even though some patients who feel unwell on LT4 monotherapy may have low serum T_3 levels, thyroid hormone treatment adjustments based on serum total or free T_3 levels are not currently routinely recommended.[13] Similarly, no indications exist for measurement of reverse T_3 levels, a metabolically inactive byproduct of thyroid hormone metabolism, in the management of patients with hypothyroidism.[13]

The fact that the interindividual variation in serum thyroid parameters is larger than intraindividual variation suggests that every individual may have a unique hypothalamic-pituitary-thyroid axis setpoint. Studies have estimated that most of this interindividual variation is determined by genetic factors.[14] While over the last 25 years many genetic variants have been identified, including variants in the gene encoding type 2 deiodinase (among others responsible for converting T_4 to T_3), these variants do not yet have a proven role in the management of patients with hypothyroidism.[14]

Clinical Case Vignettes

Case 1

A 35-year-old woman on LT4, 100 mcg daily, seeks help to manage persistent symptoms of fatigue and brain fog. While discussing her symptoms, she states that she is sometimes so tired she has a hard time getting out of bed in the morning. In addition, she feels that she has not been able to think clearly for the past several months and often feels sluggish and is unable to focus. She has been unable to lose weight despite changing her diet and adhering to a regular exercise regimen. She has no other relevant medical history. Thyroid function tests in the past year have repeatedly shown serum TSH and free T$_4$ values in the reference range.

Most recent laboratory test results:

TSH = 2.70 mIU/L
Free T$_4$ = 1.7 ng/dL (SI: 21.9 pmol/L)

She is upset and tearful. She asks if adjusting her LT4 dosage may help with her symptoms.

Which of the following is the best initial step in addressing this patient's concerns?

A. Rule out other possible etiologies of symptoms, including other autoimmune diseases

B. Increase the LT4 dosage while maintaining euthyroidism

C. Increase the LT4 dosage to suppress TSH

D. Consider switching to LT4/LT3 combination therapy

E. Consider switching to DTE

Answer: A) Rule out other possible etiologies of symptoms, including other autoimmune diseases

This patient is biochemically euthyroid with several persistent symptoms. After acknowledging the patient's symptoms, the first step is to exclude other possible etiologies, including other autoimmune diseases, depression, etc (Answer A). If additional etiologies of the persistent symptoms are ruled out, optimizing health habits, such as sleep, exercise, and nutrition, is also imperative before considering thyroid hormone regimen adjustments. Subsequently, small adjustments to the LT4 dosage may be attempted to see if the patient feels better at a different TSH concentration in the normal range (possible individual setpoint). Increasing

the LT4 dosage to suppress TSH would be inappropriate and should be avoided, as iatrogenic hyperthyroidism has been associated with adverse cardiovascular and skeletal effects.[15]

Case 2

A 40-year-old man with hypothyroidism due to Hashimoto thyroiditis is referred by his primary care provider for persistent, severe tiredness heavily affecting his work productivity and social life. He has been on a stable dosage of LT4, 125 mcg daily, for years, and he is biochemically euthyroid (also confirmed in the endocrine outpatient clinic). His primary care provider already tried multiple small adjustments in the LT4 dosage without any success in relieving the patient's symptoms. An extensive evaluation excluded other causes of tiredness. The patient's wife is a renowned endocrinologist who frequently attends the annual meeting of the Endocrine Society and has listened to various debates on the use of synthetic LT4/LT3 combination therapy and DTE. The patient would like to try one of these treatments.

Which of the following is an appropriate response to this patient's request?

A. Neither synthetic LT4/LT3 combination therapy nor DTE should be prescribed

B. Synthetic LT4/LT3 combination therapy should not be prescribed; DTE could be considered, starting with 1 grain daily

C. Synthetic LT4/LT3 combination therapy should not be prescribed; DTE could be considered, starting with 2 grains daily

D. Synthetic LT4/LT3 combination therapy could be considered, starting with a 5:1 ratio; DTE should not be prescribed

E. Synthetic LT4/LT3 combination therapy could be considered, starting with a 16:1 ratio; DTE should not be prescribed

Answer: E) Synthetic LT4/LT3 combination therapy could be considered, starting with a 16:1 ratio; DTE should not be prescribed

Two randomized controlled trials have evaluated the efficacy of DTE and did not find any improvements in QoL or symptom scores.[16,17] However, as these studies have various limitations, such as limited sample size and no targeted inclusion of patients with persistent symptoms, these results should be interpreted with caution, and future large studies are needed to provide a definitive answer as to whether DTE is effective in the management of hypothyroidism. For these reasons, DTE is not endorsed by international guidelines for the management of hypothyroidism, including in select cases.

As randomized controlled trials of synthetic LT4/LT3 combination therapy show conflicting results and have important limitations (see above), international guidelines recommend against the routine use of synthetic LT4/LT3 combination therapy, but state that a trial could be considered in select patients who are adherent to their regimen and are biochemically well-controlled, but have persistent symptoms despite LT4 treatment and after ruling out other etiologies for symptoms. This 3-month trial should be discontinued if the patient does not experience clinical improvement.[1] The European Thyroid Association guideline on combination therapy provides guidance for clinicians when calculating the combined LT4/LT3 dosing regimen.[11] Although systematically collected long-term safety data are needed, retrospective data analyses suggest that there is no increased risk of long-term adverse effects as long as physiological LT4 to LT3 ratios are used and TSH is kept within the reference range.[18]

Case 3

A 47-year-old woman with longstanding hypothyroidism due to Hashimoto thyroiditis presents with significant fatigue and hair loss. These symptoms are causing substantial distress, and she describes feeling very unhappy. She has been on a stable LT4 dosage, 75 mcg daily. Weight is stable. Her TSH and free T_4 levels have been in the reference range for the past several years (most recent measurement 2 weeks ago). She states that she read on social media that some people do not appropriately convert T_4 to T_3, and she would like to be tested for this to see if it is contributing to her symptoms.

Which of the following is an appropriate response to this patient's request?

A. Measure reverse T_3

B. Measure serum free T_3 and adjust the LT4 dosage accordingly

C. Repeat TSH and free T_4 measurements

D. No further testing is necessary

E. Evaluate for genetic variations in genes involved in thyroid hormone metabolism (eg, in *DIO2*)

Answer: D) No further testing is necessary

This patient has been biochemically euthyroid on LT4 replacement for years, confirmed by recent TSH and free T_4 measurements. Therefore, repeating TSH and free T_4 measurements would not be useful. Furthermore, there is no proven role for titrating LT4 based on serum T_3 or reverse T_3 levels. For example, it has been shown that in LT4-treated thyroidectomized patients, there is no relation between thyroid hormone parameters (including serum T_3 and reverse T_3) and QoL.[13] Genetic variation in type 2 deiodinase had been shown to impair T_4 to T_3 conversion. Various clinical studies have therefore investigated these variants in LT4-treated patients and found conflicting results regarding their relationship with QoL and benefit from LT4/LT3 combination therapy.[1,14] This is likely because these studies had several limitations, including small sample sizes and heterogeneity in methodology. Instead of focusing on a single genetic variant, Kus et al tested a panel of genetic variants (polygenic score), showing that this panel was able to provide personalized TSH reference ranges, with substantial effects on diagnosis reclassification and LT4 prescription behavior.[19] However, such panels need to be further refined and tested clinically before considering their routine use in clinical practice.

Key Learning Points

- Clinicians should acknowledge hypothyroid patients' report of continued symptoms despite biochemical euthyroidism and further investigate for possible etiologies.

- While studies have shown no benefit of LT4 dosage adjustments to low-normal or high-normal TSH levels on a population level, it remains to be determined whether such adjustments may be beneficial on an individual patient level.

- A trial of combination synthetic LT4/LT3 therapy may be cautiously considered in select patients.

References

1. Taylor PN, Medici MM, Hubalewska-Dydejczyk A, Boelaert K. Hypothyroidism. Lancet. 2024;404(10460):1347-1364. PMID: 39368843

2. Peterson SJ, Cappola AR, Castro MR, et al. An online survey of hypothyroid patients demonstrates prominent dissatisfaction. Thyroid. 2018;28(6):707-721. PMID: 29620972

3. Wiersinga WM. Paradigm shifts in thyroid hormone replacement therapies for hypothyroidism. Nat Rev Endocrinol. 2014;10(3):164-174. PMID: 24419358

4. Perros P, Nagy EV, Papini E, et al. Hypothyroidism and somatization: results from E-mode patient self-assessment of thyroid therapy, a cross-sectional, international online patient survey. Thyroid. 2023;33(8):927-939. PMID: 37134204

5. Walsh JP, Ward LC, Burke V, et al. Small changes in thyroxine dosage do not produce measurable changes in hypothyroid symptoms, well-being, or quality of life: results of a double-blind, randomized clinical trial. J Clin Endocrinol Metab. 2006;91(7):2624-2630. PMID: 16670161

6. Samuels MH, Kolobova I, Niederhausen M, Janowsky JS, Schuff KG. Effects of altering levothyroxine (L-T4) doses on quality of life, mood, and cognition in L-T4 treated subjects. J Clin Endocrinol Metab. 2018;103(5):1997-2008. PMID: 29509918

7. Fish LH, Schwartz HL, Cavanaugh J, Steffes MW, Bantle JP, Oppenheimer JH. Replacement dose, metabolism, and bioavailability of levothyroxine in the treatment of hypothyroidism. The role of triiodothyronine in pituitary feedback in humans. N Engl J Med. 1987;316(13):764-770. PMID: 3821822

8. Jonklaas J, Davidson B, Bhagat S, Soldin SJ. Triiodothyronine levels in athyreotic individuals during levothyroxine therapy. JAMA. 2008;299(7):769-777. PMID: 18285588

9. Escobar-Morrelae, del Rey FE, Obregon MJ, de Escobar GM. Only the combined treatment with thyroxine and triiodothyronine ensures euthyroidism in all tissues of the thyroidectomized rat. Endocrinology. 1996;137(6):2490-2502. PMID: 8641203

10. Nassar M, Hassan A, Ramadan S, Desouki MT, Hassan MA, Chaudhuri A. Evaluating the effectiveness of combined T4 and T3 therapy or desiccated thyroid versus T4 monotherapy in hypothyroidism: a systematic review and meta-analysis. BMC Endocr Disord. 2024;24(1):90. PMID: 38877429

11. Wiersinga WM, Duntas L, Fadeyev V, Nygaard B, Vanderpump MPJ. 2012 ETA guidelines: the use of L-T4 + L-T3 in the treatment of hypothyroidism. Eur Thyroid J. 2012;1(2):55-71. PMID: 24782999

12. Esfandiari NH, Reyes-Gastelum D, Hawley ST, Haymart MR, Papaleontiou M. Patient requests for tests and treatments impact physician management of hypothyroidism. Thyroid. 2019;29(11):1536-1544. PMID: 31436135

13. Massolt ET, van der Windt M, Korevaar TIM, et al. Thyroid hormone and its metabolites in relation to quality of life in patients treated for differentiated thyroid cancer. Endocrinol (Oxf). 2016;85(5):781-788. PMID: 27175823

14. Kus A, Chaker L, Teurner A, Peeters RP, Medici M. The genetic basis of thyroid function: novel findings and new approaches. J Clin Endocrinol Metab. 2020;105(6):dgz225. PMID: 32271924

15. Evron JM, Hummel SL, Reyes-Gastelum D, Haymart MR, Banerjee M, Papaleontiou M. Association of thyroid hormone treatment intensity with cardiovascular mortality among US veterans. JAMA Netw Open. 2022;5(5):e2211863. PMID: 35552725

16. Hoang TD, Olsen CH, Mai VQ, Clyde PW, Shakir MKM. Desiccated thyroid extract compared with levothyroxine in the treatment of hypothyroidism: a randomized, double-blind, crossover study. J Clin Endocrinol Metab. 2013;98(5):1982-1990. PMID: 23539727

17. Shakir MKM, Brooks DI, McAninch EA, et al. Comparative effectiveness of levothyroxine, desiccated thyroid extract, and levothyroxine+liothyronine in hypothyroidism. J Clin Endocrinol Metab. 2021;106(11):e4400-e4413. PMID: 34185829

18. Gottwald-Hostalek U, Tayrouz Y. A review of the safety of triiodothyronine in combination with levothyroxine for the management of hypothyroidism. Curr Med Res Opin. 2024;40(12):2109-2116. PMID: 39625345

19. Kus A, Sterenborg RBTM, Haug EB, et al. Towards personalized TSH reference ranges: a genetic and population-based approach in three independent cohorts. Thyroid. 2024;34(8):969-979. PMID: 38919119

Navigating Thyroid Eye Disease: From Diagnosis to Management

Marius N. Stan, MD. Division of Endocrinology, Mayo Clinic, Rochester, MN; Email: Stan.marius@mayo.edu

Educational Objectives

After reviewing this chapter, learners should be able to:

- Identify the important elements needed for thyroid eye disease (TED) evaluation.

- Identify TED activity and severity status.

- Recommend appropriate TED medical management choices.

Significance of the Clinical Problem

TED is present in 25% to 40% of individuals with Graves disease, and its management requires a combination of medical and surgical therapy. Medical management of this condition has been dominated by steroids for many years, but recently an IGF-1 receptor blocker, teprotumumab, has significantly changed the field. Both of these therapies, and others less commonly used (eg, tocilizumab, rituximab, mycophenolate), are generating many systemic health implications and adverse effects that should be carefully considered. These therapies would best be carried out in a multidisciplinary TED clinic, yet that approach rarely materializes.

Practice Gaps

- Endocrinologists are insufficiently familiar with the evaluation of TED.

- Medical management of TED requires skills that are the domain of endocrinology, but care for patients with this condition is typically provided by ophthalmologists.

Corollary: Endocrinologists would be ideal partners to ophthalmologists in guiding medical management of TED, if they would familiarize themselves with TED evaluation.

Clinical Case Vignettes and Discussion

Case 1

A 48-year-old woman develops palpitations associated with weight loss and increased sweatiness over the last month. She also has difficulty sleeping and notes a sense of discomfort over her eyes. Her eyes are watering more and are irritated and red. Her primary care physician diagnoses Graves disease, prescribes a β-adrenergic blocker, and refers her to an endocrinologist.

Laboratory test results:

TSH = <0.01 mIU/L
Free T_4 = 3.8 ng/dL (SI: 48.9 pmol/L)
Total T_3 = 430 ng/dL (SI: 6.6 nmol/L)
Thyrotropin antibodies = 7 IU/L (<1.75 IU/L)
White blood cell count, normal
Liver function tests, normal

On physical examination, she has an enlarged thyroid gland (about 25 g) and slight tachycardia (92 beats/min). Overall, she is feeling better since starting propranolol. Her eyes have injected conjunctiva and mild lid edema but no other abnormalities. Extremities, nails included, are unremarkable.

The diagnosis of Graves disease is confirmed, and she is informed that the eye changes are consistent with TED. After a conversation about antithyroid drugs, radioactive iodine, and surgery, she concludes that she would like to start methimazole, 10 mg twice daily, and continue propranolol.

Which of the following elements in the patient's history is NOT necessary for TED evaluation?

A. Cigarette smoking status

B. Thyroid hormone levels

C. TED recent progression

D. Her main concern about TED

E. Selenium levels

Answer: E) Selenium levels

Cigarette smoking (Answer A) is associated with a higher likelihood of TED progression and poor response to most therapies.[1] Thyroid hormone levels (Answer B) are important to determine, as dysthyroidism has a negative impact on TED.[2] Progression in eye changes over the last 3 months (Answer C) likely reflects ongoing inflammation and possible responsiveness to medical therapy. Knowing which TED element the patient considers most troublesome (Answer D) is useful to understand when determining the main goal of management/therapy. Selenium levels (Answer E) are not known to affect TED disease course, and the data on the benefits of selenium therapy are not based on serum levels.[7] Thus, knowing the patient's selenium levels is not necessary in her TED evaluation.

Case Follow-Up

The patient has smoked 10 cigarettes per day for 15 years. We know she has elevated thyroid hormone levels, but her TED has been stable over recent weeks and months, and her main concern is local discomfort (pain, redness, and swelling). She is counseled regarding the negative impact of smoking on TED.

Disease Stage and Severity

To determine disease stage, or disease activity, it is still useful to consider the Rundle curve[3] and evaluate the clinical activity score (CAS)[4]. This assessment guides the provider toward the appropriate set of therapeutic options. Disease severity is most important for deciding on the aggressiveness of potential therapies from the subset of choices based on the disease stage identified earlier (ie, after disease activity was established). The main symptoms and signs useful for evaluating inflammation and severity are the following:

- Diplopia
- Pain in primary vision and pain with extraocular movements
- Changes in clarity and accuracy of vision
- Changes in color perception (reds and blues)
- Assess conjunctiva: edema (ie, what is chemosis?), injection
- Assess globe position (ie, what is proptosis?)
- Assess lids: edema, erythema, closure (ie, what is lagophthalmos?)
- Assess caruncles
- Changes in quality of life

Diplopia is the presence of double vision, and it typically relates to dysfunction of the extraocular muscles. Muscles that are inflamed or enlarged by infiltration with glycosaminoglycans lack normal mobility and, consequently, they no longer synchronize their action with the corresponding muscles in the pair eye. This results in the brain receiving 2 separate images. When the images are relatively close, the brain can still fuse them and restore single vision (with an effort). When the images are far apart, the brain can ignore 1 image and attain single vision. The problem is most challenging when the images are in between these scenarios and the optical cortex continues to struggle with 2 images and is unable to perceive reality clearly and safely. This is when patients give up driving and are unable to operate various appliances/machines, which may require them to change jobs or alter their day-to-day activities.

Diplopia should resolve when patient closes one eye (binocular diplopia), given the mechanism described earlier. If diplopia persists in that case (monocular diplopia) then the problem is one of corneal surface and not extraocular muscle dysfunction. This is best addressed by an ophthalmologist.

The change in vision clarity is usually due to corneal dryness (increased palpebral aperture with increased dryness). In that situation, vision should become clearer with repeated blinking, and this can be proactively aided by aggressive eye lubrication. If these steps do not improve vision clarity, then there should be a concern about optic nerve dysfunction. An early sign of this is the inability to distinguish various hues of red and blue. Testing for optic nerve dysfunction is certainly the domain of ophthalmology, but a quick assessment for the presence of relative afferent pupillary defect is helpful to ascertain likely optic nerve compression and can be performed in the endocrinology office.

Pain could be a sign of inflammation in TED and should be inquired about both in primary gaze ("straight out") when pain reflects increased intraorbital pressure, as well as in the patient looking at different angles (pain with extraocular muscles movements) when pain likely indicates inflammation of the muscles that are being stretched.

Case 1, Continued

Which of the following best describes the benefit of defining the patient's clinical activity score?

A. Establishing potential benefit of medical therapy

B. Indicating need for medical therapy

C. Understanding risk of adverse effects from medical therapy

D. Understanding the complications of surgical therapy

E. Defining which medical therapy would be best

Answer: A) Establishing potential benefit of medical therapy

Disease Activity and Severity

Clinical Activity Score

Disease activity is meant to reflect the presence or absence of orbital inflammation as opposed to fibrosis. This distinction is based on the Rundle curve[3] combined with the work of the Amsterdam group,[4,5] which deemed that the first phase of TED is one of inflammatory changes (dolor, rubor, tumor, calor) and thus they quantified it through an instrument called the Clinical Activity Score (CAS). At the first encounter, this score can take a value between 0 and 7 (*Box*), and at subsequent visits, the score can be between 0 and 10, adding the assessment of changes in severity measures to the evaluation of inflammation. This instrument has been found useful in identifying patients with high probability of responding to glucocorticoids if they have a CAS score of 3 or higher. Unfortunately, the use of CAS has expanded and it has been used as a trial outcome, with improvement in CAS value below 3 deemed to reflect a good overall result. This approach has been taken by many clinical trials, without validation of its significance from the perspective of patients.

Box. Clinical Activity Score

1. Spontaneous retrobulbar pain
2. Pain with eye movement
3. Redness of the eyelids
4. Redness of the conjunctiva
5. Swelling of the eyelids
6. Inflammation of the caruncle
7. Conjunctival edema

Clinical activity score = sum of all items present in each eye (1 point/item present); score might be different for left vs right; use highest score for decision-making.

Therefore, the CAS is useful to indicate whether medical therapy could help to control inflammation (if CAS >2) (Answer A), but it will not determine the need for such therapy (Answer B) or which specific agent to use (Answer E). That decision derives from TED severity and TED dominant features. CAS will also not give any information on the potential adverse effects of medical therapy (Answer C) or provide information on potential surgical complications (Answer D).

Assessing Disease Severity

Disease severity has been practically defined by the European Group on Graves Orbitopathy (EUGOGO) into 3 categories: mild, moderate-to-severe, and sight-threatening disease.[6]

Sight-threatening disease is more obvious to identify and is characterized by the presence of TED complications that can, as the name implies, lead to rapid loss of vision if untreated: dysthyroid optic neuropathy, globe subluxation (the displacement of the eyeball in front of the lids, which are thus unable to protect it anymore), and corneal ulceration with potential infection (globe infection is extremely difficult to eradicate). The distinction between mild and moderate-to-severe (a name I dislike for its length and difficulty in using in conversation with patients and colleagues) is based on extent of eye parameter changes (eg, degree of diplopia, proptosis, soft-tissue changes) and the impact TED has on patients' daily activities. The information presented in the *Table* can be used as a guide for severity assessment.

Potential Differential Diagnosis

TED is, in most cases, the obvious diagnosis when there is symmetric inflammation and proptosis in patients with an ongoing history of Graves disease. However, asymmetric presentation should raise the question of a possible intraorbital mass masquerading as TED (eg, orbital lymphoma, meningioma, arteriovenous fistula/aneurysm).

This is particularly challenging when the patient is not hyperthyroid (eg, remote history of radioactive iodine therapy or thyroidectomy, euthyroid TED, or TED with Hashimoto thyroiditis). Documenting thyroid autoimmunity markers (thyrotropin receptor antibodies—TRAb and/or thyroid-stimulating immunoglobulins) and imaging the orbit is necessary in these cases. Rarely, biopsy from the extraocular muscles is needed to clarify the diagnosis.

TED Management—Mild Disease

General Measures

For all patients, normal thyroid hormone levels should be pursued, along with smoking cessation (including eliminating secondary smoking) and adequate lubrication of the cornea (artificial tears during the day and gel or ointment at night). Additional measures can include the use of wraparound glasses or glasses with lateral shield that limit draft in front of the eyes, sleeping with the head of the bed elevated (decreasing lid edema), cold compresses (beneficial for pain), and minimizing stress (expected to minimize autoimmune response). The more specific TED approach taken beyond these basic measures depends on disease activity and severity.

Mild TED

The patient in this vignette has mild disease and therefore general measures will represent the bulk of therapy. Additionally, there are data that selenium (200 mcg daily for 6 months) can improve local discomfort in mild TED, with persistent effect up to 6 months.[7]

Table. TED Severity per EUGOGO Guidelines

Degree of severity	Lid retraction	Soft-tissue involvement	Proptosis	Diplopia	Cornea exposure	Optic nerve status	Globe prolapse/subluxation
Mild (≥1)	<2 mm	Mild	<3 mm	Absent or Intermittent	Absent	Normal	Absent
Moderate-to-severe (≥1)	≥2 mm	Moderate or severe	≥3 mm	Inconstant or constant	Mild	Normal	Absent
Sight-threatening (≥1)	N/A	N/A	N/A	N/A	Ulcer	Affected	Present

Case Follow-Up
Despite normalization of thyroid hormone levels, the patient describes progressive pain associated with more eye bulging and double vision upon looking to the sides (worse when looking up and to the right). She has been consuming Brazil nuts (rich in selenium) for past 2 months without benefit. Upon reevaluation, her CAS is determined to be 5 with excess proptosis of 4 mm in the right eye and 2 mm in the left eye. Diplopia is indeed inducible at the angle described.

Case 1, Continued

Which of the following is the best recommendation in this patient's management at this stage?

A. Intravenous steroids

B. Teprotumumab

C. Orbital decompression

D. Strabismus surgery (for diplopia)

E. Observation

Answer: B) Teprotumumab

TED Management—Moderate-to-Severe Disease
The patient now has moderate-to-severe disease, and consultation with ophthalmology is mandatory. Understanding the perspective of ophthalmologists on eye health is essential to confirm the active disease stage and to rule out sight-threatening elements. At our multidisciplinary TED clinic, patients are seen same morning by endocrinology, ophthalmology, and otolaryngology. Cases are discussed at the noon conference by all these teams, and a joint decision is made about therapy. That decision is communicated to the patient in a brief recap visit in early afternoon performed jointly by the endocrinologist and ophthalmologist. For the patient in this vignette, we concluded that she has active disease of moderate severity with no sight-threatening elements. This is best managed with medical therapy, mostly with immunomodulatory action. As the disease has progressed and is still active, neither observation

(Answer E) nor surgical management (Answer D) is appropriate. Medical choices that can mitigate inflammation include teprotumumab (Answer B) and steroids. However, teprotumumab can significantly improve proptosis and potentially improve diplopia, which are features unlikely to change significantly with intravenous steroid therapy (Answer A). Therefore, I would endorse teprotumumab if no significant contraindications were present.

Medical Management
The most common therapeutic approach used to be steroids for inflammation control. This is still a favored therapy if other agents are not available. Steroids have proved their efficacy in a number of trials, with intravenous steroids being superior to oral steroids regarding efficacy (a composite index of eye parameters) and safety (better tolerated regarding the gastrointestinal tract and bone health to name a few).[8] Many other agents have been tried over the years (including somatostatin analogues, B-cell depleter [eg, rituximab], interleukin-6 blockers, azathioprine, mycophenolate, TNF-α blockers) with inconsistent or minimal efficacy.[9] However, the agent that has been introduced most recently, teprotumumab, an IGF-1 receptor blocker, is likely to be most effective. The data available about this agent reveal significant improvement in proptosis (primary outcome in 2 randomized controlled trials), CAS/inflammation and quality of life, while diplopia responded less consistently.[10] The benefit on proptosis was about 3 mm on average, which is equivalent to the expected result of orbital decompression surgery targeting 1 orbital wall (implicitly, more aggressive reduction in proptosis can be achieved with more aggressive surgery). If the patient in this vignette had struggled with only inflammatory features (without significant proptosis or diplopia), steroids would be a very reasonable choice. Notably, no head-to-head trial has compared teprotumumab with steroids, either intravenous or oral. In this patient's case, however, I would consider teprotumumab as the best agent to achieve a good result with respect to proptosis

and inflammation and, possibly, improvement in double vision as well. To proceed with therapy, it is important to review the logistics of treatment (8 intravenous infusions every 3 weeks, administered at an infusion therapy center) and the patient's comorbidities to understand if there are any contraindications or potential conditions that could be aggravated by teprotumumab. I am particularly interested in patients' hearing acuity and discuss with them their concerns/perspective on potential local ear discomfort (eg, tinnitus, fullness, autophonia) and possible sensorineural hearing loss. I obtain a baseline audiogram since occasionally preexisting hearing loss might not have been apparent to the patient, and it is important to establish a baseline for later assessing the impact of therapy. I also discuss contraindications regarding inflammatory bowel disease and uncontrolled diabetes. If patients have diabetes, then a hemoglobin A_{1c} value less than 8.0% (64 mmol/mol) should be pursued. Furthermore, it is important to ensure that these aspects are monitored during therapy. For patients with diabetes, I request a glucose measurement after the first 2 infusions, and I repeat audiography after the fourth infusion. That is also the time when we reassess the TED response to therapy with the knowledge that most patients have a very rapid response, usually noticeable after the first 2 infusions. Several other adverse effects of therapy, including amenorrhea, should be considered when discussing teprotumumab. Multiple review articles are available for those seeking a more thorough review of teprotumumab's adverse effects, their putative mechanism, and their management.[11]

Case Follow-Up

Due to concerns for hearing loss related to teprotumumab, the patient elects therapy with intravenous glucocorticoids. The patient initiates the EUGOGO regimen of methylprednisone, 500 mg weekly for 6 weeks, followed by a dosage of 250 mg weekly for another 6 weeks. In this case, close monitoring of glucose and blood pressure is required, and other adverse effects should be considered during follow-up. For an extensive overview of the benefits and risks associated with different medical treatments, see the American Thyroid Association consensus statement on TED.[12] She patient achieves a decrease in CAS to a score of 1 (conjunctival injection persisted), but has no changes in proptosis or diplopia.

At this point, it is important to understand the patient's perception of these results. She is still affected on a functional level by diplopia and on a social level by significant proptosis. Her evaluation with ophthalmology is again important to establish the new baseline and rule out (consistently, at every visit) the possibility of sight-threatening disease. The findings arere confirmed, and a discussion takes place about the potential benefit of rehabilitative surgery. This entails the spectrum of orbital decompression (removing retro-orbital fat, as well as some of the orbital bone, to create space for globe recession into the orbit), strabismus surgery (extraocular muscle adjustments to synchronize the globe movements and ensure single vision in primary gaze—main goal), and lid surgery to repair excess retraction and troublesome globe exposure. The sequence of these interventions must start with decompression if proptosis is significant, followed by strabismus surgery (if diplopia is present up-front or induced by orbital decompression [15%-25% of cases]), and conclude with lid adjustments, if needed. These procedures are only performed after there is evidence of stability for a minimum of 3 months, ideally 6 months. The experience of the ophthalmologist in performing these interventions should be considered a primordial factor for success. The role as endocrinologists at this stage is to ensure that thyroid parameters remain stable, cigarette smoking is eliminated if possible, and other comorbidities are well controlled.

Alternative scenario: had the patient selected therapy with teprotumumab, my expectation is that we would have achieved good improvement in proptosis and inflammation but probably not complete resolution of diplopia. I also expect that we would have encountered prediabetes (around 60% general risk), which I tackle early with metformin. This issue is rarely a significant problem and after completion of therapy, we are often able to discontinue metformin. There are frequent complaints of muscle cramps, which I target with aggressive hydration, daily multivitamins and minerals, and occasionally muscle relaxants. Muscle cramps tend to resolve within couple months after therapy. Ear-related changes are common, and a variety of symptoms are encountered: ear pain, pressure, autophonia, and occasionally diminished hearing from sensory-neural injury, manifesting itself as hearing loss at high frequencies. While most of the non–hearing loss symptoms are reversible, it seems that sensory-neural hearing loss is a persistent problem and may sometimes lead to the use of hearing aids.

Can the disease progress despite therapy? Development of sight-threatening disease is quite rare. Compressive optic neuropathy (dysthyroid optic neuropathy) occurs in 3% to 5% of persons with TED and is initially treated with intravenous glucocorticoids (my preferred regimen is 1g-0.5g-0.5 g for 3 consecutive days, repeated 2 weeks later, and reevaluated in another 1 to 2 weeks). If no improvement is noted, then emergent orbital decompression should be pursued. The other 2 sight-threatening complications—orbital subluxation and corneal ulceration—are ophthalmological emergencies and should be entirely the prerogative of that specialty.

Additional Case Follow-Up
The patient undergoes bilateral orbital decompression and achieves nice improvement in proptosis. Unfortunately, her diplopia remains clinically significant, and she is following up with the strabismus experts for planned further interventions.

Future Directions to Share With Patients
TED is an area of active research, and, fortunately for many patients, there is no urgency for immediate intervention. Multiple agents are currently being developed, targeting the IGF-1 receptor, interleukin-6 and interleukin-6 receptor, TRAb (through neonatal Fc receptor targeting), TSH receptor, and a few others that have different targets. Some of these agents are already in phase 2/3 of evaluation, and I expect our therapeutic choices will likely include some of them in the coming years. Their potential benefits could be improved efficacy in comparison with available drugs, simultaneous targeting of TED and hyperthyroidism (if present), and a better adverse effect profile, allowing us to more effectively individualize TED therapy.

Key Learning Points

- For all patients with Graves disease, risk factors for TED development/progression should be identified (eg, cigarette smoking, radioactive iodine, dysthyroidism) with the aim to minimize them.

- When TED is present, the patient's CAS and disease severity should be defined as a necessary step toward therapy selection.

- In general, the inflammatory phase of TED should be addressed with medical therapy and the chronic, inactive phase should be addressed with surgical management.

References

1. Bartalena L, Marcocci C, Tanda ML, et al. Cigarette smoking and treatment outcomes in Graves ophthalmopathy. *Ann Intern Med.* 1998;129(8):632-635. PMID: 9786811

2. Prummel MF, Wiersinga WM, Mourits MP, Koornneef L, Berghout A, van der Gaag R. Effect of abnormal thyroid function on the severity of Graves' ophthalmopathy. *Arch Int Med.* 1990;150(5):1098-1101. PMID: 1691908

3. Rundle FF, Wilson CW. Development and course of exophthalmos and ophthalmoplegia in Graves' disease with special reference to the effect of thyroidectomy. *Clin Sci.* 1945;5(3-4):177-194. PMID: 21011937

4. Mourits MP, Prummel MF, Wiersinga WM, Koornneef L. Clinical activity score as a guide in the management of patients with Graves' ophthalmopathy. *Clin Endocrinol.* 1997;47(1):9-14. PMID: 9302365

5. Prummel MF, Mourits MP, Berghout A, et al. Prednisone and cyclosporine in the treatment of severe Graves' ophthalmopathy. *N Engl J Med.* 1989;321(20):1353-1359. PMID: 2519530

6. Bartalena L, Kahaly GJ, Baldeschi L, et al. The 2021 European Group on Graves' orbitopathy (EUGOGO) clinical practice guidelines for the medical

management of Graves' orbitopathy. *Eur J Endocrinol.* 2021;185(4):G43-G67. PMID: 34297684

7. Marcocci C, Kahaly GJ, Krassas GE, et al. Selenium and the course of mild Graves' orbitopathy. *N Engl J Med.* 2011;364(20):1920-1931. PMID: 21591944

8. Kahaly GJ, Pitz S, Hommel G, Dittmar M. Randomized, single blind trial of intravenous versus oral steroid monotherapy in Graves' orbitopathy. *J Clin Endocrinol Metab.* 2005;90(9):5234-5240. PMID: 15998777

9. Stan MN, Salvi M. Management of endocrine disease: rituximab therapy for Graves' orbitopathy - lessons from randomized control trials. *Eur J Endocrinol.* 2017;176(2):R101-R109. PMID: 27760790

10. Douglas RS, Kahaly GJ, Patel A, et al. Teprotumumab for the treatment of active thyroid eye disease. *N Engl J Med.* 2020;382(4):341-352. PMID: 31971679

11. Stan MN, Krieger CC. The adverse effects profile of teprotumumab. *J Clin Endocrinol Metab.* 2023;108(9):e654-e662. PMID: 37071658

12. Burch HB, Perros P, Bednarczuk T, et al. Management of thyroid eye disease: a consensus statement by the American Thyroid Association and the European Thyroid Association. *Thyroid.* 2022;32(12):1439-1470. PMID: 36480280

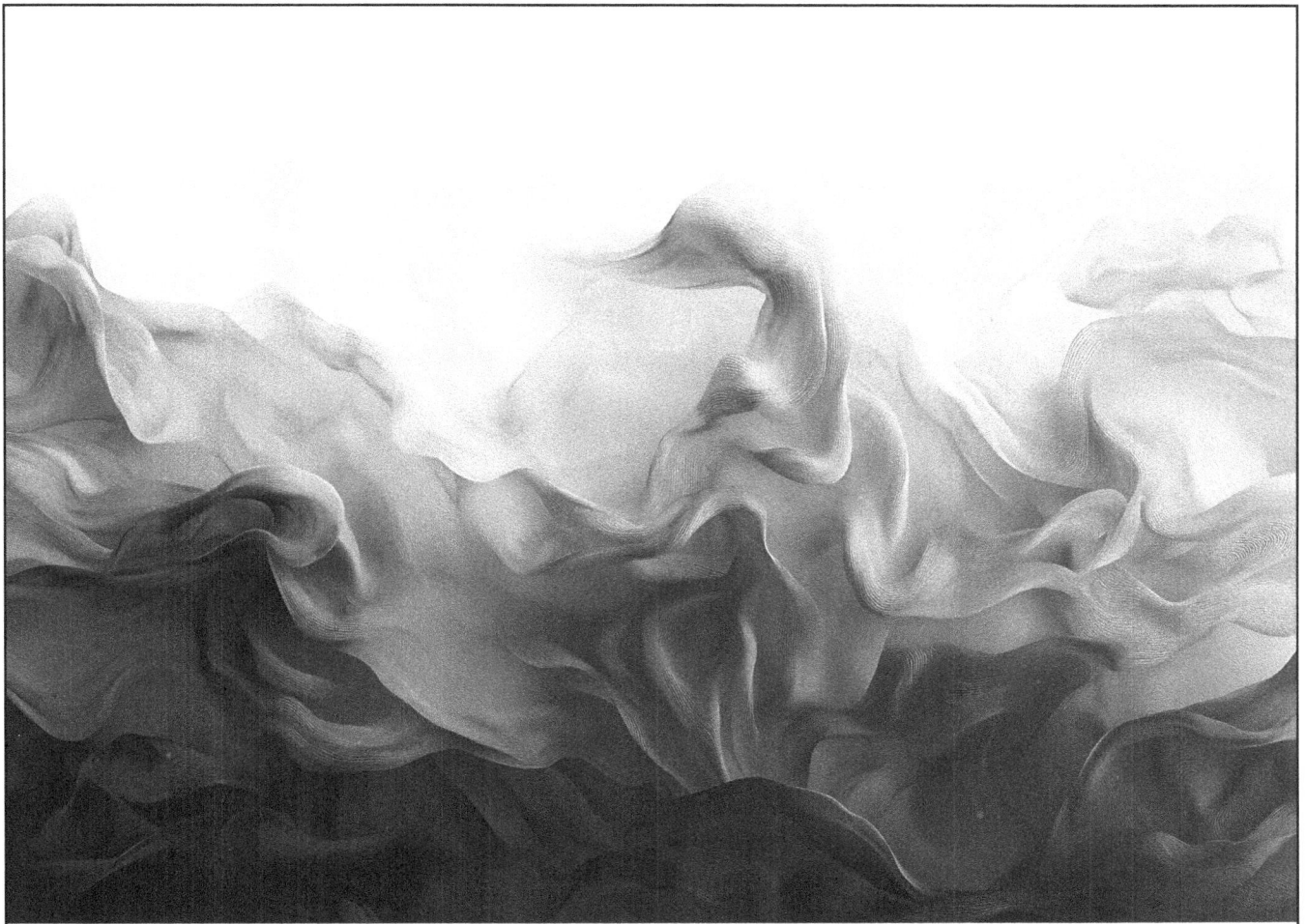

TUMOR BIOLOGY

Landscape of Genetic Alterations in Well-Differentiated Thyroid Cancer in Pediatric Patients

Andrew J. Bauer, MD. The Thyroid Center, Division of Endocrinology and Diabetes, Children's Hospital of Philadelphia and Perelman School of Medicine, University of Pennsylvania, Philadelphia, PA; Email: bauera@chop.edu

Educational Objectives

After reviewing this chapter, learners should be able to:

- Describe the oncogenic drivers associated with thyroid cancer and recognize the spectrum of invasive disease associated with each oncogenic driver.

- Describe the opportunities to incorporate oncogenic drivers into stratifying and optimizing surgical and medical management of thyroid nodules and thyroid carcinoma.

- Apply new knowledge to create an evaluation process for thyroid nodules in children and adolescents that optimizes outcomes.

Significance of the Clinical Problem

Thyroid nodules in pediatric patients carry a higher risk for thyroid carcinoma, and the risk of malignancy in indeterminate thyroid nodules is higher in children than in adults. Thyroid ultrasonography is recommended as the best radiological exam for evaluation of thyroid nodules. However, there is less experience within pediatrics with a high degree of interobserver and intraobserver variability in interpretation of malignant sonographic features, as well as incomplete evaluation for cervical neck lymph node metastasis. The variability in interpretation for malignancy carries over in the cytological interpretation of FNA reflected by the broad risk of malignancy within the indeterminate categories of The Bethesda System for Reporting Thyroid Cytopathology (TBSRTC): 0% to 50% for atypia of undetermined significance; 20% to 100% for follicular neoplasm; and 40% to 100% for suspicious for malignancy. There is a higher surgical resection rate for benign nodules in children than in adults, and there are a substantial number of patients with metastatic thyroid carcinoma who require additional surgery for persistent disease after initial tumor resection.

Practice Gaps

- There is a lack of training and experience in completing and interpreting thyroid ultrasonography with reduced stratification of nodules selected for FNA.

- There is an increased risk of malignancy in nodules with TBSRTC indeterminate categories with a broader risk range for children compared with adults within the same categories.

- It is critical to train providers involved in the evaluation and management of pediatric patients with thyroid nodules.

Discussion

Thyroid tumorigenesis is driven by well-described oncogenic driver alterations. In 2014, The Cancer Genome Atlas Program published the "integrated genomic characterization of papillary thyroid carcinoma" in adults, which suggests that compared with traditional histopathological classification, reclassification of thyroid cancers into molecular subtypes better reflects differentiation and invasive potential. Similar data in pediatrics have been accumulating over the last decade, supporting incorporation of oncogenic drivers to increase the accuracy of identifying thyroid malignancy in nodules with indeterminate cytology, and, potentially, to optimize stratification of surgery. With the availability of FDA-approved oncogene specific inhibitors, there is also more research evaluating how to incorporate these oral chemotherapeutic agents in both the neoadjuvant and adjuvant settings. This chapter provides an update on current research focusing on the use of somatic oncogenic driver alterations in an effort to improve stratification of care in pediatric patients with thyroid nodules and differentiated thyroid carcinoma.

Compared with papillary thyroid carcinoma (PTC) in adults, PTC in children has a higher prevalence of kinase fusions, especially in patients 10 years or younger. The presence of a fusion oncogene involving *RET, NTRK, ALK,* or *BRAF* (most common; *RET*-like) is associated with an increased risk for extrathyroidal invasion and distant metastasis in children compared with disease associated with *RAS*-like variants or the *BRAF* V600E pathogenic variant. Since the publication of the 2015 American Thyroid Association pediatric guidelines, there are accumulating data on the potential utility of integrating ultrasound features with cytology to increase the accuracy of predicting thyroid malignancy with the addition of somatic oncogene analysis, which ultimately provides objective data to help stratify the surgical approach. Most nodules with the designation TBSRTC category III (atypia of unknown significance) and IV (follicular neoplasm) cytology have low-risk to indeterminate sonographic features (solid or complex composition with smooth margins and no punctate echogenic foci) and harbor oncogenic alterations associated with a low risk for invasive behavior (*RAS, DICER1, PTEN,* non-V600E *BRAF* pathogenic variants or fusions involving *PAX8::PPARG*). For patients with these features who are undergoing surgical intervention, lobectomy without prophylactic central neck lymph node dissection may be considered with additional surgical intervention based on histological features. In contrast, nodules with TBSRTC category V (suspicious for malignancy) or VI (malignant) cytology typically have sonographic features suspicious for malignancy (solid composition, hypoechoic echogenicity, irregular, lobulated or infiltrative margin, and punctate echogenic foci) and harbor oncogenic alterations associated with intermediate or high risk for invasive behavior (*BRAF* V600E pathogenic variant or *RET*-like kinase fusions). Total thyroidectomy with prophylactic central neck lymph node dissection is recommended for most patients harboring a thyroid nodule/lesion with these features, with lobectomy and ipsilateral prophylactic central neck lymph node dissection considered in select patients with no evidence of lymph node metastasis on preoperative ultrasonography (AJCC N0b).[1]

After total thyroidectomy, the decision to use radioiodine (RAI) therapy is based on the extent of extrathyroidal disease. For patients with distant metastasis, most commonly to the lungs, a significant percentage develop persistent, stable disease with a smaller number of patients developing structurally progressive disease despite single or repeated RAI treatments. Recent advances in molecular profiling and clinical use of next-generation sequencing have led to increasing recognition of targetable oncogenic drivers in pediatric thyroid carcinoma. In parallel, multiple molecularly targeted therapies for the treatment of thyroid carcinoma have been studied, primarily in adult patients, and have received FDA approval. Approval for some of these agents now extends into the pediatric age range. With molecular therapy for pediatric thyroid carcinoma in its nascency, questions remain regarding the timing for initiation of these agents (neoadjuvant, adjuvant), indications (disease not amenable to surgery/radiation, systemic disease, differentiation therapy for increasing RAI efficacy), durability of response and duration of treatment, and combination with other agents or modalities (especially RAI and surgery).[2]

Clinical Case Vignettes

Case 1

A 15-year-old girl is found to have a right neck swelling during routine physical examination. Ultrasonography confirms a 3.5-cm solid, hypoechoic intrathyroidal nodule with a wider-than-tall shape, smooth margins, and no punctate echogenic foci. No abnormal lymph nodes are identified in the central or right lateral neck. Findings from FNA of the left thyroid nodule are compatible with TBSRTC atypia of unknown significance. Somatic oncogene testing reveals an *NRAS* pathogenic variant (Q61R [c.182A>G]).

Which of the following is the best surgical option associated with the highest likelihood of remission and lowest risk of potential complications for this patient?

A. Total thyroidectomy

B. Right lobectomy

C. Total thyroidectomy with ipsilateral central neck lymph node dissection

D. Right lobectomy with ipsilateral central neck lymph node dissection

Answer: B) Right lobectomy

This patient underwent right thyroid lobectomy (Answer B) with an uneventful recovery. Histopathologic examination revealed a unifocal, minimally invasive follicular thyroid carcinoma (FTC) measuring 3.6 cm. Two lymph nodes were incidentally removed from right level VI (central) and were negative for malignancy. TNM staging was T2N0aM0(clinical), placing the patient in the American Thyroid Association pediatric low-risk category for persistent postinitial surgical disease. Postoperative thyroid function testing 6 weeks after surgery revealed a TSH value in the low-mid reference range. Thyroid ultrasonography surveillance 1 year postoperatively showed a normal left thyroid lobe without evidence of persistent/recurrent disease in the right thyroid bed.

Thyroid nodules with smooth margins are typically encapsulated tumors associated with a higher likelihood of benign cytology (adenoma or noninvasive follicular thyroid neoplasm with papillary-like nuclear features [NIFTP]) or a carcinoma with a lower-risk for metastasis (invasive encapsulated follicular variant PTC or minimally invasive FTC). Based on this, total thyroidectomy (Answers A and C) and prophylactic central neck lymph node dissection (Answers C and D) are not necessary to achieve remission. After lobectomy, if the lesion displays low or no mitotic activity, no extrathyroidal extension, and either no evidence of capsular angioinvasion or invasion in fewer than 3 blood vessels, lobectomy should be adequate to achieve remission. If histology reveals extensive angioinvasion or high-grade histological features, completion thyroidectomy should be considered to provide an opportunity to evaluate and initiate surveillance for distant metastasis that may be present at the time of initial surgery or present 5 to 10 years after initial diagnosis. Because of the paucity of data on angioinvasive FTC in the pediatric population, the flow diagram (*Figure, following page*) suggests more than 2 vessels to raise consideration and discussion regarding the benefit of completion thyroidectomy. High-grade histologic features include solid, trabecular, or insular growth patterns, mitotic index of 3 or more per 10 high-power field, necrosis, and convoluted nuclei.[1]

Figure. Integrative Analysis of a Thyroid Nodule

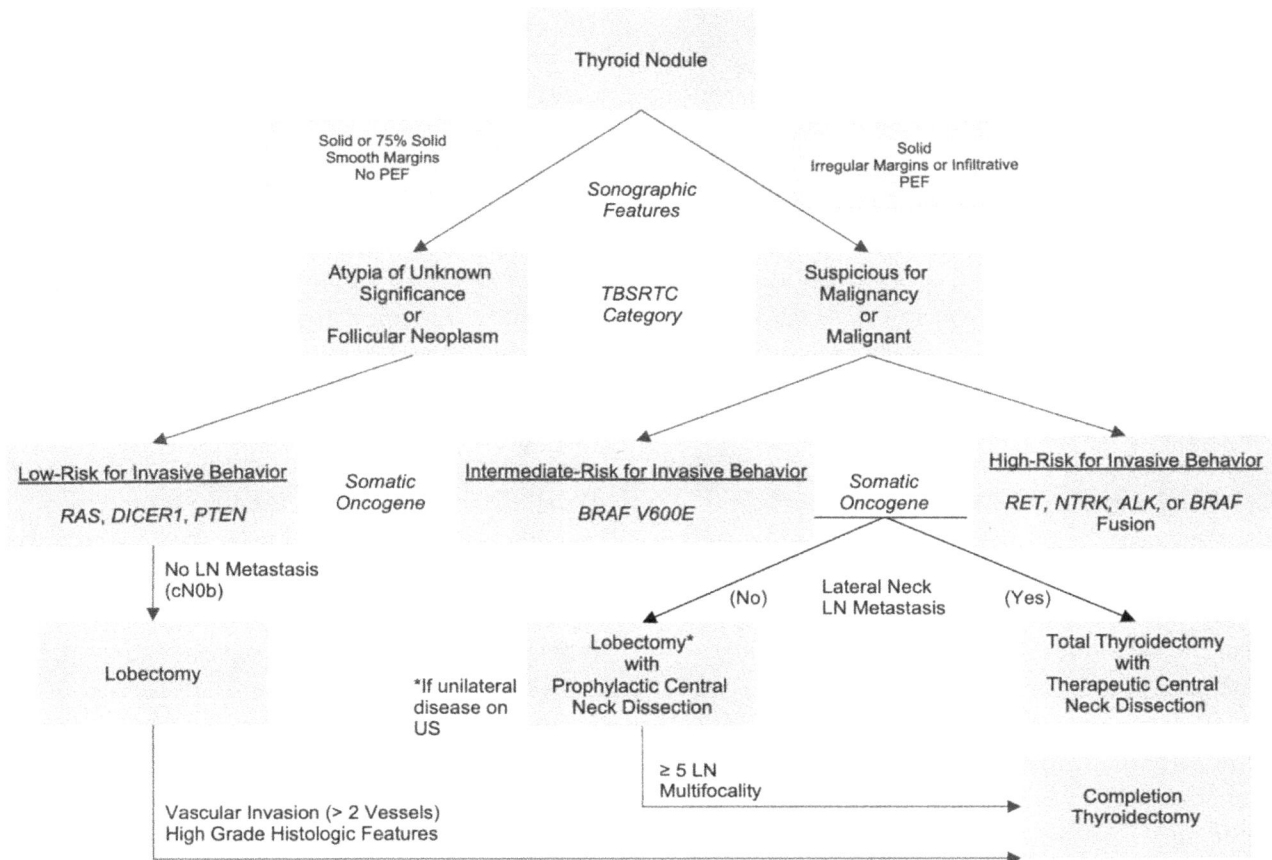

Incorporation of preoperative oncogene data across the 3-tiered pediatric risk of invasive behavior of differentiated thyroid carcinoma to stratify surgical management of a thyroid nodule. High-grade histologic features include solid, trabecular, or insular growth patterns, mitotic index ≥3 per 10 high power fields, necrosis, and convoluted nuclei.

Reprinted from Lai STT & Bauer AJ. JCEM, 2025; Published online ahead of print: 1–14. © The Authors. Published by Oxford University Press on behalf of the Endocrine Society

[Color—Print (Color Gallery page CG22) or web & ePub editions]

Case 2

A 16-year-old previously girl is noted to have a left neck swelling. Thyroid ultrasonography identifies a 4-cm, solid, very hypoechoic infiltrative lesion with wider-than-tall shape, irregular margins, and punctate echogenic foci in the left lobe. Multiple enlarged, round hypoechoic cervical lymph nodes with peripheral blood flow are identified in the right central neck (levels VI and VII). There are no abnormal lymph nodes in the lateral neck (levels 2, 3, 4, or 5). FNA of the thyroid nodule is compatible with TBSRTC category VI (malignant) cytology.

Which of the following is the best surgical option associated with the highest likelihood of remission and lowest risk of potential complications for this patient?

A. Total thyroidectomy

B. Left lobectomy

C. Total thyroidectomy with ipsilateral central neck lymph node dissection

D. Left lobectomy with ipsilateral central neck lymph node dissection

Answer: C) Total thyroidectomy with ipsilateral central neck lymph node dissection

This patient underwent total thyroidectomy with left-sided central neck dissection (Answer C). Pathology revealed a 4.2-cm classic PTC without extrathyroidal extension but with lymphatic invasion, including intrathyroidal psammomatous metastasis in the right lobe (primary tumor in the left lobe). PTC was present in 9 of 25 central lymph nodes. AJCC TNM staging was pT2N1aM0, and she was at pediatric intermediate risk for persistent postinitial surgical disease by American Thyroid Association criteria. A diagnostic whole-body scan revealed residual activity in the thyroid bed; single-photon emission computed tomography (SPECT)/CT was not sensitive enough to determine whether the activity was thyroid remnant and/or residual lymph node metastasis. The patient received ^{131}I therapy (1 mCi/kg) with an excellent response at 1 and 3 years after initial therapy. Although there was no clinical indication for somatic oncogene testing (ie, the patient did not have progressive disease where systemic therapy was being considered), a research-based somatic next-generation sequencing panel was performed and was positive for a *BRAF* V600E pathogenic variant.

The sonographic features of PTC associated with a *BRAF* V600E pathogenic variant and *RET*-like kinase fusion oncogenic alterations are similar, including solid composition, hypoechoic to very hypoechoic echogenicity, irregular margin or infiltrative pattern, increased rate of extrathyroidal extension, and punctate echogenic foci. Central and lateral neck lymphadenopathy are common, so pre-FNA ultrasonography must include sonographic assessment of the central neck (below the thyroid and above the clavicle; levels 6 and 7), as well as the lateral neck (levels 2, 3, 4, and 5) to optimize the surgical plan. Cytology is typically TBSRTC category V or VI. In the presence of bilateral disease and/or lateral neck involvement, total thyroidectomy with therapeutic central neck dissection is warranted with the extent of the lateral neck dissection based on preoperative ultrasonography and FNA confirmation of lateral neck compartment metastasis. Conversely, a more conservative surgical approach with lobectomy and prophylactic central neck dissection may be sufficient to achieve remission in patients with unilateral disease and tumors smaller than 4 cm and without lateral neck lymph node involvement on preoperative ultrasonography. Prophylactic central neck dissection is recommended for all patients harboring a *BRAF* V600E pathogenic variant or *RET*-like fusion oncogenic alteration secondary to the increased risk of central neck lymph node metastasis (thus, Answers A and B are incorrect). In patients who undergo lobectomy as the initial surgical approach, completion thyroidectomy should be considered if histology reveals multifocal disease or 5 or more positive central neck lymph nodes are identified on prophylactic central neck lymph node dissection. Based on the tumor size, total thyroidectomy would be recommended rather than lobectomy (Answer D). Last, the data on tumor size are limited[3] and until additional data are available, lobectomy should only be considered in patients with unifocal tumors smaller than 1 cm with no preoperative evidence of lymph node disease (AJCC N0b).[4]

Case 3

A 12-year-old girl with a history of radiation exposure presents with cervical neck lymphadenopathy. Ultrasonography reveals an infiltrative lesion occupying both lobes with bilateral lateral neck lymph node metastases. FNA is positive for malignancy (TBSRTC category VI) to include a lymph node from both right and left levels 2 and 4. Totally thyroidectomy with central and bilateral lateral dissection is performed. Histology confirms diffuse sclerosing PTC with extensive angioinvasion and lymphatic invasion with 33 of 82 positive lymph nodes (AJCC T3aN1b). A therapeutic dose of RAI is administered, and the posttreatment whole-body scan shows uptake in the neck, lungs, and skull (M1). Over the next 18 months, serial chest CT shows structural progression of diffuse micronodular metastasis, and the patient begins to develop mild shortness of breath during aerobic activities.

Which of the following is the best option for this patient based on the current data?

A. Continued surveillance with serial laboratory tests and imaging every 6 months

B. Repeated ^{131}I therapy

C. Multityrosine kinase inhibitor therapy with lenvatinib

D. Oncogene-specific inhibitor therapy

Answer: D) Oncogene-specific inhibitor therapy

Most pediatric patients with structural PTC lung metastasis do not achieve complete remission (excellent response), even with repeated RAI therapy (Answer B). While many have stable, persistent disease (the PTC metastasis does not progress, remaining present in a dormant state), a percentage of patients develop progressive disease with an increasing number and size of PTC lesions detected on serial, noncontrast chest CT. Structural progression with or without RAI avidity is one of several forms of RAI-refractory disease and may be associated with up to 10% disease-specific mortality in pediatric patients.[2]

Continued surveillance (Answer A) may be considered based on the extent of pulmonary disease, as structural progression occurs slowly (months to years). However, patients may develop signs and symptoms, most commonly during high-effort aerobic activity or associated with an acute respiratory illness. If the somatic oncogene can be identified, oncogene-specific inhibitory therapy (Answer D) is preferred over multityrosine kinase inhibitor therapy (Answer C), as the drugs result in both tumor regression and increased expression of the sodium-iodide symporter, raising the possibility for additional RAI therapy. Compared with multityrosine kinase inhibitors, oncogene-specific inhibitors have a lower adverse effect profile.

For this patient, somatic oncogene testing identified a *NCOA4::RET* alteration (RET/PTC3). Based on these findings, selpercatinib was initiated. Subsequent chest CT showed near-complete structural response after 6 months on systemic therapy. Under a multicenter, prospective protocol, a second treatment with RAI was administered, and selpercatinib was stopped 5 days later. Chest CT 1 year later displayed near-complete structural response in the lungs. While this single case highlights the potential benefit of oncogene-specific inhibitory therapy, prospective, multicenter clinical trials are needed to better define the use of systemic therapy in pediatric patients, including those with RAI-refractory disease and those who present with morbidly invasive regional disease (neoadjuvant therapy).[2]

Key Learning Points

- Over the past 2 decades, significant progress has been made in the understanding the molecular landscape of thyroid neoplasms.

- The incorporation of an integrated, multimodal approach to the evaluation of pediatric thyroid nodules into clinical practice, including the use of somatic oncogene testing, has the potential to improve the diagnostic accuracy and reliability of preoperative evaluation to optimize the surgical approach.

- Knowledge of the somatic oncogene provides opportunities to incorporate oncogene-specific inhibitor therapy both in adjuvant and neoadjuvant settings.

References

1. Lai S-TT, Bauer AJ. Approach to the pediatric patient with thyroid nodules. *J Clin Endocrinol Metab*. 2025 [Online ahead of print]. PMID: 39943817

2. Yang AT, Lai S-TT, Laetsch TW, et al. Molecular landscape and therapeutic strategies in pediatric differentiated thyroid carcinoma. *Endocr Rev*. 2025 [Online ahead of print]. PMID: 39921216

3. Sugino K, Nagahama M, Kitagawa W, et al. Risk stratification of pediatric patients with differentiated thyroid cancer: is total thyroidectomy necessary for patients at any risk? *Thyroid*. 2020;30(4):548-556. PMID: 31910105

4. Sudoko CK, Jenks CM, Bauer AJ, et al. Thyroid lobectomy for T1 papillary thyroid carcinoma in pediatric patients. *JAMA Otolaryngol Head Neck Surg*. 2021;147(11):943-950. PMID: 34554217

ENDO 2025
COLOR GALLERY CONTENTS

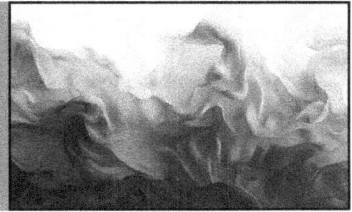

ADIPOSE TISSUE, APPETITE, OBESITY, AND LIPIDS

ADRENAL

BONE AND MINERAL METABOLISM

DIABETES AND VASCULAR DISEASE

GENERAL ENDOCRINOLOGY

NEUROENDOCRINOLOGY AND PITUITARY

PEDIATRIC AND ADOLESCENT ENDOCRINOLOGY

THYROID BIOLOGY AND CANCER

TUMOR BIOLOGY

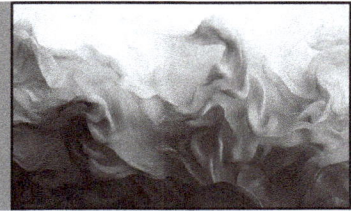

ADIPOSE TISSUE, APPETITE, OBESITY, AND LIPIDS

Weight-Loss Pharmacotherapy in the Spectrum of Obesity Care
José O. Alemán, MD, PhD

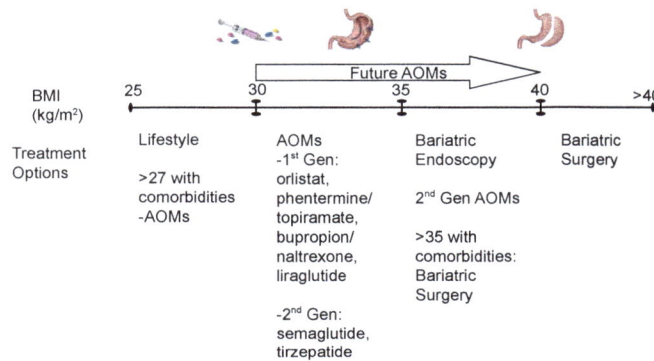

The spectrum of care for obesity by BMI reflects increasing overlap between AOMs and procedures, including bariatric endoscopy and bariatric surgery.

Metabolic Dysfunction-Associated Steatotic Liver Disease: Tips for Endocrinologists
Eveline Bruinstroop, MD, PhD, and A. G. (Onno) Holleboom, MD, PhD

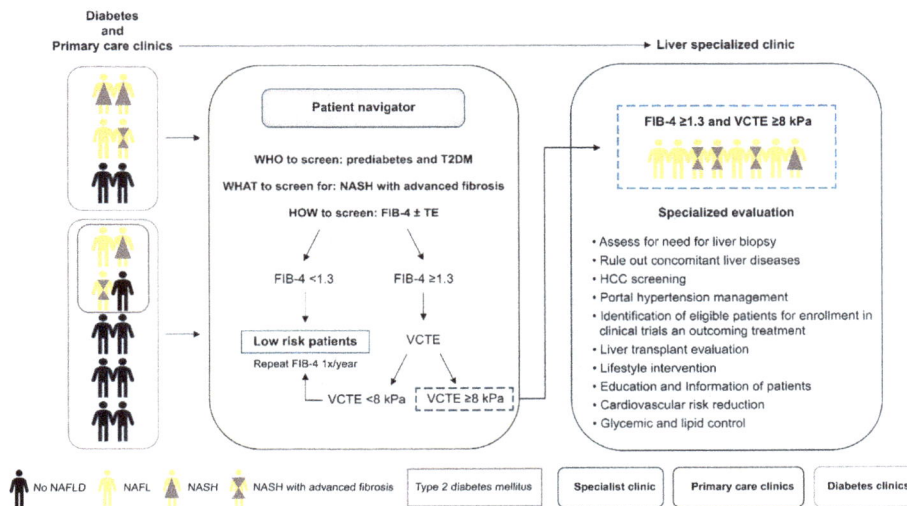

Screening strategy for MASLD, formerly known as nonalcoholic fatty liver disease (NAFLD) and nonalcoholic steatohepatitis (NASH). The strategy is based on a 2-tier testing approach starting with FIB-4 and, when necessary, vibration-controlled transient elastography (VCTE). Patients with high suspicion of advanced fibrosis should be referred to a specialized liver clinic for further evaluation.[10]

Reprinted with permission from Vieira Barbosa J &, Lai M. *Hepatol Commun*, 2020; 5(2): 158-167. © The Authors. Published by Wiley Periodicals LLC on behalf of American Association for the Study of Liver Diseases.

Atypical and Secondary Etiologies of Obesity
Andrew T. Kraftson, MD

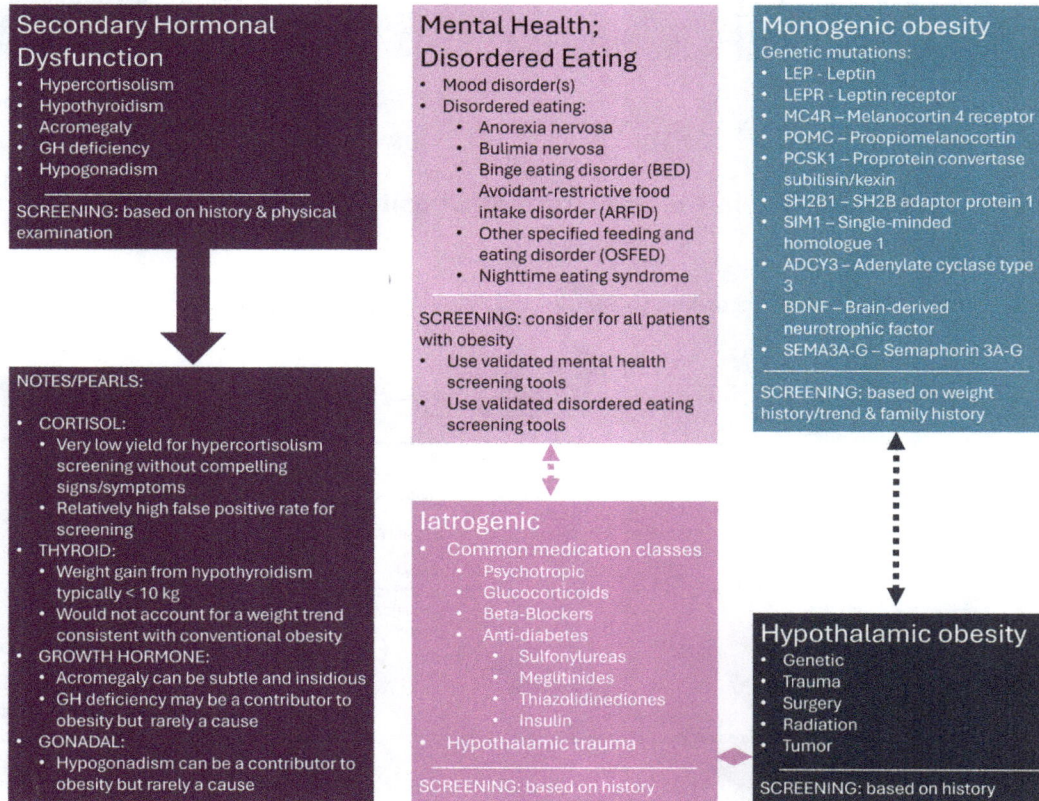

Secondary Hormonal Dysfunction
- Hypercortisolism
- Hypothyroidism
- Acromegaly
- GH deficiency
- Hypogonadism

SCREENING: based on history & physical examination

NOTES/PEARLS:
- CORTISOL:
  - Very low yield for hypercortisolism screening without compelling signs/symptoms
  - Relatively high false positive rate for screening
- THYROID:
  - Weight gain from hypothyroidism typically < 10 kg
  - Would not account for a weight trend consistent with conventional obesity
- GROWTH HORMONE:
  - Acromegaly can be subtle and insidious
  - GH deficiency may be a contributor to obesity but rarely a cause
- GONADAL:
  - Hypogonadism can be a contributor to obesity but rarely a cause

Mental Health; Disordered Eating
- Mood disorder(s)
- Disordered eating:
  - Anorexia nervosa
  - Bulimia nervosa
  - Binge eating disorder (BED)
  - Avoidant-restrictive food intake disorder (ARFID)
  - Other specified feeding and eating disorder (OSFED)
  - Nighttime eating syndrome

SCREENING: consider for all patients with obesity
- Use validated mental health screening tools
- Use validated disordered eating screening tools

Iatrogenic
- Common medication classes
  - Psychotropic
  - Glucocorticoids
  - Beta-Blockers
  - Anti-diabetes
    - Sulfonylureas
    - Meglitinides
    - Thiazolidinediones
    - Insulin
- Hypothalamic trauma

SCREENING: based on history

Monogenic obesity
Genetic mutations:
- LEP - Leptin
- LEPR - Leptin receptor
- MC4R – Melanocortin 4 receptor
- POMC – Proopiomelanocortin
- PCSK1 – Proprotein convertase subilisin/kexin
- SH2B1 – SH2B adaptor protein 1
- SIM1 – Single-minded homologue 1
- ADCY3 – Adenylate cyclase type 3
- BDNF – Brain-derived neurotrophic factor
- SEMA3A-G – Semaphorin 3A-G

SCREENING: based on weight history/trend & family history

Hypothalamic obesity
- Genetic
- Trauma
- Surgery
- Radiation
- Tumor

SCREENING: based on history

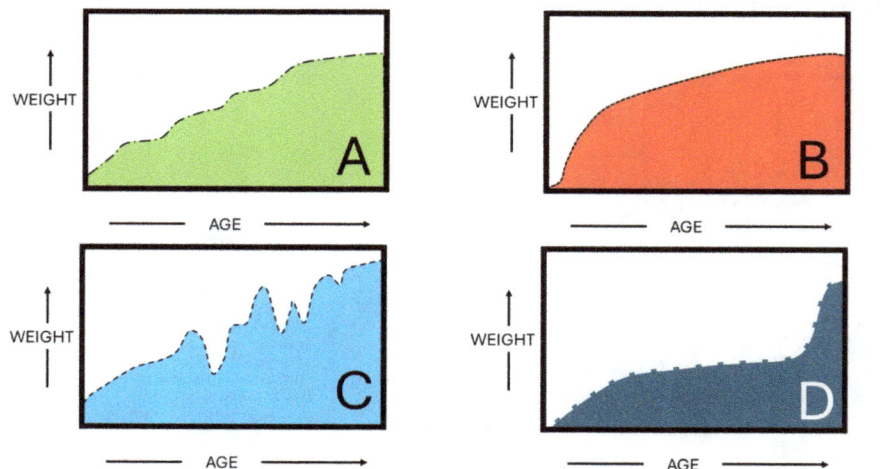

A: gradual weight gain associated with typical, polygenic obesity
B: early-onset, significant obesity associated with monogenic obesity
C: gradual weight gain with repeated weight loss attempts associated with typical obesity
D: sudden onset weight escalation associated with a medical change

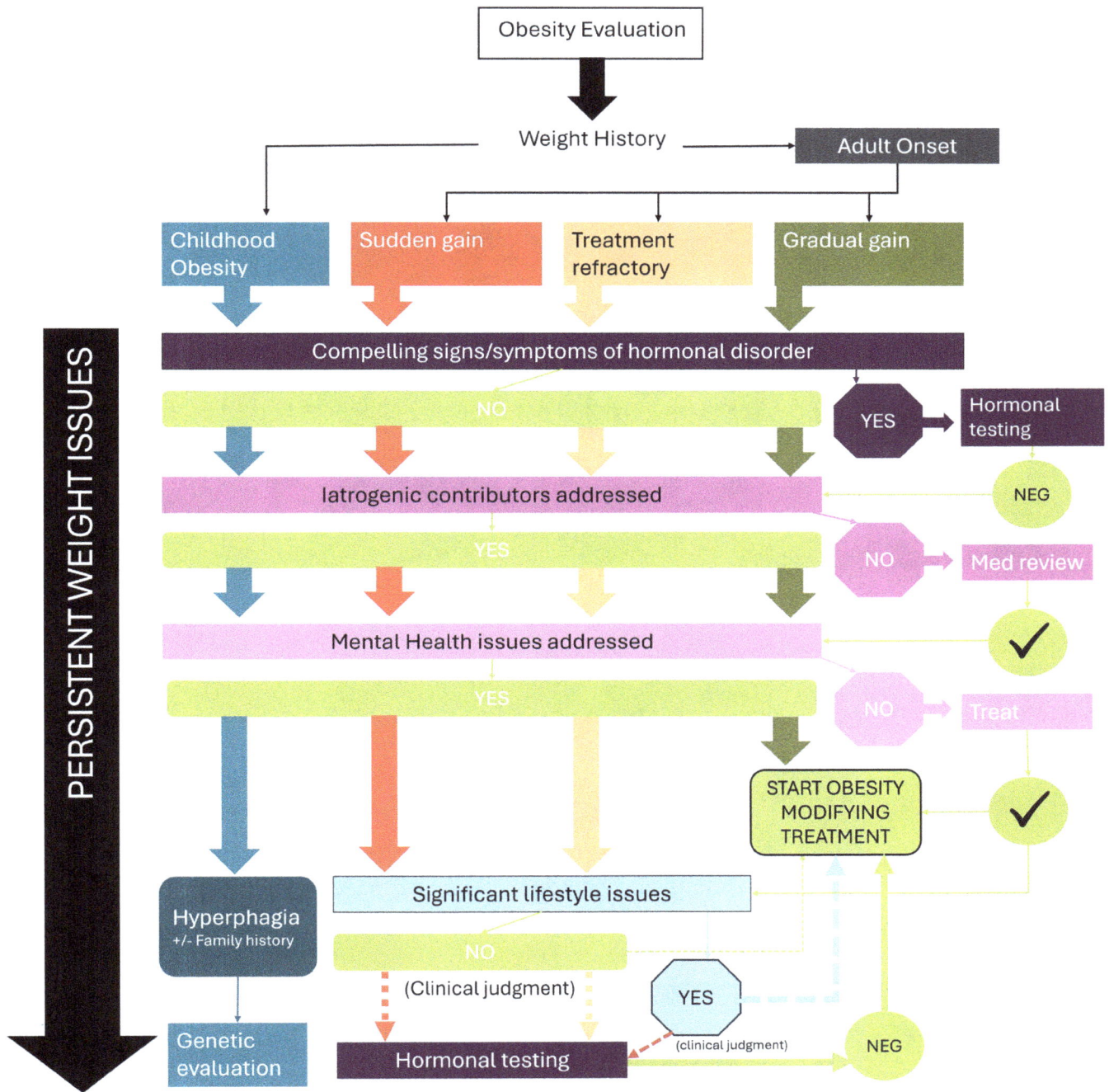

ADRENAL

How to Manage Bilateral Adrenal Masses
Jérôme Bertherat, MD, PhD

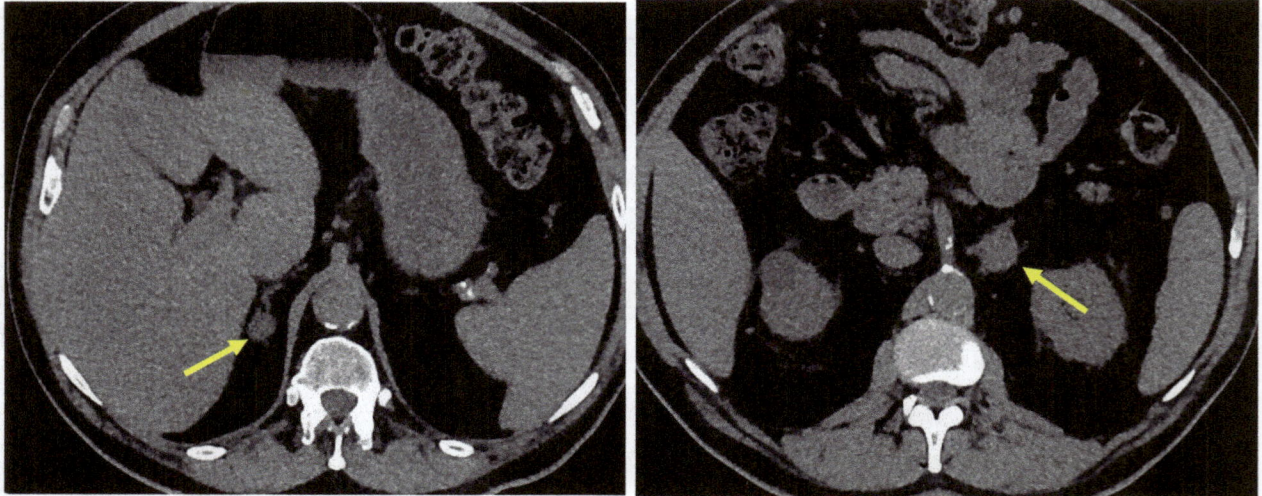

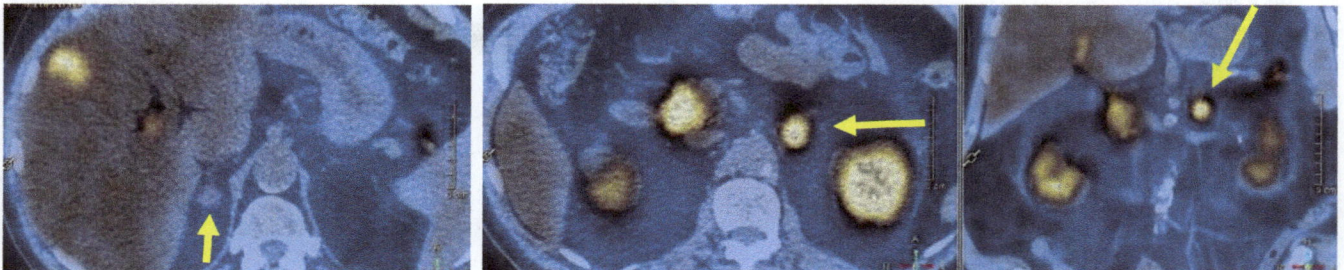

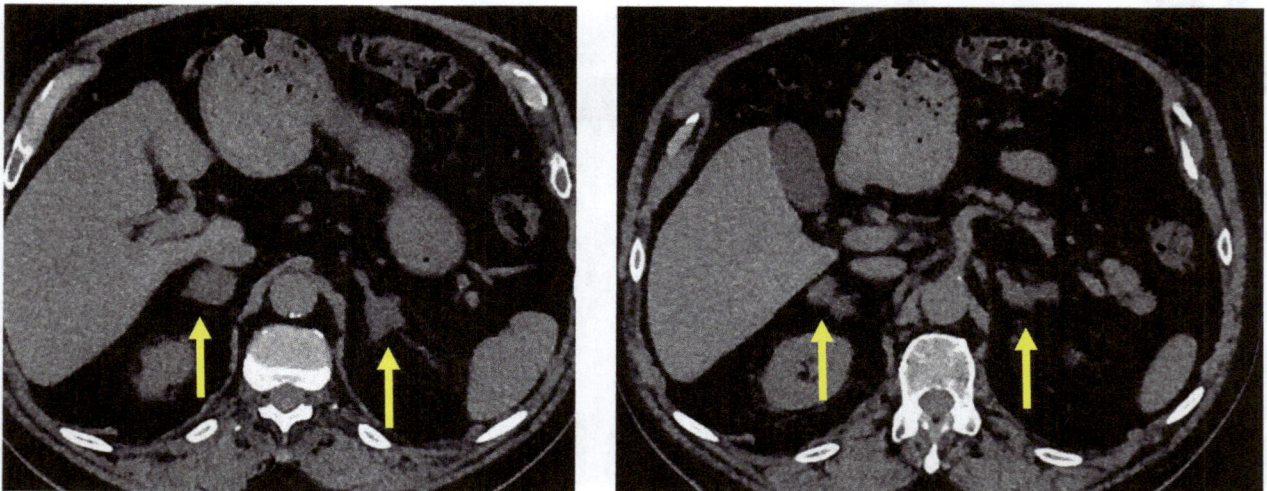

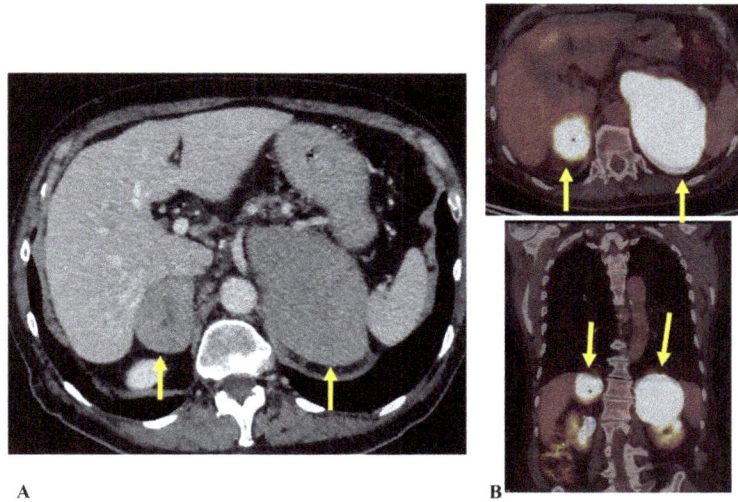

A   B

Evaluation and Management of Postmenopausal Androgen Excess

Michael W. O'Reilly, MD, PhD, and Wiebke Arlt, MD, DSc

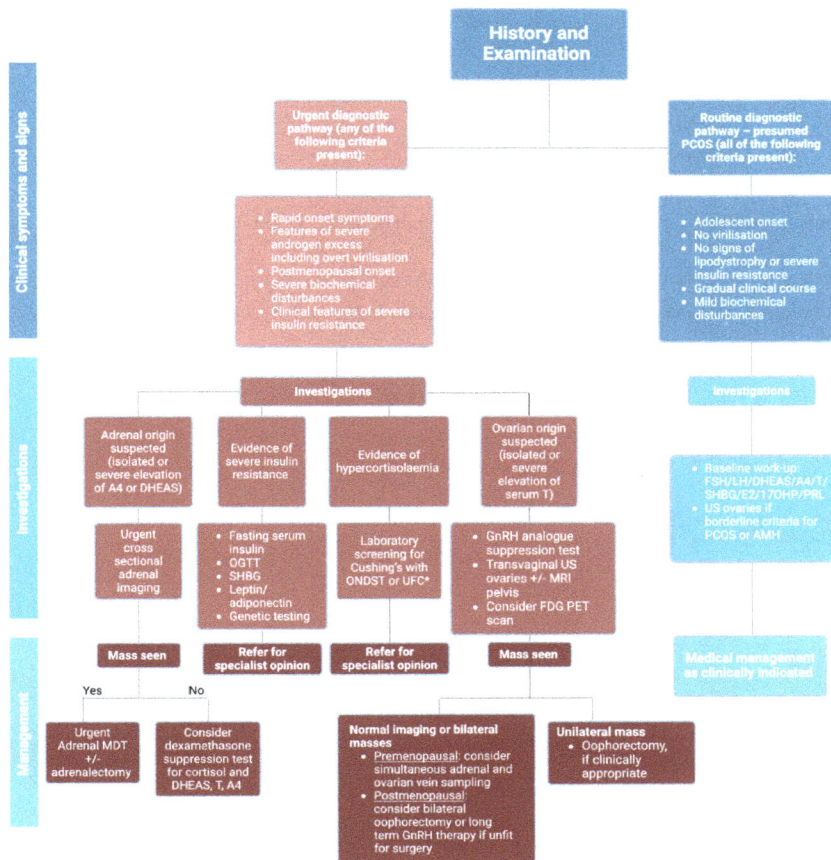

Reprinted from Elhassan YS et al. Clinical Endocrinology, 2025, 1-27. https://doi.org/10.1111/cen.15265 © The Authors. Clinical Endocrinology is published by John Wiley & Sons Ltd.

BONE AND MINERAL METABOLISM

Long-Term Complications of Mild Asymptomatic Primary Hyperparathyroidism: To Treat or Not to Treat?

Ghada El-Hajj Fuleihan, MD, MPH

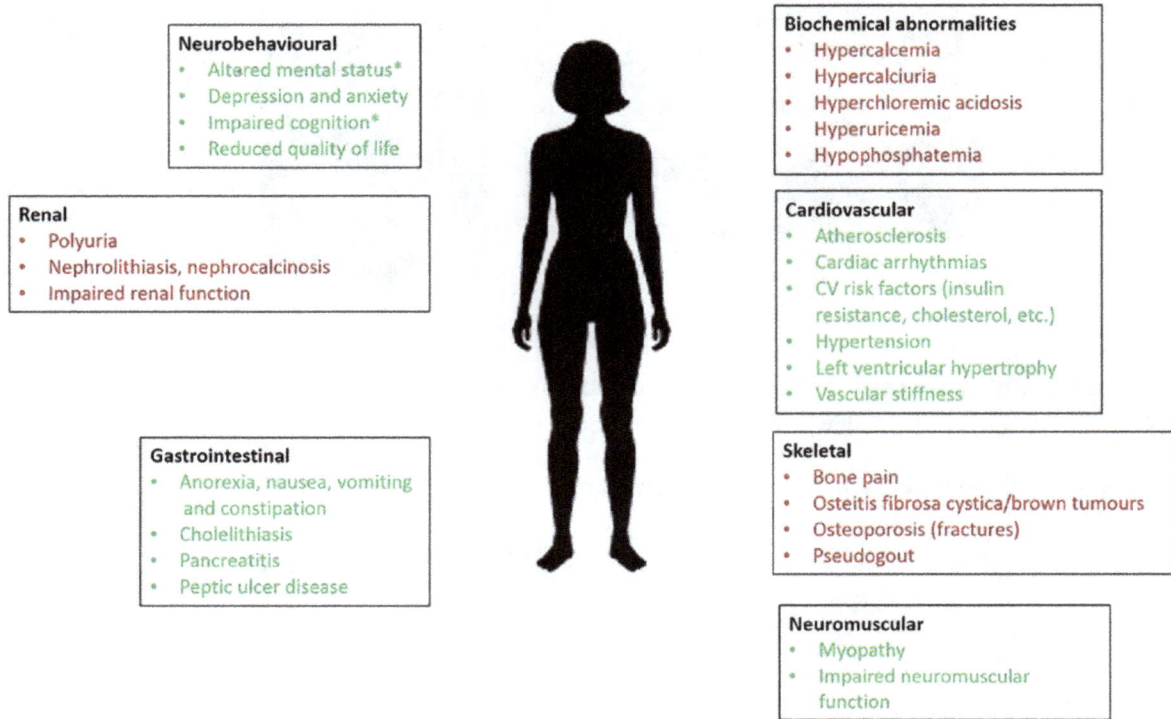

Neurobehavioural
- Altered mental status*
- Depression and anxiety
- Impaired cognition*
- Reduced quality of life

Renal
- Polyuria
- Nephrolithiasis, nephrocalcinosis
- Impaired renal function

Gastrointestinal
- Anorexia, nausea, vomiting and constipation
- Cholelithiasis
- Pancreatitis
- Peptic ulcer disease

Biochemical abnormalities
- Hypercalcemia
- Hypercalciuria
- Hyperchloremic acidosis
- Hyperuricemia
- Hypophosphatemia

Cardiovascular
- Atherosclerosis
- Cardiac arrhythmias
- CV risk factors (insulin resistance, cholesterol, etc.)
- Hypertension
- Left ventricular hypertrophy
- Vascular stiffness

Skeletal
- Bone pain
- Osteitis fibrosa cystica/brown tumours
- Osteoporosis (fractures)
- Pseudogout

Neuromuscular
- Myopathy
- Impaired neuromuscular function

Symptoms and complications depend on disease severity. Causality is implied from evidence by reversal with surgery or from mechanistic studies. Causal in is red, and association in green.

*Moderate to severe hypercalcemia may cause changes in mental status or cognitive function that are often reversible with correction of the serum calcium.

Reprinted from El-Hajj Fuleihan G et al. J Bone Miner Res, 2022; 37(11): 2330-2350. © The Authors. Published by Wiley Periodicals LLC on behalf of American Society for Bone and Mineral Research

Complex Cases in Hypophosphatemia: Navigating Diagnostic and Treatment Challenges of Low Phosphate

Eva S. Liu, MD

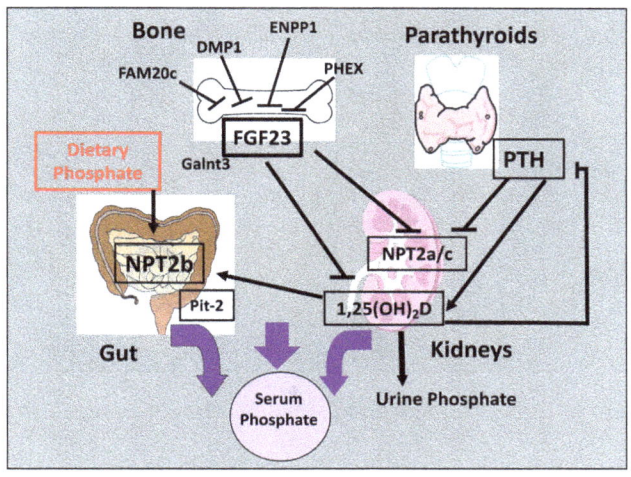

Dietary phosphate is absorbed in the gut by sodium phosphate transporter (NPT) 2b (NPT2b) and filtered by the kidneys. In the small intestine, phosphate transport is predominantly regulated by NPT2b. 1,25-dihydroxyvitamin D (1,25[OH]$_2$D) increases Pit-2 expression in the small intestine, which also leads to phosphate absorption. PTH binds to the PTHR1 to reduce NPT2a and NPT2c protein levels, resulting increased renal loss of phosphate. FGF-23 is predominantly expressed in bone and binds to the FGFR with α-Klotho (KL) as coreceptor in the kidneys. Urinary phosphate excretion increases with decreased renal proximal tubule expression of NPT2a and NPT2c. FGF-23 also stimulates 24-hydroxlase expression, and it reduces 1α-hydroxylase. The combined net effects of the actions of FGF-23 in the proximal renal tubules are decreased serum levels of phosphate and 1,25-(OH)$_2$D. FGF-23 expression is reduced by *PHEX, DMP1, ENPP1,* and *FAM20C.* Consequently, lack of these negative regulators leads to increased secretion of biologically active FGF-23, resulting in hypophosphatemia. GALNT3 glycosylates and thus stabilizes FGF-23; lack of this enzyme enhances FGF-23 degradation, thereby reducing urinary phosphate excretion.

Reprinted from Liu ES and Juppner H "Chapter 20: Disorders of Phosphate Homeostasis" in Radovich S and Misra M, Eds. *Pediatric Endocrinology,* 4th Edition: Springer 2024; 499-526.

DIABETES AND VASCULAR DISEASE

Monitoring Diabetes Control Using Hemoglobin A$_{1c}$ and Continuous Glucose Monitoring: Advantages and Pitfalls

Shichun Bao, MD, PhD

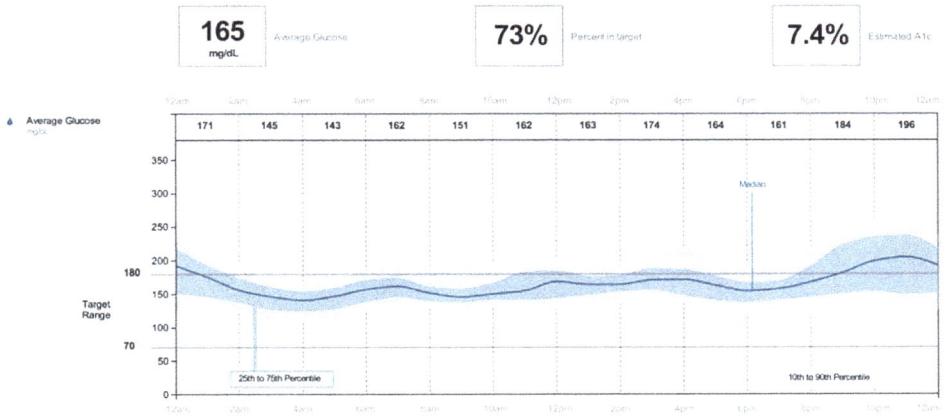

LibreView daily patterns report shows ambulatory glucose profile with average sensor glucose of 165 mg/dL (9.2 mmol/L), 73% readings within the target range of 70 to 180 mg/dL (3.9-10.0 mmol/L), and an estimated HbA$_{1c}$ of 7.4% (57 mmol/mol). Dark and light shading shows 25th-75th and 10th-90th percentiles, respectively.

Integrating Quality Improvement into Inpatient Diabetes Care
Sonali Thosani, MD

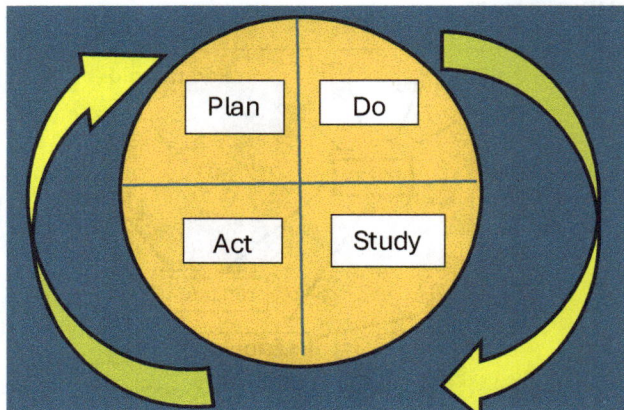

Reprinted from Barr E. & Brannan, GD. Quality Improvement Methods (LEAN, PDSA, SIX SIGMA), in *StatPearls*. 2025: Treasure Island (FL). © StatPearls Publishing LLC.

GENERAL ENDOCRINOLOGY

Complications of Novel Nonimmunotherapy Cancer Treatments
Afreen Shariff, MD, and Randol Kennedy, MD

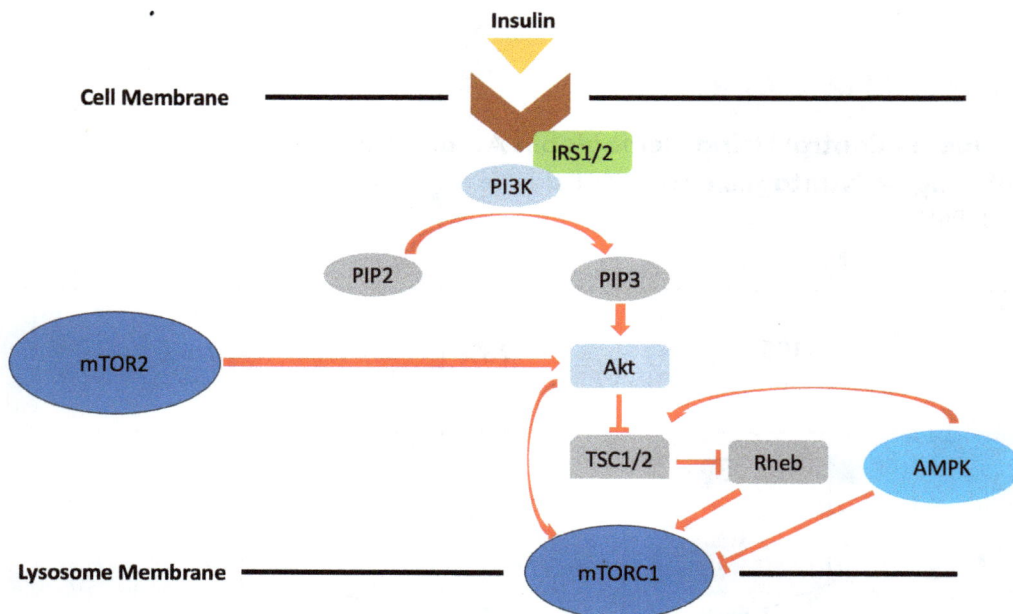

Insulin binding initiates autophosphorylation and activation of the tyrosine kinase component of the β domain. The activated tyrosine kinase phosphorylates IRS1, which, when triggered, activates PI3K that generates PIP3 from PIP2. PIP3 phosphorylates Akt/protein kinase B, which when activated, either indirectly affects mTORC1 through TSC2 or directly through PRAS40 (proline-rich Akt substrate of 40 kDa), leads to regulation of cellular metabolism and growth/proliferation. Activation is shown by arrowhead lines, whereas inhibition is indicated by 'T'-shaped lines. Abbreviations: AMPK, AMP-activated protein kinase; IRS1/2, insulin receptor substrate 1 and 2; mTORC1/2, mechanistic target of rapamycin complex 1 and 2; PI3K, phosphatidylinositide-3 kinase; PIP2, phosphatidylinositol 4,5-bisphosphate; PIP3, phosphatidylinositol 3,4,5-triphosphate; Rheb, Ras homolog enriched in brain; TSC1/2, tuberous sclerosis protein complex 1 and 2.

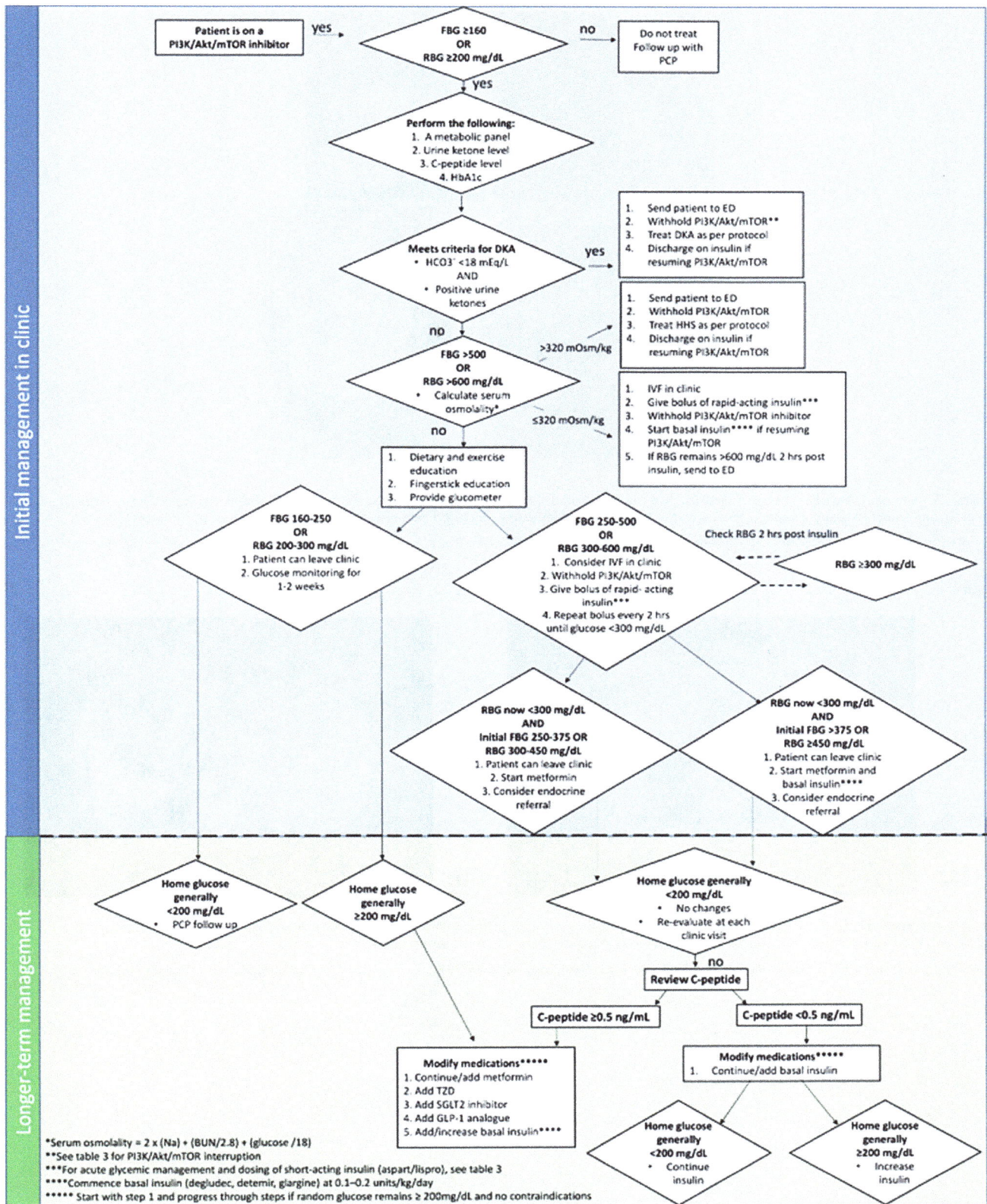

Abbreviations: DKA, diabetic ketoacidosis; ED, emergency department; eGFR, glomerular filtration rate; HCO3, bicarbonate; HHS, hyperglycemic hyperosmolar syndrome; IVF, intravenous fluids; MF, metformin; PCP, primary care provider; Na, serum sodium; TZD, thiazolidinediones; BUN, serum urea nitrogen.[6]

Reprinted from Cheung YM et al. *Curr Probl Cancer*, 2022; 46(1): 100776. © Elsevier Inc.

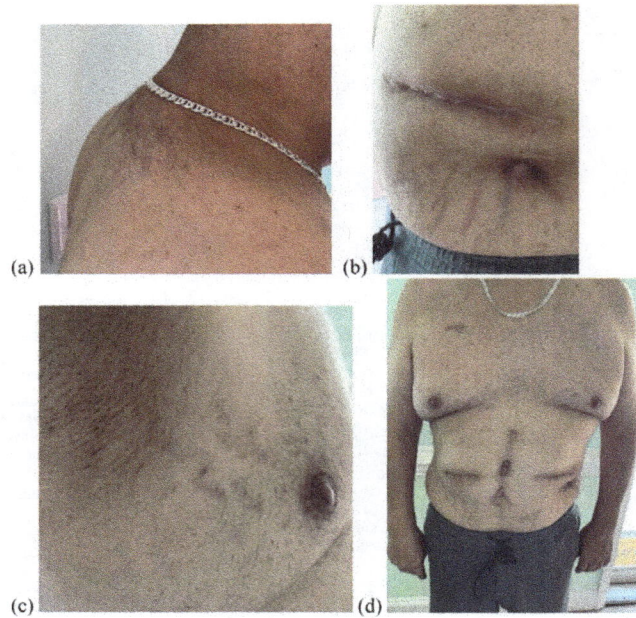

Physical exam findings include a dorsocervical fat pad ("buffalo hump") (*Panel A*), purple abdominal striae on the abdomen (*Panel B*) and under the armpit (*Panel C*), and truncal obesity 2 years after starting HIAP with dexamethasone, pictured here roughly 30 months after therapy initiation.[25]

Reprinted from Ferreira MS & Shariff AI. *Current Problems in Cancer: Case Reports*, 2022; 7(1): 100177. © The Authors. Published by Elsevier Inc.

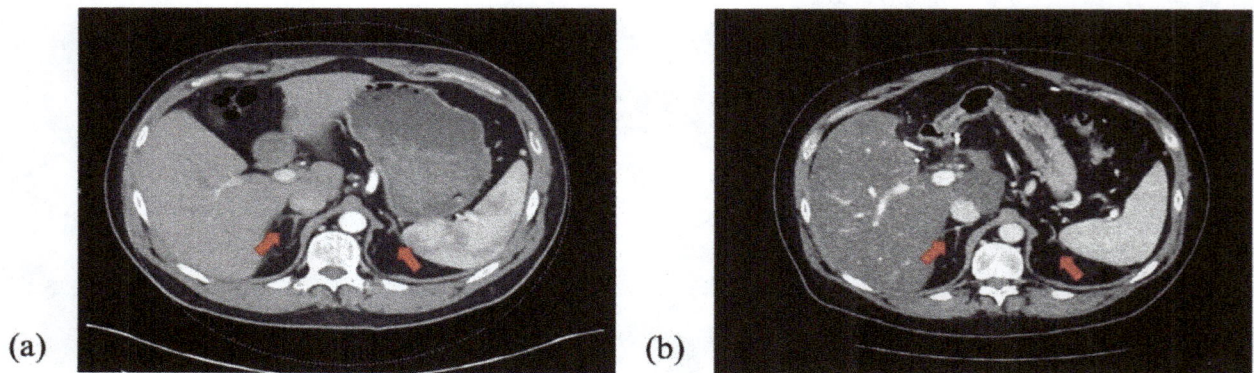

Contrast-enhanced abdominal CT of normal adrenal glands before initiation of floxuridine (FUDR) via HIAP (*Panel A*), and significant adrenal atrophy approximately 64 weeks after receiving 20 mg HIAP dexamethasone every 2 to 3 weeks (*Panel B*).

Reprinted from Ferreira MS & Shariff AI. *Current Problems in Cancer: Case Reports*, 2022; 7(1): 100177. © The Authors. Published by Elsevier Inc.

Challenging Cases of Hyponatremia
Mirjam Christ-Crain, MD

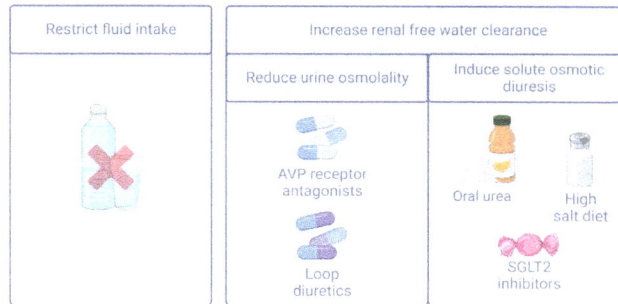

Management of Pituitary Tumors During Pregnancy
Andrea Glezer, MD, PhD

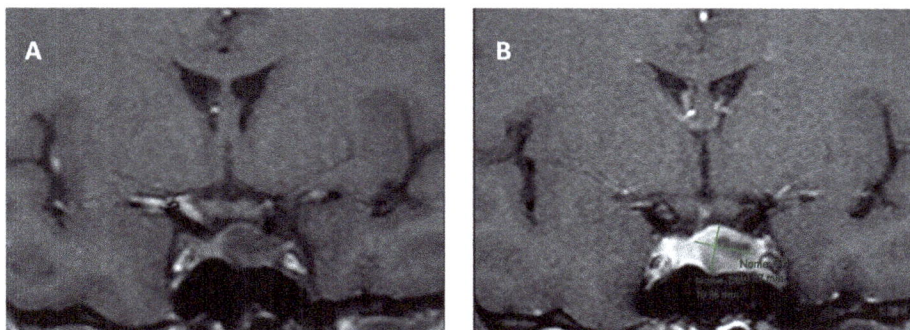

Sellar MRI, T1 coronal views, without contrast (*Panel A*) and with contrast (*Panel B*), showing a pituitary macroadenoma on the left with suprasellar expansion, not reaching the optical chiasma and in contact with the left cavernous sinus.

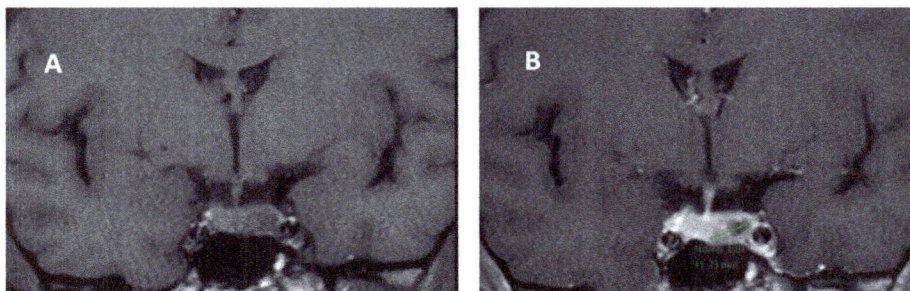

Sellar MRI, T1 coronal views without contrast (*Panel A*) and with contrast (*Panel B*), showing reduction of tumor dimensions and no suprasellar expansion.

Craniopharyngiomas in Adults: Modern Management and Changes in the Paradigm

Emmanuel Jouanneau, MD, PhD, and Gerald Raverot, MD, PhD

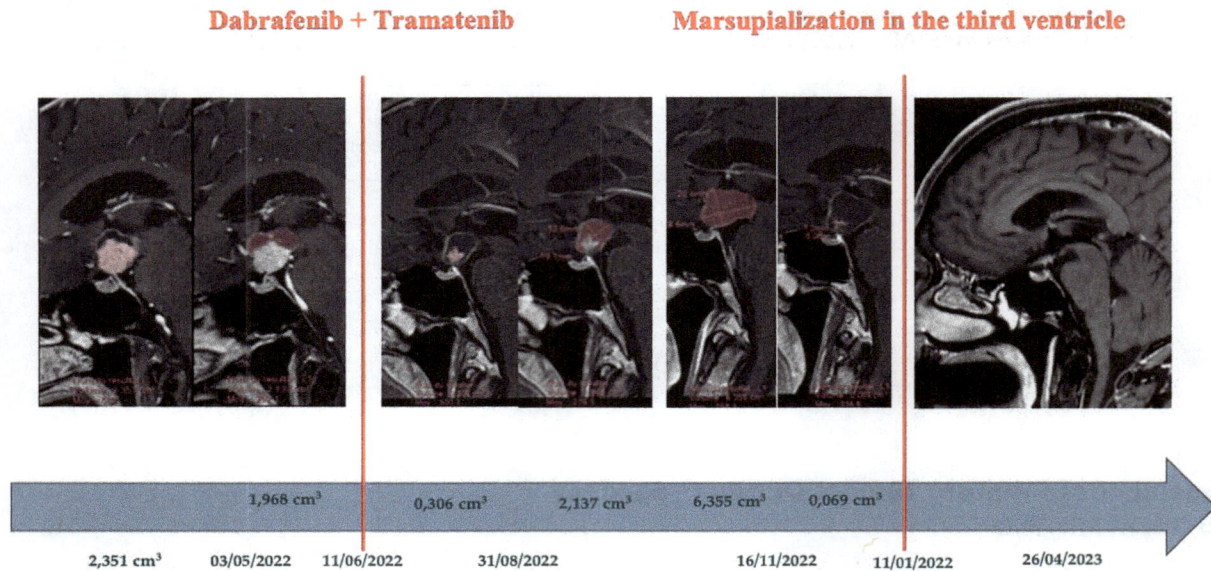

Reprinted from De Rosa A et al. *Annales d'Endocrinologie*, 2023; 84(6):727–733. © Elsevier Masson SAS.

Perioperative Management of Pituitary Tumors

Whitney W. Woodmansee, MD, MA

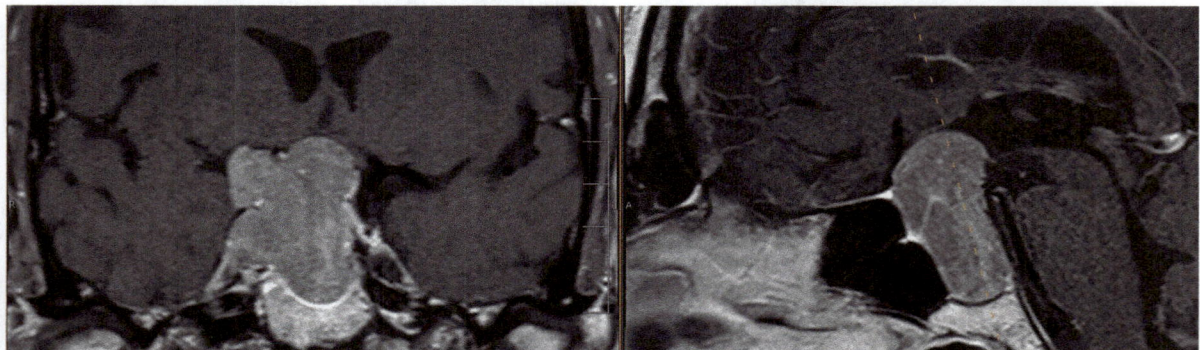

T1 postcontrast MRI demonstrating a large lobulated sellar mass invading the right cavernous sinus and compressing the optic chiasm.

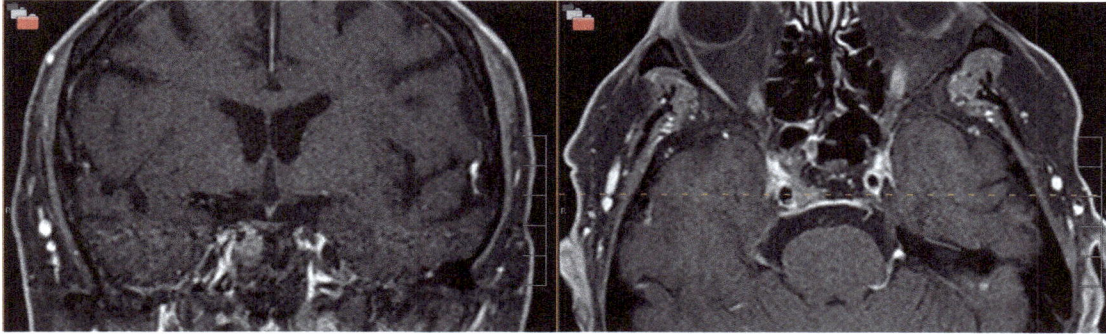

T1 postcontrast MRI demonstrating recurrent tumor invading the right cavernous sinus.

PEDIATRIC AND ADOLESCENT ENDOCRINOLOGY

How to Approach Children With Short Stature Not Responding to Growth Hormone Treatment
Stefano Cianfarani, MD

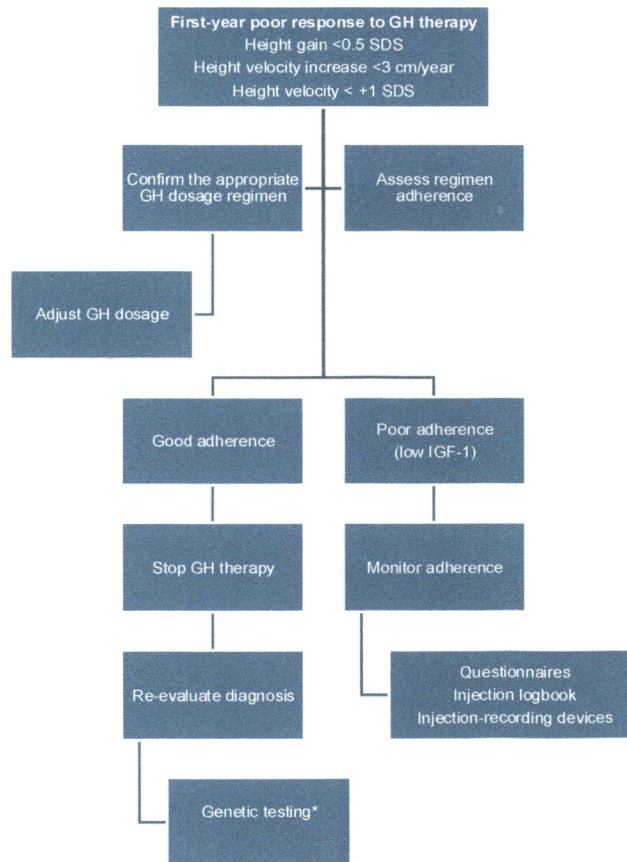

* Genetic testing includes karyotype analysis, comparative genomic hybridization array, single-nucleotide polymorphism array, whole-exome sequencing, whole-genome sequencing, and DNA methylation analysis.[21] More than one-third of children diagnosed as being small-for-gestational age or having idiopathic short stature have pathogenic variants, mainly in genes involved in growth cartilage physiology, such as ACAN, COL2A1, FBN1, FGFR3, IHH, NPPC, NPR2, and SHOX.[14,22,23] Some polymorphisms located in GHR, IGFBP3, and SOCS2 reduce responsiveness to GH treatment.[24]

Update on the Management of Nonhereditary Medullary Thyroid Carcinoma

Rossella Elisei, MD

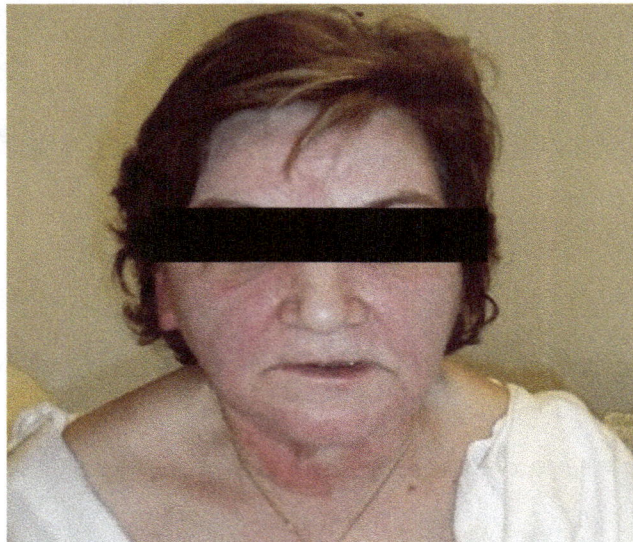

Patient with advanced MTC and flushing syndrome.

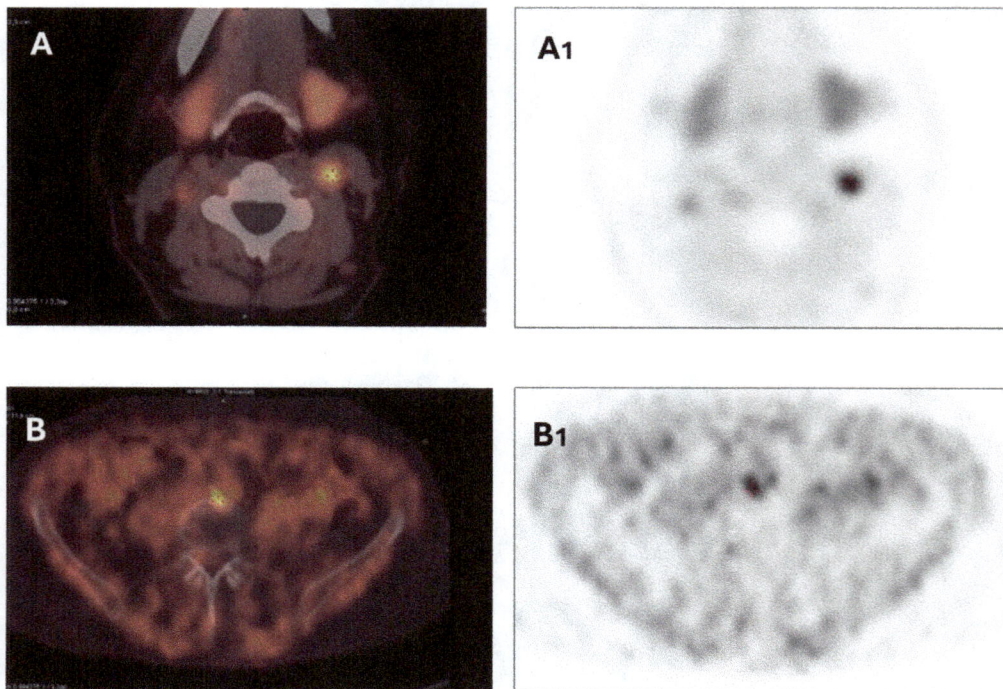

[18]DOPA PET showing a left latero-cervical lymph node (*Panel A*) and lesion in the anterior border of L4 (*Panel B*) and their CT coregistrations (*Panels A1 and B1*). Neither lesion had been previously identified on other imaging.

Oncocytic Thyroid Cancer

Ian Ganly, MD, MS, PhD

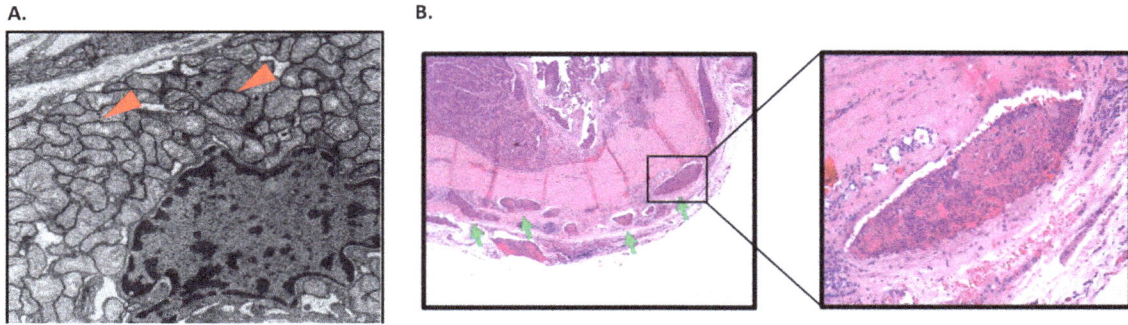

Panel A, Electron microscopy showing nucleus of cell surrounded by abundant mitochondria. Panel B, Hematoxylin and eosin slide showing vascular invasion in vessels surrounding a widely invasive OTC.

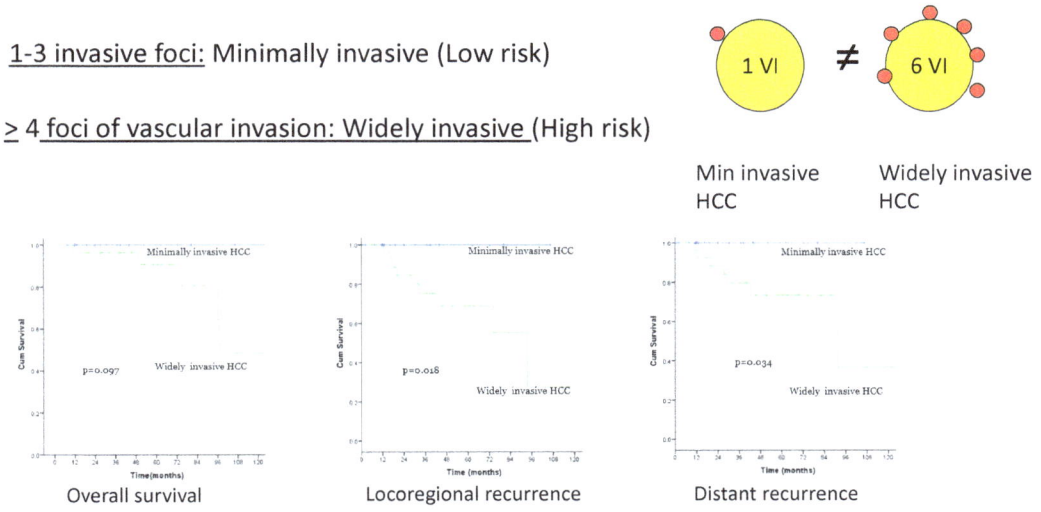

Panel A, Classification of OTC into minimally invasive and widely invasive by extent of vascular invasion. Panel B, Outcomes stratified by extent of vascular invasion showing poorer outcome with widely invasive carcinoma.

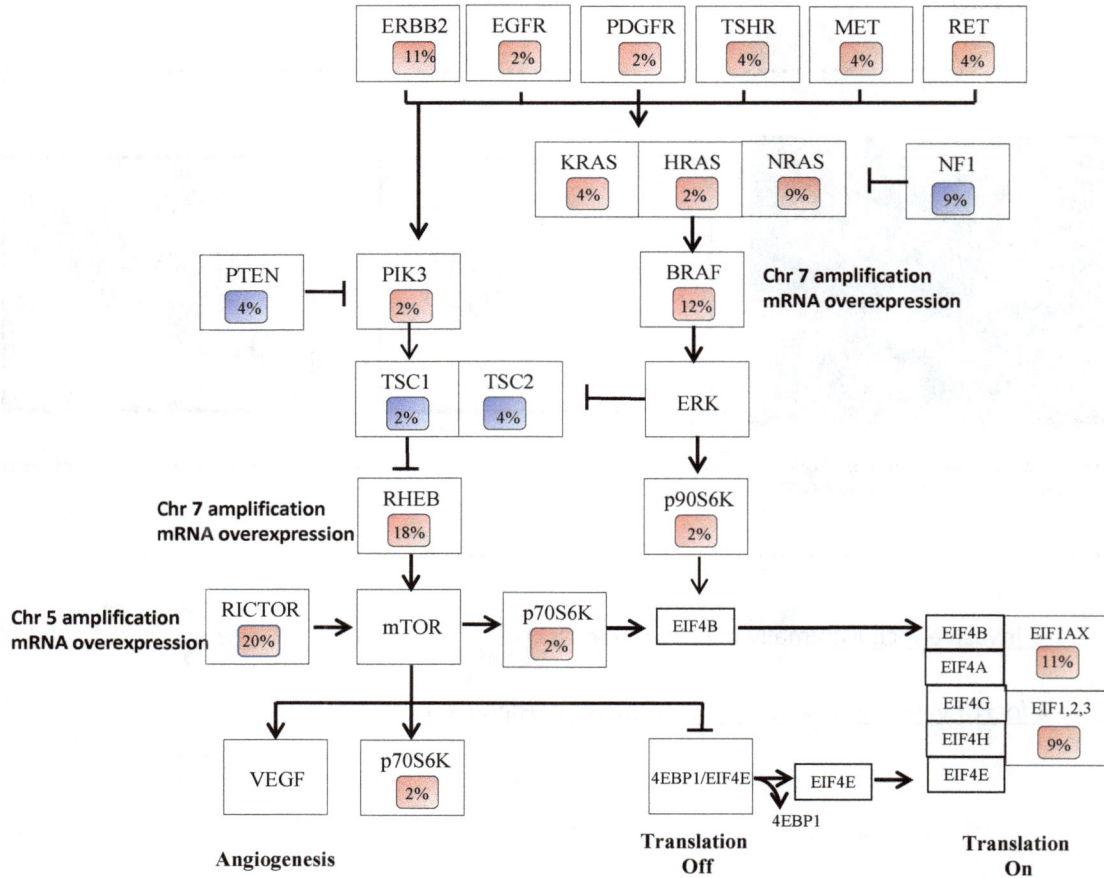

RTK/PIK3/RAS Pathway showing alterations in 60% of cancers

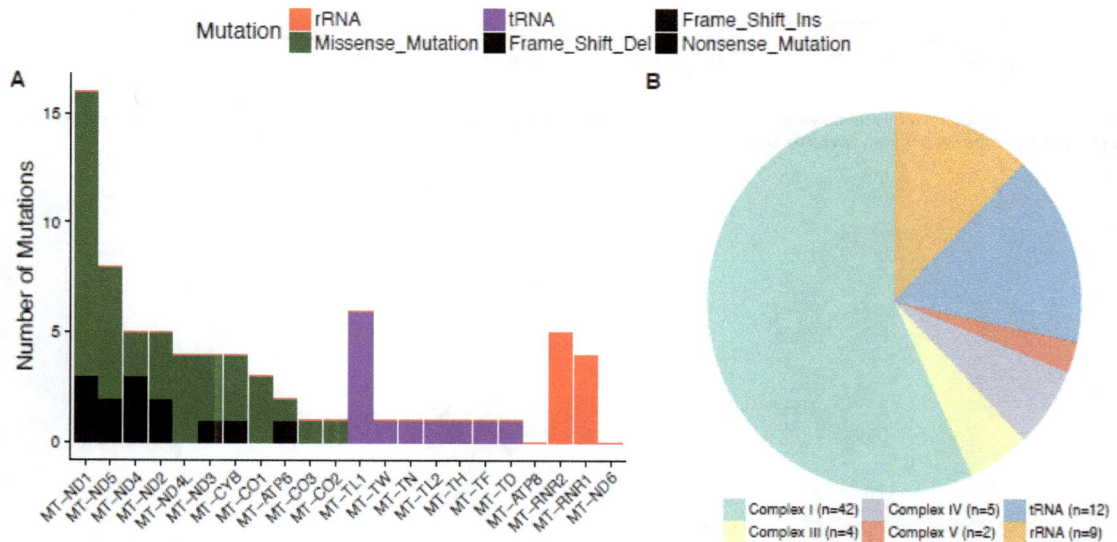

Panel A, Types of mitochondrial pathogenic variants observed in 56 OTCs.[2] *Panel B*, Mitochondrial variants categorized by electron transport complexes.

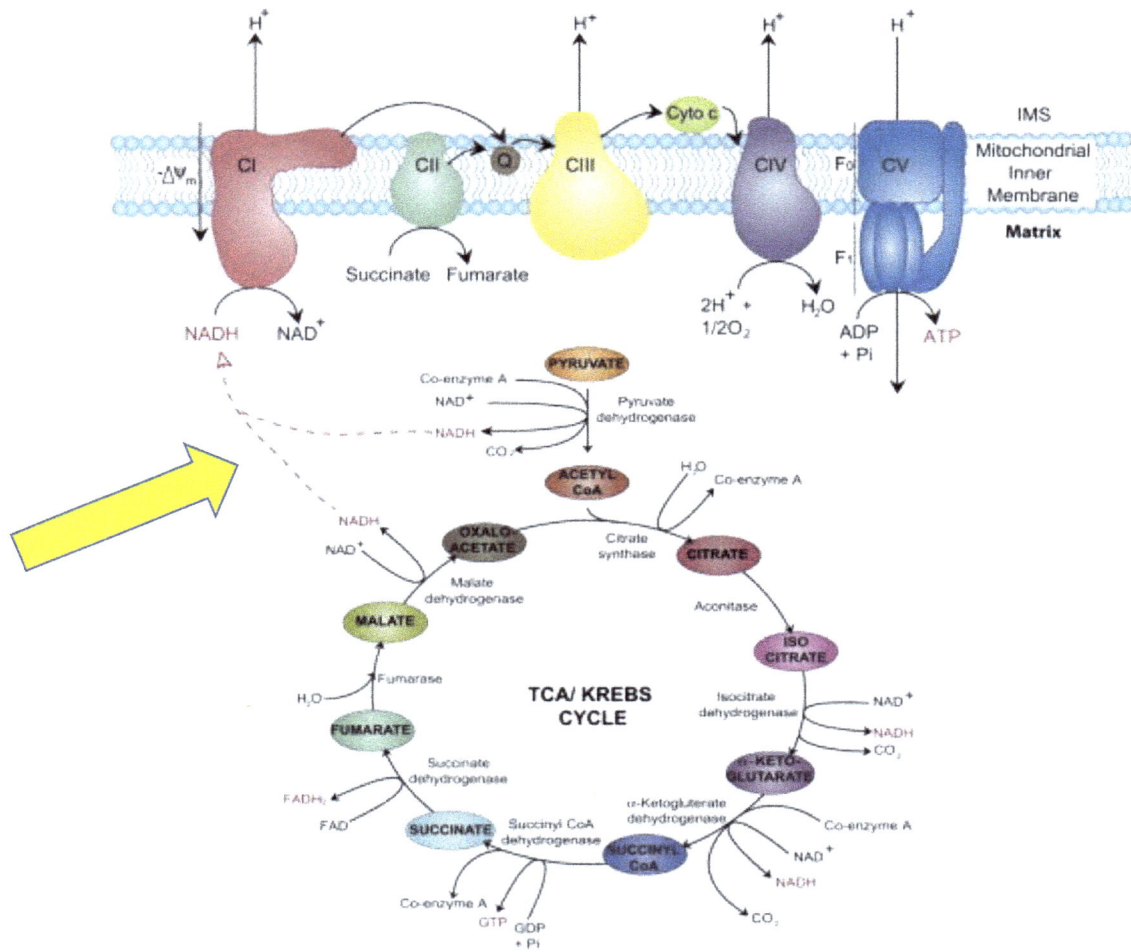

Electron transport chain showing interaction of complexes with Krebs cycle. The arrow indicates complex I is the first site of electron transport chain. Pathogenic variants in complex I disrupt electron transport chain, which in turn disrupts the TCA cycle.

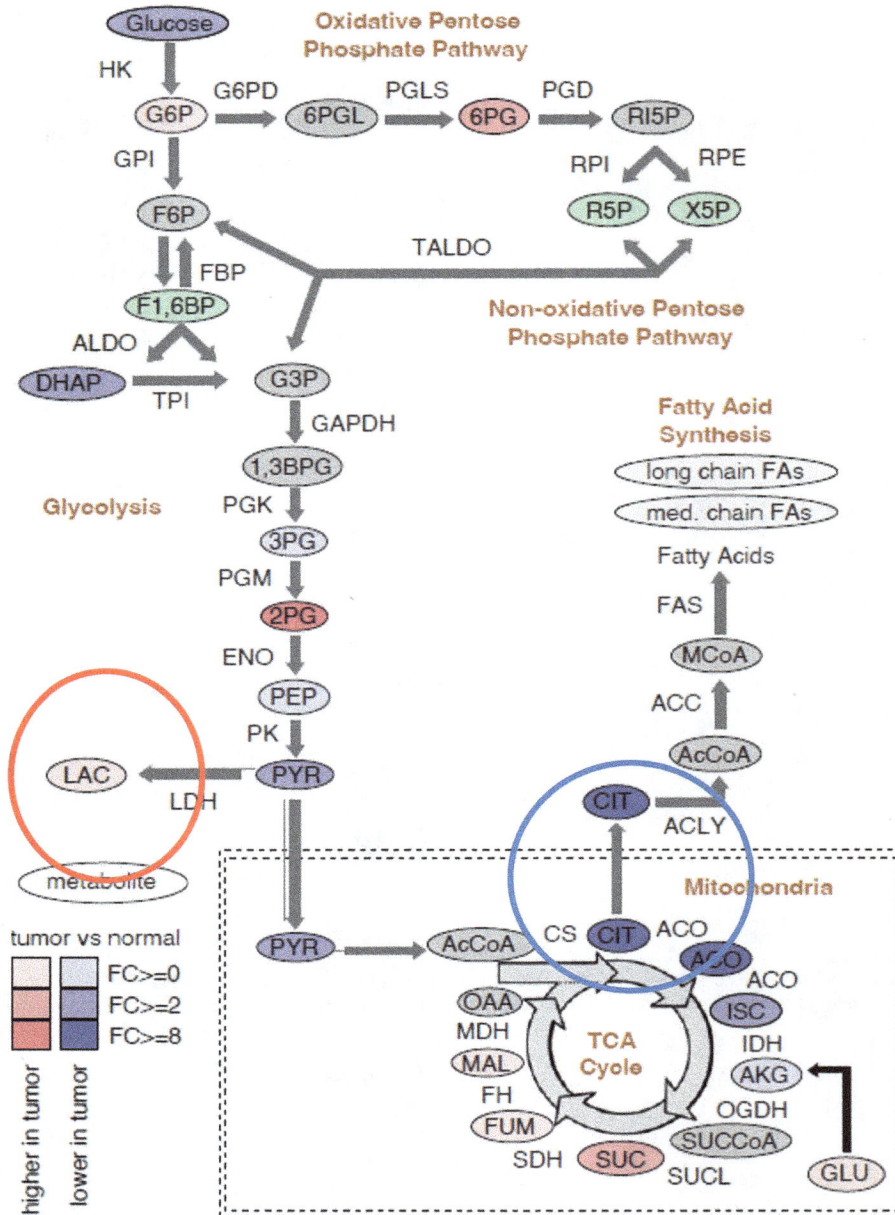

Metabolic alterations in 40 OTCs. Metabolites with less abundance to normal are shown in *blue* and those greater than normal are shown in *red*. The *blue* circle indicates the large decrease in citrate in the TCA cycle. The red circle indicates the increase in lactate due to increased aerobic glycolysis.

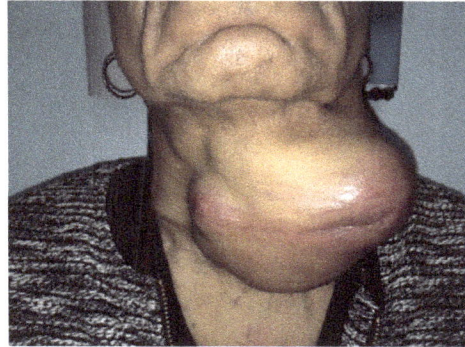

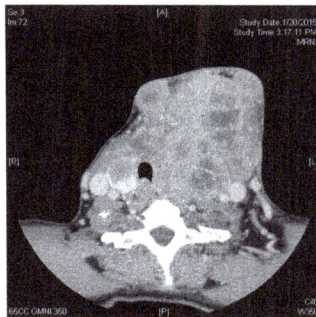
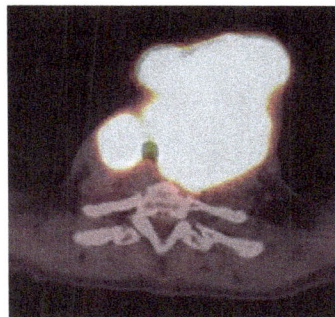
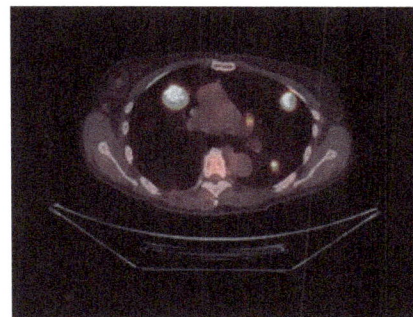

CT neck   PET/CT neck   PET/CT lung metastases

OTCs are hypermetabolic on FDG PET due to increased aerobic glycolysis. Imaging shows a large left thyroid lobe mass on CT and PET. The patient has multiple hypermetabolic lung metastases.

Figure 8. 298

A.

Haploid phenotype

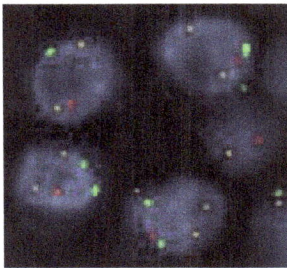

Chr 2 haploid (1 copy arrowed)
Chr 5 diploid
Chr 7 diploid

B.

Polysomic phenotype

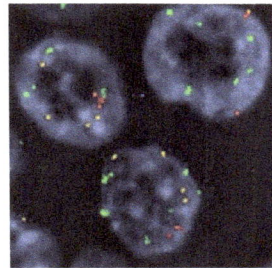

Chr 2 diploid
Chr 5 WCD (4 copies per cell)
Chr 7 WCD (>4 copies per cell)

C.

Global LOH

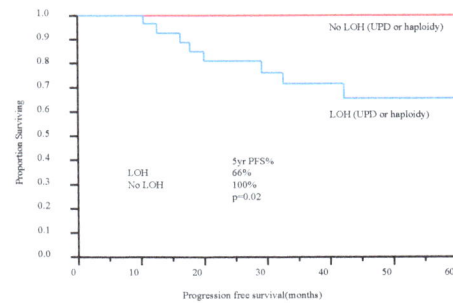

•chr2   •chr5   •chr7

Panel A, Fluorescent in situ hybridization (FISH) staining of a haploid cancer showing 1 copy of chromosome 2 and 2 copies of chromosome 5 and 7. Panel B, FISH staining of a polysomic cancer showing 2 copies of chromosome 2 and 4 copies of chromosome 5 and 7. Panel C, Loss of chromosomes results in a global loss of heterozygosity (LOH). Cancers with global LOH have a poorer outcome as shown by the Kaplan Meier plot.

A.

B.

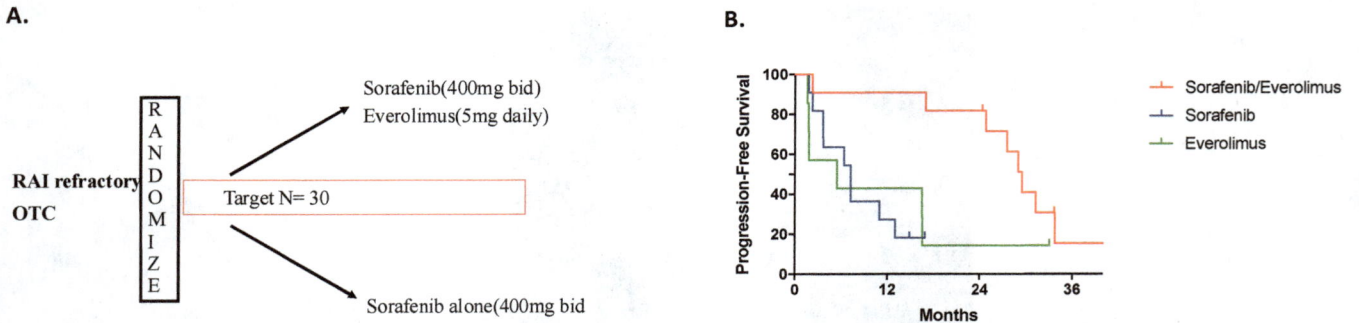

Panel A, Clinical phase 2 trial of patients with RAI-refractory OTC randomly assigning patients to sorafenib alone vs sorafenib/everolimus. Panel B, Patients treated with sorafenib/everolimus had increased progression-free survival.

TUMOR BIOLOGY

Landscape of Genetic Alterations in Well-Differentiated Thyroid Cancer in Pediatric Patients
Andrew J. Bauer, MD

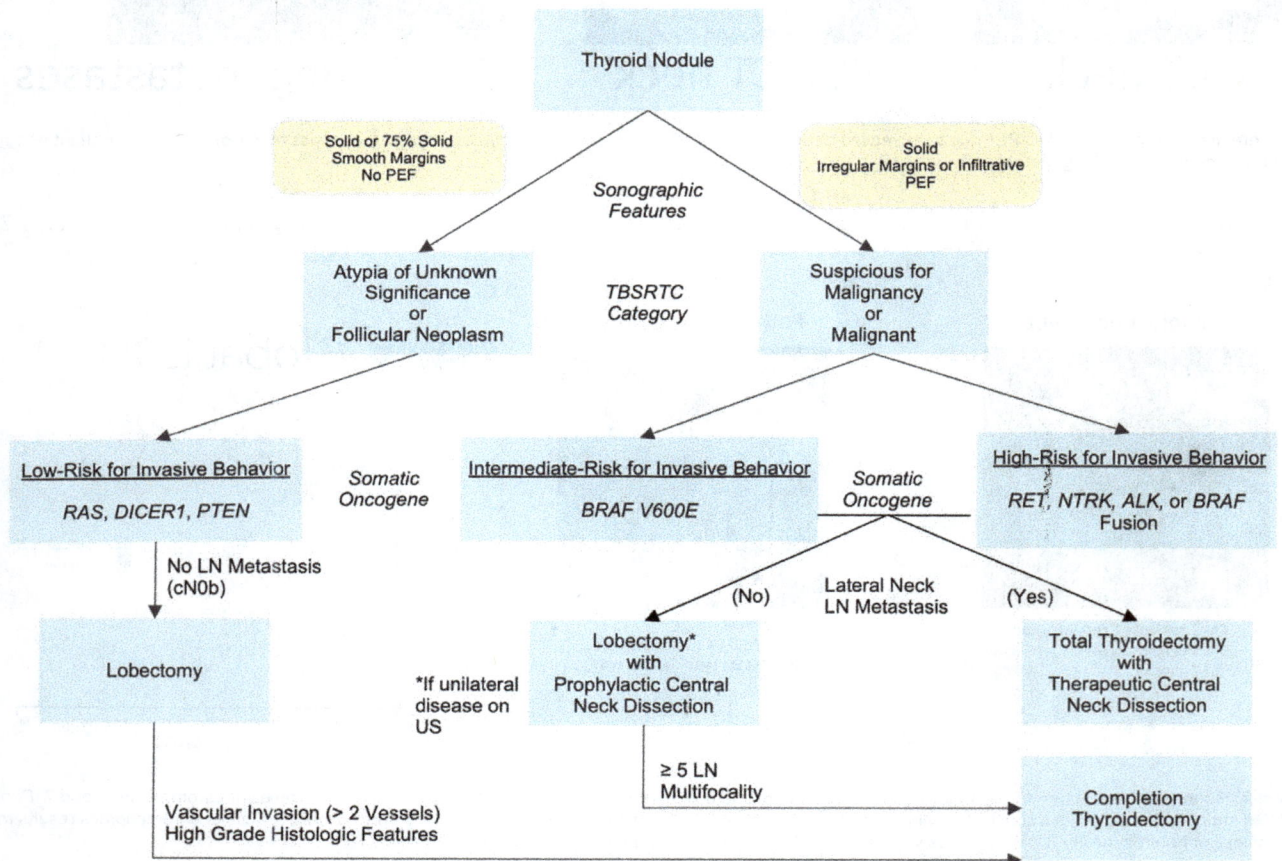

Incorporation of preoperative oncogene data across the 3-tiered pediatric risk of invasive behavior of differentiated thyroid carcinoma to stratify surgical management of a thyroid nodule. High-grade histologic features include solid, trabecular, or insular growth patterns, mitotic index ≥3 per 10 high power fields, necrosis, and convoluted nuclei.

Reprinted from Lai STT & Bauer AJ. JCEM, 2025; Published online ahead of print: 1–14. © The Authors. Published by Oxford University Press on behalf of the Endocrine Society